Y0-ASQ-422

Imaging of the spine in clinical practice

Imaging of the spine in clinical practice

Adam Greenspan, MD
Professor of Radiology and Orthopedic Surgery
University of California–Davis School of Medicine
Chief, Orthopedic Radiology
UCD Medical Center
Sacramento, California

Pasquale Montesano, MD
Assistant Clinical Professor of Orthopedic Surgery
University of California–Davis School of Medicine
Spine Surgeon: Mercy and Sutter Hospitals
Sacramento, California
Consultant in Spinal Disorders
Meadowlands Hospital
Meadowlands, New Jersey

WOLFE
London St. Louis Baltimore Boston Chicago Philadelphia Sydney Toronto

Copyright © 1993 Mosby Europe Limited. All rights reserved. No part of this publication may be reproduced, stored in a retrieval system, or transmitted in any form or by any means electronic, mechanical, photocopying, recording, or otherwise without prior permission of the publisher.

Published in 1993 by Wolfe Publishing, an imprint of Mosby Europe Limited.

For full details of all Mosby Europe Limited titles please write to:
   Mosby Europe Limited
   Brook House
   2–16 Torrington Place
   London WC1E7LT
   England

Library of Congress Cataloging-in-Publication Data

Greenspan, Adam.
   Imaging of the spine in clinical practice / Adam Greenspan, Pasquale Montesano.
      p.   cm.
   Includes bibliographical references and index.
   ISBN 1-56375-014-7
   1. Spine—Imaging. Montesano, Pasquale, 1953– . II. Title.
   [DNLM: 1. Diagnostic Imaging. 2. Spinal Cord Diseases—diagnosis.
3. Spinal Cord Injuries—diagnosis. 4. Spinal Diseases—diagnosis.
5. Spinal Injuries—diagnosis.   WE 725 G815i]
RD768.G73   1993
617.4'820754—dc20   92–48322

British Library Cataloguing-in-Publication Data.
A catalogue record for this book is available from the British Library.

Printed in Singapore by Imago

10 9 8 7 6 5 4 3 2 1

Editor/Project Manager: Tim Condon
Illustrators: Laura Pardi Duprey, Carol Kalafatic, and Nick Guarracino
Line Drawings: Patricia Gast and Kimberley Connors
Art Director: Kathryn Armstrong
Design and Layout: Enrique Sevilla
Typesetting Supervisor: Erick Rizzotto

Dedications

- To my son Michael with love

  —A.G.

- To the loving memory of my parents

  Pasquale Montesano, MD, and Maria T. Montesano

  and

  to my aunt Grace for always being there

  —P.X.M.

Preface

Imaging of the Spine in Clinical Practice is intended primarily for clinicians who either deal with disorders of the vertebral column or merely have an interest in them. Its goal is to present the most effective use of currently available imaging modalities (listed in Chapter 1) in the diagnosis and treatment of spinal disorders. To this end, the book is richly illustrated with radiographs, CT scans, and MR images, among other modalities, with liberal use of line drawings to delineate features of the images, schematic diagrams, and tables—features that residents training in either radiology or orthopedic surgery may find useful to complement the more comprehensive texts currently available. Traditionally, in the radiology literature the spine is viewed from the front, that is, the left side of the patient is on the right-hand side of the reader. In orthopedic literature, however, the spine is viewed from the back, so the sides of the patient coincide with the sides of the reader. In this text we decided to follow the radiologic approach, and all radiographs and MRIs of the spine are presented in the front view.

As the most common problem facing the treating physician, spinal trauma forms a good portion of the text. Emphasis in the chapters dealing with trauma (Chapters 2 and 3) has been placed on the implications of radiologic findings with regard to treatment options. In addition, preoperative imaging studies are, whenever possible, accompanied by images of the postoperative vertebral column. The remainder of the text is devoted to arthritides affecting the spine (Chapters 4–7), tumors and tumor-like lesions of the vertebral column (Chapters 8–10), together with an important chapter on the diagnostic workup and treatment of spinal tumors (Chapter 11), infections (Chapters 12 and 13), metabolic and endocrine disorders (Chapters 14–17), congenital and developmental anomalies (Chapter 18), and, finally, scoliosis and anomalies with general effects on the skeleton (Chapter 19).

To provide the practicing physician with more than a discussion of radiologic appearance, we chose to broaden our focus to include the pathogenesis of many disorders affecting the spine and discussion of the choices of an appropriate diagnostic approach. We therefore include some general information and clinical background pertinent to the various disorders, and occasionally, as in the chapters on the arthritides and the metabolic diseases, discuss their presentation in anatomic regions other than the vertebral column. In addition, by including certain systemic diseases affecting the spine, such as hyperparathyroidism and osteopetrosis, and some rare conditions, such as the mucopolysaccharidoses and alkaptonuria, we sought to produce a volume that would encompass a wide spectrum of spinal disorders and offer quick reference and helpful hints for radiologists and orthopedic surgeons alike.

We have not attempted to be encyclopedic, however. We hope instead that this book will ignite interest in spine diseases and prompt the reader to explore the field in the more detailed texts and monographs on the subjects. Imaging of the Spine in Clinical Practice should prove to be a useful resource for radiologists, orthopedic surgeons, and other practicing physicians, as well as for residents training in radiology or orthopedic surgery.

ADAM GREENSPAN, MD • PASQUALE MONTESANO, MD
Sacramento, California

ACKNOWLEDGMENTS

This book reflects the collective efforts and contribution of many individuals. In particular, we would like to thank our colleagues from the departments of Radiology and Orthopedic Surgery—the faculty and residents alike—for their valuable comments and suggestions during the production of this text. We also wish to express our gratitude to Peter G. Bullough, MB, ChB, and Oheneba Boachie-Adjei, MD, as well as Javier Beltran, MD, for their permission to use some of the illustrations from their respective books, *Atlas of Spinal Diseases* and *MRI: Musculoskeletal System*. Many members of the publisher's production staff have coped effortlessly with the work on this book. Tim Condon, the editor and project manager, did a wonderful job at every step of this endeavor, meticulously polishing the format and style of this project. The copyeditor Sharon Rule was able to effectively refine the rough form of our writing. Designer Enrique Sevilla and illustrators Laura Pardi Duprey, Carol Kalafatic, Nick Guarracino, Patricia Gast, and Kimberley Connors created a beautiful and artistic piece of work, and Daniel Benevento should be complimented for the outstanding quality reproduction of the radiographs. Finally, special thanks to Valerie Anderson and Carol Harris for their invaluable secretarial assistance.

Forewords

Recent years have witnessed significant advances in the technology of medical imaging. Some of the most important advances have occurred with regard to imaging of the vertebral column and spinal cord. *Imaging of the Spine in Clinical Practice* is an excellent text that addresses the needs of the clinician and radiologist who must deal with patients with vertebral and spinal cord disease. It is written by Adam Greenspan, MD, a world-renowned musculoskeletal radiologist, and Pasquale Montesano, MD, a well-respected spine surgeon.

The book follows the formula used by Dr. Greenspan in his previous text, *Orthopedic Radiology*, combining an easy-to-understand text with excellent images, many of which are accompanied by line drawings as well as functional and practical tables. In addition, there are many drawings on mechanisms of disease. Although the text is not encyclopedic, there is enough information for the reader as well as lists of current references at the end of each chapter for those in need of more in-depth information.

The book is divided into 19 chapters. Chapter 1 discusses imaging modalities in the evaluation of spinal disorders. Each of the main types of imaging studies is briefly discussed and illustrated. The remaining 18 chapters each discuss a related group of abnormalities. Chapters 2 and 3 deal with injury to the cervical and thoracolumbar spine, respectively. These chapters begin by covering anatomic and radiologic consideration and classification by mechanisms of injury and by stability. Specific injuries and/or complexes of injuries are then discussed from the standpoint of mechanism and treatment.

Chapter 4 is a generic chapter on the radiologic evaluation of the arthritides affecting the spine. This is followed by separate chapters on degenerative diseases (Chapter 5), inflammatory arthritides (Chapter 6), and miscellaneous arthropathies (Chapter 7). The next four chapters deal with tumors and tumor-like lesions that affect the vertebral column. These include Chapter 8, "The Radiologic Evaluation of Tumors and Tumor-like Lesions," a general introductory chapter that is followed by benign lesions (Chapter 9), malignant tumors (Chapter 10), and the diagnostic workup and treatment of spinal tumors (Chapter 11). This last chapter also deals with the differential diagnosis of back pain.

The next two chapters discuss infectious diseases that affect the vertebral column. Chapter 12 is of an introductory nature; Chapter 13 discusses pyogenic and nonpyogenic infections.

The next four chapters cover metabolic and endocrine disorders. Chapter 14 is introductory, covering radiologic evaluation of metabolic and endocrine disorders. This is followed by Chapter 15 on osteoporosis, osteomalacia, rickets, and hyperparathyroidism. Chapter 16 is devoted to Paget disease, and Chapter 17 discusses a variety of miscellaneous metabolic and endocrine disorders.

The final two chapters deal with congenital and developmental abnormalities as well as scoliosis. Chapter 18 provides a brief introduction to the radiologic evaluation of congenital and developmental abnormalities. This is followed by a very thorough and understandable Chapter 19 dealing with scoliosis and spinal abnormalities with general effects on the skeleton.

The authors are to be commended for their work. They have provided a book that represents both the practical and systematic approach to the evaluation of spinal disorders by multimodal imaging. The writing is clear and concise; the illustrations, drawings, and tables are superb and should easily hold the reader's attention. I am pleased to have been asked to write a foreword to this practical book.

Richard H. Daffner, MD, FACR *Professor of Radiologic Sciences*
Allegheny General Hospital and
The Medical College of Pennsylvania
Allegheny Campus
Pittsburgh, Pennsylvania

Diagnosis and treatment of spinal disorders are among the most challenging problems facing the clinician in the 1990s. One contributing factor is the technological advances in diagnostic imaging of the vertebral column. We can now see the spinal column and its contents in ways not possible just a few years ago. For this reason, a book such as Greenspan and Montesano's *Imaging of the Spine in Clinical Practice* is an important resource for those who treat spinal problems.

The approach taken by the authors is practical and effective. Because a radiologist has joined forces with a spinal surgeon, the text speaks clearly to those in both disciplines. The first chapter of this book discusses the imaging modalities specifically, and the 18 subsequent chapters describe how the techniques are used in pathologic conditions. Roentgenographic and MRI technology are succinctly described and explained. In many cases the radiographs are schematically reconstructed, making interpretation easy and meaningful. Similarly, the treatment options as determined by the imaging studies are presented to demonstrate the capabilities of the equipment rather than to delineate the role of the surgeon.

We have waited too long for this practical approach to the understanding of spinal column imaging. Although we have been amazed by what new imaging methods show us, our knowledge of how to apply this information has often remained vague. Drs. Greenspan and Montesano effectively teach the reader what radiographs and MRIs mean and how to use the information these methods provide.

This book is written at a level that is useful for both medical students and advanced spinal surgeons. Other readers to whom it is addressed are radiologists and any practitioner who has to interpret imaging tests and give opinions on spinal disorders, including resident physicians in specialities such as orthopedic surgery, neurosurgery, and physical medicine and rehabilitation. All of us will be better able to use the imaging information now available, thanks to the authors' efforts in providing this richly illustrated book.

DANIEL R. BENSON, MD *Professor of Orthopaedic Surgery*
University of California, Davis, School of Medicine
Sacramento, California

Contents

1 Imaging Modalities in Evaluation of Spinal Disorders — 1.1

Plain Film Radiographs — 1.2
Tomography — 1.2
Computed Tomograpy (CT) — 1.2
Angiography — 1.3
Myelography — 1.4
Diskography — 1.4
Ultrasonography (US) — 1.6
Scintigraphy (Radionuclide Bone Scan) — 1.6
Single Photon Emission Computed Tomography (SPECT) — 1.8
Magnetic Resonance Imaging (MRI) — 1.8

2 Injury to the Cervical Spine — 2.1

Anatomic and Radiologic Considerations — 2.2
Classification by Mechanism of Injury and by Stability — 2.15
Fractures of the Occipital Condyles — 2.17
Occipito-cervical Dislocations — 2.19
Fractures and Dislocations of the C1 and C2 Vertebrae — 2.20
Fractures of the Mid and Lower Cervical Spine — 2.29

3 Injury to the Thoracolumbar Spine — 3.1

Anatomic and Radiologic Considerations — 3.2
Injury to the Thoracolumbar Spine — 3.10
Spondylolysis and Spondylolisthesis — 3.27
Injury to the Diskovertebral Junction — 3.31

4 Radiologic Evaluation of the Arthritides Affecting the Spine — 4.1

Clinical Findings — 4.3
Radiologic Evaluation — 4.3
Radiographic Features of the Arthritides — 4.7

5 Degenerative Diseases of the Spine — 5.1

Degenerative Diseases of the Spine — 5.3
Complications of Degenerative Diseases of the Spine — 5.6
Treatment — 5.11

6 Inflammatory Arthritides of the Spine — 6.1

Rheumatoid Arthritis — 6.2
Seronegative Spondyloarthropathies — 6.3

7 Miscellaneous Arthropathies Affecting the Spine — 7.1

Alkaptonuria (Ochronosis) — 7.2
Hyperparathryoidism Arthropathy — 7.2
Gout — 7.3
CPPD Crystal Deposition Disease — 7.4
Hemochromatosis — 7.4
Arthritis Associated with AIDS — 7.5
Infectious Arthritis — 7.5

8 Radiologic Evaluation of Tumors and Tumor-like Lesions — 8.1

Classification — 8.2
Radiologic Imaging Modalities — 8.2
Tumors and Tumor-like Lesions of the Spine — 8.7

9 Benign Lesions of the Vertebral Column — 9.1

Osteoid Osteoma — 9.2
Osteoblastoma — 9.3
Osteochondroma — 9.4
Multiple Osteocartilaginous Exostoses — 9.6
Enchondroma (Chondroma) — 9.6
Enchondromatosis (Ollier Disease) — 9.6
Chondroblastoma — 9.7
Chondromyxoid Fibroma — 9.7
Aneurysmal Bone Cyst — 9.8
Giant-cell Tumor — 9.9

Hemangioma	*9.11*
Lymphangioma	*9.12*
Lipoma	*9.12*
Non-neoplastic Lesions Simulating Tumors	*9.12*

10 Malignant Tumors of the Vertebral Column   10.1

Osteosarcoma	*10.2*
Chondrosarcoma	*10.5*
Ewing Sarcoma	*10.7*
Lymphoma of Bone	*10.7*
Myeloma	*10.8*
Fibrosarcoma	*10.10*
Chordoma	*10.11*
Radiation-induced Sarcoma	*10.13*
Skeletal Metastases	*10.13*

11 Diagnostic Workup and Treatment of Spinal Tumors   11.1

Differential Diagnosis of Back Pain	***11.2***

12 Radiologic Evaluation and Treatment of Infections of the Spine   12.1

Musculoskeletal Infections	***12.2***
Infections of the Spine	***12.2***

13 Pyogenic and Nonpyogenic Infections of the Spine   13.1

Pyogenic Infections	***13.2***
Tuberculosis of the Spine	***13.5***
Fungal Infections	***13.7***
Soft Tissue Infections	***13.8***

14 Radiologic Evaluation of Metabolic and Endocrine Disorders   14.1

Composition and Production of Bone	***14.2***
Evaluation of Metabolic and Endocrine Disorders	***14.2***

15 Osteoporosis, Osteomalacia, Rickets, and Hyperparathyroidism   15.1

Osteoporosis	*15.2*
Rickets and Osteomalacia	*15.4*
Renal Osteodystrophy	*15.5*
Hyperparathyroidism	*15.5*

16 Paget Disease   16.1

Pathophysiology	*16.2*
Radiographic Evaluation	*16.2*
Differential Diagnosis	*16.3*
Complications	*16.3*
Orthopedic Management	*16.5*

17 Miscellaneous Metabolic and Endocrine Disorders   17.1

Familial Idiopathic Hyperphosphatasia	*17.2*
Acromegaly	*17.2*
Gaucher Disease	*17.4*

18 Radiologic Evaluation of Congenital and Developmental Anomalies   18.1

Classification	*18.2*
Radiologic Imaging Modalities	*18.2*

19 Scoliosis and Anomalies with General Effects on the Skeleton   19.1

Scoliosis	*19.2*
Anomalies with General Effects on the Skeleton	*19.18*

Index   I.1

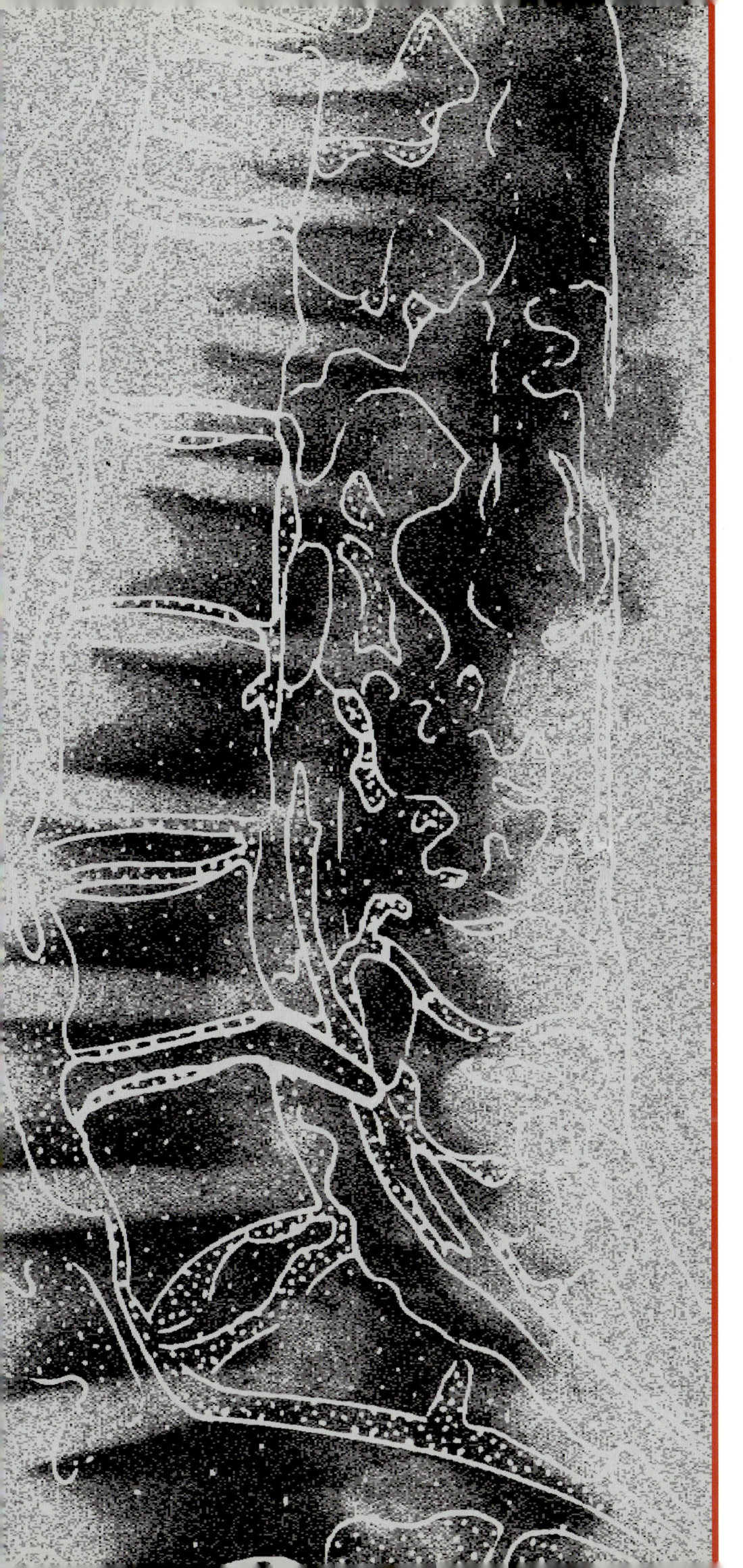

Imaging Modalities in Evaluation of Spinal Disorders

1

This chapter will describe the principles and limitations of current imaging modalities. At present, a vast number of imaging modalities are available for diagnosing many commonly encountered disorders of the spine. An understanding of these techniques can help the physician to select the most effective radiologic modality, with a view to minimizing the cost of examination as well as the exposure of patients to radiation. To this end, it is important to match the most effective imaging technique to the specific type of spine abnormality in question and, when the more conventional techniques are used (eg, plain radiography), to be familiar with the particular views and techniques that will best demonstrate the abnormality. It should be stressed that plain film radiography remains the most effective means for demonstrating bone and joint abnormalities of the vertebral column. Both the radiologist and the orthopedic surgeon must be familiar with a variety of radiologic techniques, since they have different uses in evaluating the presence, type, and extent of involvement for various spinal abnormalities. These practitioners should also be aware of the indications and limitations of each imaging method, and familiar with all the possible imaging approaches to an abnormality at specific sites.

Plain Film Radiography

The most frequently used modality for evaluation of spinal disorders, and particularly of traumatic conditions, is plain film radiography. In the standard radiographic approach, at least two views of the spine are obtained at 90° angles to each other. Usually these films comprise the anteroposterior (posteroanterior) and lateral views; occasionally an oblique or other special view is necessary. Special projections are sometimes required to demonstrate a particular abnormality of the spine to greater advantage (Fig. 1.1).

Tomography

Tomography is a form of body section radiography that permits more accurate visualization of lesions that are too small to be seen on conventional radiographs or of anatomic detail that is obscured by overlying structures. This technique employs continuous motion of the radiographic tube and film cassette in opposite directions during exposure, with the fulcrum of the motion located in the plane of interest. Because this motion blurs the structures above and below the area being examined, the area of study is sharply outlined on a single plane of focus. The newer tomographic units can localize the image more precisely and have greatly enhanced the ability to detect lesions as small as 1 mm. The simplest tomographic motion is linear, with the radiographic tube and film cassette moving on a straight line in opposite directions. This linear movement has little application in the study of bony structures because it creates streaks that often interfere with radiologic interpretation. Resolution of the plane of focus is much clearer when there is more uniform blurring of undesired structures. This requires a multidirectional movement, as used in zonography or circular tomography. In this type of tomography, the radiographic tube makes one circular motion at a preset angle of inclination. More complex multidirectional hypocycloidal or trispiral movements increase the distance of excursion of the tube and create a varying angle of projection of the x-ray beam during the exposure. These complex movements are more advantageous because they produce even greater blurring and yield the sharpest images. Trispiral tomography is an important radiographic technique in the diagnosis and management of a variety of problems of the bones and joints. It continues to be a basic tool for examining patients who have sustained trauma to the spine. The advantages of trispiral tomography over conventional radiography include the visualization of subtle fractures with delineation of the fracture line and demonstration of its extent (Fig. 1.2), and evaluation of the healing process, of post-traumatic complications, and of bone grafts in treatment of nonunions. It is also invaluable for evaluation of various tumor and tumor-like lesions (eg, to demonstrate a nidus of osteoid osteoma or to delineate the extent of an aneurysmal bone cyst). Small cystic and sclerotic lesions, as well as subtle erosions, can be better demonstrated. As a rule, a tomogram should be interpreted together with a plain radiograph for comparison.

Computed Tomography (CT)

The essential components of a CT system include a circular scanning gantry which houses the x-ray tube and image sensors, a table for the patient, an x-ray generator, and a computerized data processing unit. The patient lies on the table and is placed inside the gantry. The x-ray tube is rotated 360° around the patient while the computer collects the data and formulates an axial image or "slice." Each cross-sectional slice represents a thickness between 0.3 and 1.5 cm of body tissue.

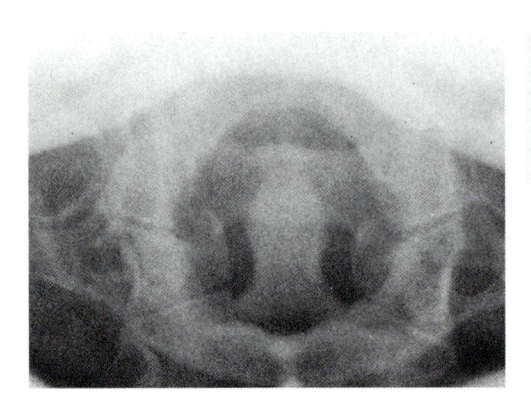

FIGURE 1.1 Special projection of the odontoid (Fuchs view) is frequently necessary to visualize the dens without overlapping structures.

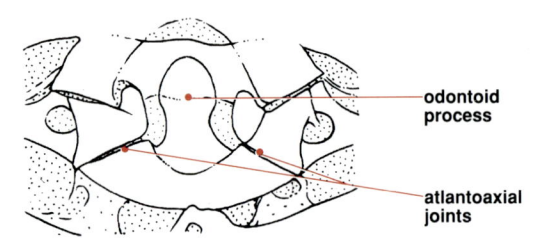

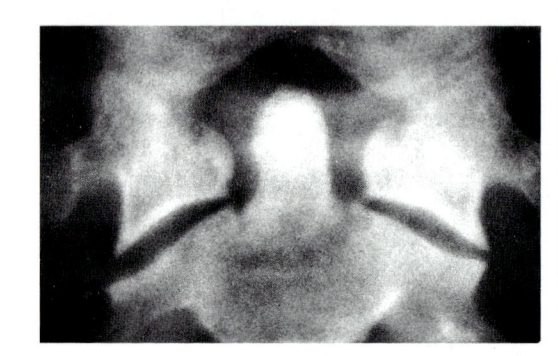

FIGURE 1.2 A 62-year-old man sustained a flexion injury of the cervical spine in an automobile accident. Thin-section trispiral tomogram in this anteroposterior projection confirms the fracture at the base of the dens. This is a Type II (unstable) fracture.

CT is indispensable in the evaluation of many traumatic conditions of the spine and of various spinal tumors because of its cross-sectional imaging capability. In cases of trauma to the vertebral column, CT is extremely useful because it can define the presence and extent of fracture and can delineate the adjacent soft tissues. CT is particularly important in the detection of small, displaced fragments of a fractured vertebral body (Fig. 1.3) and in the assessment of concomitant injury to the cord or thecal sac. The advantage of CT over conventional radiography is its ability to provide excellent contrast resolution and accurate measurement of the tissue attenuation coefficient, and to obtain direct transaxial images. A further advantage is its ability, through data obtained from the thin, contiguous sections, to image the spine in coronal, sagittal, and oblique planes, using reformation technique. This multiplanar reconstruction is particularly helpful in evaluation of vertebral alignment (Fig. 1.4), demonstration of horizontally oriented fractures of the vertebral body, and evaluation of complex fractures. Modern CT scanners employ collimated fan beams directed only at the tissue layer under investigation. Recent advances in development of sophisticated software enable three-dimensional (3-D) reconstruction, which is helpful in analysis of the vertebral column. The rapid development of new computer systems has now made it possible to construct plastic models of the area of interest based on these 3-D images. Such models facilitate operative planning and allow "rehearsal" in advance of surgery involving complex reconstructive procedures.

CT plays a significant role in evaluation of the spinal tumors, owing to its superior contrast resolution and its ability to measure accurately the tissue attenuation coefficient (Hounsfield units). Although CT by itself is rarely helpful in making a specific diagnosis, it can provide a precise evaluation of the extent of the bone lesion and may demonstrate extension through the cortex and involvement of surrounding soft tissues. It is also useful for monitoring the results of treatment, evaluating recurrence of resected tumor, and demonstrating the effect of nonsurgical treatment, such as radiation therapy and chemotherapy. Intravenously injected iodinated contrast agents are sometimes used to enhance CT imaging. These injected agents directly alter image contrast by increasing the x-ray attenuation, and thus display increased brightness in the CT images. CT with contrast can help to identify a suspected soft tissue mass when the initial CT is unremarkable, or to assess the vascularity of a paravertebral soft tissue or spinal tumor.

CT is also a very useful adjunct to successful aspiration or biopsy of vertebral or paravertebral soft tissue lesions, since it provides visual guidance for precise placement of the instrument within the lesion (Fig. 1.5).

CT has a crucial role in bone mineral analysis. The ability of CT to measure the attenuation coefficients of each pixel provides a basis for accurate, quantitative analysis of bone minerals in cancellous and cortical bone (see Fig. 14.6).

Among the disadvantages of CT is the so-called average volume effect, which results from the lack of homogeneity in the composition of a small volume of tissue. In particular, the measurement of Hounsfield units results in average values for the different components of the tissue. This *partial volume effect* becomes particularly important when normal and pathologic processes interface within a section under investigation. Another disadvantage of CT is poor tissue characterization. Despite its ability to discriminate among certain differences in tissue density, a simple analysis of attenuation values does not permit precise histologic characterization. Moreover, any movement of the patient will produce artefacts that degrade the image quality. Similarly, an area that contains metal (eg, various rods and screws) will produce significant artefacts. Finally, the radiation dose to the patient may occasionally be high, particularly when contiguous and overlapping sections are obtained.

Angiography

The use of contrast material injected directly into selected branches of both the arterial and venous circulation has aided greatly in assessing the involvement of the circulatory system in various conditions, and has provided a precise method for defining local pathology. Arteriography employs injection of contrast agent into the arteries, after which a rapid sequence of films is obtained. Venography employs injection of contrast into the veins.

In evaluation of spinal tumors, arteriography is used mainly to delineate bone lesions, to demonstrate their vascularity, and to assess the extent of disease. It is also used to demonstrate the vascular supply of a tumor and to locate vessels suitable for preoperative intraarterial chemotherapy. Angiography is very useful for demonstrating the area suitable for open biopsy, since the most vascular parts of a tumor represent its

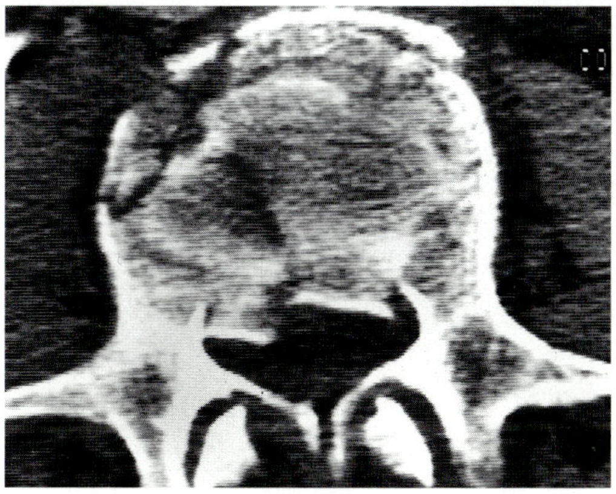

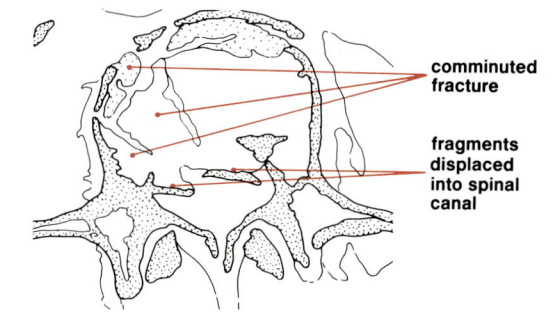

FIGURE 1.3 A 56-year-old merchant seaman fell from a 60-foot-high ladder on a ship. The severity of the injury is shown on this CT section through the body of L3. There is comminution of the vertebral fracture and displacement of the two bony fragments into the spinal canal, with compression of the thecal sac.

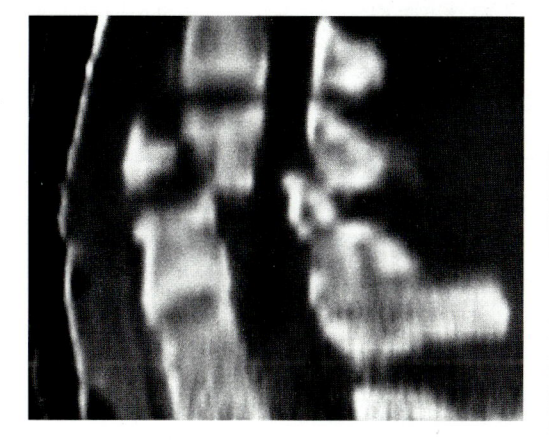

FIGURE 1.4 Sagittal CT reformation image demonstrates the flexion "tear-drop" fracture of C5. It also effectively shows malalignment of the vertebral body and narrowing of the spinal canal. (Reproduced with permission from Greenspan A: Imaging modalities in orthopaedics. In Chapman MW (ed): *Operative Orthopaedics*, 2nd ed. Philadelphia, J B Lippincott, in press)

most aggressive component. Arteriography can sometimes be used to demonstrate abnormal tumor vessels, corroborating findings of plain film radiography and tomography. It can also be combined with an interventional procedure such as embolization of hypervascular tumors before further treatment is undertaken (see Fig. 8.5).

MYELOGRAPHY

During this procedure, water-soluble contrast agents are injected into the subarachnoid space, mixing freely with the cerebral spinal fluid to produce a column of opacified fluid with a higher specific gravity than the nonopacified fluid. By tilting the patient, the opacified fluid can be made to travel up or down the thecal sac under the influence of gravity (Fig. 1.6). The injection is usually done in the lumbar area at the L2–L3 or L3–L4 level. For examination of the cervical segment, injection is performed at C1–C2 level (Fig. 1.7). Since the development of high resolution CT and high-quality MRI, myelography has been almost completely replaced by these newer techniques.

DISKOGRAPHY

Diskography is a technique that involves injection of contrast material into the nucleus pulposus. Although this is a controversial procedure and has been abandoned by many investigators, under tightly restricted indi-

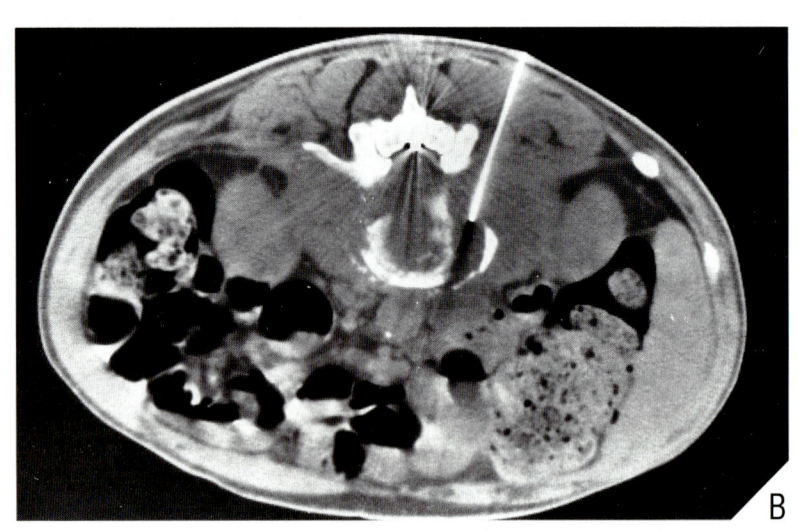

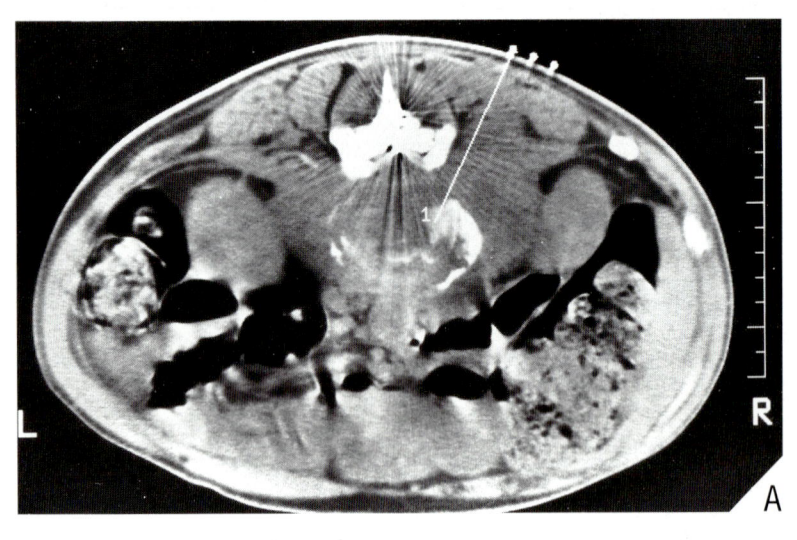

FIGURE 1.5 Aspiration biopsy of an infected disk is performed under CT guidance. **(A)** Measurement is obtained from the skin surface to the area of interest (intervertebral disk). **(B)** The needle is advanced under CT guidance and placed at the site of the destructive lesion.

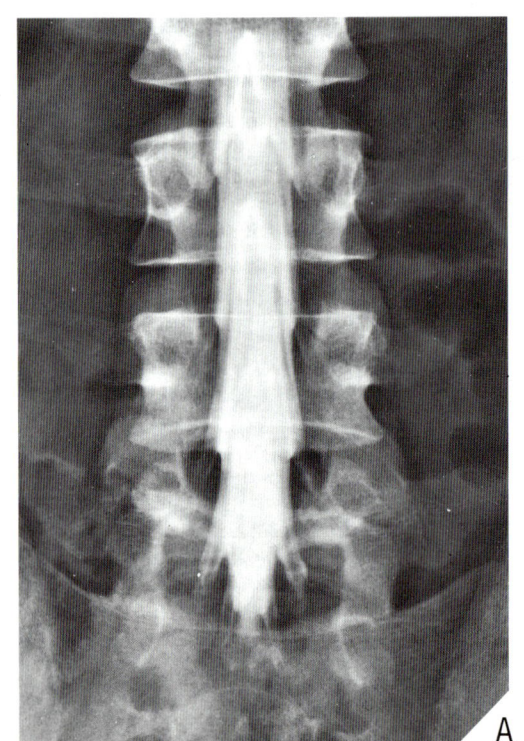

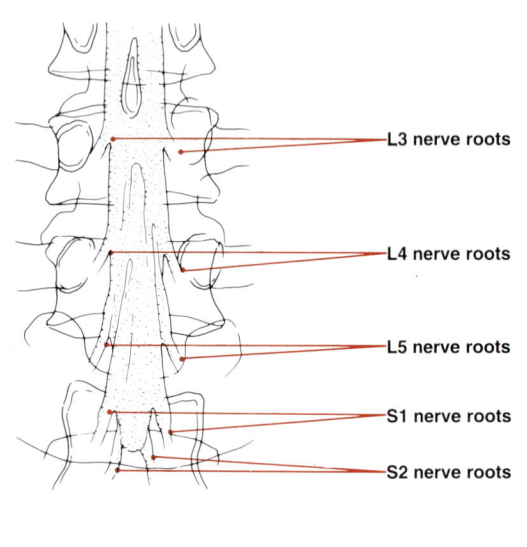

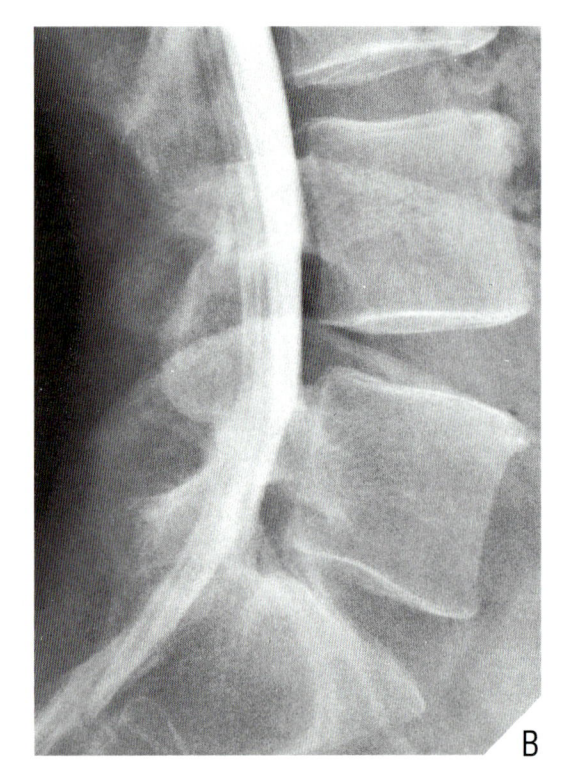

FIGURE 1.6 For myelographic examination of the lumbar spine, the patient is prone on the table. The puncture site, usually at the L3–L4 or L2–L3 level, is marked under fluoroscopic control. A 22-gauge needle is inserted into the subarachnoid space, and free flow of spinal fluid indicates proper placement. Fifteen milliliters of Iohexol in a concentration of 180 mg iodine/ml is slowly injected, and films are obtained in the posteroanterior **(A)** and cross-table lateral **(B)** projections. In these normal studies, contrast is seen outlining the subarachnoid spaces of the thecal sac, as well as the cul-de-sac or most caudal part of the subarachnoid space. The nerve roots appear symmetric on both sides of the contrast column. A linear filling defect represents a nerve root in its contrast-filled sleeve. The length of the root pocket may vary from one patient to another, but in each patient, all roots are approximately equal in length.

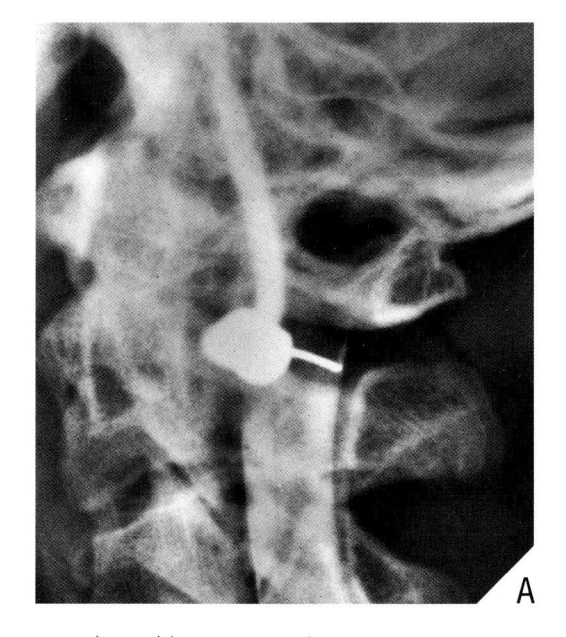

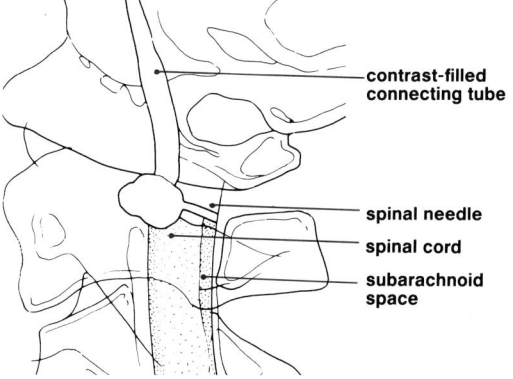

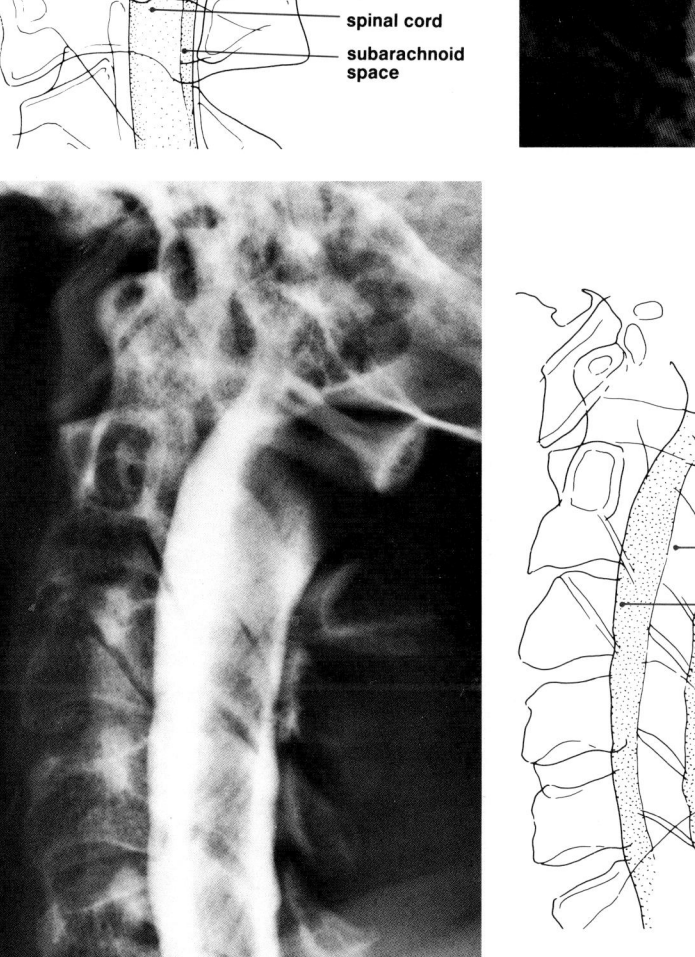

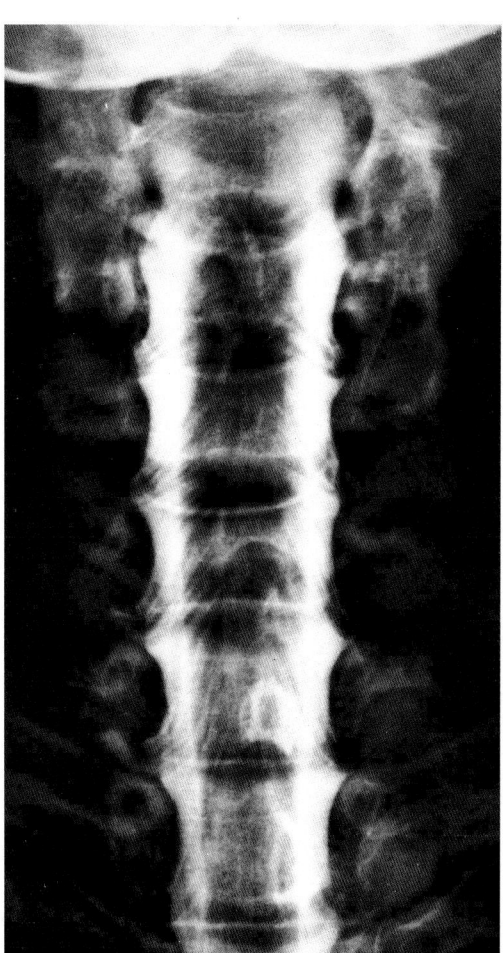

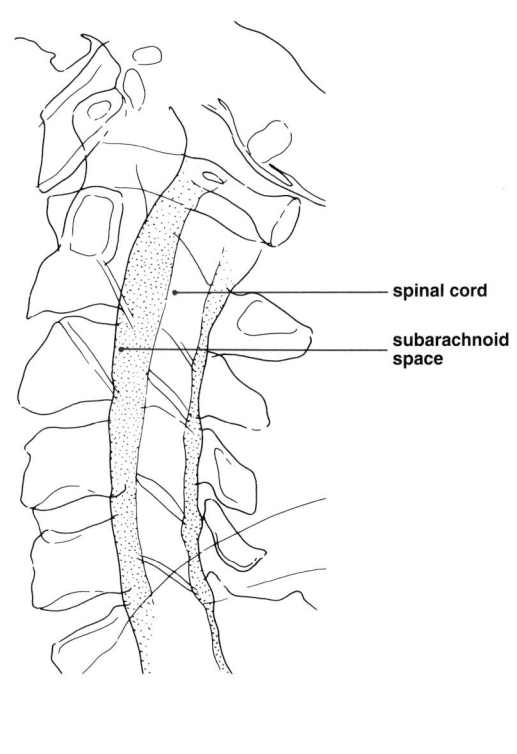

FIGURE 1.7 For myelographic examination of the cervical spine, the patient is recumbent on the table, lying on the left side. Using fluoroscopy, the point of entrance of the needle is marked at the C1–C2 level, and a 22-gauge needle is inserted vertically, the tip being directed to the dorsal aspect of the subarachnoid space, above the lamina of C2. Free flow of spinal fluid indicates the correct position of the needle. **(A)** About 10 ml of Iohexol, a water-soluble nonionic iodinated contrast agent, at a concentration of 240 mg iodine/ml, is slowly injected. Films are obtained in the posteroanterior **(B)**, cross-table lateral **(C)**, and oblique projections. (Oblique projections, however, are obtained not by rotating the patient but by angling the radiographic tube 45°.) If the lower segment of the cervical spine is not satisfactorily demonstrated or if the upper thoracic segment needs to be visualized, a film may also be obtained in the swimmer's position. Myelography demonstrates the thecal sac filled with contrast and the outline of the normal nerve roots and nerve root sleeves.

Imaging Modalities in Evaluating Spinal Disorders

cations and with impeccable technique a diskogram can yield valuable information. Diskography is valuable in determining the source of low back pain. It is not solely an imaging technique, since the symptoms produced during the procedure (pain during the injection) are considered to have even greater diagnostic value than the radiographs obtained. Diskography should always be combined with CT examination (the so-called CT diskography) (Fig. 1.8). According to the official position statement on diskography by the Executive Committee of the North American Spine Society in 1988, this procedure is indicated in the evaluation of patients with unremitting spinal pain, with or without extremity pain, of greater than four months duration, when the pain has been unresponsive to all appropriate methods of conservative therapy. According to the same statement, before diskography is performed the patient should have undergone investigation by other modalities (eg, CT, MRI, myelography), and the surgical correction of the problem should be anticipated.

Ultrasonography (US)

Over the past several years ultrasound has made an enormous impact in the field of radiology. However, it is rarely used in skeletal radiology, and only in exceptional cases for evaluation of the spine. It is a very safe and noninvasive modality, relying on the interaction of propagated sound waves with tissue interfaces in the body. When the directed pulse of sound waves encounters an interface between tissues of different acoustic impedance, reflection or refraction occurs; the sound waves reflected back to the ultrasound transducer are recorded, then converted into images. The advantage of this technique is it does not use ionized radiation, and is therefore safe for use in pregnant women and infants. Modern probe technology, development of real-time imaging, and color Doppler imaging have extended to some degree the use of ultrasound in orthopedic radiology. Higher-frequency transducers of 7.5 and 10 MHz have excellent spatial resolution. Applications of ultrasound in spine surgery include the assessment of reduction of some spinal fractures and occasional evaluation of soft tissue masses (eg, hemangioma).

Scintigraphy (Radionuclide Bone Scan)

One of the major advantages of skeletal scintigraphy over all other imaging techniques is its ability to image the entire skeleton at once. Bone scanning provides useful information in that it can confirm the presence of disease, demonstrate the distribution of the lesion, and help to evaluate the activity of the pathologic process. The indications for skeletal scintigraphy include traumatic conditions, tumors (primary and metastatic), various arthritides, infections, and metabolic bone disease. The abnormality detected may manifest either as decreased uptake of a bone-seeking radiopharmaceutical (eg, in most cases of myeloma) or as increased uptake, such as in the case of fracture, primary or metastatic neoplasm, or focus of osteomyelitis (Fig. 1.9). Some structures, such as sacroiliac joints or normal pedicle, may show increased activity under normal conditions.

Although scintigraphy is a very sensitive imaging modality, it is not very specific, and it is impossible to distinguish among the various processes that can cause increased uptake. Occasionally, however, the bone scan can yield very specific information and may even suggest a diagnosis (eg, in multiple myeloma or osteoid osteoma). Scintigraphy is helpful for distinguishing between similar-appearing lesions of myeloma and bone metastases, because in most cases of myeloma there is no significant increase in the uptake of the radiopharmaceutical, whereas in skeletal metastasis the uptake of the tracer is invariably significantly elevated. In osteoid osteoma, the radionuclide bone scan typically demonstrates the so-called double density sign: uptake is increased in the center of the lesion, related to the nidus, and is less increased at the periphery, related to the reactive sclerosis surrounding the nidus.

Radionuclide bone scanning is an indicator of mineral turnover and, because there is usually enhanced deposition of bone-seeking radiophar-

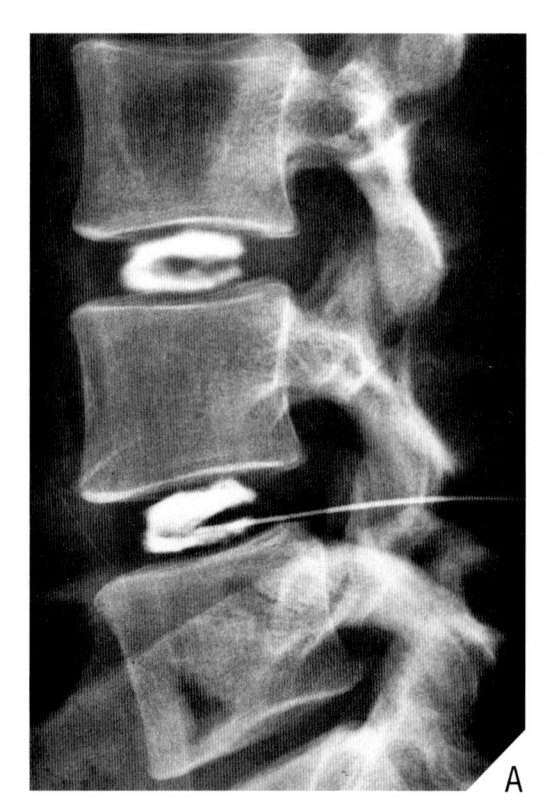

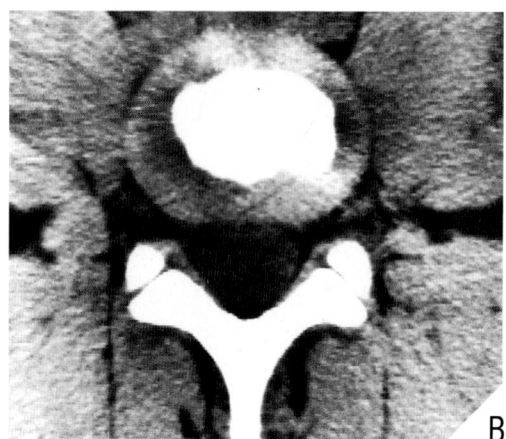

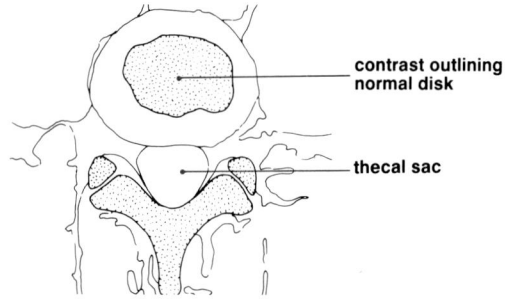

FIGURE 1.8 For diskographic examination of the lumbar spine, the patient is prone on the table, and the level of the injection, depending on the indication, is marked. The needle is inserted into the center of the nucleus pulposus, and 2 to 3 ml of metrizamide is injected. **(A)** Lateral view of a normal diskogram shows a concentration of contrast in the nucleus pulposus outlining the disk; there should be no extradural leak of contrast medium while the needle is in place. **(B)** CT section through the L3–L4 disk space following diskography shows the normal appearance of this structure.

maceuticals in areas of bone undergoing change and repair, this technique is useful for localizing tumors and tumor-like lesions in the spine. It is particularly helpful in conditions such as eosinophilic granuloma and metastatic cancer, in which more than one lesion is present, and some may represent a "silent" site of involvement. Scintigraphy also plays an important role in localizing small lesions (eg, osteoid osteoma) that may not always be seen on plain film studies. Although in most instances radionuclide bone scanning cannot distinguish benign lesions from malignant tumors, since increased blood flow with consequently increased isotope deposition and increased osteoblastic activity occurs in both these conditions, it can occasionally make such a differentiation in benign lesions that may not absorb the radioactive isotope (eg, bone island).

In traumatic conditions, scintigraphy is extremely helpful in the early diagnosis of stress fractures, which may not be visible on conventional radiographs or even tomographic studies. It is also valuable for diagnosis of vertebral fractures in elderly patients when the routine radiographic examinations may appear normal.

In metabolic bone disorders, bone scintigraphy is helpful in establishing the extent of skeletal involvement (eg, in Paget disease) and assessing the response to treatment. Although it has no value in the evaluation of patients with generalized osteoporosis, it is occasionally helpful in differentiating osteoporosis from osteomalacia, and in differentiating multiple vertebral fractures caused by osteoporosis from those associated with metastatic carcinoma.

Skeletal scintigraphy is frequently used in evaluation of infections. In particular, 99m technetium (^{99m}Tc) MDP and Indium-111 (^{111}In) labeled white blood cells are highly sensitive in detecting early and occult osteomyelitis. In chronic osteomyelitis, imaging with ^{67}Ga-citrate is more accurate in detecting the response or lack of response to treatment than ^{99}Tc-phosphate bone imaging. For detecting recurrent active infection in patients with chronic osteomyelitis, ^{111}In appears to be the radiopharmaceutical of choice. A three-phase technique (see below) can be effectively used to distinguish between soft tissue infection (cellulitis) and osseous infection (osteomyelitis).

In neoplastic conditions, probably the most common indication for skeletal scintigraphy is the detection of skeletal metastases. However, this is not the method of choice to determine the extent of the lesion in the bone. Scintigraphy alone cannot diagnose the type of the tumor, but it may be useful in detection and localization of some primary tumors as well as multifocal lesions (eg, multicentric osteosarcoma).

Scintigraphy with ^{99m}Tc MDP is used primarily to determine whether a lesion is monostotic or polyostotic, and is therefore essential in staging of bone tumors. It is important to remember that although the degree of abnormal uptake may be related to the aggressiveness of the lesion, this does not correlate well with the histologic grade. Scintigraphy with ^{67}Ga may show increased uptake in a soft tissue sarcoma and may help to differentiate a sarcoma from a benign soft tissue lesion.

Although radionuclide bone scan may be useful in demonstrating the extent of the primary malignant tumor in bone, it is not as accurate as CT or MRI. It can be helpful in the detection of local recurrence of tumor and can occasionally indicate the response or lack of response to treatment (radiotherapy or chemotherapy).

Several bone-seeking tracers are available for scintigraphic imaging.

Diphosphonates

In recent years there has been remarkable progress in the development of new gamma-emitting diagnostic agents for radionuclide imaging. The radiopharmaceuticals presently used in bone scanning include organic diphosphonates, ethylene diphosphonates (HEPD), methylene diphosphonates (MDP), and methane hydroxydiphosphonates (HNDP), all labeled with ^{99m}Tc, a pure gamma-emitter with a 6-hour half-life. MDP is the agent most often used, particularly in adults, typically at a dose that provides 15 mCi (555 MBq) of ^{99m}Tc. After intravenous injection of the radiopharmaceutical, approximately 50% of the dose localizes in bone. The remainder circulates freely in the body and is eventually excreted by the kidneys. A gamma-camera can then be used in a procedure known as *three-phase isotope bone scanning*. The first phase, the *radionuclide*

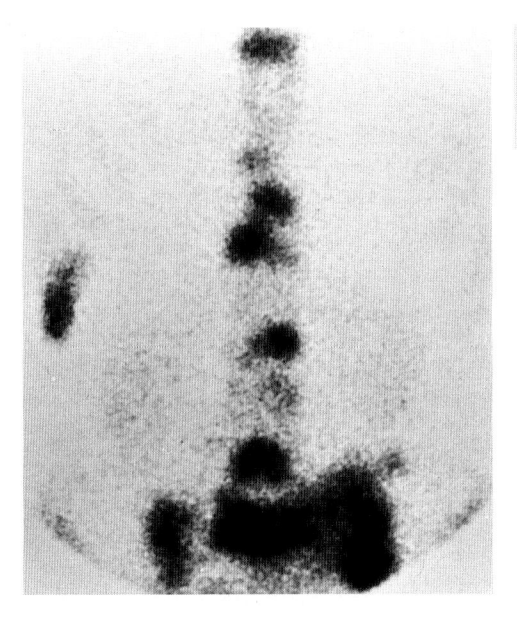

FIGURE 1.9 A radionuclide bone scan was performed on a 68-year-old woman with metastatic breast carcinoma to determine the distribution of metastases. After an intravenous injection of 15 mCi (555 MBq) of technetium-99m diphosphonate, an increased uptake of the radiopharmaceutical is seen in the lumbar spine and pelvis, localizing the multiple metastases.

angiogram, occurs during first minute after injection, when the serial images demonstrate the radioactive tracer in the major blood vessels. In the second phase, the *blood pool scan*, which lasts from 1 to 3 minutes after injection, isotope is detected in the vascular system and in the extracellular space in the soft tissues before being taken up by bone. The third phase, or *static bone scan*, usually occurs 2 to 3 hours after injection and discloses radiopharmaceutical in the bone. This phase can be divided into two stages. In the first, the isotope diffuses passively through the bone capillaries. In the second stage, the radionuclide is concentrated in bone. The most intense localization occurs in the first and second phases in areas with increased blood flow, and in the third phase in areas with increased osteogenic activity, increased calcium metabolism and active bone turnover.

Gallium-67

Gallium-67 (^{67}Ga) citrate is frequently used to diagnose infectious processes in bone and joints. The sensitivity of ^{67}Ga for abscess detection varies from 58% to 100% and the specificity from 75% to 99%. The images are usually obtained 6 and 24 hours after the injection of 5 mCi (185 MBq) of this radiopharmaceutical. These images have been shown to be extremely accurate for following the response to therapy of chronic osteomyelitis. In particular, the changing activity of ^{67}Ga uptake parallels the patient's clinical course in disk infection more closely than the images obtained after injection of ^{99m}Tc-labeled diphosphonate. Gallium scanning is also used to differentiate a sarcoma from a benign soft tissue lesion.

Indium

The diagnostic advantage of ^{111}In-oxine-labeled white blood cells over other bone-seeking radiopharmaceuticals for detection of inflammatory abnormalities in the skeletal system is still a controversial issue. Because ^{111}In leukocytes are not usually incorporated into areas of increased bone turnover, indium imaging presumably reflects inflammatory activity only, and early experience has shown it to be specific in the detection of abscesses or acute infectious processes including osteomyelitis and disk infection. The sensitivity varies from 75% to 90% and the specificity, as recently reported, is around 91%. False-negative results were often seen in patients with chronic infections in which there was reduced inflow of circulating leukocytes. False-positive results were seen in patients who had an inflammatory process without infection (such as rheumatoid arthritis mistaken for septic arthritis).

"Nanocolloid"

Recently, in Europe, very small particles of ^{99}Tc-labeled colloid of human serum albumin were tried as a bone marrow imaging agent. About 86% of these particles are 30 nm or smaller, and the remainder between 30 and 80 nm. This "nanocolloid" has a sensitivity for detection of osteomyelitis equal to that of indium-labeled leukocytes.

SINGLE PHOTON EMISSION COMPUTED TOMOGRAPHY (SPECT)

With the recent development of single photon emission tomography (SPET) and single photon emission computed tomography (SPECT), diagnostic precision in evaluating bone and joint abnormalities has increased tremendously. The efficiency of instrumentation for SPECT is improving with multiple crystal detectors, fan beam and cone beam collimators, detection of a greater fraction of photons, and improved algorithms. In comparison with planar images, SPECT provides increased contrast resolution, utilizing a tomographic mode that eliminates the noise from tissue outside the plane of imaging, similar to conventional tomography. It provides not only qualitative information on the uptake of bone-seeking radiopharmaceuticals but also quantitative data.

MAGNETIC RESONANCE IMAGING (MRI)

MRI is based on the re-emission of an absorbed radiofrequency signal while the patient is in a strong magnetic field. An external magnetic field is usually generated by a magnet with field strengths of 0.2–1.5 Tesla. The system includes magnet, radiofrequency coils (transmitter and receiver), gradient coils, and a computer display unit with digital storage facilities. The physical principles of MRI cannot be discussed in detail because of space limitations, and only a brief overview will be given.

The ability of MR to image body parts depends on the intrinsic spin of atomic nuclei with an odd number of protons and/or neutrons (eg, hydrogen), thus generating a magnetic moment. Nuclei of tissues placed within the main magnetic field tend to align along the direction of that field. Application of radiofrequency (rf) pulses induces resonance of particular sets of nuclei. The required frequency of the pulse is determined by the strength of the magnetic field and the particular nucleus under investigation. The energy absorbed during the transition from a high-energy state to a low-energy state is subsequently released and can be recorded as an electrical signal, which provides the data from which digital images are derived. On the images produced by MR, the intensity of a given tissue is a function of the concentration of hydrogen atoms (protons) resonating within the imaged volume and of the longitudinal and transverse relaxation times which, in turn, depend on the biophysical state of the tissue's water molecules. Two relaxation times are described, namely T1 and T2. The T1 relaxation time (longitudinal) is characterized by the return of protons to equilibrium after application and removal of the rf pulse. T2 relaxation time (transverse) is characterized by the associated loss of coherence or phase between individual protons immediately after application of the rf pulse.

A variety of radiofrequency pulse sequences can be used to enhance the differences in tissue relaxation times T1 and T2, thus providing the necessary image contrast. The most commonly used sequences are spin-echo (SE), partial saturation recovery (PSR), inversion recovery (IR), chemical selective suppression (CHESS), and fast-scan (FS) technique. Spin-echo (SE) pulse sequences, utilizing short repetition times (TR) (0.5 sec or less) and short echo delay times (TE) (40 msec or less)—known as T1 weighting—provide good anatomic detail. Long repetition times (TR) (1.5 sec or more) and long echo delay times (TE) (90 msec or more) pulse sequences (or T2), on the other hand, provide good contrast sufficient for evaluation of pathologic processes. Inversion recovery (IR) sequences can be combined with multiplanar imaging to shorten scanning time. With a short inversion time (TI) in the range of 100 to 150 msec, the effects of prolonged T1 and T2 relaxation times are cumulative and the signal from fat is suppressed. This technique, called STIR (short tau inversion recovery) has been useful for evaluation of bone tumors. CHESS is a sequence also used for fat signal suppression. In this sequence, the chemical shift artefacts are removed, and high-intensity fat signal is suppressed; thus, the effective dynamic range of signal intensities is increased, and contrast depiction of anatomic details is improved. Fast imaging techniques have become increasingly popular because of their advantages compared with much slower SE imaging. In particular, so-called gradient recalled echo (GRE) pulse sequences using variable flip angles (5° to 90°), have gained rapid acceptance in orthopedic radiology, since they represent the most effective means of performing fast MR imaging. Several different types of GRE methods are in clinical use. Each of these relies on the use of a reduced flip angle to enhance signal with short TR. These techniques are known by a variety of acronyms such as FLASH (fast low-angle shot), FISP (fast imaging with steady procession), GRASS (gradient-recalled acquisition), and MPGR (multiplanar gradient recalled).

In most examinations, at least two orthogonal planes should be obtained (axial and either coronal or sagittal), and on many occasions all three planes are necessary. Surface coils are necessary for adequate MRI, since they provide improved spatial resolution. Most surface coils are designed specifically for different areas of the body.

The musculoskeletal system is ideally suited for evaluation by MRI, since different tissues display different signal intensity on T1- and T2-

weighted images. The images displayed may have a low signal intensity, intermediate signal intensity, high signal intensity or variations of these. *Low signal intensity* can be subdivided into (a) signal void (black) and (b) signal lower than that of normal muscle (dark). *Intermediate signal intensity* can be subdivided into (a) signal equal to that of normal muscle and (b) signal higher (brighter) than muscle but lower (darker) than subcutaneous fat. *High signal intensity* can be subdivided into (a) signal equal to normal subcutaneous fat (bright) and (b) signal higher than substance fat (extremely bright). High signal intensity of fat planes and differences in signal intensity of various structures allow separation of the different tissue components including muscles, tendons, ligaments, vessels, nerves, hyaline cartilage, fibrocartilage, cortical bone, and trabecular bone (Fig. 1.10). For instance, fat, bone marrow, and hematoma display relatively high signal intensity on T1-weighted images; cortical bone, air, ligaments, tendons, and fibrocartilage display low signal intensity on T1- and T2-weighted images; muscle, nerves and hyaline cartilage display inter-

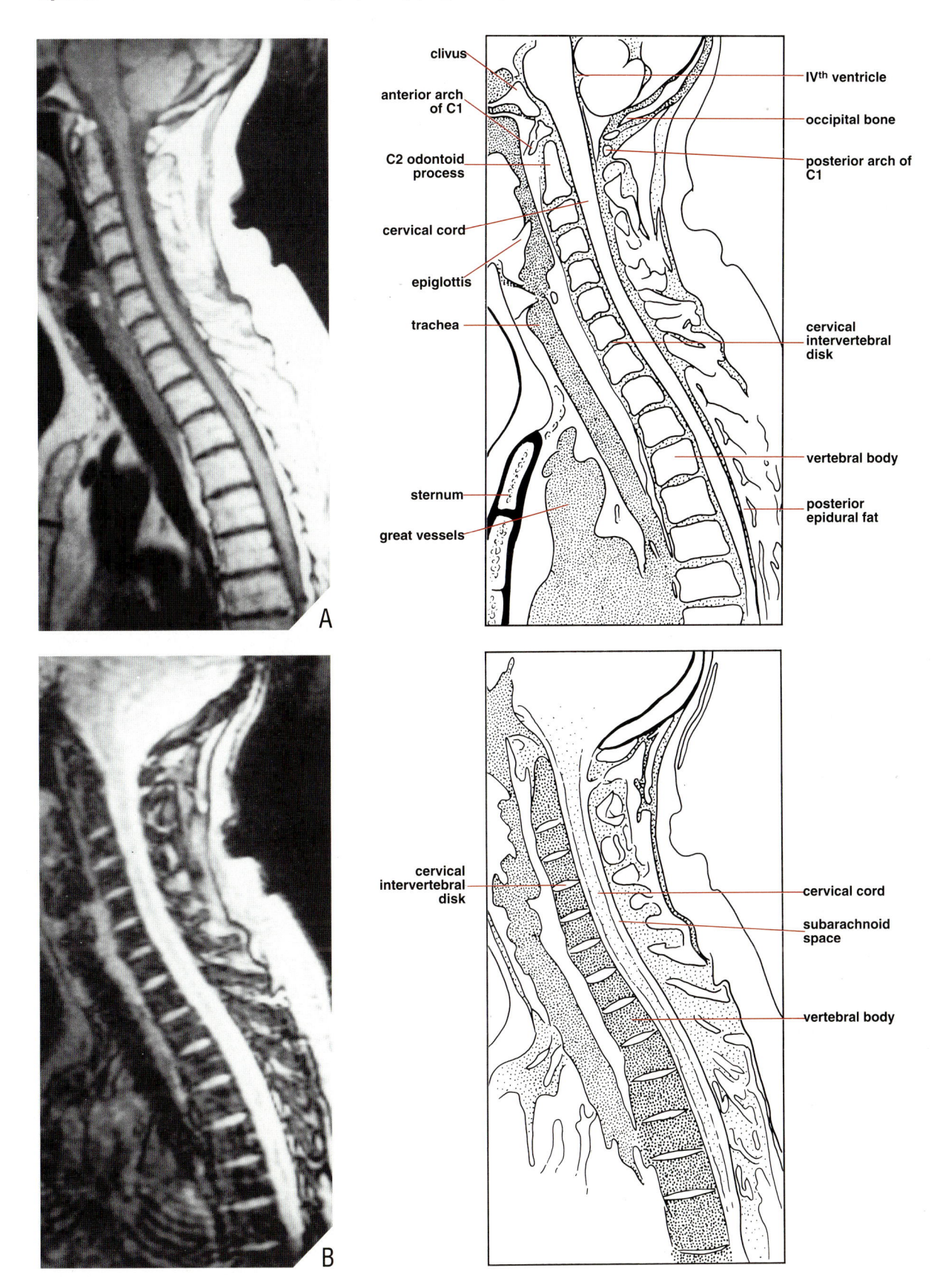

FIGURE 1.10 Magnetic resonance image of a normal cervical spine. **(A)** On a sagittal midline T1-weighted section (SE, TR 800/TE 20), the craniocervical junction is well outlined. The foramen magnum is defined by the fat within the occipital bone and clivus. The anterior and posterior arches of C1 appear as small oval marrow-containing structures of the upper cervical spine. The spinal cord displays intermediate signal intensity outlined by lower signal intensity of CSF. The cervical and thoracic intervertebral disks are imaged as relatively low signal intensity structures. **(B)** On sagittal midline gradient echo section (GRASS, TR 1000/TE 12, flip angle 22°), the high water content of the intervertebral disks produces very high signal, similar to that of CSF. The cervical cord is outlined within the much higher intensity of CSF. The vertebral bodies exhibit a more uniformly low signal intensity. (Reproduced with permission from Beltran J: *MRI:Musculo. Skeletal System*. New York, Gower, 1990)

Imaging Modalities in Evaluating Spinal Disorders

mediate signal intensity on T1- and T2-weighted images. Most tumors display low to intermediate signal intensity on T1-weighted images and high signal intensity on T2-weighted images.

MR images may be enhanced by intravenous injection of gadopentate dimeglumine (Gd-DTPA), known as *gadolinium*. The mechanism by which gadolinium produces enhancement in MRI is different from the mechanism of contrast enhancement by CT. Unlike iodine in CT, gadolinium itself produces no MR signal. Instead, it acts by shortening the T1-relaxation times of tissue into which it extravasates, resulting in an increase in signal intensity on T1-weighted (short TR/TE) imaging sequences.

At present the use of MRI in spine radiology is mainly confined to two areas: trauma and tumors. MRI is particularly effective in evaluation of traumatic conditions of the spinal cord, thecal sac, and nerve roots, as well as in evaluation of disk herniation (Fig. 1.11) and spinal ligament injury. Demonstration of the relationship of vertebral fragments to the spinal cord with direct sagittal imaging is extremely helpful, particularly for evaluation

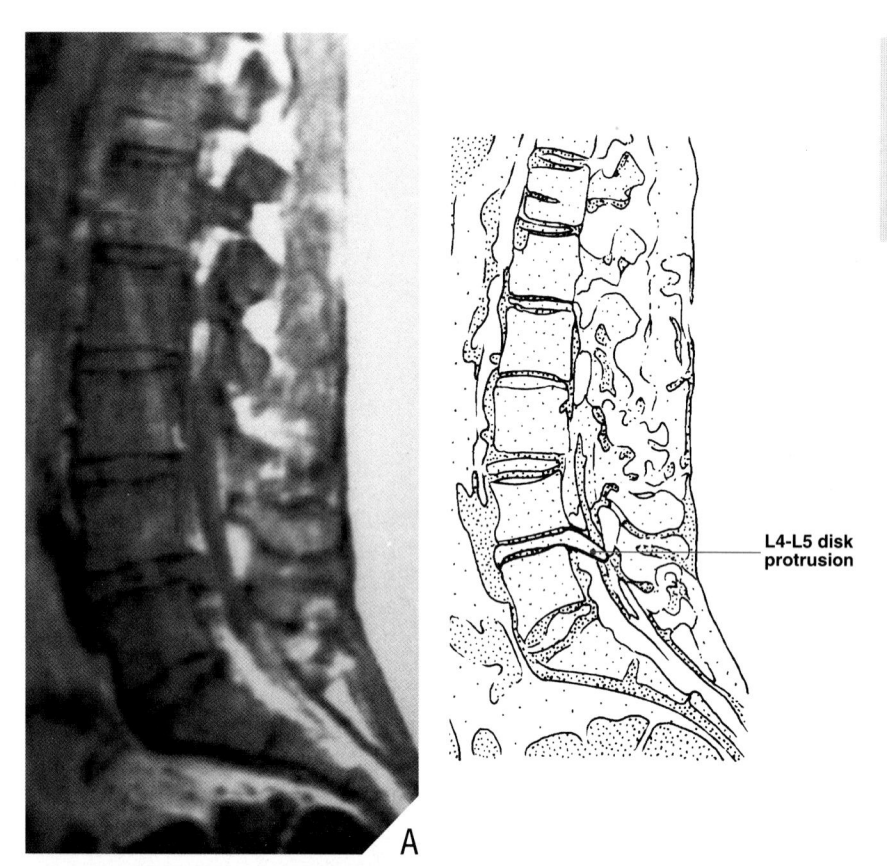

FIGURE 1.11 (A) On this parasagittal proton-density-weighted section (SE, TR 1500/TE 20), a large central focal disk herniation is seen at the L4–L5 interspace. The herniated disk displaces the epidural fat and comes in contact with the thecal sac. **(B)** Axial T1-weighted image (SE, TR 800/TE 20) shows a large central disk protrusion obliterating the epidural fat, anterior to the dural sac. The signal intensity of the disk is moderately different than that of the CSF. The dura is slightly compressed on the right. The fat surrounding the nerve roots remains intact.

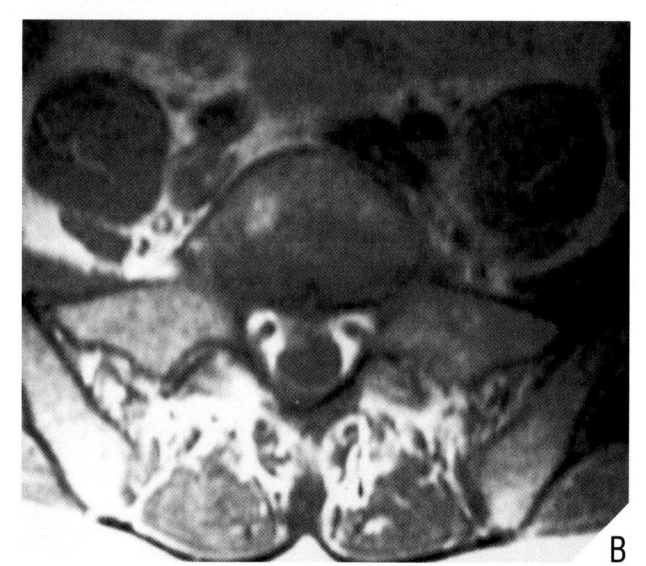

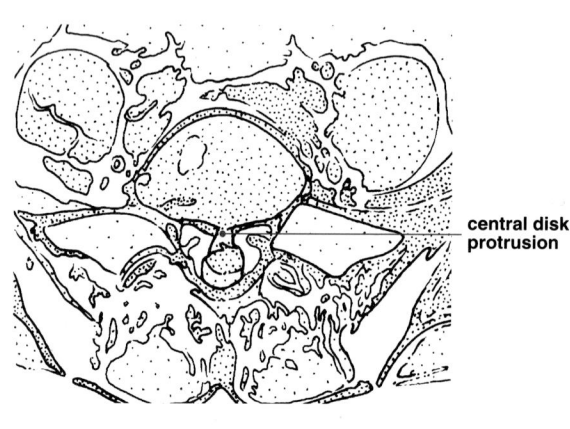

of injury in the cervical and thoracic area. MRI is also indispensable in evaluation of vertebral and soft tissue tumors. Particularly in the case of paravertebral soft tissue masses, MRI offers distinct advantages over CT. There is improved visualization of tissue planes surrounding the lesion, and neurovascular involvement can be evaluated without the use of intravenous contrast. In comparison with CT, however, MR images do not clearly depict or allow characterization of calcification in the tumor matrix; in fact, large amounts of calcification or ossification may be occasionally almost undetectable. Moreover, MRI has shown itself less satisfactory than CT, or even plain films and tomography, for demonstration of cortical destruction.

Although MRI has many advantages, disadvantages exist as well. These include the typical contraindications of scanning patients with cardiac pacemakers, cerebral aneurysm clips, and claustrophobia. The presence of metallic objects, such as ferromagnetic surgical clips, causes focal loss of signal with or without distortion of image. Metallic objects create "holes" in the image, but ferromagnetic objects cause more distortion. Another disadvantage is that MRI still lacks high resolution in evaluation of osseous anatomy and fractures as compared with CT and conventional tomography. Similar to CT, average volume effect may be observed in MR images, leading to occasional problems in interpretation.

SUGGESTED READING

Aisen AN, Martel W, Braunstein EM, et al: MRI and CT evaluation of primary bone and soft tissue tumors. *Am J Radiol* 146:749, 1986.

Al Sheikh, W, Sfakianakis GN, Mnaymneh W, et al: Subacute and chronic bone infections: Diagnosis using In-111, Ga-67, and Tc99m MDP bone scintigraphy and radiography. *Radiology* 155:501, 1985.

Baker LL, Goodman SB, Perkash I, Lane B, Enzmann DR: Benign versus pathologic compression fractures of vertebral bodies: Assessment with conventional spin-echo, chemical-shift, and STIR MR imaging. *Radiology* 174:495, 1990.

Ballinger PW: *Merrill's Atlas of Radiographic Positrons and Radiologic Procedures,* 6th ed, vol. 1. St. Louis, C V Mosby, 1986.

Beck RN: Radionuclide imaging principles. In Taveras JM, Ferrucci JT (eds.): *Radiology–Diagnosis, Imaging, Intervention,* vol I. Philadelphia, J B Lippincott, 1990.

Borders J, Kerr E, Sartoris DJ, et al: Quantitative dual-energy radiographic absorptiometry of the lumbar spine: In vivo comparison with dual-photon absorptiometry. *Radiology* 170:129, 1989.

Dalinka MK, Boorstein JM, Zlatkin MB: Computed tomography of musculoskeletal trauma. *Radiol Clin North Am* 27:933, 1989.

Derchi LE, Balconi G, DeFlaviis L, et al: Sonographic appearance of hemangiomas of skeletal muscle. *J Ultrasound Med* 8:263, 1989.

Deutsch AL, Mink JH: Magnetic resonance imaging of musculoskeletal injuries. *Radiol Clin North Am* 27:983, 1989.

Erlemann R, Vasallo P, Bongartz G, et al: Musculoskeletal neoplasms: Fast low-angle shot MR imaging with and without Gd-DTPA. *Radiology* 176:489, 1990.

Errico TJ: The Role of diskography in the 1980s. *Radiology* 162:285, 1989.

Fuchs AW: Cervical vertebrae (Part I). *Radiogr Clin Photogr* 16:2, 1940.

Genant HK, Cann CE, Chafetz NI, et al: Advances in computed tomography of the musculo-skeletal system. *Radiol Clin North Am* 19:645: 1981.

Haughton VM: MR imaging of the spine. *Radiology* 166:297, 1988.

Ho C, Sartoris DJ, Resnick D: Conventional tomography in musculoskeletal trauma. *Radiol Clin North Am* 27:929, 1989.

Magid D, Fishman EK: Imaging of musculoskeletal trauma in three dimensions. *Radiol Clin North Am* 27:945, 1989.

McAfee JG: Update on radiopharmaceuticals for medical imaging. *Radiology* 171:593, 1989.

McAfee JG, Samin A: Indium-111 labelled leukocytes: A review of problems in image interpretation. *Radiology* 155:221, 1985.

Negendank WG, Crowley MG, Ryan JR, et al: Bone and soft-tissue lesions: Diagnosis with combined H-1 MR imaging and P-31 MR spectroscopy. *Radiology* 173:181, 1989.

Sartoris DJ, Resnick D: Current and innovative methods for noninvasive bone densitometry. *Radiol Clinics North Am* 28:257, 1990.

Sartoris DJ, Sommer, FG: Digital film processing: Applications to the musculoskeletal system. *Skeletal Radiol* 11:274, 1984.

Schmalbrock P, Beltran J: Principles of magnetic resonance imaging. In Beltran J (ed.): *MRI Musculoskeletal System.* Philadelphia, J B Lippincott, 1990.

Shapiro R: Current status of lumbar diskography (Letter). *Radiology* 159:815, 1986.

Sundaram M, McLeod RA: MR imaging of tumor and tumorlike lesions of bones and soft tissues. *AJR* 155:817, 1990

Vanharanta H, Guyer RD, Ohnmeiss DD, et al: Disc deterioration in low-back syndromes. A prospective, multi-center CT/discography study. *Spine* 13:1249, 1988.

Zucherman J, Derby R, Hsu K, et al: Normal magnetic resonance imaging with abnormal discography. *Spine* 13:1355, 1988.

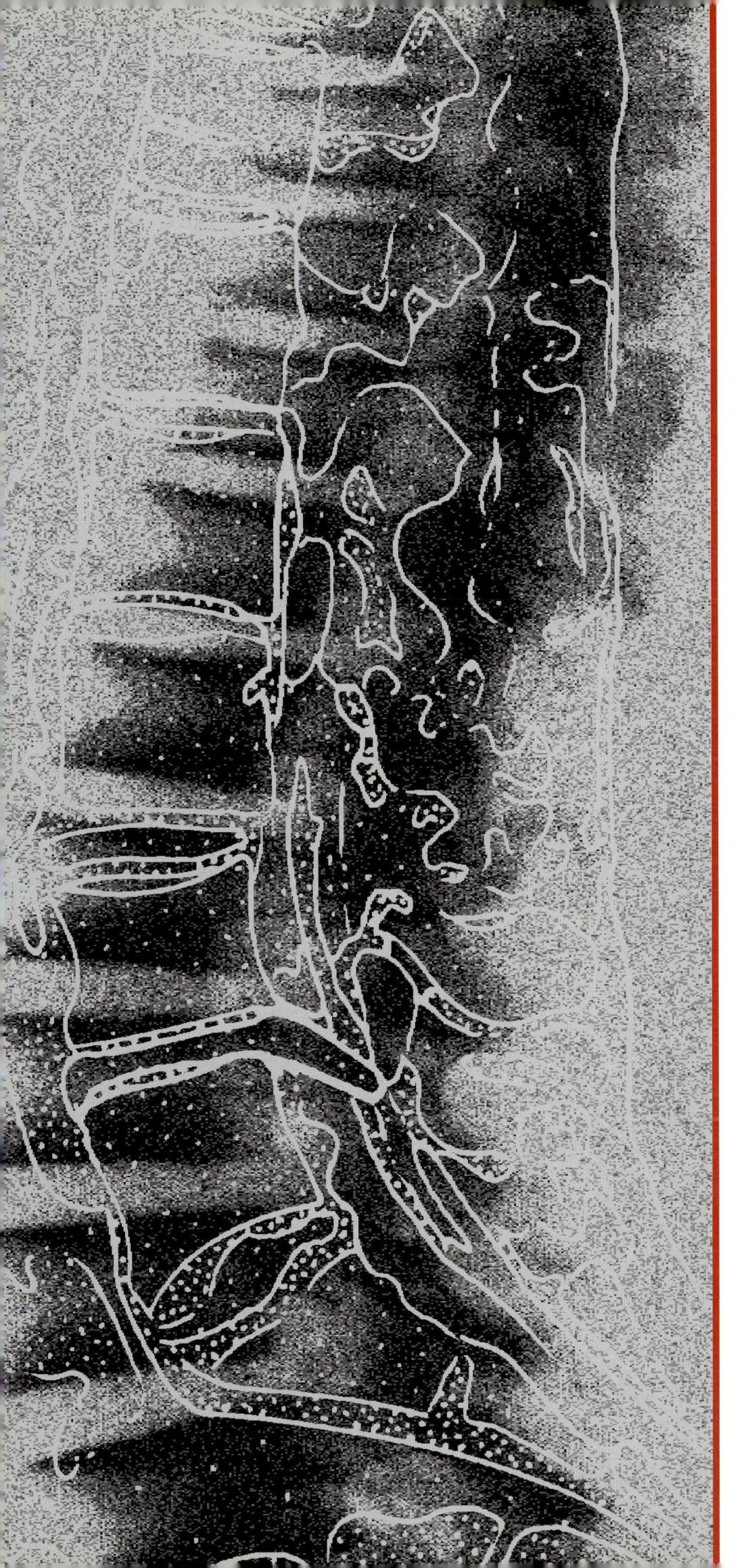

Injury to the Cervical Spine

2

Fractures of the vertebral column are important not only because of the structures involved but because of the potential for complications that may affect the spinal cord. Constituting about 3% to 6% of all skeletal injuries, fractures of the vertebral column are most common in people between the ages of 20 and 50 years, the great majority of cases (80%) involving males. Automobile accidents, sports-related activities (eg, diving, skiing), and falls from heights are the most common cause of spinal injuries. Most spinal fractures occur at the thoracic or lumbar level, but injury to the cervical area has a greater potential risk for spinal cord damage. Neurologic complications occur in 40% of patients with cervical level injury and in 15% to 20% of patients with thoracolumbar level injury.

ANATOMIC AND RADIOLOGIC CONSIDERATIONS

The spine is composed of 33 vertebrae: 7 cervical, 12 thoracic, 5 lumbar, a sacrum of 5 fused segments, and a coccyx of 4 fused segments. With the exception of the first and second cervical vertebrae (C1 and C2), the vertebral bodies are separated from each other by intervertebral disks.

The first and second cervical vertebrae possess anatomic features distinct from those of the remaining five cervical vertebrae (Fig. 2.1). The first vertebra, C1 or *atlas* (so called because it supports the globe of the head), is a bony ring consisting of anterior and posterior arches connected by two lateral masses. The atlas has no body; its main weight-bearing structures are the lateral masses, also called *articular pillars*. In many ways, C1 functions as an ossified meniscus. The second vertebra, C2 or *axis*, is a more complex structure whose distinguishing feature is the odontoid process also known as the *dens* (tooth), projecting cephalad from the anterior surface of the body. The odontoid process actually represents the body of C1 which, during embryonal development, becomes separated from C1 and united to C2. The space between the odontoid process and the anterior arch of the atlas, called the *atlantal–dens interval*, should not exceed 3 mm in adults, whether the head is flexed or extended. In children under 8 years of age, this distance can be as much as 4 mm, particularly in flexion, because of greater laxity of the associated ligaments.

The vertebrae C3–C7 exhibit almost identical anatomic features and are more uniform in appearance, consisting of a vertebral body and a posterior neural arch, including the right and left pedicles and laminae

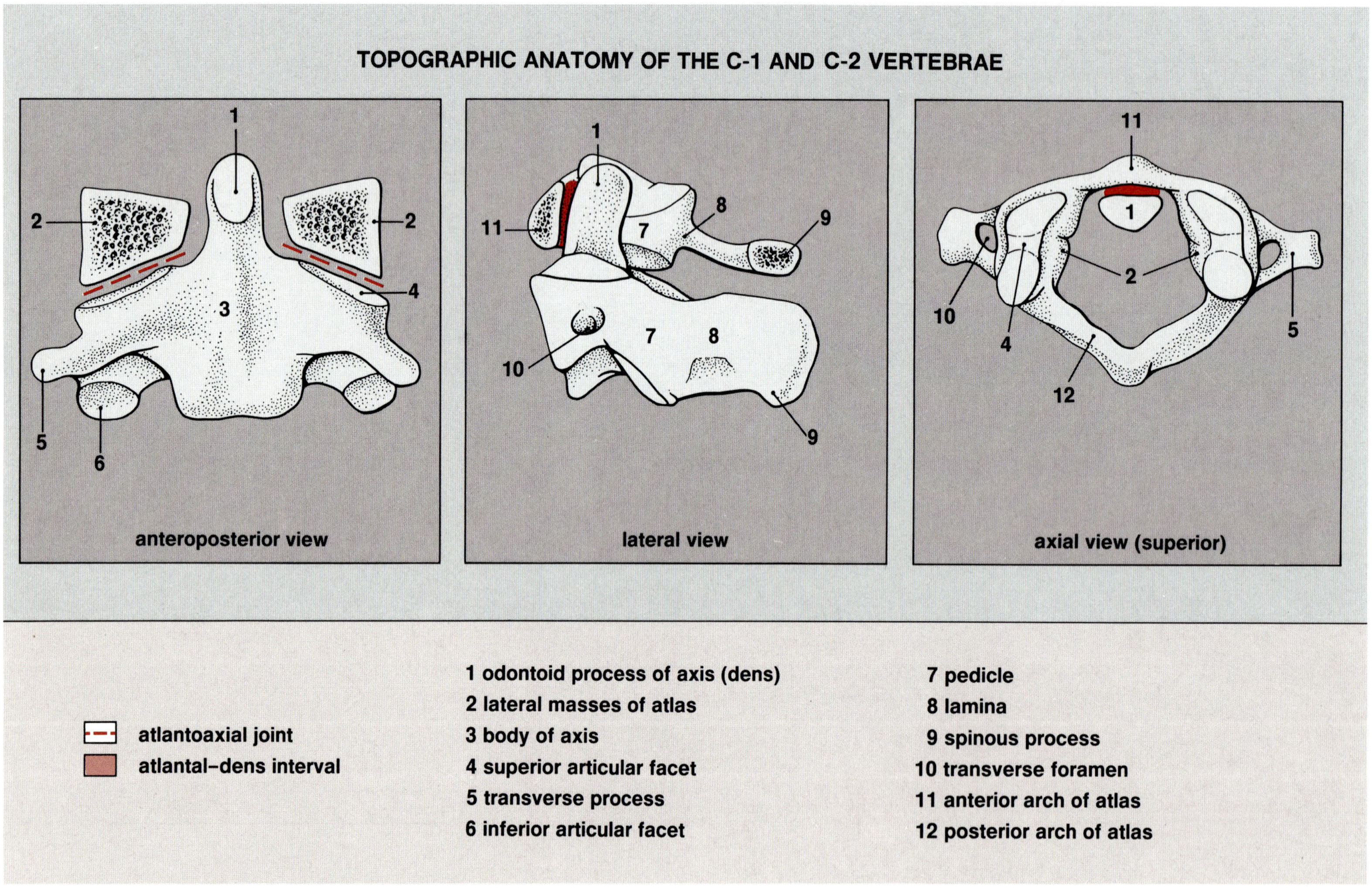

TOPOGRAPHIC ANATOMY OF THE C-1 AND C-2 VERTEBRAE

1 odontoid process of axis (dens)	7 pedicle
2 lateral masses of atlas	8 lamina
3 body of axis	9 spinous process
4 superior articular facet	10 transverse foramen
5 transverse process	11 anterior arch of atlas
6 inferior articular facet	12 posterior arch of atlas

atlantoaxial joint
atlantal–dens interval

FIGURE 2.1 Topographic anatomy of the C1 and C2 vertebrae.

Imaging of the Spine in Clinical Practice

which, together with the posterior aspect of the body, enclose the spinal canal (Fig. 2.2). Extending caudad and cephalad from the junction of the pedicle and lamina on each side are superior and inferior articular processes, which form the apophyseal joints between the successive vertebrae. Extending laterally from the pedicle on each side is a transverse process, and in the posterior portion a spinous process (frequently bifid) extends from the junction of the laminae in the midline. On the cephalad surface of the transverse process is a groove (*sulcus*) for the spinal nerve, which runs posterior to the vertebral artery. The vertebral arteries pass through the transverse foramina located in the transverse processes. Vertebra C7, in addition, is distinguished by its long spinous process and large transverse processes. Like C1–C6, C7 has a transverse foramen; however, the vertebral artery does not pass through it.

Radiographic examination of a patient with cervical spine trauma may be difficult and must usually be limited to one or two projections because (1) the patient is often unconscious, (2) associated injuries may be present, and (3) unnecessary movement risks damage to the cervical cord. The single most valuable projection in such a case is the *lateral view*, which can be obtained in the standard fashion or in the supine position, depending on the patient's condition (Fig. 2.3). This projection demonstrates most traumatic conditions of the cervical spine, including injuries involving the anterior and posterior arches of C1, the odontoid process (which is seen in profile), and the anterior atlantal–dens interval. The bodies and spinous processes of C2–C7 are fully visualized, and the intervertebral disk spaces and prevertebral soft tissues can be adequately evaluated.

The lateral view may also be obtained in flexion of the neck, which is particularly effective in demonstrating suspected instability at C1–C2 by allowing evaluation of the atlanto–odontoid space. An increase in this space to more than 3 mm indicates atlanto–axial subluxations. On the lateral projection of the cervical spine it is extremely important to visualize C7 and T1 vertebrae, as this is the most commonly overlooked site of injury.

The lateral view of the cervical spine, including the lower part of the skull, is very useful for evaluation of vertical subluxation involving the

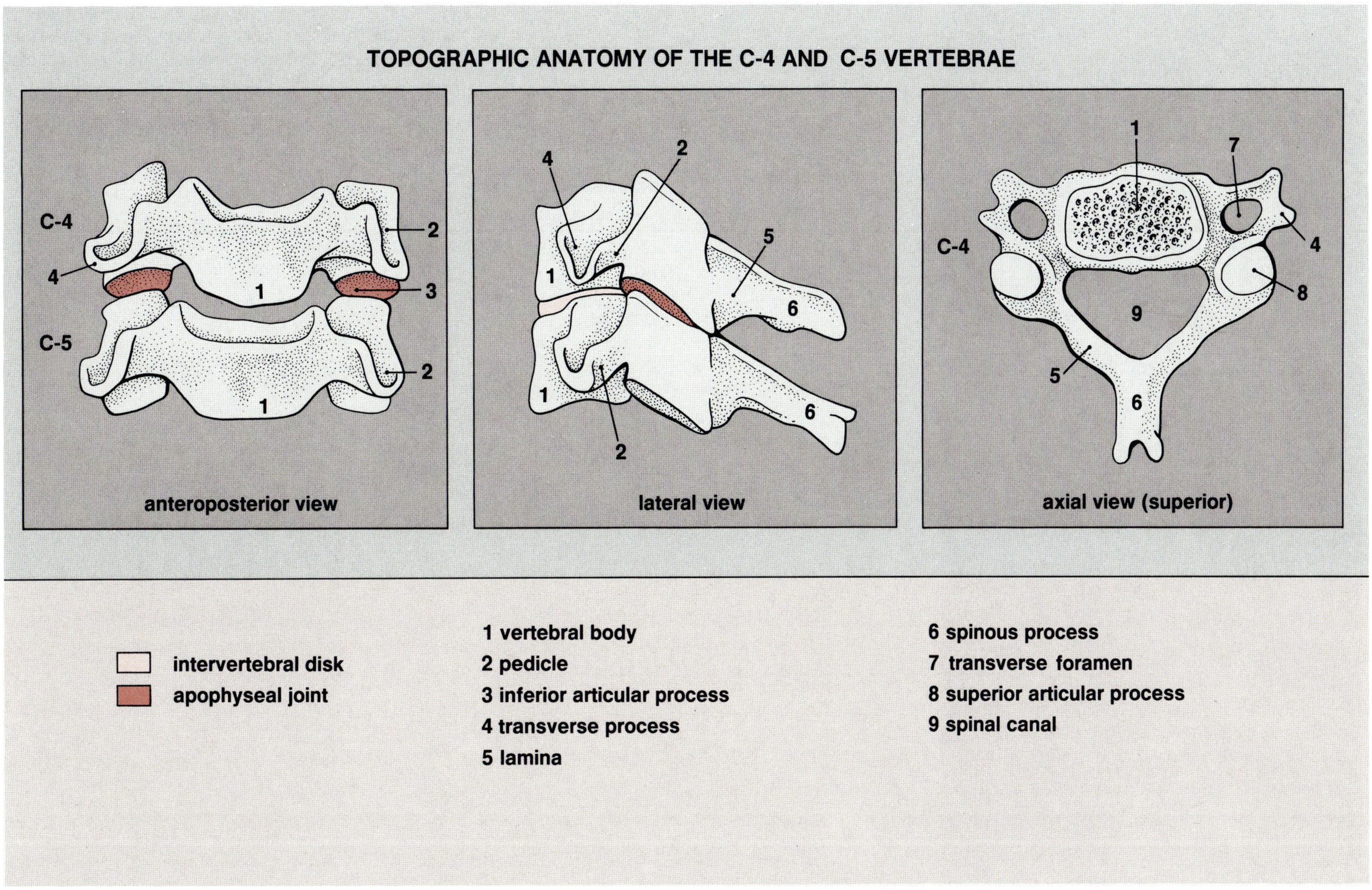

FIGURE 2.2 Topographic anatomy of the C4 and C5 vertebrae, representing the mid and lower cervical vertebrae.

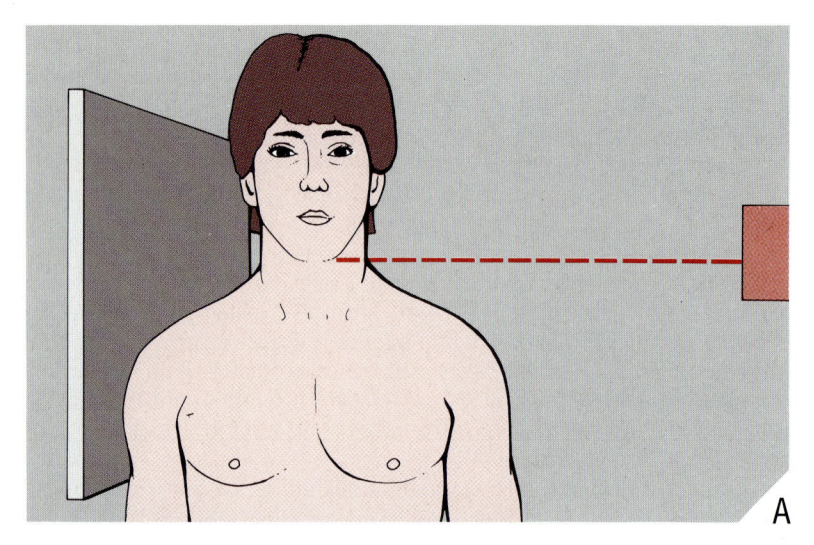

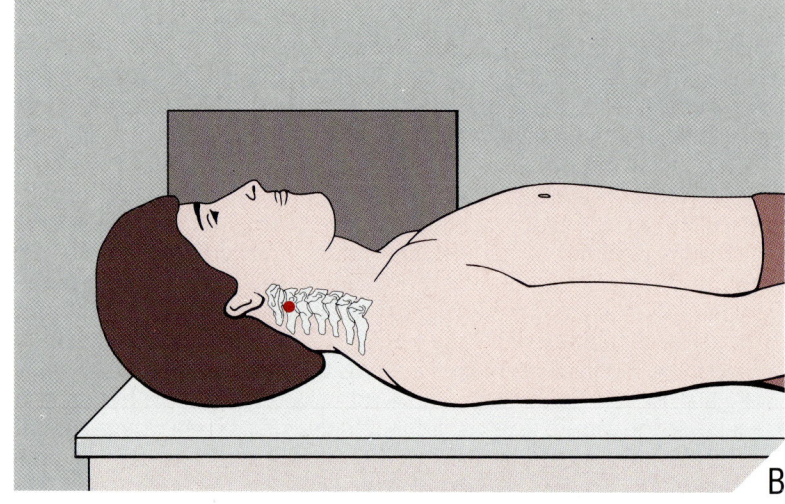

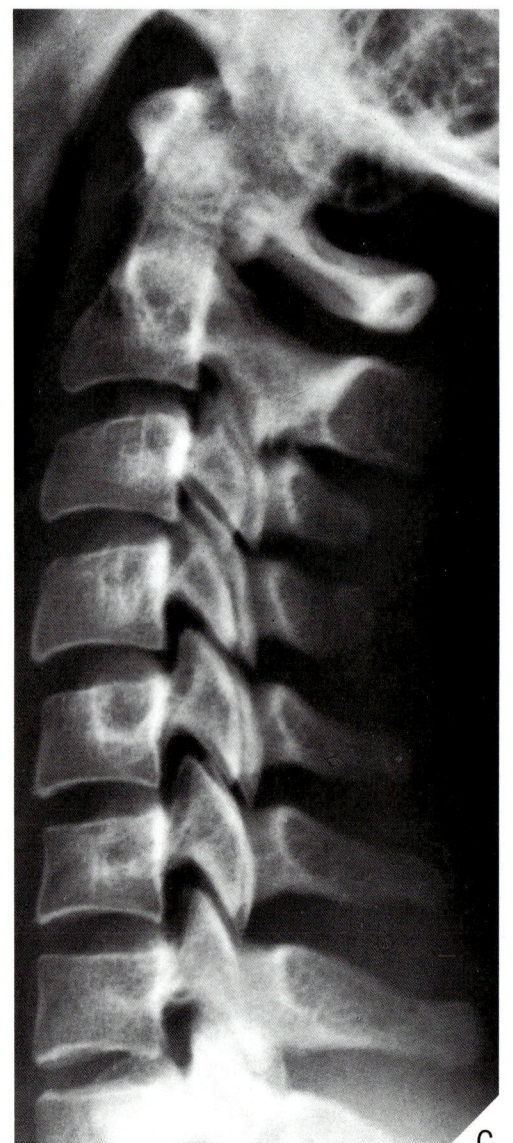

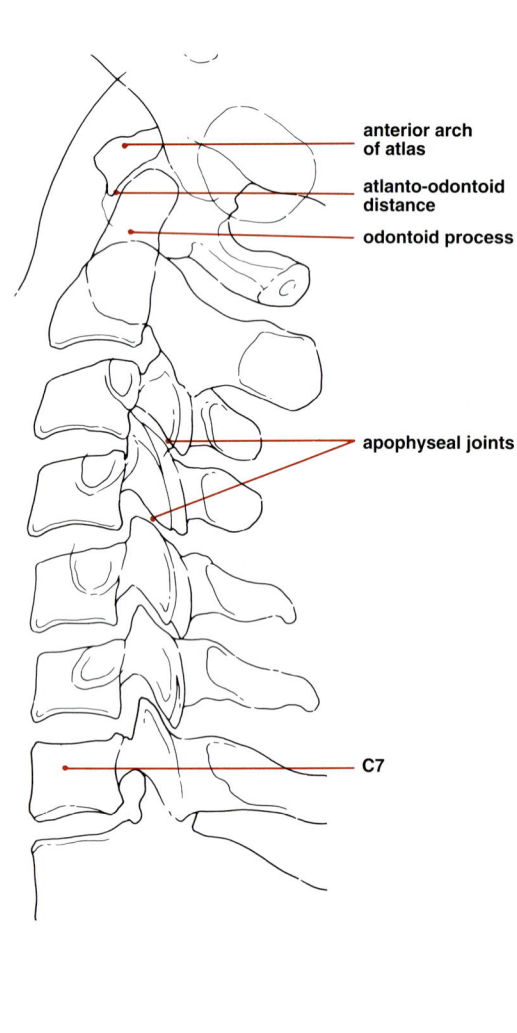

FIGURE 2.3 (A) For the erect lateral view of the cervical spine, the patient is standing or seated, with the head straight in the neutral position. The central beam is directed horizontally to the center of the C4 vertebra (at the level of the chin). **(B)** For the cross-table lateral view, the patient is supine on the radiographic table. The radiographic cassette (a grid cassette to obtain a clearer image) is adjusted to the side of the neck, and the central beam is directed horizontally to a point (*red dot*) about 2.5 to 3 cm caudal to the mastoid tip. **(C)** The lateral radiograph clearly shows the vertebral bodies, apophyseal joints, spinous processes, and intervertebral disk spaces. It is mandatory to demonstrate the C7 vertebra.

- anterior arch of atlas
- atlanto-odontoid distance
- odontoid process
- apophyseal joints
- C7

2.4 *Imaging of the Spine in Clinical Practice*

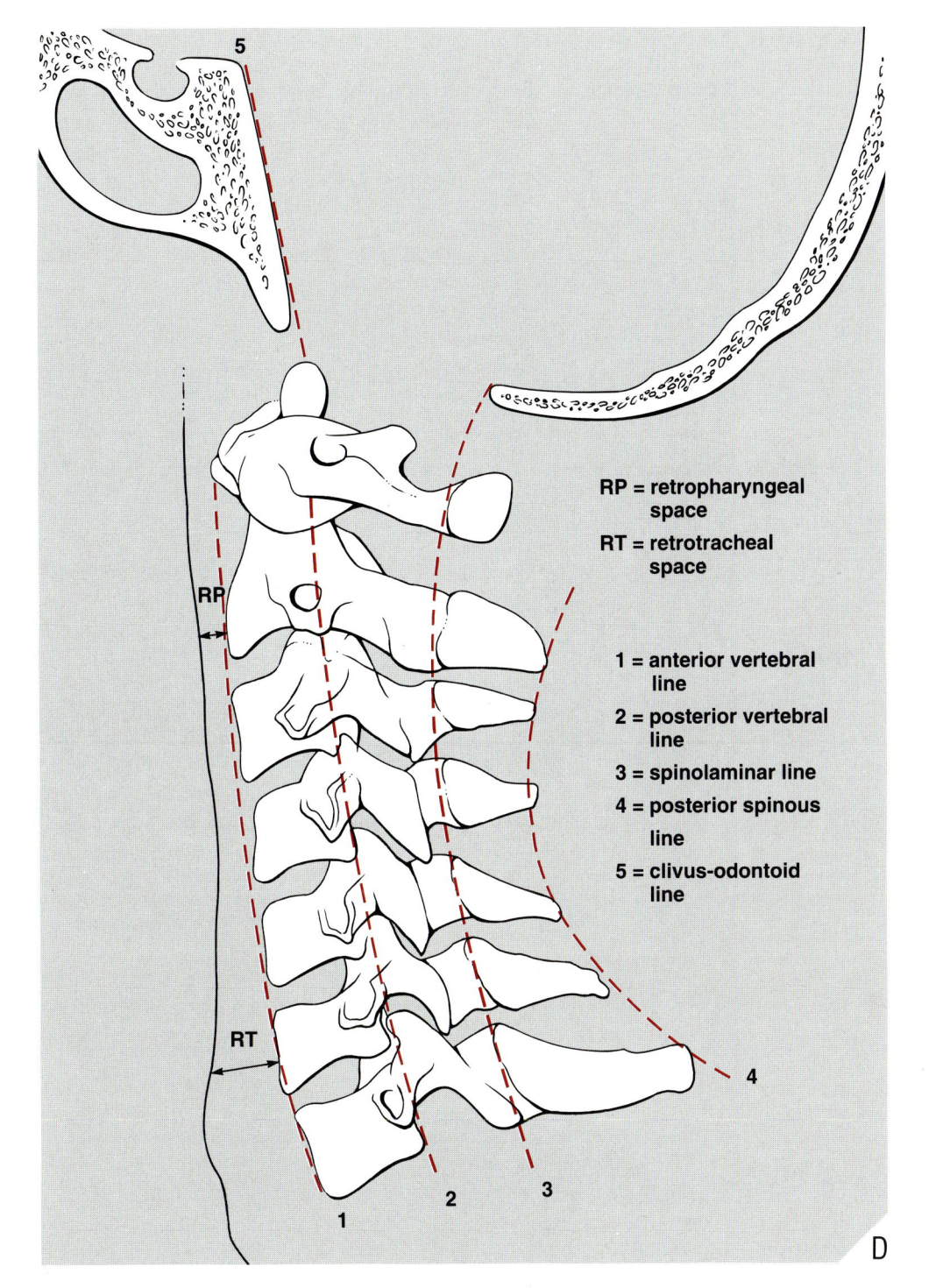

FIGURE 2.3 (cont.) **(D)** With this lateral view the four contour lines of the normal cervical spine can be demonstrated: (1) anterior vertebral line drawn along anterior margins of the vertebral bodies; (2) posterior vertebral line (outlines anterior margin of spinal canal), drawn along posterior margins of the vertebral bodies; (3) spinolaminar line (outlines posterior margin of the spinal canal), drawn along the anterior margins of the bases of the spinous processes at the junction with lamina; (4) posterior spinous line drawn along the tips of the spinous processes from C2–C7; all four lines should be running smoothly, without angulation or interruption; (5) the clivus–odontoid line, drawn from the dorsum sellae along the clivus to the anterior margin of the foramen, should point to the tip of the odontoid process at the junction of the anterior and middle thirds. The retropharyngeal space (the distance from the posterior pharyngeal wall to the anteroinferior aspect of C2) should measure 7 mm or less; the retrotracheal space (the distance from the posterior wall of the trachea to the anteroinferior aspect of C6) should measure no more than 22 mm in adults and 14 mm in children.

Injury to the Cervical Spine

atlanto–axial articulation and the migration of the odontoid process into the foramen magnum. Several measurements are helpful to identify atlanto–axial impaction or cranial settling resulting in superior migration of the odontoid process (Figs. 2.4–2.7).

On the *anteroposterior view* of the cervical spine, the bodies of the C3–C7 vertebrae (and occasionally, in young persons, even C1 and C2) are well demonstrated, as are the uncovertebral (Luschka) joints and the intervertebral disk spaces (Fig. 2.8). The spinous processes are seen

FIGURE 2.4 Chamberlain's line is drawn from the posterior margin of the foramen magnum (opisthion) to the dorsal (posterior) margin of the hard palate. The odontoid process should not project above this line more than 3 mm. Odontoid process 6.6 mm (± 2 SD) above this line strongly indicates cranial settling.

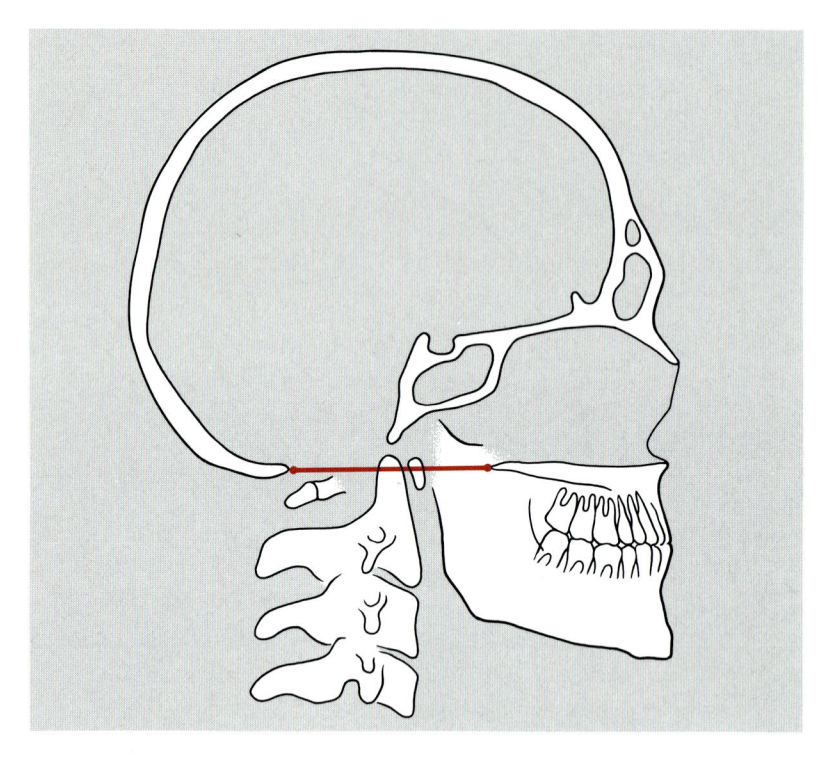

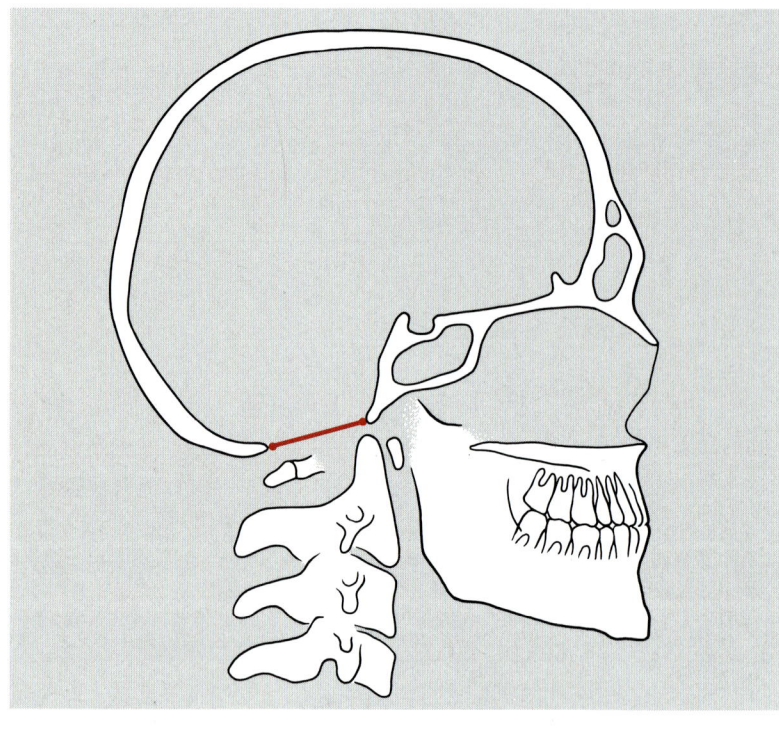

FIGURE 2.5 McRae's line defines the opening of the foramen magnum and connects the anterior margin (basion) with posterior margin (opisthion) of the foramen magnum. The odontoid process should be just below this line or the line may intersect only the tip of the odontoid process. In addition, a perpendicular line drawn from the apex of the odontoid to this line should intersect it in its ventral quarter.

almost on end, casting oval shadows resembling teardrops. A variant of the anteroposterior projection, known as the *open-mouth view* (Fig. 2.9), may also be obtained as part of the standard examination. This view effectively visualizes the structures of the first two cervical vertebrae. The body of C2 is clearly imaged, as are the atlanto–axial joints, the odontoid process, and the lateral spaces between the odontoid process and the articular pillars of C1. If the open-mouth view is difficult to obtain or if the odontoid process is not clearly visualized (particularly its upper half), *Fuchs view* (1940) may be helpful (Fig. 2.10). *Oblique projections* of the cervical spine (Fig. 2.11) are not routinely obtained, although at times

FIGURE 2.6 McGregor's line connects the posterosuperior margin of the hard palate to the most caudal part of the occipital curve of the skull. The tip of the odontoid normally does not extend more than 4.5 mm above the line.

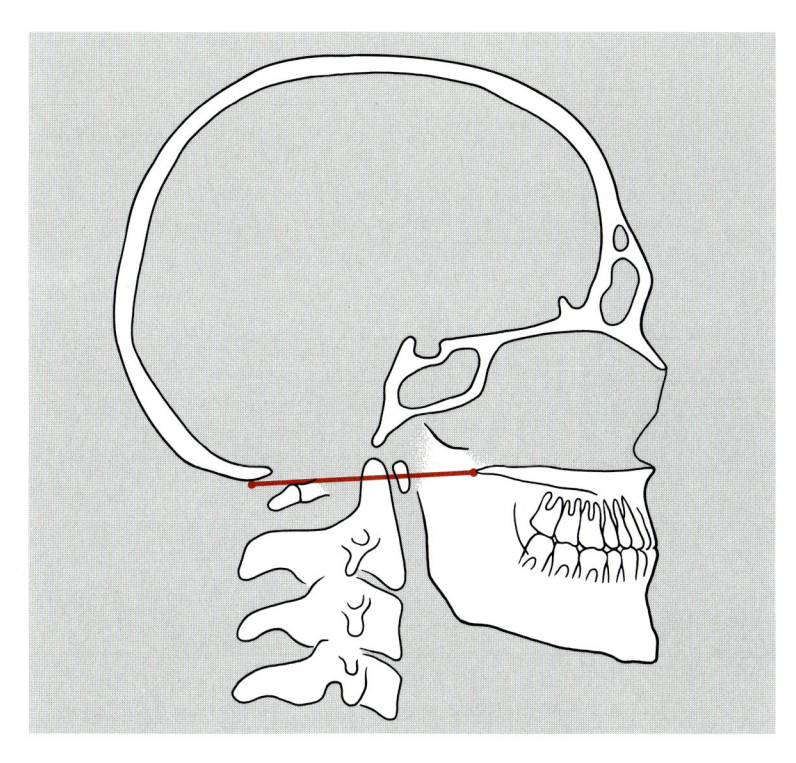

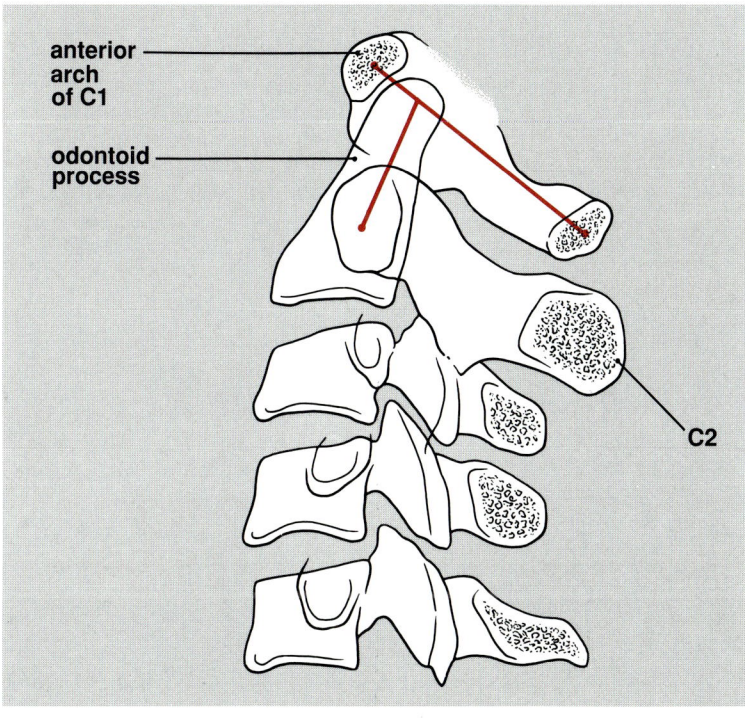

FIGURE 2.7 Ranawat and associates developed a new method for determining the extent of the superior margin of the odontoid process, since the hard palate often is not identifiable on the radiographs of the cervical spine. The coronal axis of C1 is determined by connecting the center of the anterior arch of the first cervical vertebra with its posterior ring. The center of the sclerotic ring in C2, representing pedicles, is marked. The line is drawn along the axis of the odontoid process to the first line. The normal distance between C1 and C2 in men averages 17 mm (± 2 mm SD), and in women, 15 mm (± 2 mm SD). Decrease in the distance indicates cephalad migration of C2.

Injury to the Cervical Spine

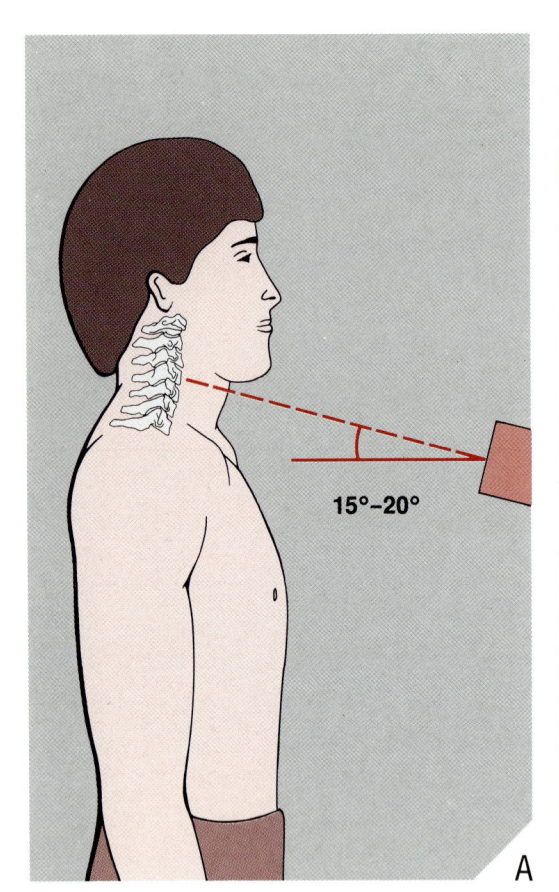

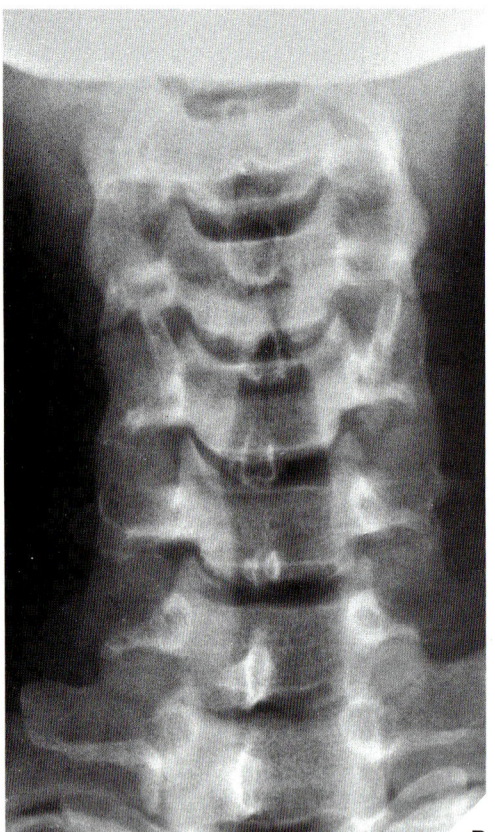

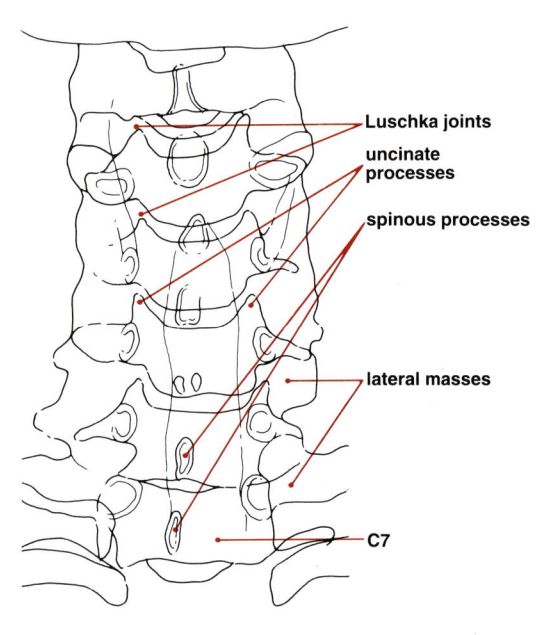

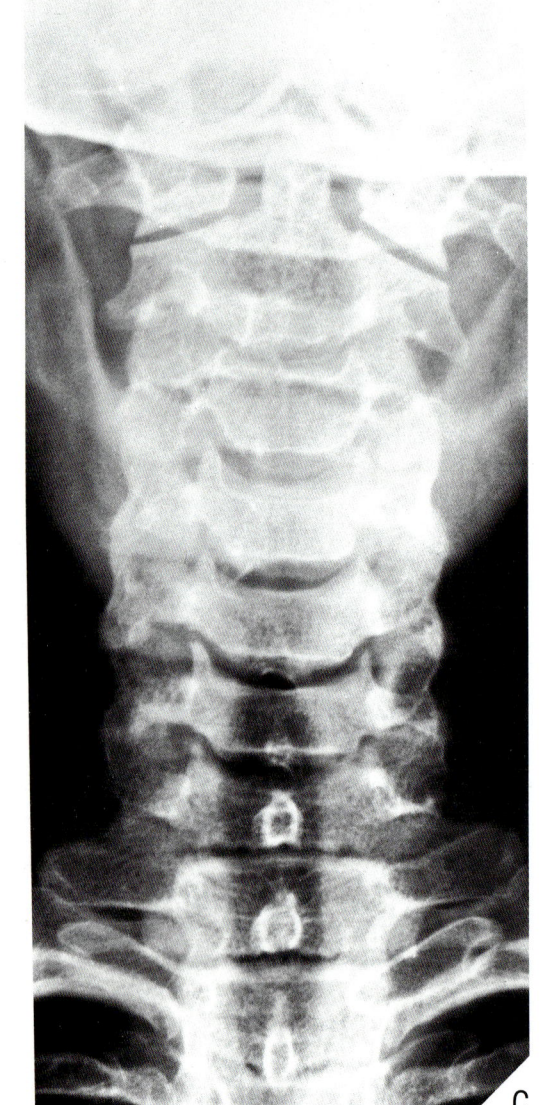

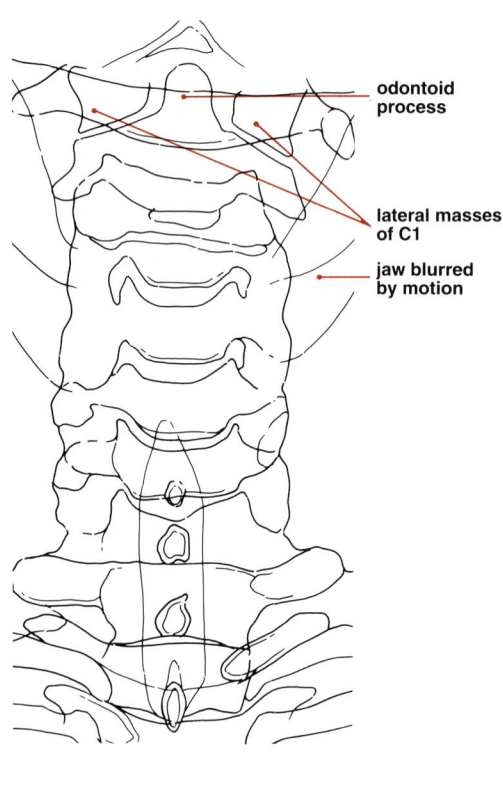

FIGURE 2.8 (A) For the anteroposterior view of the cervical spine, the patient is either erect or supine. The central beam is directed toward the C4 vertebra (at the point of the Adam's apple) at an angle of 15° to 20° cephalad. **(B)** The film in this projection demonstrates the C3 through C7 vertebral bodies and the intervertebral disk spaces. The spinous processes are seen superimposed on the bodies, resembling teardrops. The C1 and C2 vertebrae are not adequately seen. For their visualization, the patient is instructed to open and close the mouth rapidly. Motion of the mandible blurs this structure, and C1 and C2 become visible **(C)**.

2.8 *Imaging of the Spine in Clinical Practice*

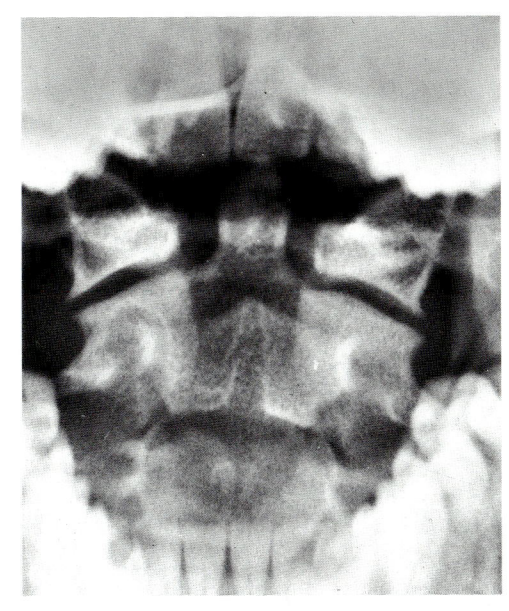

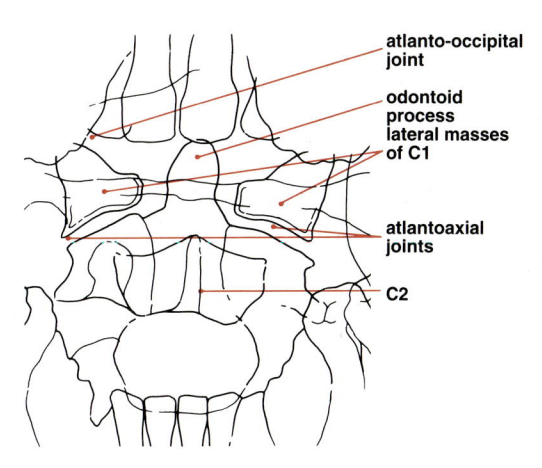

FIGURE 2.9 For the open-mouth view, the patient is positioned in the same manner as for the supine anteroposterior projection; the head is straight, in the neutral position. With the patient's mouth open as widely as possible, the central beam is directed perpendicular to the midpoint of the open mouth. During the exposure, the patient should softly phonate "ah" to affix the tongue to the floor of the mouth so that its shadow is not projected over C1 and C2. On the radiograph, the odontoid process, the body of C2, and the lateral masses of the atlas are well demonstrated; the atlantoaxial joints are seen to best advantage.

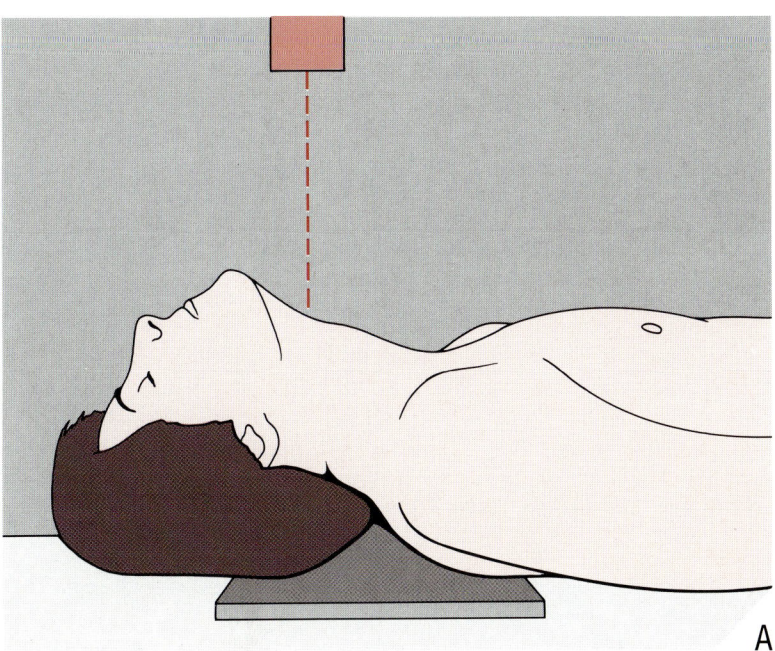

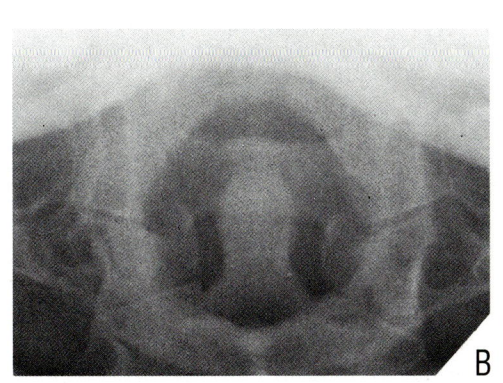

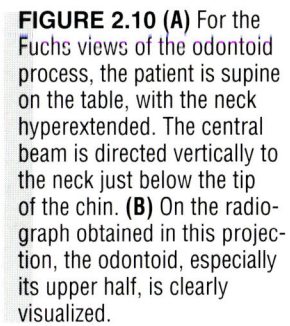

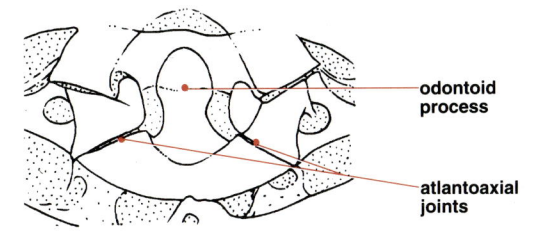

FIGURE 2.10 (A) For the Fuchs views of the odontoid process, the patient is supine on the table, with the neck hyperextended. The central beam is directed vertically to the neck just below the tip of the chin. **(B)** On the radiograph obtained in this projection, the odontoid, especially its upper half, is clearly visualized.

Injury to the Cervical Spine **2.9**

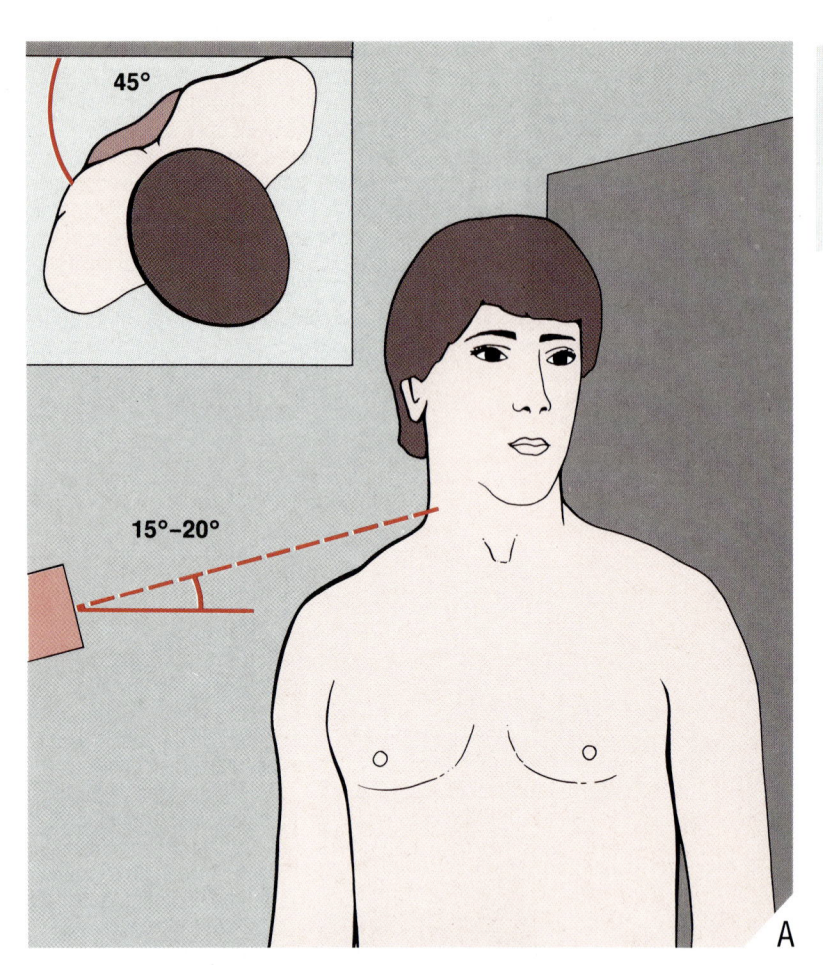

FIGURE 2.11 (A) An oblique view of the cervical spine may be obtained in the anteroposterior, as shown here, or posteroanterior projection. The patient may be erect or recumbent, but the erect position (seated or standing) is more comfortable. The patient is rotated 45° to one side—to the left, as shown here, to demonstrate the right-sided neural foramina and to the right to demonstrate the left-sided neural foramina. The central beam is directed to the C4 vertebra with 15° to 20° cephalad angulation. **(B)** The film in this projection is effective primarily for demonstrating the intervertebral neural foramina.

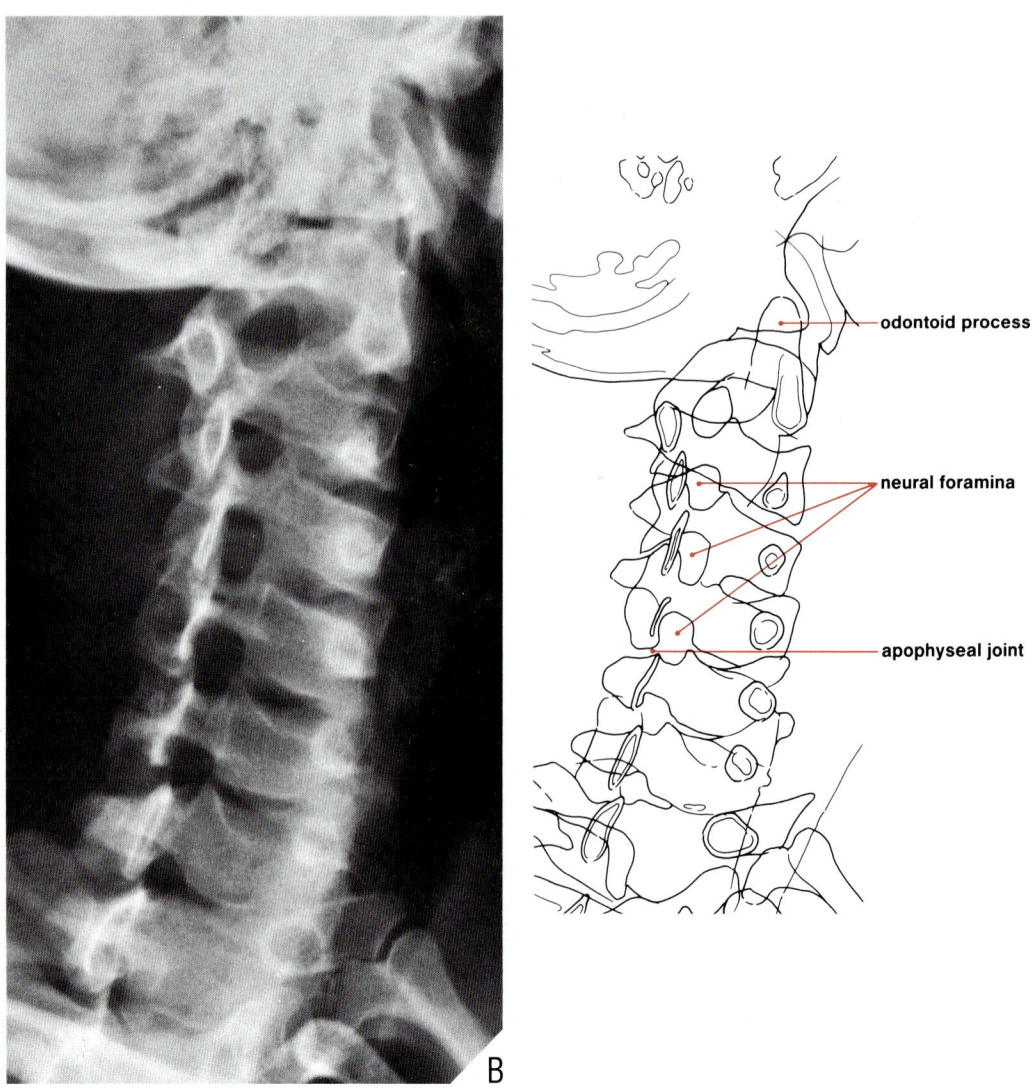

- odontoid process
- neural foramina
- apophyseal joint

2.10 *Imaging of the Spine in Clinical Practice*

they can help to visualize obscure fractures of the neural arch or abnormalities of the neural foramina and apophyseal joints.

Special projections are occasionally required for sufficient evaluation of the structures of the cervical spine. The *pillar view* (Fig. 2.12), which can be obtained in the anteroposterior or oblique projection, demonstrates the lateral masses of the cervical vertebrae. The *swimmer's view* (Fig. 2.13) can be employed for better demonstration of C7, T1, and T2, which on the standard lateral or oblique projection are obscured by the overlapping clavicle and the soft tissues of the shoulder girdle. Fluoroscopy and videotaping are usually of little help in acute injuries because pain may prevent the movement necessary to position the patient.

Ancillary imaging techniques play an important role in the evaluation of suspected spinal trauma. Conventional tomography and computed tomography (CT) are commonly employed. In the evaluation of fractures

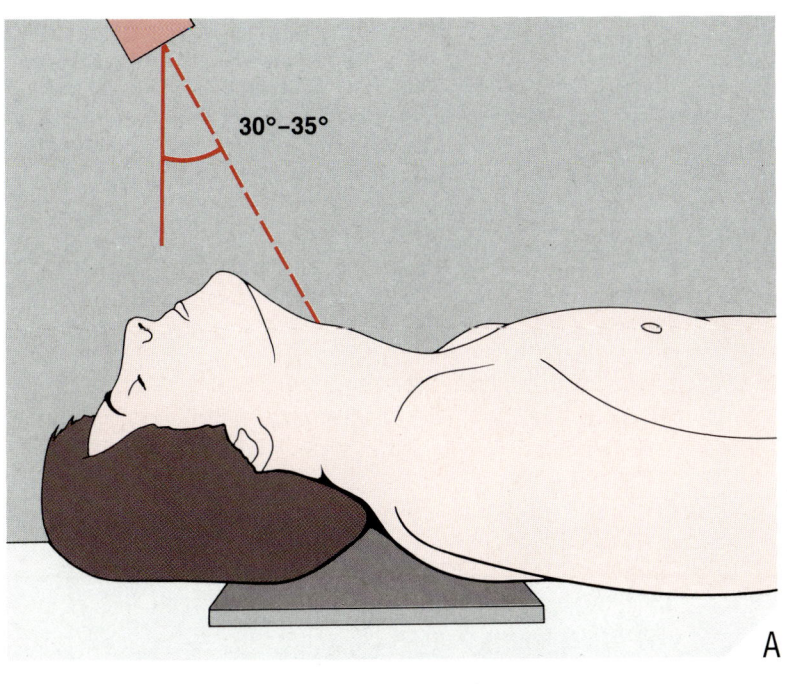

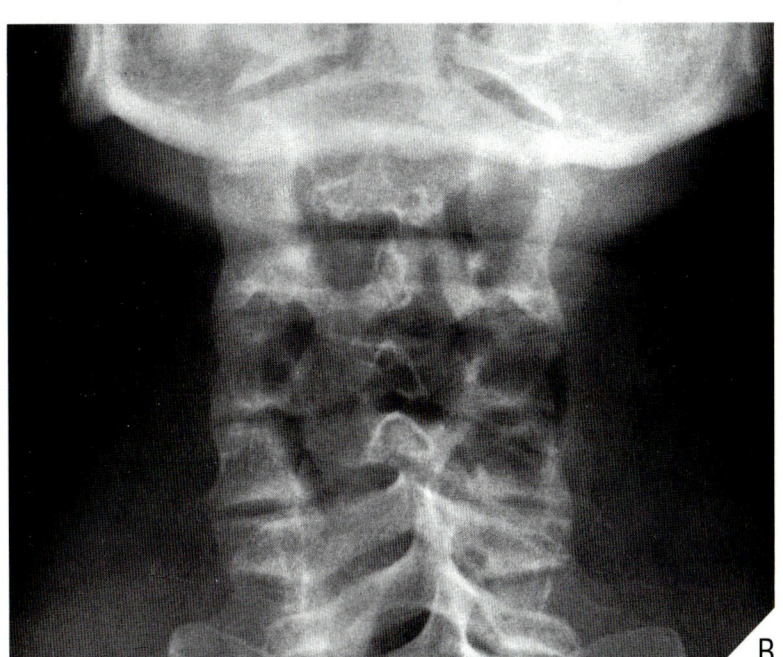

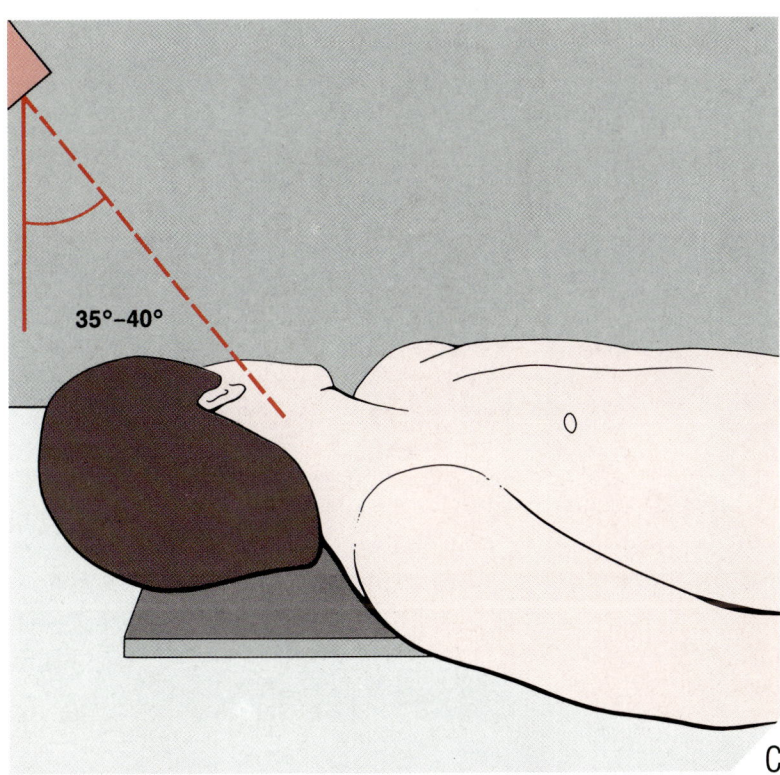

FIGURE 2.12 (A) For the pillar view of the cervical spine, the patient is supine on the table, with the neck hyperextended. The central beam is directed to the center of the neck in the region of the thyroid cartilage at a caudal angulation of 30° to 35°. **(B)** On the film in this projection, the lateral masses (pillars) of the cervical vertebrae are well demonstrated. **(C)** The pillar view can also be obtained in the oblique projection. The patient is supine on the table, with the neck hyperextended and the head rotated 45° toward the unaffected side. The central beam is directed with about 35° to 40° caudal angulation to the lateral side of the neck about 3 cm below the earlobe. **(D)** On the radiograph obtained with leftward rotation of the head, an oblique view of the right pillars is achieved.

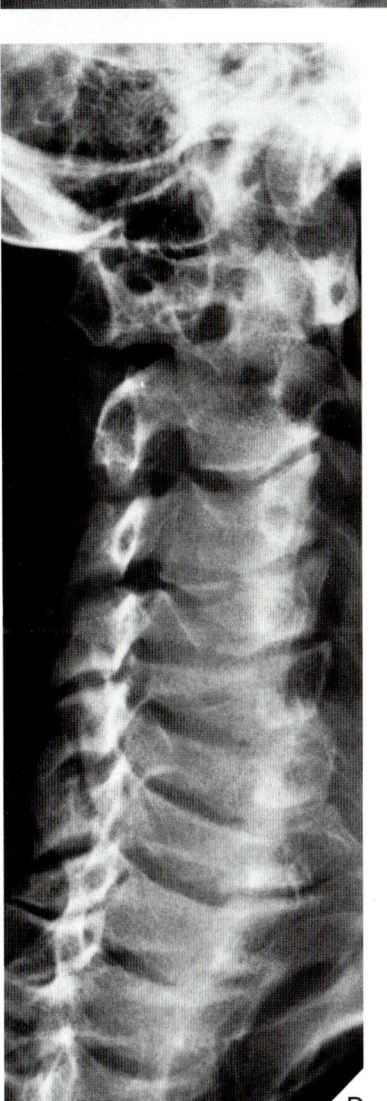

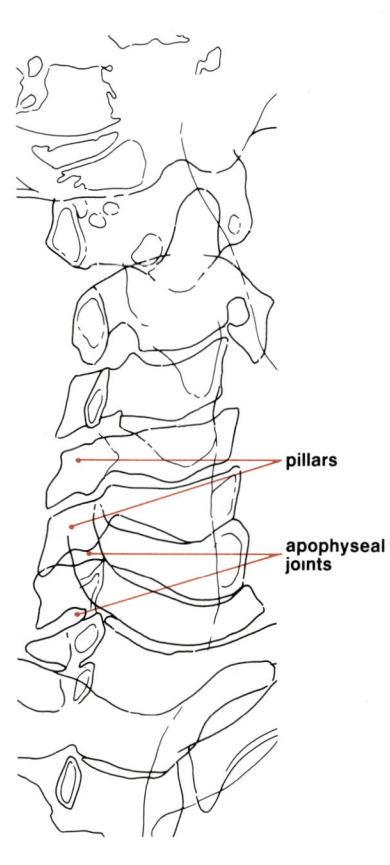

Injury to the Cervical Spine 2.11

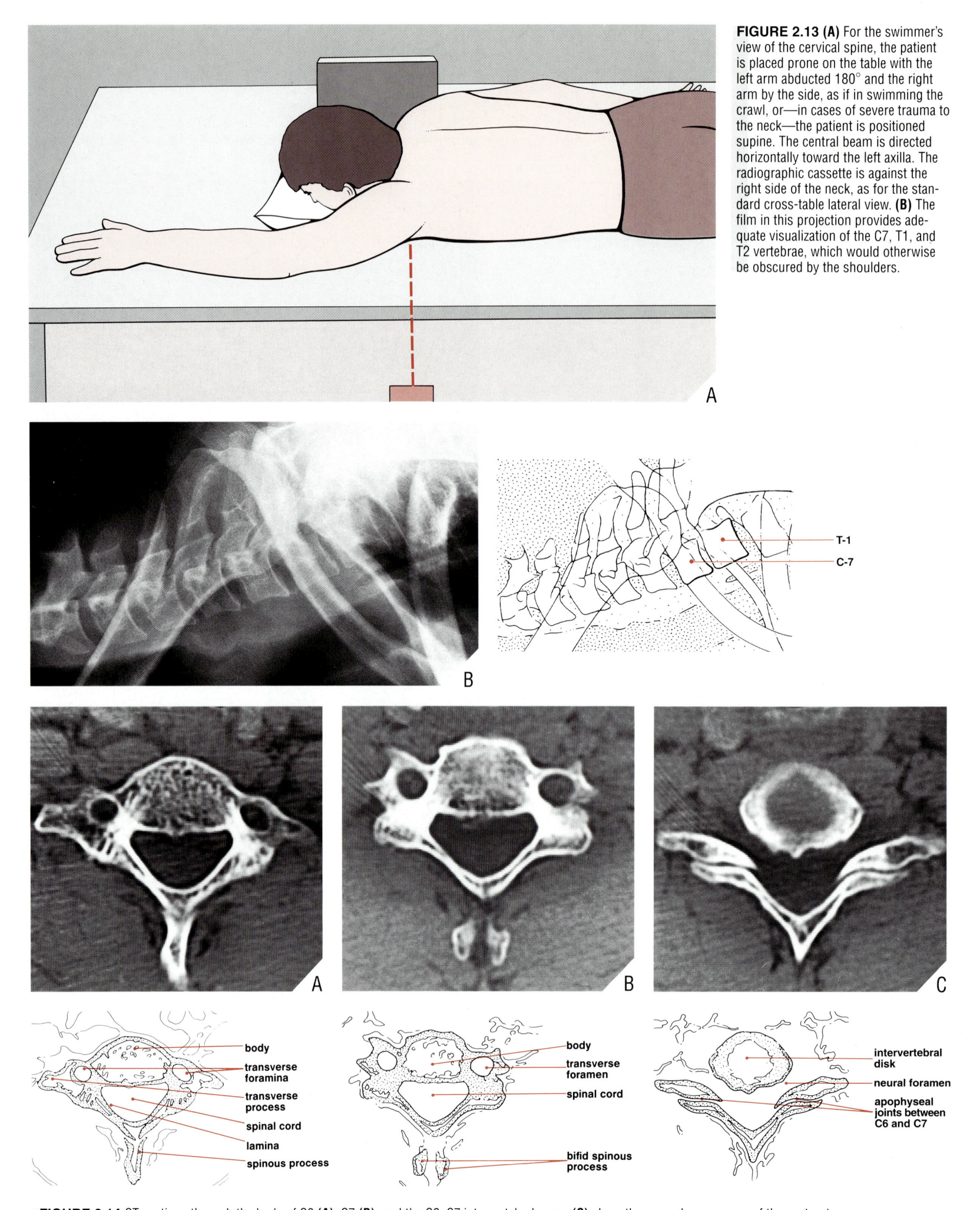

FIGURE 2.13 (A) For the swimmer's view of the cervical spine, the patient is placed prone on the table with the left arm abducted 180° and the right arm by the side, as if in swimming the crawl, or—in cases of severe trauma to the neck—the patient is positioned supine. The central beam is directed horizontally toward the left axilla. The radiographic cassette is against the right side of the neck, as for the standard cross-table lateral view. **(B)** The film in this projection provides adequate visualization of the C7, T1, and T2 vertebrae, which would otherwise be obscured by the shoulders.

FIGURE 2.14 CT sections through the body of C6 **(A)**, C7 **(B)**, and the C6–C7 intervertebral space **(C)** show the normal appearance of these structures.

2.12 *Imaging of the Spine in Clinical Practice*

of the odontoid process, for example, conventional tomography is particularly helpful. For determination of the extent of cervical spine injuries in general, including soft tissue trauma, CT (Fig. 2.14) provides valuable information regarding the integrity of the spinal canal and the localization of fracture fragments within the canal.

Over the past several years, magnetic resonance imaging (MRI) has become the most effective modality for evaluation of vertebral trauma because of its impressive quality of imaging and its multiplanar capability, which makes it possible to examine an acutely traumatized patient without the movement required for special positioning. In evaluation of fractures, MRI is useful not only to determine the relationship of bone fragments that may be displaced in the vertebral canal but also to demonstrate the full extent of injury, especially to the soft tissues and the spinal cord. The effect of the trauma on the spinal cord can be directly imaged, and spinal cord compression can be diagnosed. The superior resolution of soft tissue contrast by MRI can reveal minimal edema and small amounts of hemorrhage within the spinal cord. Injury to ligamentous structures and extradural pathology can also be readily identified. In the cervical spine, 3-mm thick sagittal sections and 5-mm thick axial sections are routinely obtained. The most effective are spin-echo (SE) images obtained in the sagittal plane (T1- and T2-weighted). Sagittal MR images permit evaluation of vertebral body alignment and integrity as well as the size of the spinal canal (Fig. 2.15A). On the parasagittal section, the articular facets are well demonstrated (Fig. 2.15B). More recently, fast scans have been advocated for demonstrating injuries in the axial plane. These fast gradient-echo pulse sequences have become a popular addition to, or replacement for, T2-weighted spin-echo sequences. Gradient-echo sequences have short acquisition times, adequate resolution, and show a satisfactory "myelographic effect" between cerebral spinal fluid and adjacent structures (Figs. 2.15C,D).

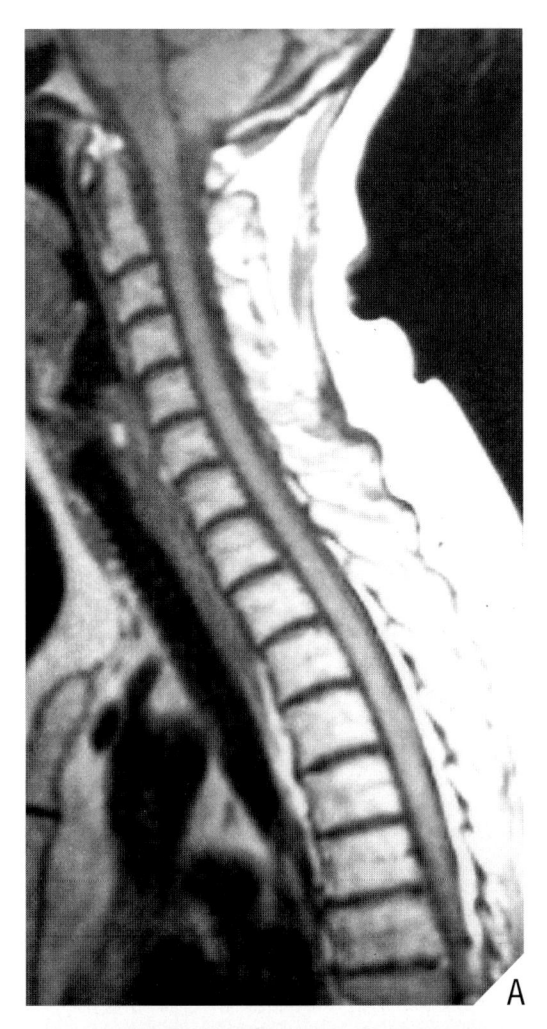

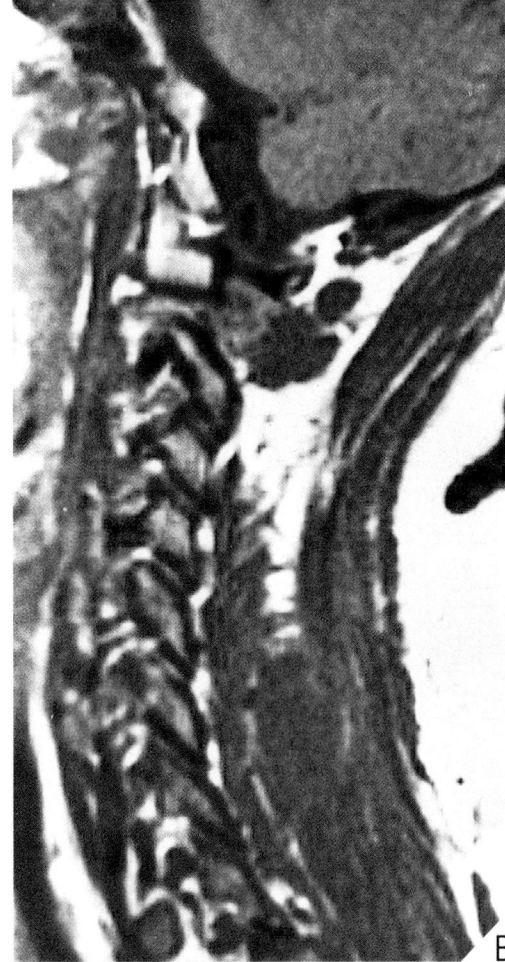

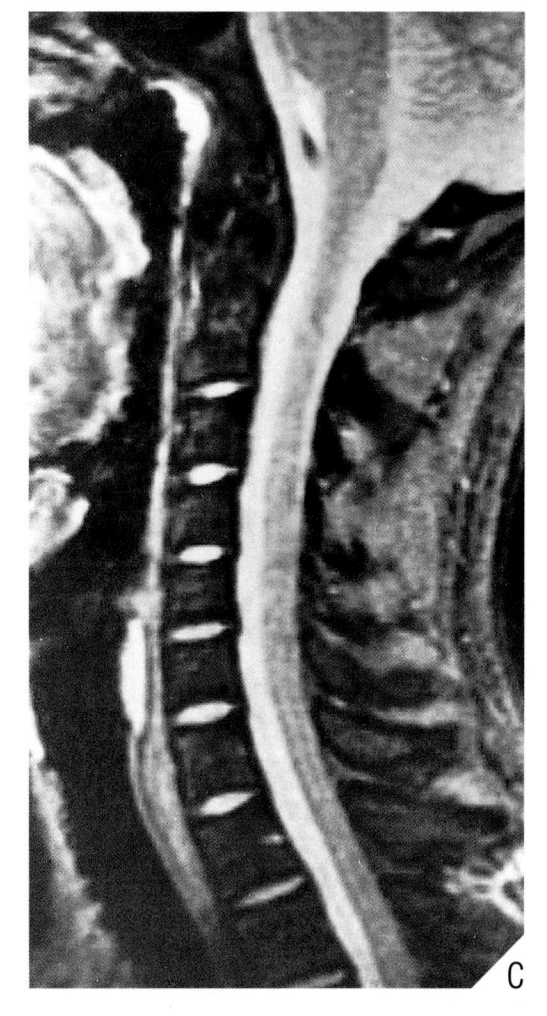

FIGURE 2.15 MR images of normal cervical spine. **(A)** T1-weighted (TR 800/TE20) spin-echo sagittal midline section demonstrates anatomic details of the bones and soft tissues. The craniocervical junction is well outlined. The foramen magnum is defined by the fat within the occipital bone and clivus. The anterior and posterior arches of C1 appear as small oval marrow-containing structures at the upper cervical spine. The spinal cord is of an intermediate signal intensity outlined by lower signal of CSF. The intervertebral disks are imaged with low signal intensity. **(B)** Parasagittal section demonstrates the apophyseal joints. **(C)** T2*-weighted MPGR sagittal image shows vertebral bodies and spinous processes to be of low signal intensity. The high water content of the intervertebral disks produces a very high signal similar to that of cerebrospinal fluid. The cord is imaged as an intermediate signal intensity structure. **(D)** Axial section demonstrates neural foramina and nerve roots. The cervical cord is faintly outlined. (Reproduced with permission from Beltran J: *MRI: Musculoskeletal System.* New York, Gower, 1990)

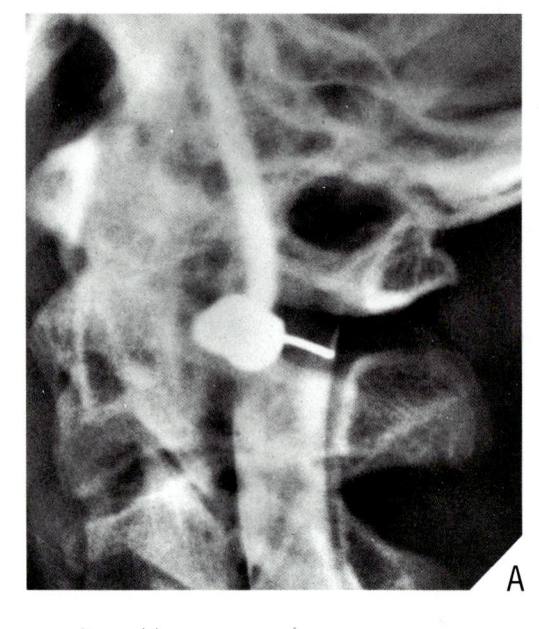

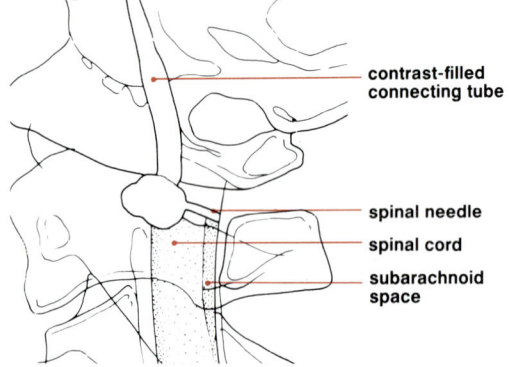

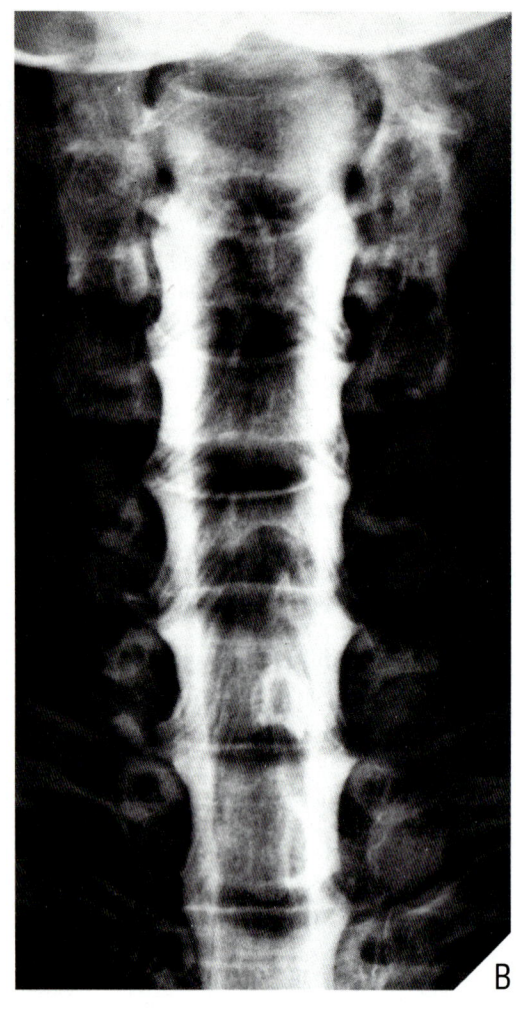

FIGURE 2.16 For myelographic examination of the cervical spine, the patient is recumbent on the table, lying on the left side. Using fluoroscopy, the point of entrance of the needle is marked at the C1–C2 level, and a 22-gauge needle is inserted vertically, the tip being directed to the dorsal aspect of the subarachnoid space, above the lamina of C2. Free flow of spinal fluid indicates the correct position of the needle. **(A)** About 10 ml of Iohexol, a water-soluble nonionic iodinated contrast agent, at a concentration of 240 mg iodine/ml, is slowly injected. Films are obtained in the posteroanterior **(B)**, cross-table lateral **(C)**, and oblique projections. (Oblique projections, however, are obtained not by rotating the patient but by angling the radiographic tube 45°.) If the lower segment of the cervical spine is not satisfactorily demonstrated or if the upper thoracic segment needs to be visualized, a film may also be obtained in the swimmer's position. Myelography demonstrates the thecal sac filled with contrast and the outline of the normal nerve roots and nerve root sleeves. **(D)** CT section at the level C3–C4 obtained following myelography demonstrates the normal appearance of contrast in the subarachnoid space.

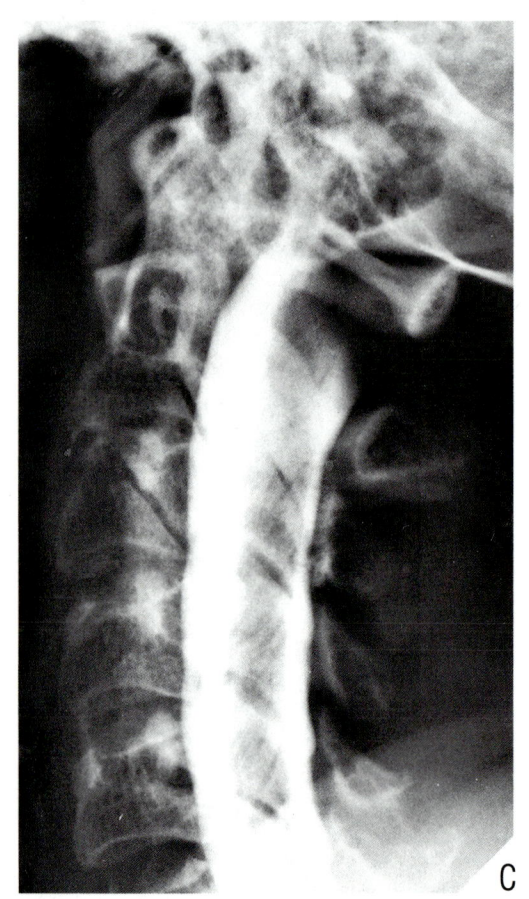

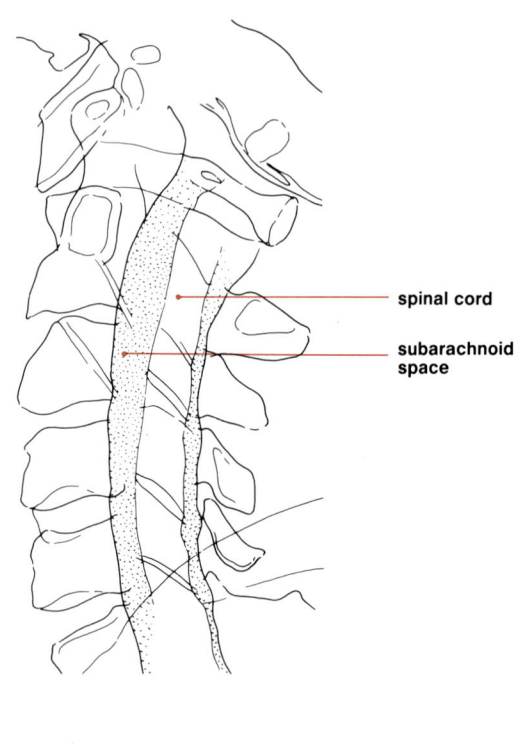

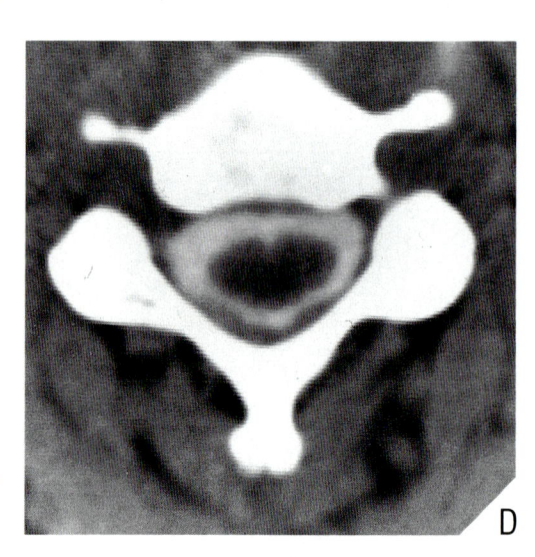

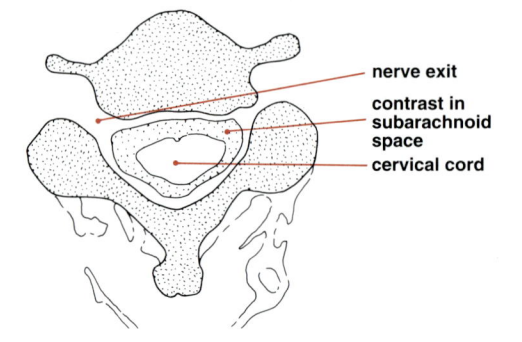

2.14 Imaging of the Spine in Clinical Practice

On T1-weighted sagittal images of the cervical spine, the vertebral bodies that contain yellow (or fatty) marrow are imaged as high signal intensity structures. The intervertebral disks demonstrate intermediate signal intensity, CSF demonstrates low signal intensity, and the cord itself intermediate signal intensity (see Fig. 2.15A).

On T2-weighted sagittal images, the vertebral bodies are imaged with intermediate signal intensity, the intervertebral disks and CSF demonstrate high signal intensity, and the cord demonstrates intermediate signal intensity.

On axial images obtained with T1 weighting, the disk demonstrates intermediate signal intensity, the spinal fluid has low signal intensity, and the cord has high to intermediate signal intensity.

On axial images obtained with T2* weighting (MPGR), both the disk and the CSF exhibit high signal intensity, in contrast to the spinal cord which images as an intermediate signal intensity structure. The bone demonstrates low signal intensity (see Fig. 2.15D).

In addition to its imaging capabilities, MRI, according to some investigators, also has a prognostic value for predicting the anticipated degree of neurologic recovery following trauma.

Since the advent of MRI, myelography is now rarely indicated in the evaluation of cervical injuries; this examination can be performed alone (Figs. 2.16A–C) or in conjunction with CT (Fig. 2.16D). It should to be stressed, however, that CT myelography remains the better choice for evaluating vertebral fractures, especially when they are nondisplaced or involve the posterior elements (lateral masses, facets, laminae, spinous processes), largely because of limitations of the spatial resolution of MRI. In addition, imaging the acutely injured patient by MRI is frequently difficult. The patient may be unstable or immobilized with either a halo or traction device unsuitable for the magnetic environment. For this reason, plain radiographs, CT, and myelography continue to play significant roles in the evaluation of the acutely traumatized spine. On the other hand, as noted by Hyman and Gorey (1988), chronic spinal cord injury is most accurately evaluated with MRI. However, regardless of whether MRI or CT myelography is chosen, the most important preoperative goal is to identify on the cross-sectional imaging studies any bone or soft tissue structures that are at risk of being displaced or pulled into the canal during reduction, with potential danger of paralysis.

For a summary of the preceding discussion in tabular form, see Figures 2.17 to 2.19.

CLASSIFICATION BY MECHANISM OF INJURY AND BY STABILITY

Traumatic conditions involving the cervical spine are almost always the result of indirect stress forces acting on the head and neck, the position of which at the time of impact determines the site and type of damage. As pointed out by Daffner (1986), vertebral fractures occur in predictable and reproducible patterns which are related to the type of force applied to the vertebral column. The same force applied to the cervical, thoracic, or lum-

---

FIGURE 2.17 TISSUE MRI SIGNAL CHARACTERISTICS

SIGNAL INTENSITY	T1-WEIGHTING	T2-WEIGHTING	GRADIENT ECHO (T2*)
Low signal	Cortical bone Vertebral endplates Degenerated disks Osteophytes Spinal vessels CSF	Cortical bone Vertebral endplates Ligaments Degenerated disks Osteophytes Spinal vessels Nerve roots	Bone marrow Verebral bodies Vertebral endplates Ligaments Osteophytes
Intermediate signal	Spinal cord Paraspinal soft tissue Intervertebral disks Nerve roots Osteophytes	Paraspinal soft tissue Osteophytes Spinal cord Facet cartilage Bone marrow Vertebral bodies	Annulus fibrosus Spinal cord Nerve roots
High signal	Epidural venous plexus Hyaline cartilage Epidural and paraspinal fat Bone marrow Vertebral bodies	Intervertebral disks CSF	Intervertebral disk CSF Facet cartilage Epidural venous plexus Arteries

(Modified from Kaiser MC, Ramos L: MRI of the Spine. A Guide to Clinical Applications. Stuttgart, Thieme Verlag, 1990)

bar spine will result in injuries that appear quite similar, producing a pattern of recognizable signs which span the spectrum from mild soft tissue damage to severe skeletal and ligamentous disruption. Daffner termed these patterns "fingerprints" of spinal injury. They depend on the mechanism of the injury, which can be an excessive movement in any direction—flexion, extension, rotation, vertical compression, shearing, distraction, or any combination of these.

Of the greatest initial importance in suspected cervical injuries, however, is the stability of a fracture or dislocation (Fig. 2.20). Stability of the vertebral column depends, as Daffner pointed out, on the integrity of the vertebrae, the intervertebral disks, the apophyseal joints, and the ligamentous structures. One of the most important factors is the integrity of the ligaments of the spine—the supraspinous and interspinous ligaments, the posterior longitudinal ligament, and the ligamentum flavum which, together with the capsule of the apophyseal joints, constitute the so-called posterior ligament complex of Holdsworth (Fig. 2.21). The more severe the damage to these structures, the more vulnerable they are to further displacement, with greater risk of sequelae involving the spinal cord.

FIGURE 2.18 STANDARD AND SPECIAL RADIOGRAPHIC PROJECTIONS FOR EVALUATING INJURY TO THE CERVICAL SPINE

PROJECTION	DEMONSTRATION
Anteroposterior	Fractures of the bodies of C3–C7
	Abnormalities of:
	Intervertebral disk spaces
	Uncovertebral (Luschka) joints
Open-mouth	Fractures of:
	Lateral masses of C1
	Odontoid process
	Body of C2
	Jefferson fracture
	Abnormalities of atlantoaxial joints
Fuchs	Fractures of odontoid process
Lateral	Occipito-cervical dislocations
	Fractures of:
	Anterior and posterior arches of C1
	Odontoid process
	Bodies of C2–C7
	Spinous processes
	Hangman's fracture
	Burst and compression fractures
	Teardrop fracture
	Clay-shoveler's fracture
	Unilateral and bilateral locked facets
	Abnormalities of:
	Intervertebral disk spaces
	Prevertebral soft tissues
	Atlanto-odontoid space
In flexion	Atlantoaxial subluxation
Oblique	Abnormalities of:
	Intervertebral (neural) foramina
	Apophyseal joints
Pillar *(anteroposterior or oblique)*	Fractures of lateral masses (pillars)
Swimmer's	Fractures of C7, T1, and T2

FIGURE 2.19 ANCILLARY IMAGING TECHNIQUES FOR EVALUATING INJURY TO THE CERVICAL, THORACIC, AND LUMBAR SPINE

TECHNIQUE	DEMONSTRATION
Tomography	Fractures, particularly of the occipital condyles and odontoid process
	Localization of displaced fracture fragments
	Progress of treatment
	Fracture healing
	Status of spinal fusion
Myelography	Obstruction or compression of the dural (thecal) sac
	Displacement or compression of the spinal cord
	Abnormalities of:
	Spinal nerve root sleeves (sheaths)
	Subarachnoid space
	Herniated disk
Diskography	Limbus vertebra
	Schmorl node
	Herniated disk
Computed Tomography *(alone or combined with myelography and/or diskography)*	Abnormalities of:
	Lateral recesses and neural foramina
	Spinal cord
	Complex fractures of the vertebrae
	Localization of displaced fracture fragments in spinal canal
	Spondylolysis
	Disk herniation
	Paraspinal soft tissue injury (eg, hematoma)
	Progress of treatment
	Fracture healing
	Status of spinal fusion
Radionuclide Imaging *(scintigraphy, bone scan)*	Subtle or obscure fractures
	Recent vs. old fractures
	Fracture healing
Magnetic Resonance Imaging	Same as myelography and computed tomography combined

Imaging of the Spine in Clinical Practice

According to Daffner, the radiographic findings that indicate instability include displacement of vertebrae, widening of the interspinous or interlaminar spaces, widening of the apophyseal joints, widening and elongation of the vertebral canal (manifesting as widening of the interpedicular distance in transverse and vertical planes), and disruption of the posterior vertebral body line. Only one of these features needs to be present for radiographic assumption of an unstable injury to be made.

These remarks on stability are also applicable to injuries of thoracic and lumbar segments.

Fractures of the Occipital Condyles

Fractures of the occipital condyles were first described in 1817 by Bell. An exhaustive review of the literature has identified only 20 cases of occipital condyles fractures. In 1974, Wachenheim described a series of six occipital condyles fractures, but no follow-up was reported: four were avulsion injuries of the occipital condyles and two were compression injuries. Since that time, several authors have reported additional cases of occipital condyles fractures. The most common clinical features were loss of con-

FIGURE 2.20 Classification of Injuries to the Cervical Spine by Mechanism of Injury and Stability

CONDITION	STABILITY
Flexion Injuries	
Occipito-cervical dislocations	Unstable
Subluxation	Stable
Dislocation in facet joints (locked facets)	
Unilateral	Stable
Bilateral	Unstable
Odontoid fractures	
Type I	Stable
Type II	Unstable
Type III	Stable
Wedge fracture	Stable
Clay-shoveler's fracture	Stable
"teardrop" fracture	Unstable
Burst fracture	Stable or unstable
Extension Injuries	
Occipito-cervical dislocations	Unstable
Fracture of posterior arch of C1	Stable
Hangman's fracture	Unstable
"Extension teardrop" fracture	Stable
Hyperextension fracture–dislocation	Unstable
Compression Injuries	
Jefferson fracture	Unstable
Burst fracture	Stable or unstable
Laminar fracture	Stable
Compression fracture	Stable
Shearing Injuries	
Lateral vertebral compression	Stable
Lateral dislocation	Unstable
Transverse process fracture	Stable
Lateral mass fracture	Stable
Rotation Injuries	
Fracture–dislocation	Unstable
Facet and pillar fractures	Stable or unstable
Transverse process fracture	Stable
Distraction Injuries	
Hangman's fracture	Unstable
Occipito-cervical dislocations	Unstable
Atlanto-axial subluxation	Stable or unstable

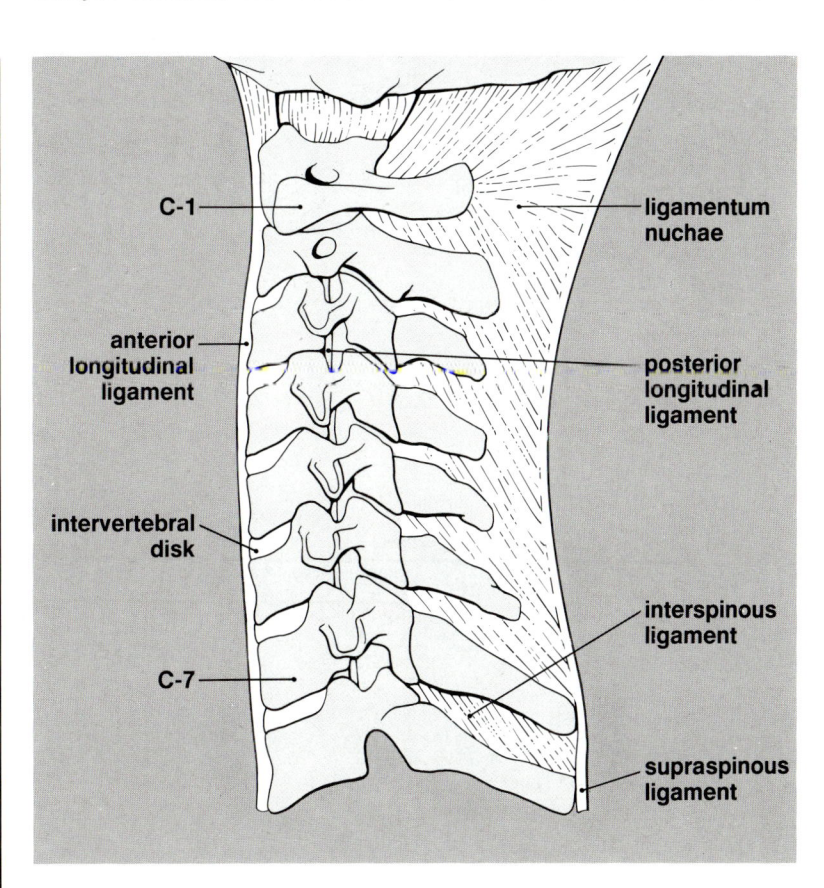

FIGURE 2.21 Anatomy of the principle ligaments of the cervical spine.

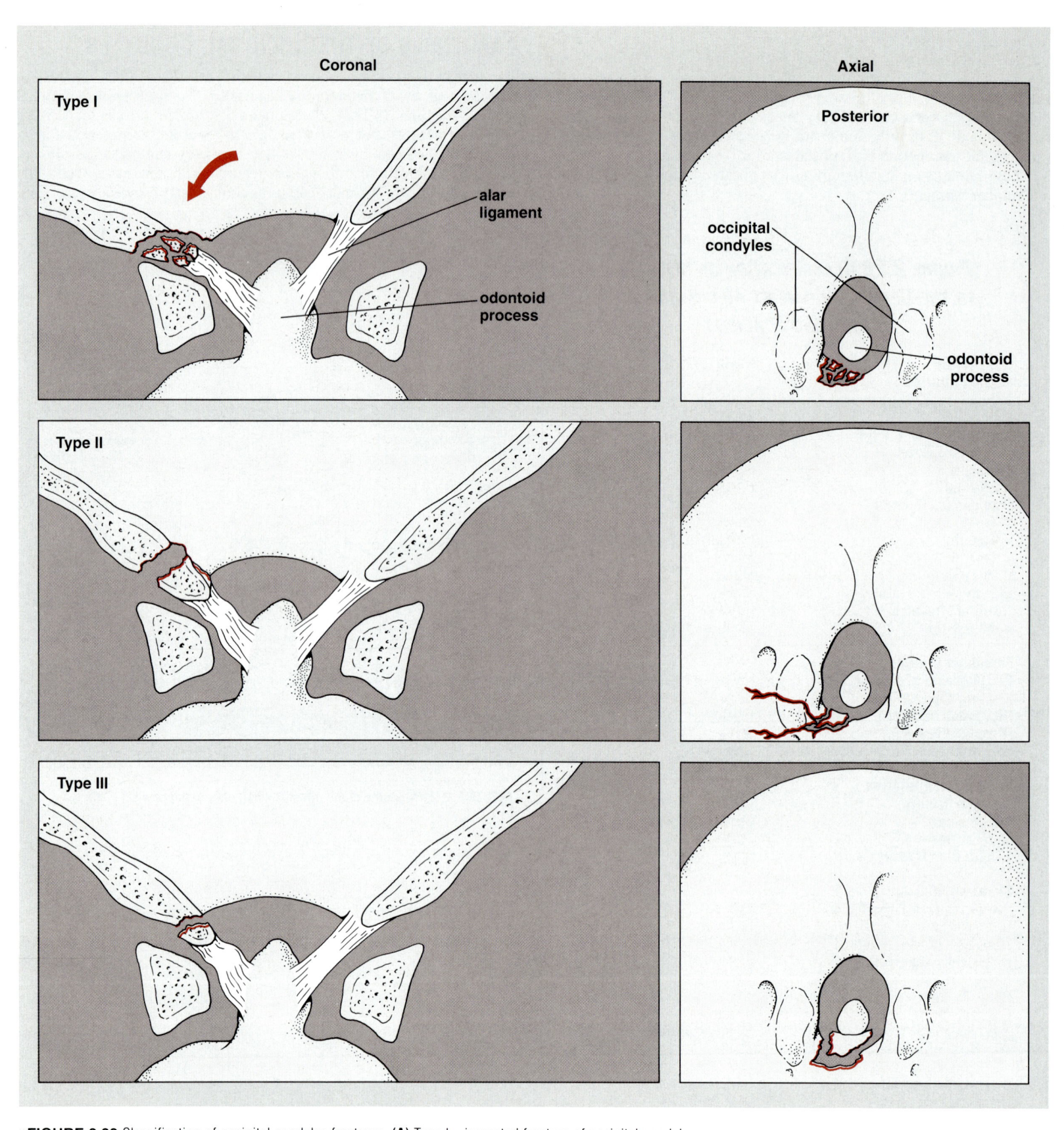

FIGURE 2.22 Classification of occipital condyles fractures. **(A)** Type I—impacted fracture of occipital condyle. **(B)** Type II—basilar skull-type fracture of occipital condyle. **(C)** Type III—avulsion fracture of occipital condyle.

sciousness and cranial nerve damage. This injury is often overlooked and is not obvious on plain films. Instead, the diagnosis requires a high index of suspicion, after which confirmation can easily be obtained by either computed tomography (CT) with coronal reformation or conventional tomography.

A classification system of occipital condyles fractures was devised by Anderson and Montesano (1988) based on fracture morphology, pertinent anatomy, and biomechanics (Fig. 2.22).

Type I

This is an impacted occipital condyle fracture occurring as the result of axial loading of the skull onto the atlas, similar to the mechanism for a Jefferson fracture. Morphologically, there is comminution of the occipital condyle with minimal or no displacement of fragments into the foramen magnum. Although the ipsilateral alar ligament may be functionally inadequate, spinal stability is assured by the intact tectorial membrane and contralateral alar ligament.

Type II

This type of occipital condyle fracture occurs as part of a basilar skull fracture. On axial CT sections of the base of the skull, a fracture line can be seen which exits the occipital condyle and enters the foramen magnum. The mechanism of injury is a direct blow to the skull. Stability is maintained by intact alar ligaments and tectorial membrane.

Type III

This is an avulsion fracture of the occipital condyle by the alar ligament. The alar ligaments are primary restraints of occipito–cervical rotation and lateral bending. Therefore, the mechanism of injury in this type is either rotation, lateral bending, or a combination of the two. After avulsion of the occipital condyle, the contralateral alar ligament and tectorial membrane are loaded. Therefore, this type of occipital condyle fracture is a potentially unstable injury. Morphologically, a small fragment from the inferior and medial aspect of the occipital condyle is displaced towards the odontoid tip.

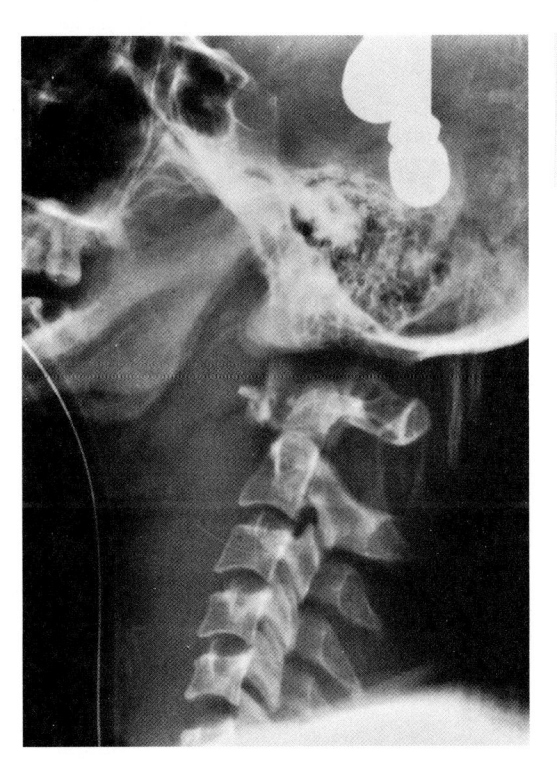

OCCIPITO–CERVICAL DISLOCATIONS

Traumatic occipito–cervical dislocations are usually fatal, and therefore, rarely present a clinical problem. With the improvement of trauma care, which now includes on-site intubation and immediate resuscitation as well as early hospital transport, more and more victims of this injury are presenting for definitive care. The radiographic diagnosis, however, still remains somewhat difficult because of the overlapping shadows of the base of the cranium and the mastoid processes. Traynelis et al. (1988) have classified occipital cervical dislocations according to the primary direction of displacement of the occiput and the C1 articulation. Anderson and Montesano (1992) have modified that classification as follows.

Type I Injuries

These are more commonly seen in patients who survive transport to the hospital. In this type of injury, both occipital condyles are translated anteriorly on their corresponding atlantal facets (Fig. 2.23). Biomechanical studies have demonstrated that for this injury to occur all major structures (alar ligaments, tectorial membrane, and occipital atlantal facet joint capsules) crossing the occipito–cervical junction must be ruptured.

Type II Injuries

There is a vertical translation of the occiput on the cervical spine, secondary to the rupture of all occipito–cervical ligaments. In Type IIA injuries there is distraction between the occiput and C1. Vertical translation of the occiput on C1 is normally less than 2 mm. Vertical displace-

FIGURE 2.23 A 24-year-old man injured his head and neck in a motorcycle accident that resulted in complete quadriplegia. The lateral view of the cervical spine shows Type I of occipito-cervical dislocation: the occipital condyles are anteriorly displaced in relation to C1 vertebra.

ment greater than this represents failure of the tectorial membrane, alar ligaments, and occipito–atlantal facet joint capsules. If, on the other hand, the occipito–atlantal facet joint capsules remain intact and failure occurs at a more distal level of the tectorial membrane (ie, at the level of the atlanto–axial facet joint ligaments), a Type IIB injury results. In this type there is also a vertical displacement of the spine which occurs, however, between C1 and C2 rather than at the atlanto–occipital level.

Type III Injuries

In these injuries, the occiput is displaced posteriorly and is translated posteriorly to the atlas.

In all types of occipito–cervical instability, associated injury to the transverse ligament and C1–C2 instability should be suspected. Radiologic examination should include a standard lateral cervical radiograph that demonstrates the region from the occiput to the cervico–thoracic junction. The articulations between occipital condyles and the atlanto–lateral masses must always be included and the clivus clearly visualized. In Type III injuries, the clivus–odontoid line, which normally points into the tip of the odontoid process (see Fig. 2.3D), points posteriorly to the odontoid.

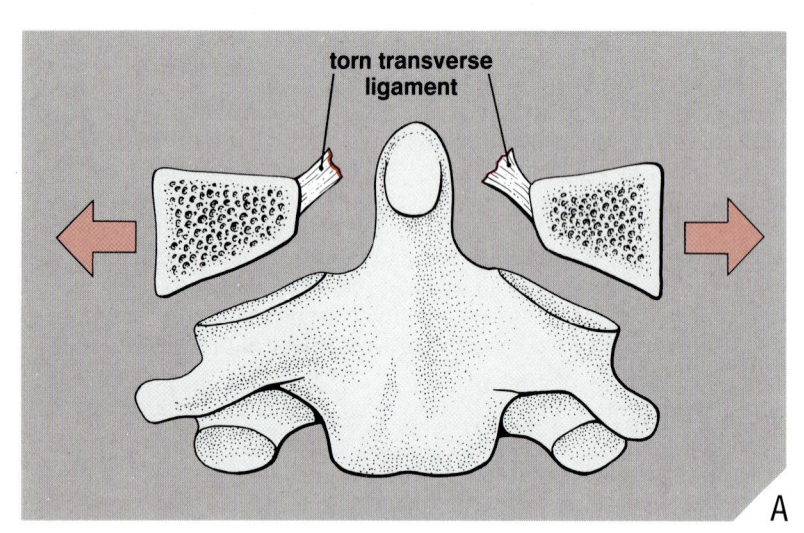

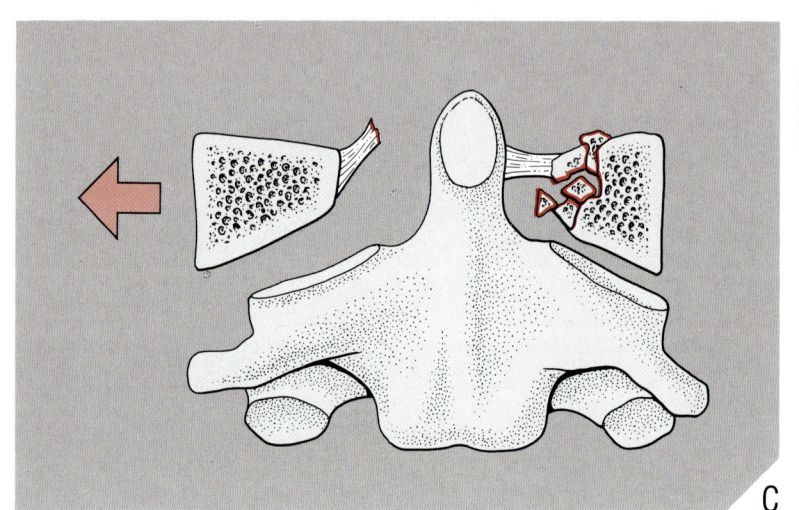

FRACTURES AND DISLOCATIONS OF THE C1 AND C2 VERTEBRAE

Jefferson Fracture

This fracture results from a blow to the vertex of the head. The axial forces transmitted symmetrically through the cranium and the occipital condyles into the superior surfaces of the lateral masses of the atlas drive the lateral masses outward, resulting in bilateral, symmetrical fractures of the anterior and posterior arches of C1, which often are associated with disruption of the transverse ligaments (Fig. 2.24). The C1 ring is most frequently separated into four fragments. Neck pain and unilateral occipital headache are characteristic clinical features of Jefferson fracture.

The best radiographic projection for demonstrating this injury is the open-mouth anteroposterior view (Fig. 2.25A); lateral view, trispiral tomography in the lateral projection using 1-mm thin cuts, as well as CT scan, may also be required for evaluation of complex fractures (Figs. 2.25B–D).

Jefferson fractures can be classified as either a stable or unstable injury. Stability is judged on the anteroposterior radiographs. If the total overhang of the lateral mass of C1 on the lateral mass of C2 from both

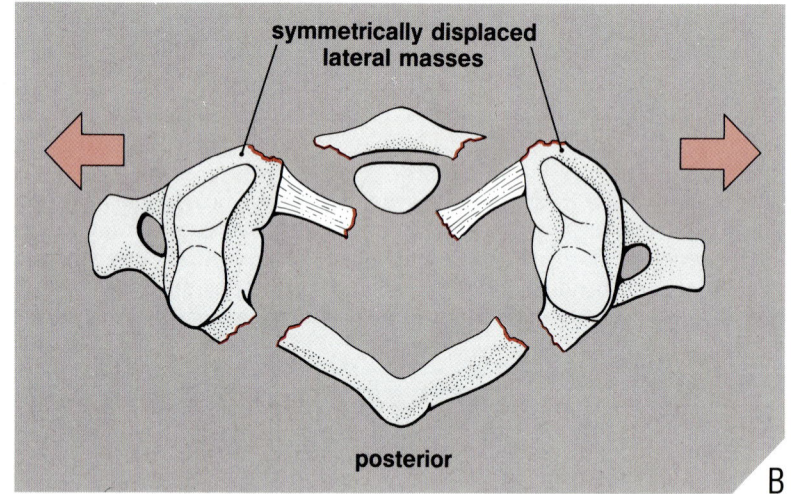

FIGURE 2.24 The classic Jefferson fracture, seen here schematically on the anteroposterior (**A**) and axial (**B**) views, exhibits a characteristic symmetric overhang of the lateral masses of C1 over those of C2. Lateral displacement of the articular pillars results in disruption of the transverse ligaments. (**C**) On occasion, only unilateral displacement of an articular pillar may be present.

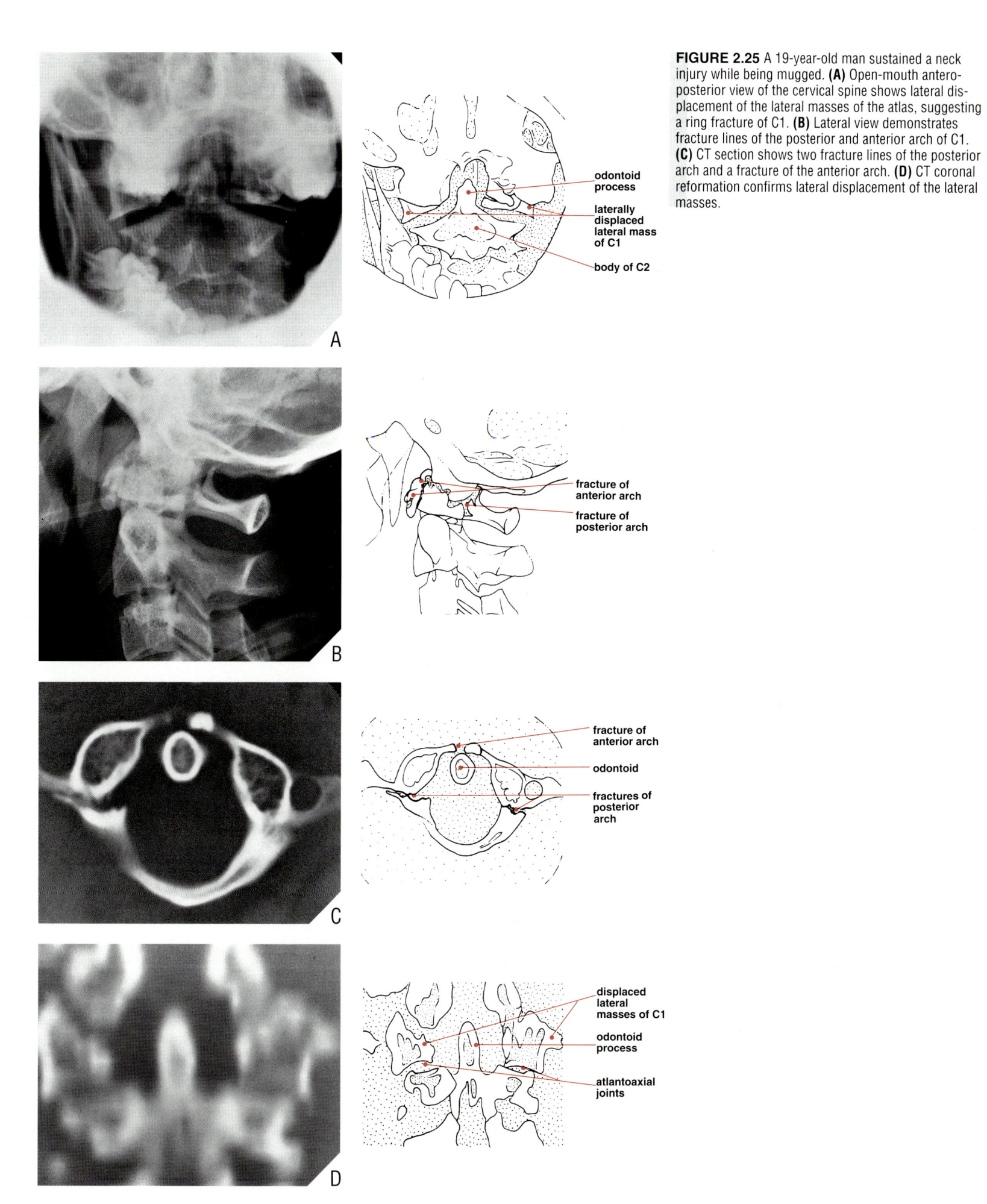

FIGURE 2.25 A 19-year-old man sustained a neck injury while being mugged. **(A)** Open-mouth anteroposterior view of the cervical spine shows lateral displacement of the lateral masses of the atlas, suggesting a ring fracture of C1. **(B)** Lateral view demonstrates fracture lines of the posterior and anterior arch of C1. **(C)** CT section shows two fracture lines of the posterior arch and a fracture of the anterior arch. **(D)** CT coronal reformation confirms lateral displacement of the lateral masses.

Injury to the Cervical Spine   2.21

sides is greater than 7 mm, there is presumably an associated rupture of the transverse ligament; hence, this is considered an unstable injury. Stable injuries are treated by halo brace immobilization for 8 to 12 weeks. Unstable injuries are treated with 8 to 12 weeks of immobilization followed by a C1–C2 fusion.

C1–C2 Dislocation

C1–C2 dislocation can be of two types: bilateral anterior translation of C1 on C2 or bilateral posterior translation of C1 on C2.

Bilateral anterior translation of C1 on C2 results from a tear of the transverse ligament. It is a highly unstable injury. Diagnosis is made on lateral radiographs, in which the atlanto–dens interval is measured; if the distance is greater than 3 mm, the diagnosis is confirmed (Fig. 2.26). Treatment of this injury consists of C1–C2 posterior arthrodesis.

Bilateral posterior translation of C1 on C2 is a rare injury which also is considered highly unstable. The transverse ligament may be torn and the facet capsules of C1–C2 are destroyed. Treatment consists of reduction by longitudinal traction, followed by posterior C1–C2 arthrodesis.

Unilateral anterior, unilateral posterior and bilateral combined anteroposterior C1–C2 dislocations are usually the result of trauma, but occasionally are caused by infection or arthritis. These are usually stable injuries, and are most readily diagnosed on CT examination. Treatment consists of closed reduction via traction or orthotic immobilization. If attempted reduction fails or if recurrent dislocation results, C1–C2 arthrodesis is recommended.

Fractures of the Odontoid Process

Fractures of the odontoid are classified as flexion injuries, although at times forces causing hyperextension of the cervical spine also result in damage to the dens. In hyperflexion injuries, the odontoid process is usually displaced anteriorly, and there may be associated forward subluxation of C1 or C2. Hyperextension injuries, on the other hand, usually cause the odontoid to be displaced posteriorly, with posterior subluxation of C1 or C2.

Several classifications of odontoid fractures have been proposed, based on the site and amount of displacement of the fracture. The system suggested by Anderson and D'Alonzo (1974) is practical and has gained wide acceptance because of its emphasis on the most important feature of such fractures—their stability (Fig. 2.27).

Type I consists of a fracture of the tip of the dens. The fracture line is usually obliquely oriented. The injury is considered stable. Type II consists of transverse fracture through the base of the odontoid, and represents an unstable injury (Fig. 2.28). Conservative treatment has been complicated

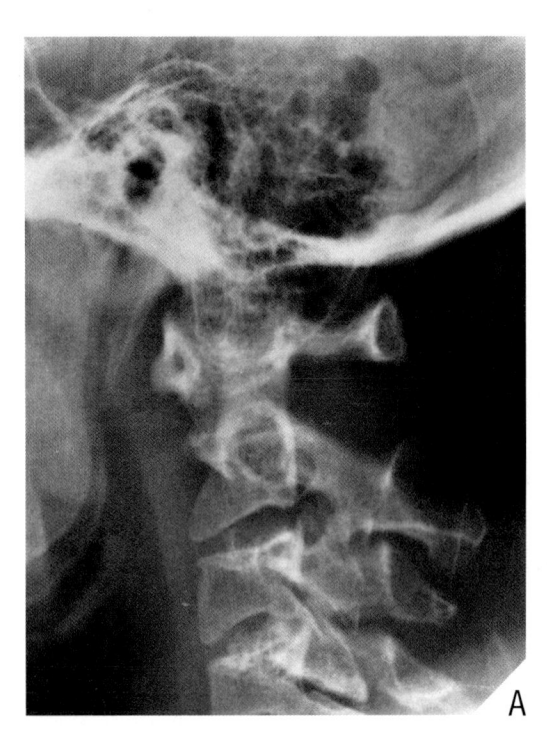

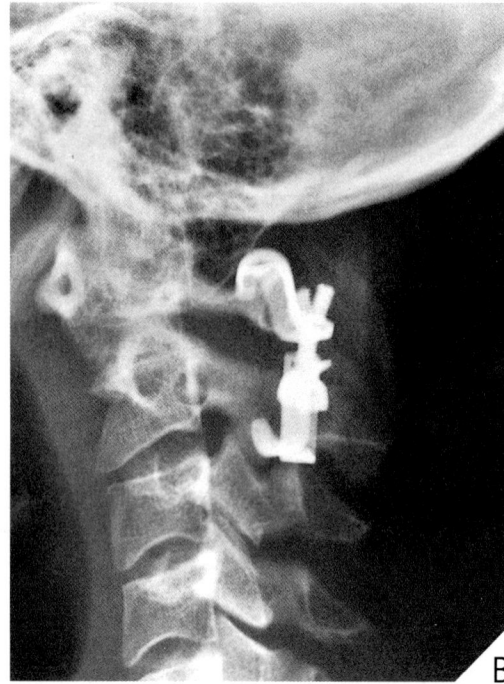

FIGURE 2.26 A 26-year-old man injured his neck in a motorcycle accident. **(A)** Lateral view shows atlanto-dens distance measuring 0.5 cm and marked widening of the interspinous distance between C1 and C2. **(B)** Treatment consisted of initial cervical traction and posterior fusion using bone graft combined with stabilization by laminar clamps. Although one of the clamps has dislodged, solid fusion has been achieved.

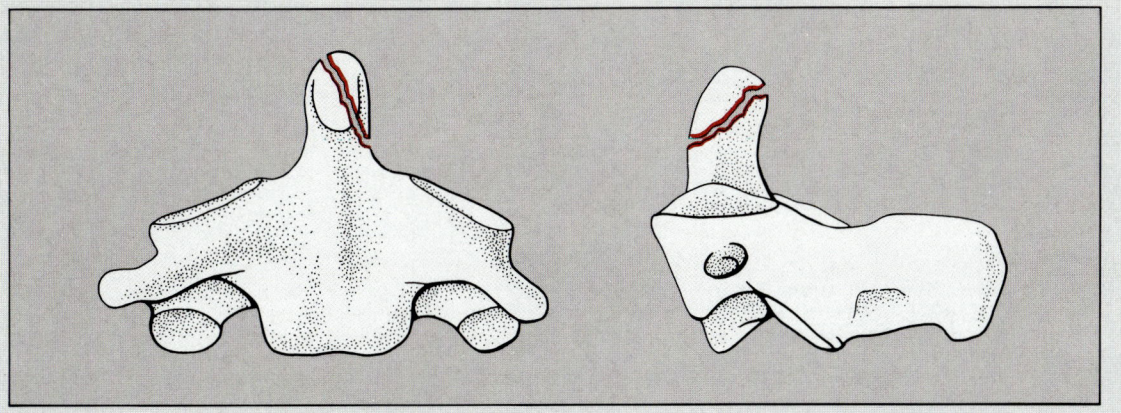

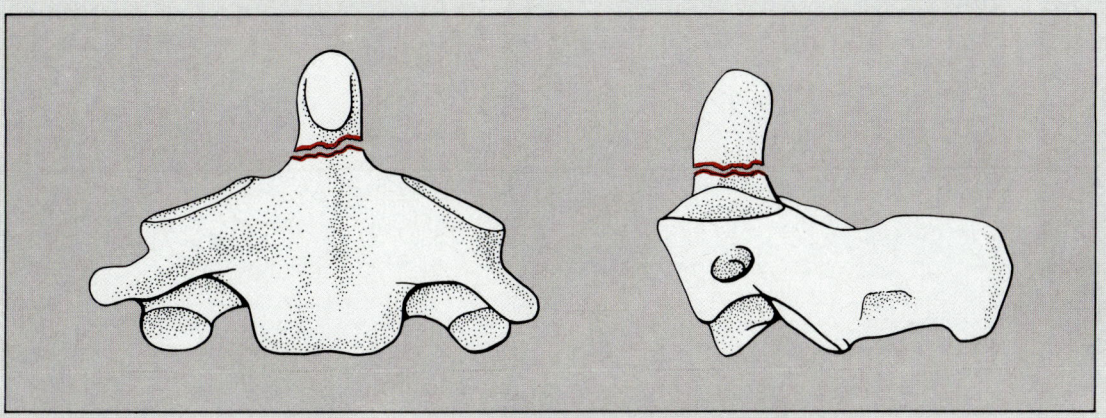

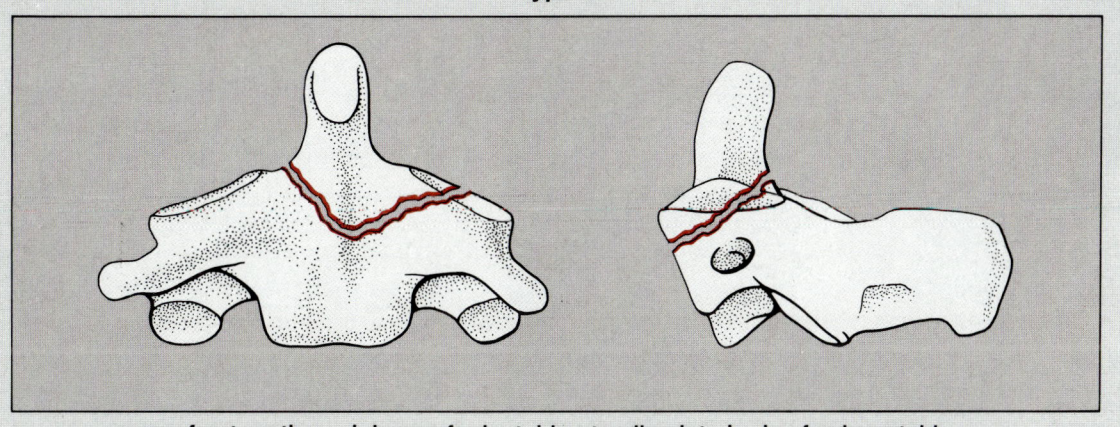

FIGURE 2.27 Classification of odontoid fractures. (Adapted from Anderson LD, D'Alonzo RT: Fractures of the odontoid process of the axis. *J Bone Joint Surg* 56A:1663, 1974)

Injury to the Cervical Spine

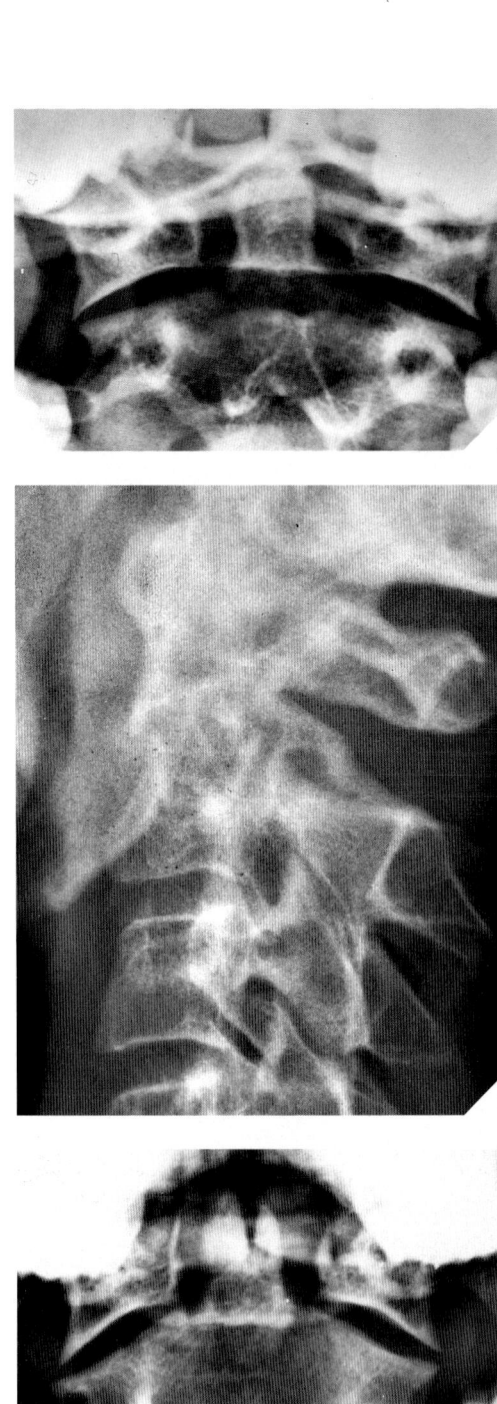

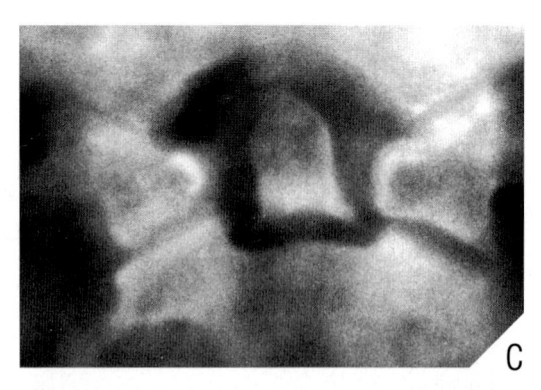

FIGURE 2.28 A 62-year-old man sustained a flexion injury of the cervical spine in an automobile accident. Open-mouth anteroposterior (A) and lateral (B) views demonstrate a fracture line at the base of the odontoid process, but the details of this injury cannot be well appreciated. Thin-section trispiral tomographic sections in the anteroposterior (C) and lateral (D) projections confirm the fracture at the base of the dens. This is a Type II (unstable) fracture.

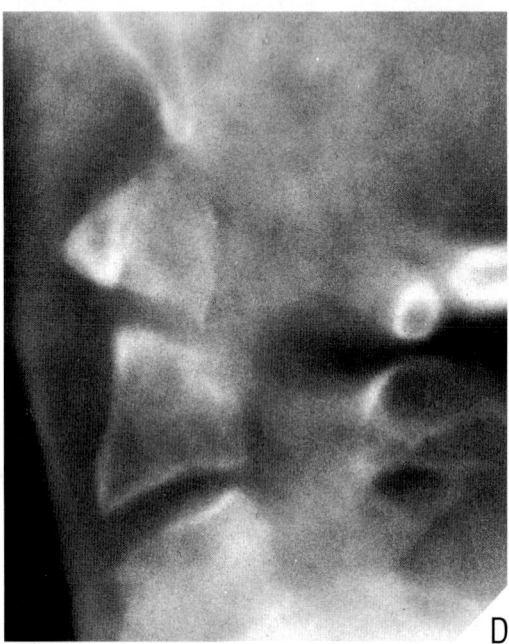

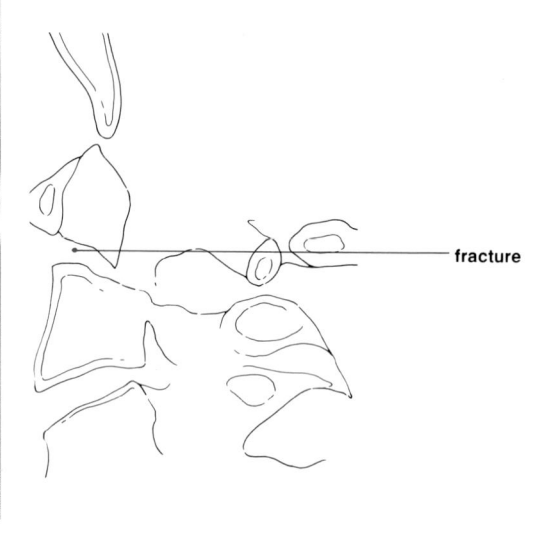

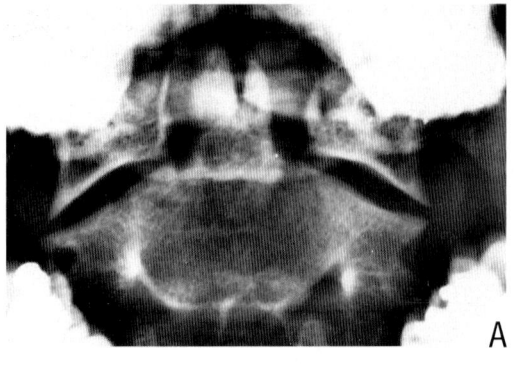

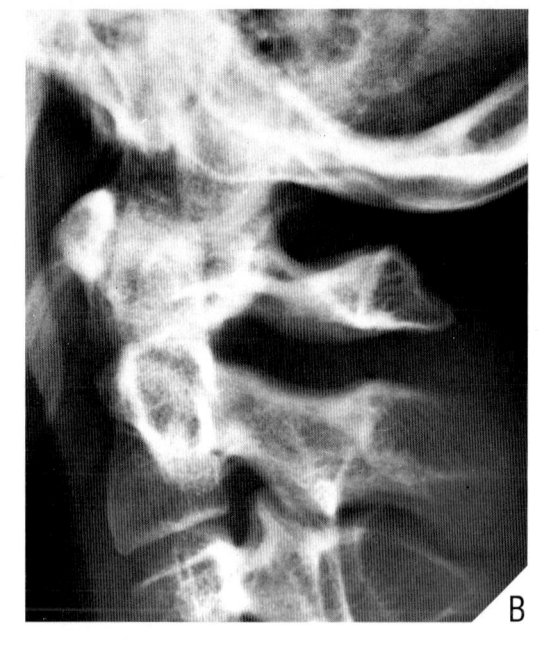

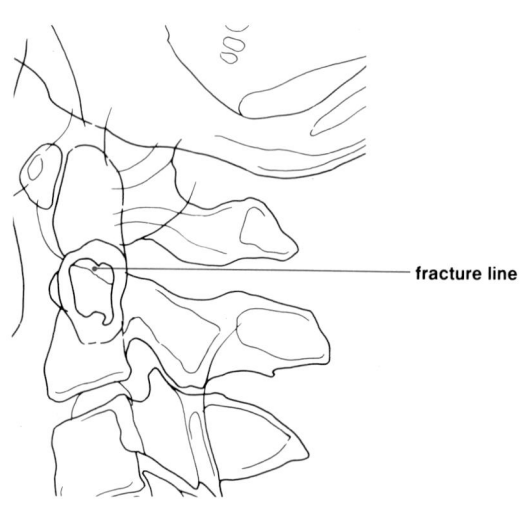

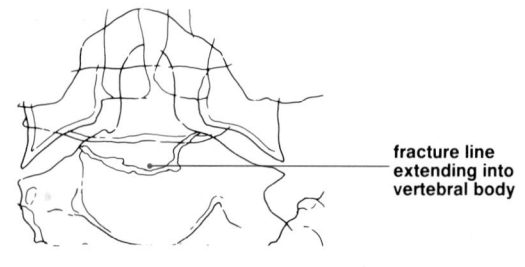

FIGURE 2.29 A 24-year-old man fell on his head in a skiing accident. Open-mouth anteroposterior (A) and lateral (B) views of the cervical spine demonstrate a fracture of the odontoid process extending into the body of C2—a Type III stable fracture. The diagnosis was confirmed by trispiral tomography in the anteroposterior projection (C).

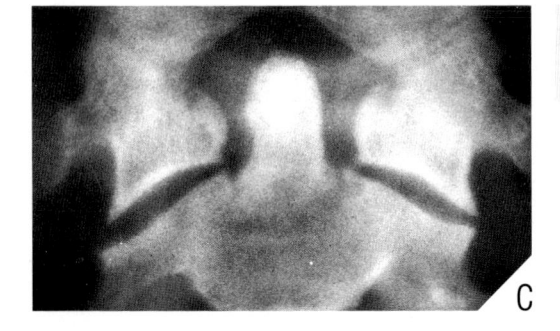

2.24   *Imaging of the Spine in Clinical Practice*

by nonunion in 35% to 85% of cases. Type III consists of a fracture through the base of the odontoid extending into the body of the axis. This is usually a stable injury (Fig. 2.29).

The best techniques for demonstrating fractures of the dens are the anteroposterior view, including the open-mouth variant or Fuchs view, and the lateral projection. Thin-section trispiral tomography may also be effective for delineating ambiguous or subtle features (see Fig. 2.28).

TREATMENT

Type I and III injuries are treated with good results by halo vest immobilization for 8 to 12 weeks. Type II injuries deserve a trial of reduction and halo immobilization; however, the results with this treatment vary. Type II odontoid fractures through the waist have a poor prognosis, with a 15% to 85% chance of nonunion (Fig. 2.30). Many factors have been associated with the failure of Type II fractures to heal. Hadley et al. (1985) have found that displacement of greater than 6 mm was associated with a 67% rate of nonunion, as compared with a 10% rate when the displacement was less than 4 mm. Other risk factors for nonunion include (1) patient age of more than 50 years, (2) posterior displacement, and (3) improper treatment methods, such as inadequate immobilization or use of prolonged traction. This poor rate of healing has led to controversies in treatment methods. Treatment options include (1) external fixation with cervical orthosis, (2) halo immobilization, and (3) primary posterior arthrodesis.

Because of the high risk of nonunion in Type II odontoid fractures, investigators have recommended primary posterior C1–C2 arthrodesis as initial treatment. This fusion compromises axial rotation by 47° and flexion–extension by 10°. Particularly difficult to manage are fractures with a concomitant ring of C1 fractures, which comprise 16% of Type II odontoid fractures. This fracture pattern precludes the initial use of C1–C2 posterior fusion. The acute operative fixation of a Type II odontoid fracture with concomitant ring of C1 fracture necessitates extension of the fusion to the occiput, resulting in a mean loss of 58° of motion in the axial plane and 23° in the coronal plane. The loss of neck motion as a result of these surgical procedures has led to the development of a direct

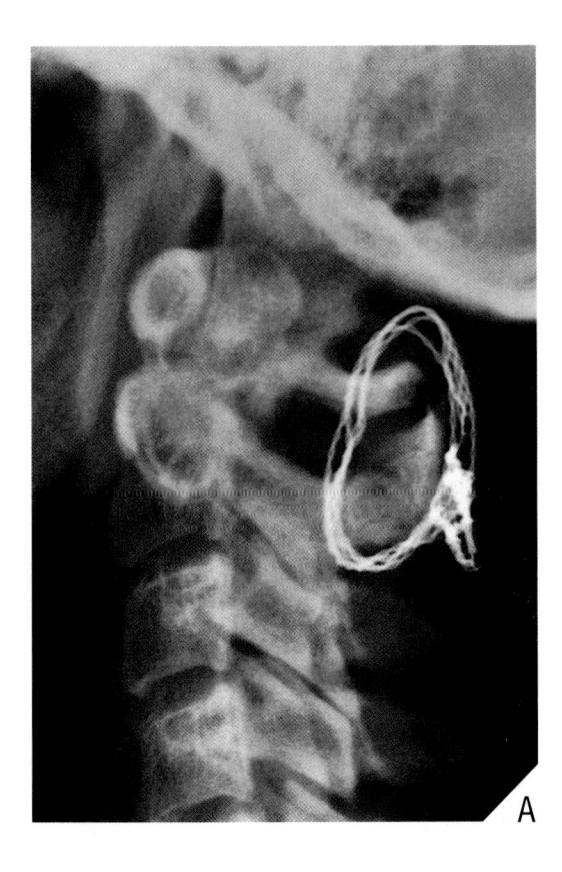

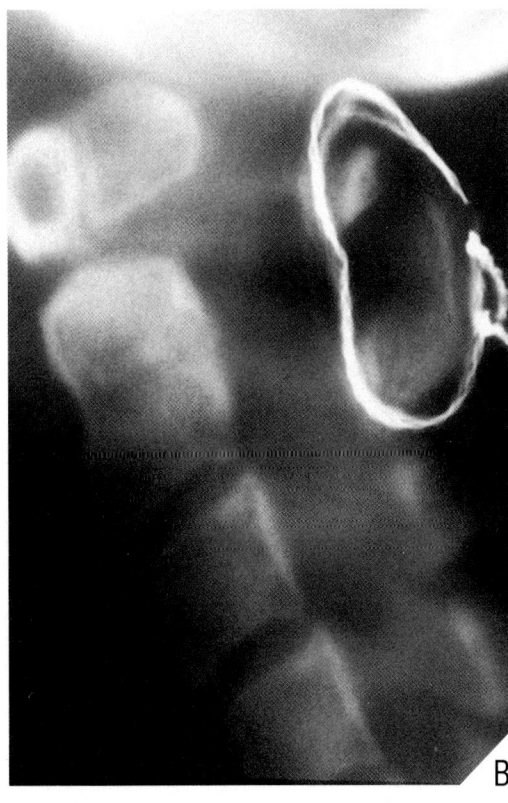

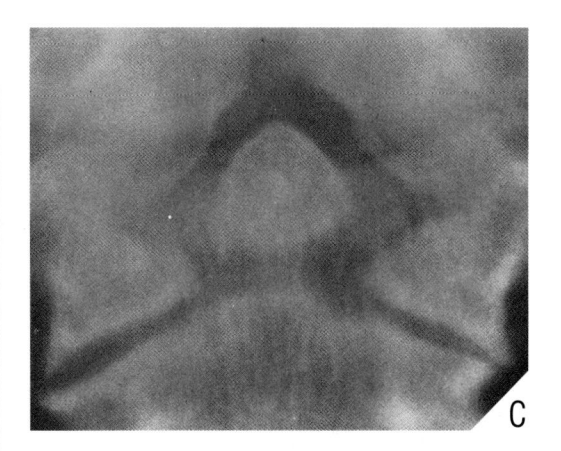

FIGURE 2.30 A 49-year-old woman sustained a Type II displaced odontoid fracture in an automobile accident. The fracture was treated with posterior fusion. Eight months after surgery there is evidence of nonunion. **(A)** Lateral view of cervical spine demonstrates bone graft over spinous processes of C1 and C2 and broken cerclage wires. There is angular deformity of odontoid and gap at the site of bony graft. **(B)** Lateral trispiral tomogram demonstrates lack of union of the odontoid, which is posteriorly angled and displaced. **(C)** Anteroposterior tomographic section demonstrates a 1-cm gap separating odontoid from body of C2.

method of open reduction and internal fixation for odontoid fractures. The treatment of odontoid fractures is evolving. More recently, direct anterior compression screw arthrodesis has been recommended.

Odontoid screw fixation is a technically demanding procedure that can be used in the treatment of odontoid fractures (Fig. 2.31). It does, however, require thorough preoperative planning. This technique is especially useful for treatment of odontoid fractures in patients with multiple injuries, patients who refuse a halo (Fig. 2.32), and in those with odontoid nonunion not associated with significant osteoporosis. Furthermore, this technique may be useful to maintain reduction in displaced fractures.

Hangman's Fracture

In 1912, Wood-Jones described the pathomechanism associated with execution by hanging. He found that hyperextension and distraction resulted in bilateral fractures through the pedicles of the axis, with anterior dislocation of the body and subsequent tearing of the spinal cord. The name "hangman's fracture" is a misnomer and it should properly be called a "hangee fracture," since the hanged man rather that his executioner sustains this injury. A similar fracture, which in fact constitutes traumatic spondylolisthesis of C2, is common in automobile accidents in which the face strikes the windshield before the vertex of the head, forcing the neck into hyperextension. This fracture is unique to this area because of the arrangement of facets at C2: unlike C3–C7, the C2 facets are not located in the same plane. Instead, the superior facet of C2 is positioned anteriorly to the inferior facet. This injury, which accounts for 4% to 7% of all cervical spine fractures and dislocations, may present as a simple, nondisplaced fracture through the pedicles of the axis or as a fracture through the arches with anterior subluxation and angulation of C2 onto C3 (Fig. 2.33). The fracture line usually lies anterior to the inferior articular facet of C2 in both variants, but displaced fractures are more often associated with ligament disruption and intervertebral disk injuries. The best projection for demonstrating this injury is the lateral view (Fig. 2.34).

Hangman's fractures have been classified into three types (Fig. 2.35):

- Type I injury includes fracture through the pedicle of C2 extending between the superior and inferior facets.
- Type II injury constitutes a Type I fracture with concomitant C2–C3 disk disruption.
- Type III injury consists of a Type II fracture with a C2–C3 facet dislocation.

TREATMENT

Type I injuries are treated with 8 to 12 weeks of immobilization in a halo jacket or rigid cervical orthosis.

Type II injuries are in treated the same way as Type I injuries. However, if there is persistent pain, the C2–C3 disk is studied by diskography or MRI. When instability is documented, a late anterior C2–C3 diskectomy and fusion are performed.

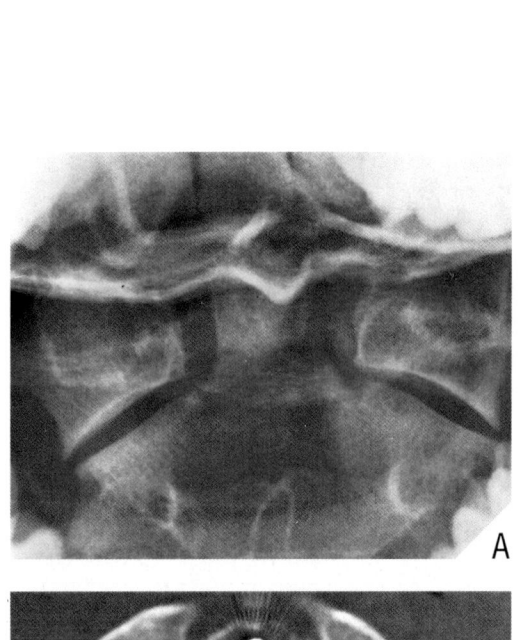

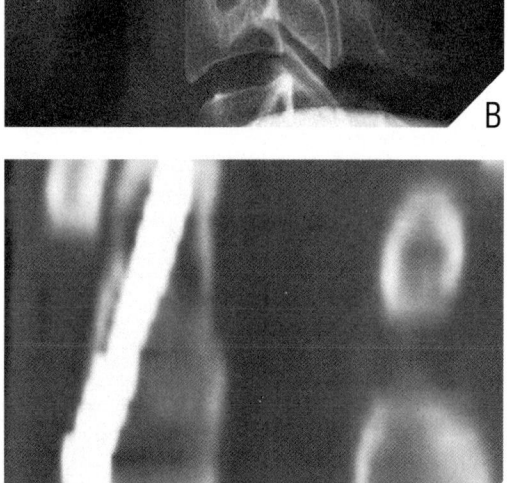

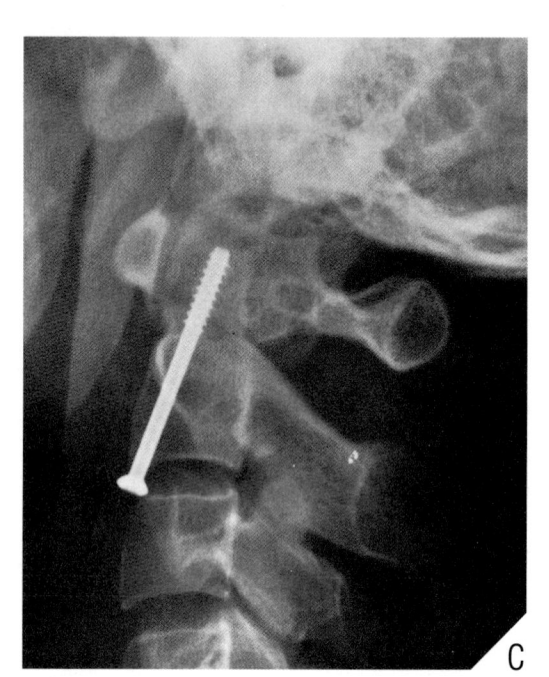

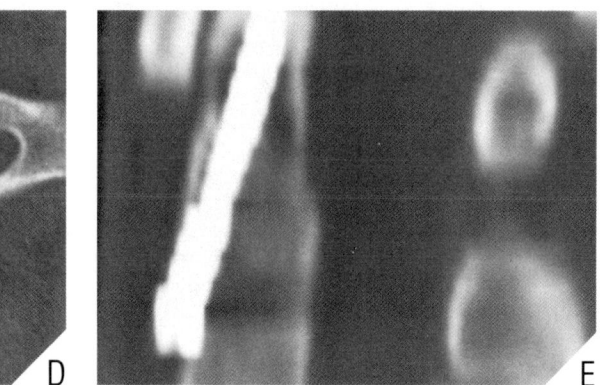

FIGURE 2.31 A 28-year-old man was injured in a motorcycle accident and sustained Type II odontoid fracture. (A) Anteroposterior open-mouth view shows a fracture line at the base of the odontoid process. (B) Lateral view shows 0.5 cm anterior displacement of odontoid with slight angulation. (C) Treatment with a single screw was elected. Note that displacement of odontoid has been reduced. Axial CT section (D) and sagittal reformation (E) show central placement of the compression screw in odontoid.

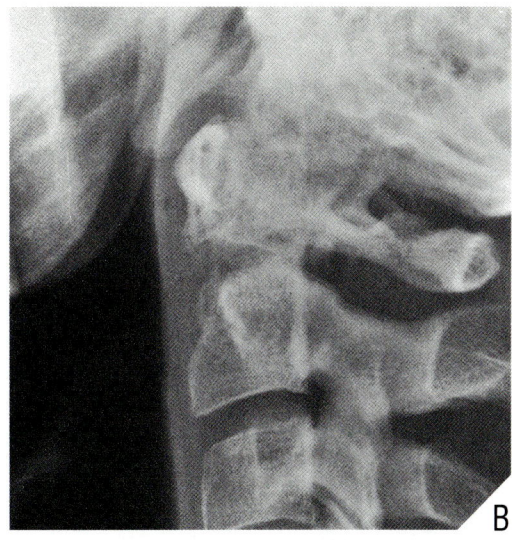

FIGURE 2.32 A 28-year-old man injured his neck in an industrial accident. He was neurologically intact. At the time of hospital admission he refused an application of halo. Anteroposterior open-mouth **(A)** and lateral **(B)** views show Type II odontoid fracture. Postsurgical open-mouth **(C)** and lateral **(D)** projections demonstrate application of two compression screws.

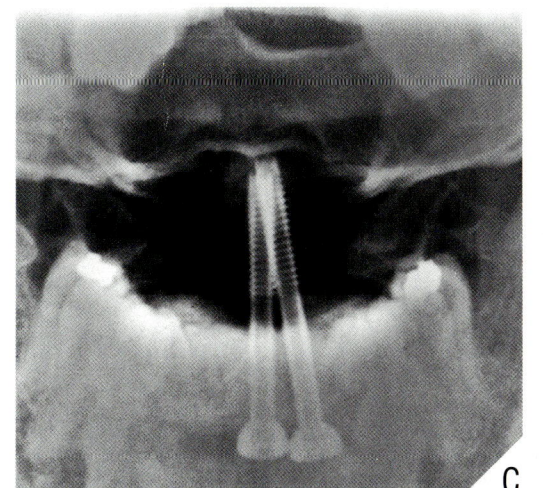

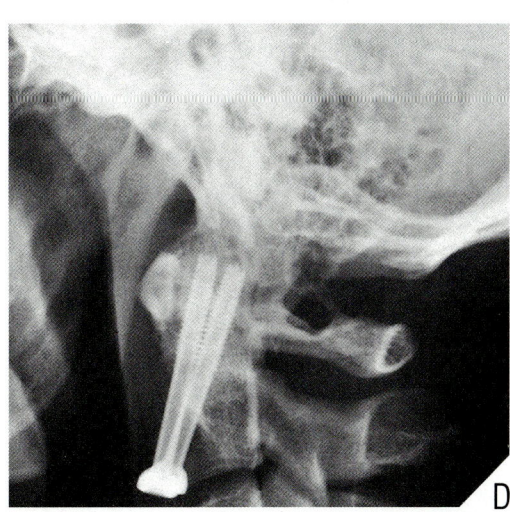

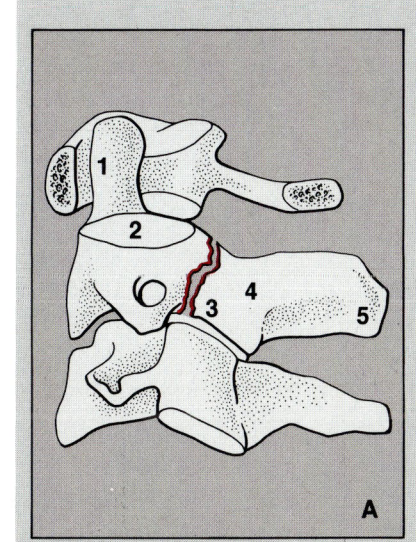

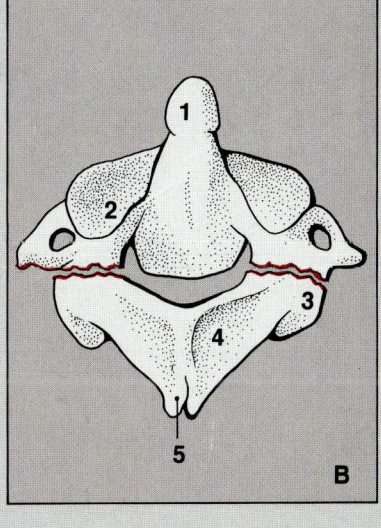

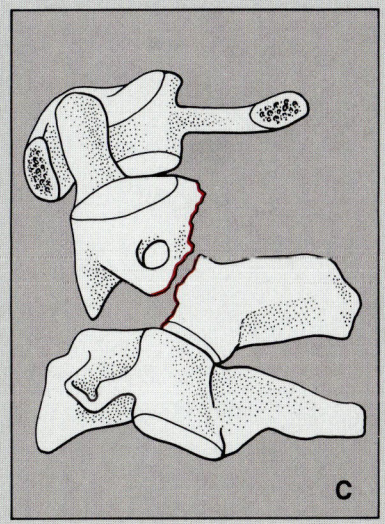

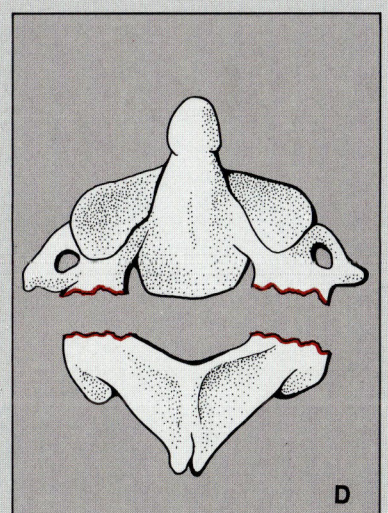

1 odontoid process
2 superior articular facet of C-2
3 inferior articular facet of C-2
4 lamina
5 spinous process

FIGURE 2.33 Hangman's fracture may present as nondisplaced fracture through the arches of C2, as seen here schematically on the lateral **(A)** and axial **(B)** views, or as displaced fractures with anterior angulation **(C,D)** associated with disruption of ligaments and the intervertebral disk.

Injury to the Cervical Spine

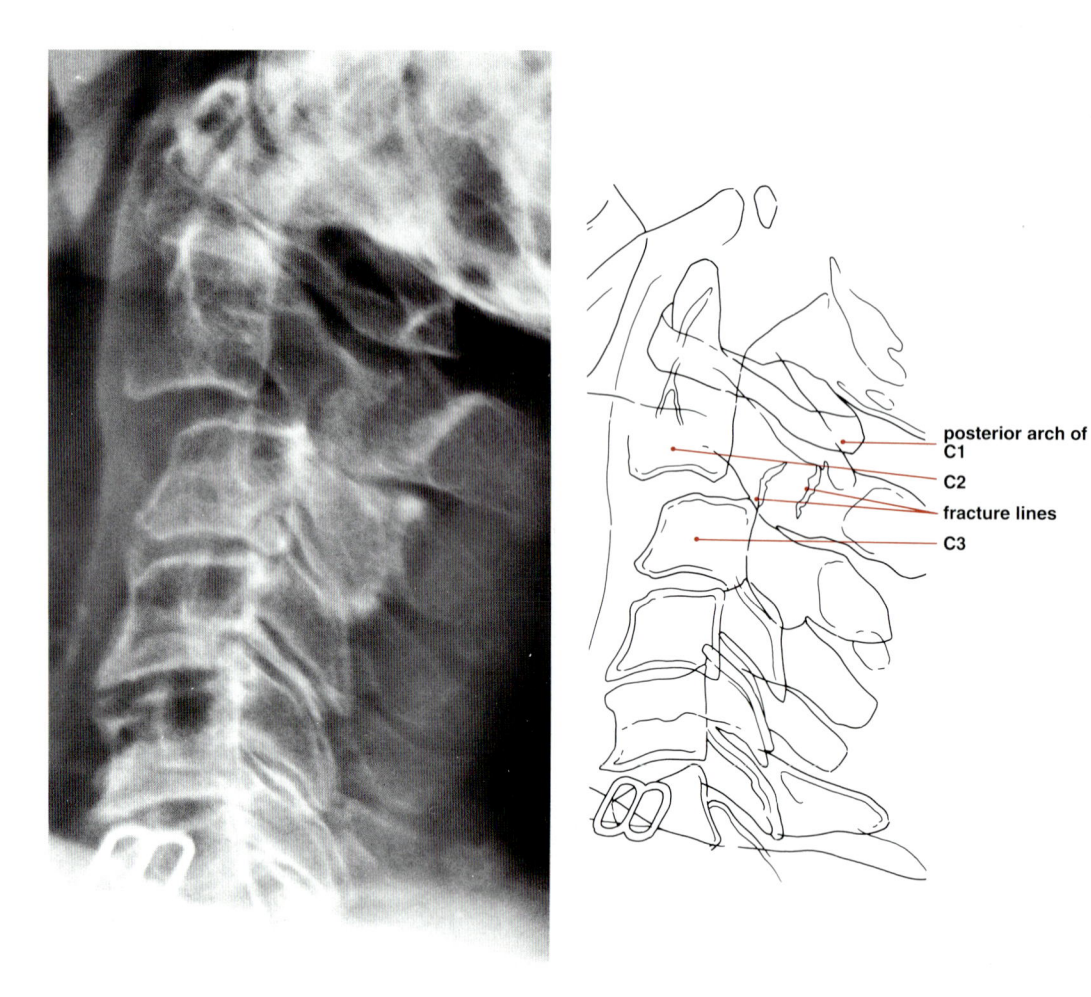

FIGURE 2.34 A 62-year-old man sustained a severe hyperextension injury to the cervical spine in an automobile accident. Lateral film shows a fracture through the pedicles of C2 associated with C2–C3 subluxation, a typical finding in hangman's fracture.

posterior arch of C1
C2
fracture lines
C3

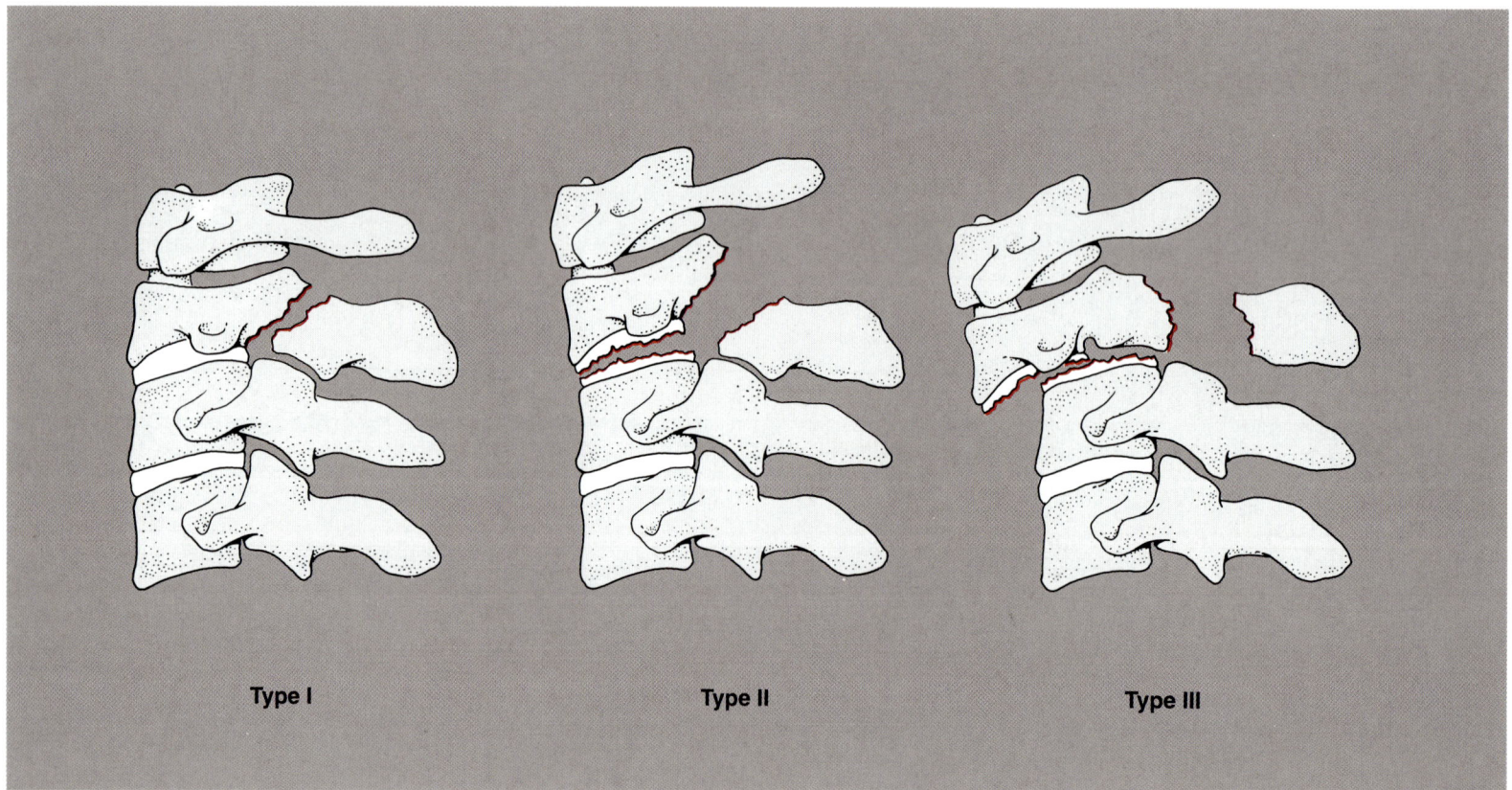

Type I   Type II   Type III

FIGURE 2.35 Classification of hangman's fractures. (Modified from Levine AM, Edwards CC: The management of traumatic spondylolisthesis of the axis. *J Bone Joint Surg* 67A:217, 1985)

Imaging of the Spine in Clinical Practice

In Type III injuries, open posterior facet reduction is performed. A compression screw can then be placed across the fracture, or the injury can then be treated as a Type I fracture.

FRACTURES OF THE MID AND LOWER CERVICAL SPINE

Burst Fracture

The mechanism of this injury is identical to that of Jefferson fracture involving C1, but burst fractures occur in the lower cervical vertebrae (C2–C7). When the nucleus pulposus, which is normally contained within the intervertebral disk, is driven through the fractured vertebral endplate into the vertebral body, the body explodes from within, resulting in a comminuted fracture. Typically, the posterior fragment is posteriorly displaced and may cause injury to the spinal cord. If the posterior ligament complex is not disrupted, a burst fracture is usually stable. Occasionally, with ligamentous disruption, the burst fracture becomes unstable. Radiographically it is characterized by a vertical split in the vertebral body, as seen on the anteroposterior view, but the plain film lateral projection (Fig. 2.36A) or lateral tomography better demonstrates the extent of comminution and posterior displacement. However, the most revealing modality in cases of burst fracture is CT, since it can demonstrate the details of the fracture of the posterior part of the vertebral body in the axial plane (Fig. 2.36B).

TREATMENT

Treatment of burst fractures depends on the presence or absence of neurologic injury. In the former instance, the patient can be treated by bracing traction or by posterior plating, depending on the severity of the injury and the need for early mobilization. The patient is then reassessed radiographically; if the vertebral body fracture is too comminuted to support weight bearing, anterior vertebrectomy and fusion may be performed.

In the presence of neurologic injury, a vertebrectomy is performed with anterior decompression. Intraoperative stability is then assessed. If the spine is felt to be unstable, anterior plating or posterior instrumentation and fusion can be performed.

"Teardrop" Fracture

The most severe and most unstable of injuries of the cervical spine, "teardrop" fracture, which represents a variant of burst fracture, is characterized by posterior displacement of the involved vertebra into the spinal canal, fracture of its posterior elements, and disruption of the soft tissues, including the ligamentum flavum and the spinal cord, at the level of injury. In addition, shear stress applied to the anterior column causes the anterior longitudinal ligament either to rupture or to avulse from the vertebral body, taking with it a piece of the anterior surface of the body. This small triangular or teardrop-shaped fragment is usually anteriorly and inferiorly displaced (Fig. 2.37). Associated spinal cord injury results in *acute anterior cervical cord syndrome,* consisting of abrupt quadriplegia

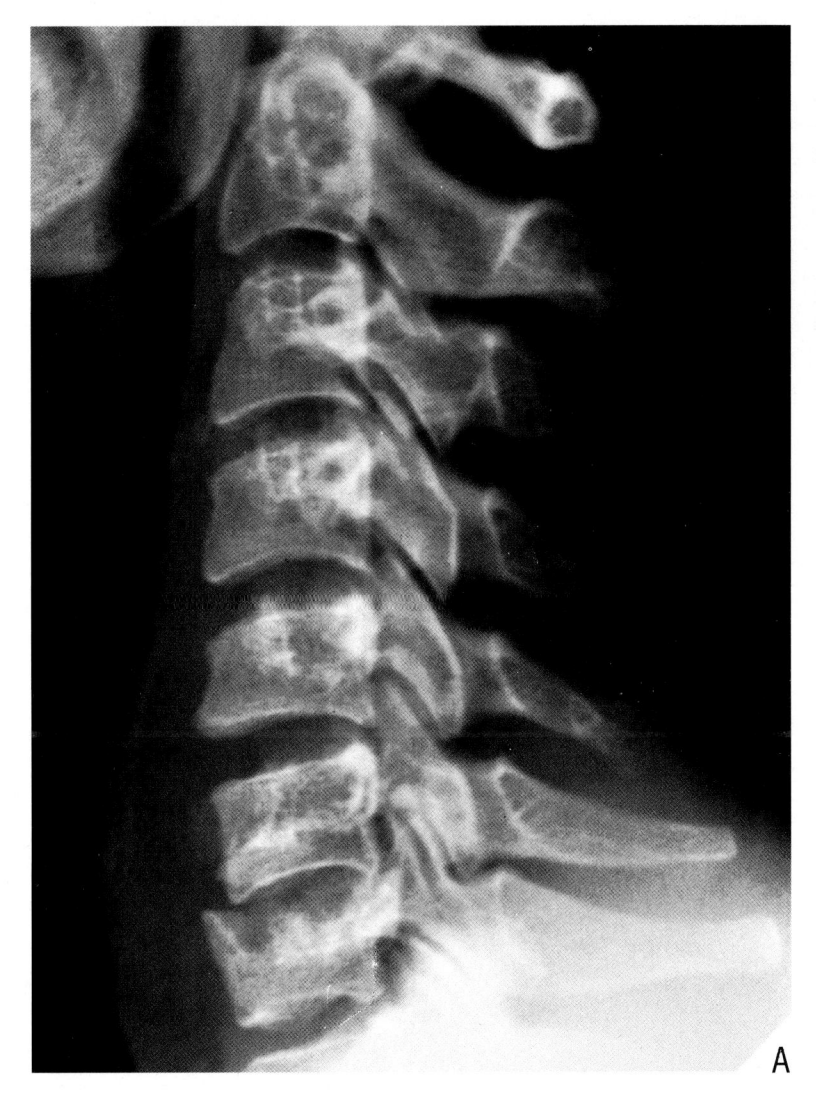

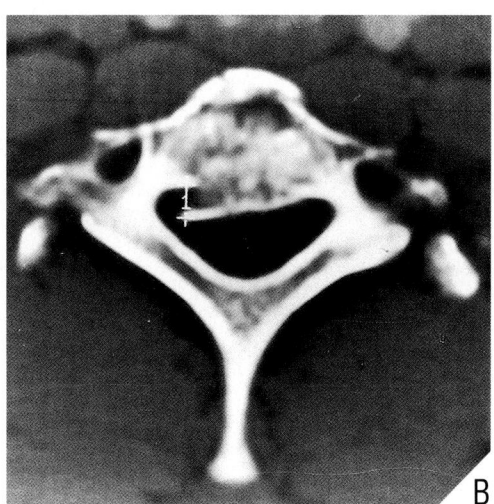

FIGURE 2.36 A 40-year-old man was ejected from a motorcycle and hit the pavement with the vertex of his head. **(A)** Lateral view of the cervical spine demonstrates a comminuted fracture of the body of C7, involving the anterior and middle columns. **(B)** A CT section confirms the burst fracture. The posterior part of the vertebral body is displaced into the spinal canal.

and loss of pain and temperature distinction; however, posterior-column senses—position, vibration, and motion—are usually preserved.

The lateral view is the best radiographic projection for demonstrating this injury; lateral tomography may also be necessary, as well as CT scan (Fig. 2.38). The evaluation of spinal cord compression requires MRI.

Occasionally a triangular fragment of bone similar in shape and location to that seen in the classic teardrop fracture may occasionally be noted in an extension type of injury. This "extension teardrop" fracture, however, is completely different; it is a stable fracture without the potentially dangerous complication of the flexion type of injury, and usually occurs at the level of C2 or C3 (Fig. 2.39).

TREATMENT

Reduction with traction is usually performed, followed by either halo application or anterior vertebrectomy combined with anterior plate stabilization (Fig. 2.40). Posterior stabilization, with plate or screws to act as a buttress, can also be performed if applied traction results in the spinal canal decompression (Figs. 2.41, 2.42).

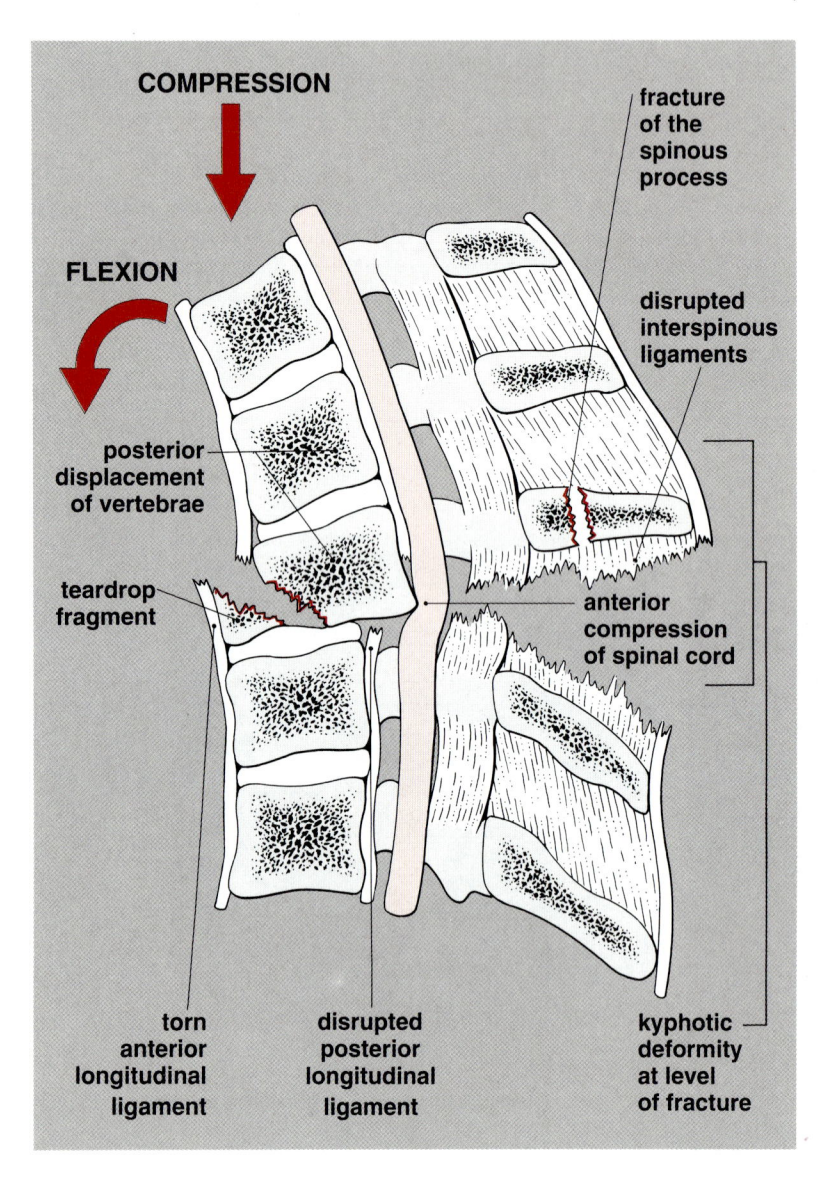

FIGURE 2.37 "Teardrop" fracture, seen here schematically in a sagittal section of the lower cervical spine, is the most serious and unstable of cervical spine injuries. Disruption of the anterior longitudinal ligament may cause avulsion of a teardrop-shaped fragment of the anterior surface of the body of C5. This fracture is also typified by posterior displacement of the involved vertebra and fracture of its posterior elements. Depending on the severity of the injury, varying degrees of spinal cord damage may result.

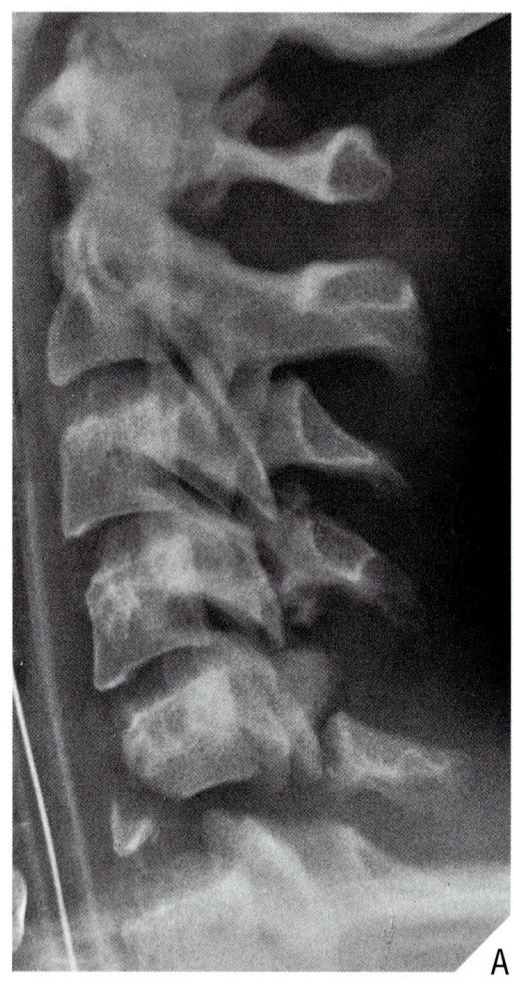

FIGURE 2.38 A 38-year-old man sustained an injury of the neck in a motorcycle accident. (A) Lateral view of the cervical spine demonstrates an avulsion fracture of the anteroinferior aspect of the body of C5 and a fracture of its spinous process. The lamina of C4 is fractured as well. There is disruption of the facets at the level of C5–C6 with marked widening. There is posterior displacement of all vertebrae including and above C5. (B) CT section demonstrates in addition a markedly comminuted fracture of the body of C5.

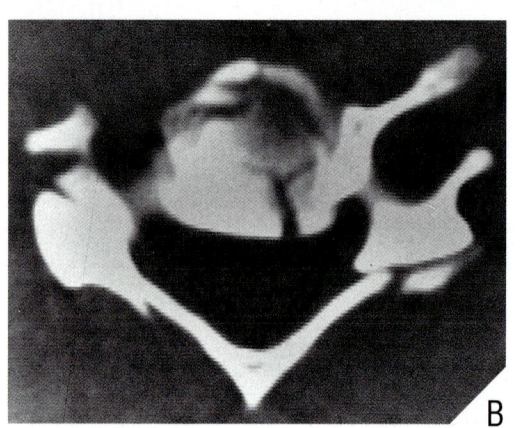

2.30 *Imaging of the Spine in Clinical Practice*

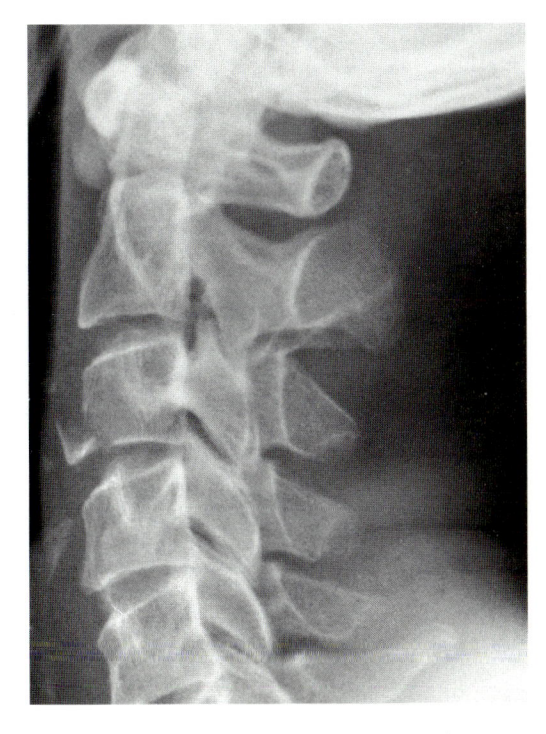

FIGURE 2.39 A 37-year-old man sustained an extension injury to the cervical spine in a fall. Lateral radiograph of the spine demonstrates an extension "teardrop" fracture of the vertebral body of C3. Note that, in contrast to a flexion-type injury, there is no subluxation, and the posterior, vertebral, and spinolaminar lines are not disrupted.

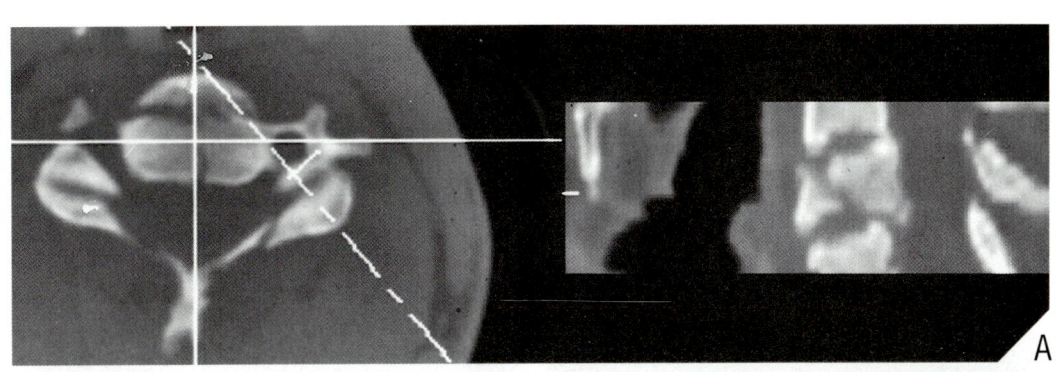

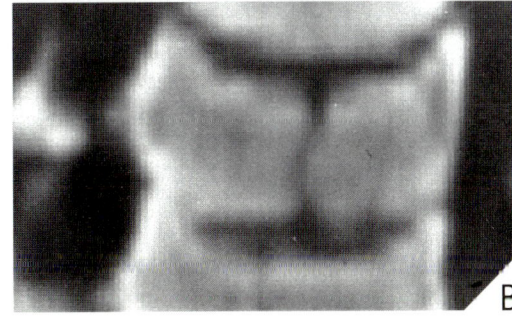

FIGURE 2.40 A 36-year-old man sustained a neck injury in a motorcycle accident. He was neurologically intact. **(A)** Computed tomography axial section and sagittal reformation demonstrate a typical "teardrop" fracture of C5. **(B)** CT coronal reformation shows the vertical fracture of body of C5 in sagittal plane. **(C)** Treatment consisted of anterior vertebrectomy, interbody fibular strut application, and anterior fusion with plate and screws.

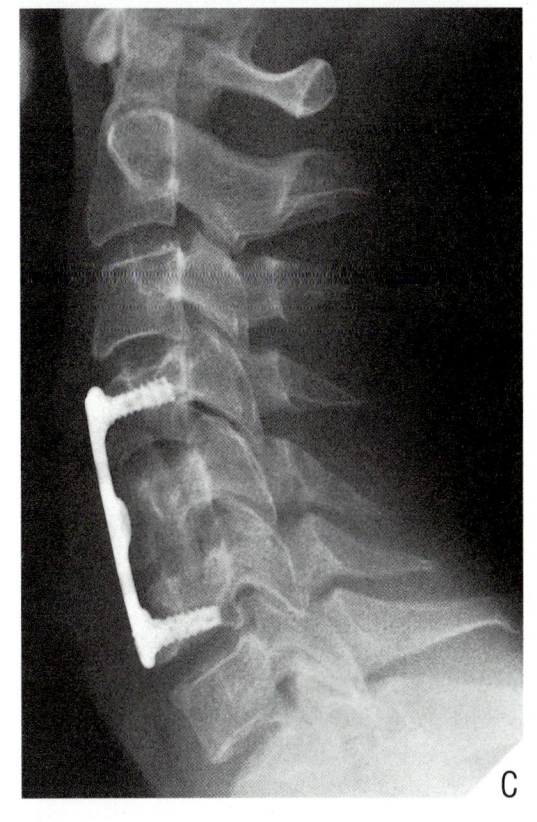

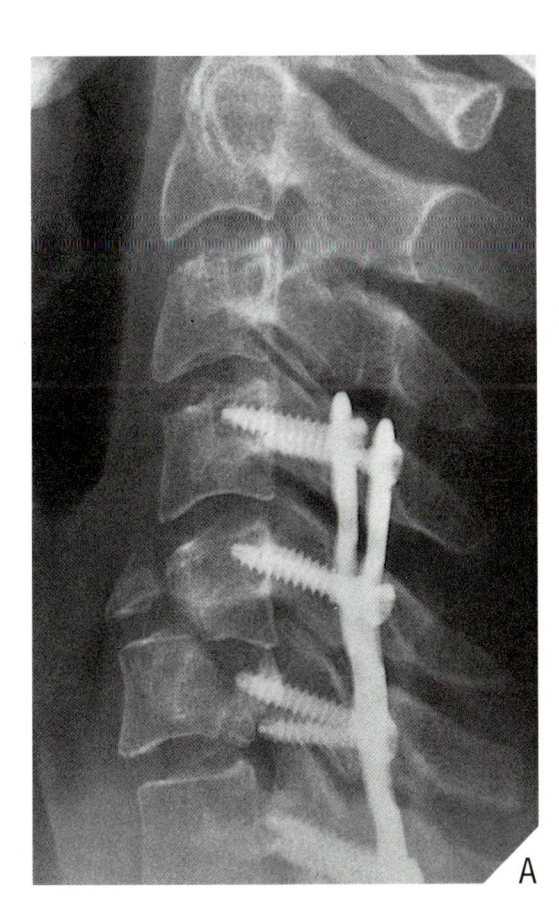

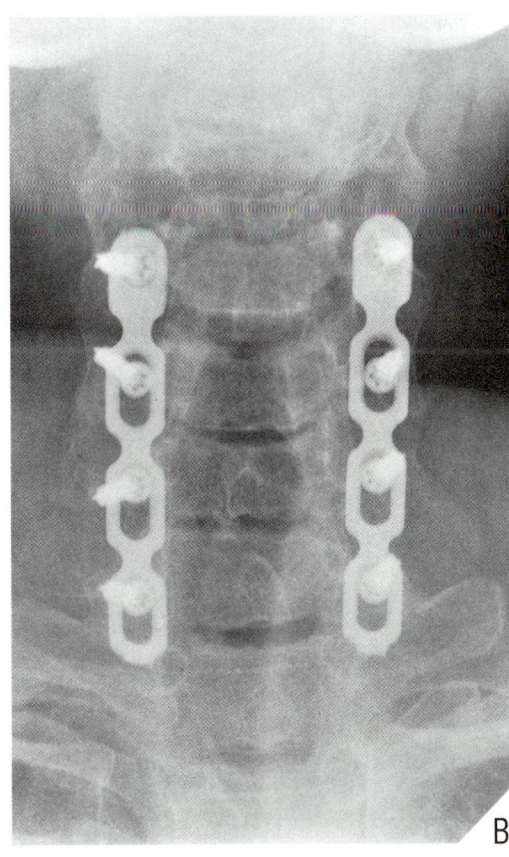

FIGURE 2.41 A 32-year-old man injured his neck in a motorcycle accident and sustained a "teardrop" fracture of C5. He was neurologically intact. Lateral **(A)** and anteroposterior **(B)** radiographs show posterior stabilization with two reconstruction plates and lateral mass screws achieved after successful decompression of the spinal canal by means of cervical traction. The C7 vertebra was included because of ligamentous damage at the C6–C7 level.

Injury to the Cervical Spine   2.31

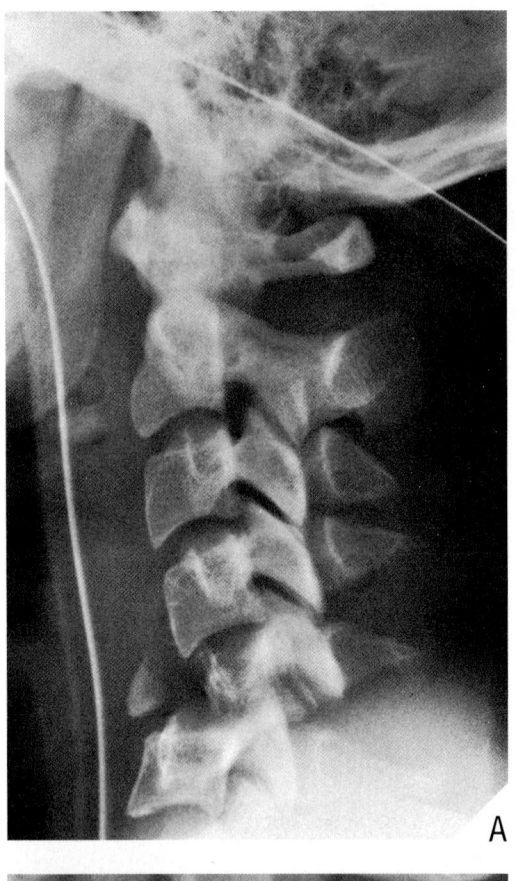

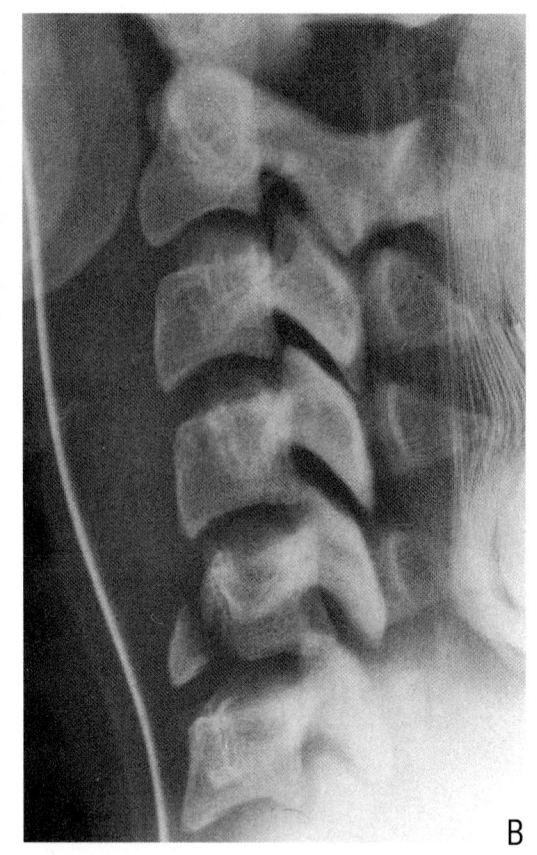

FIGURE 2.42 An 18-year-old man sustained a neck injury in a diving accident. He was neurologically intact. **(A)** Lateral view of the cervical spine shows a "teardrop" fracture of C5. Note widening of the facet joints and interspinous space of C5–C6, and significant C5–C6 subluxation. **(B)** After application of 45 lbs of traction there is adequate reduction of subluxation and decompression of the spinal canal. Lateral **(C)** and anteroposterior **(D)** radiographs show evidence of posterior fusion using bone graft and cerclage wire together with two facet screws.

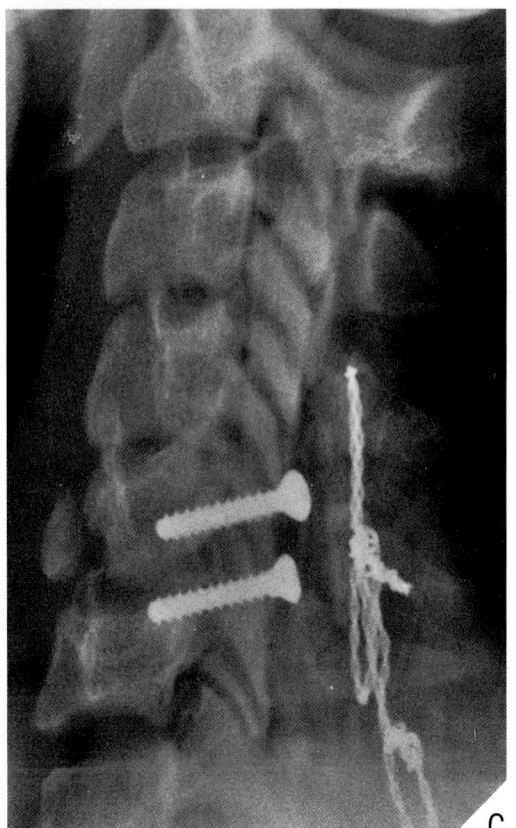

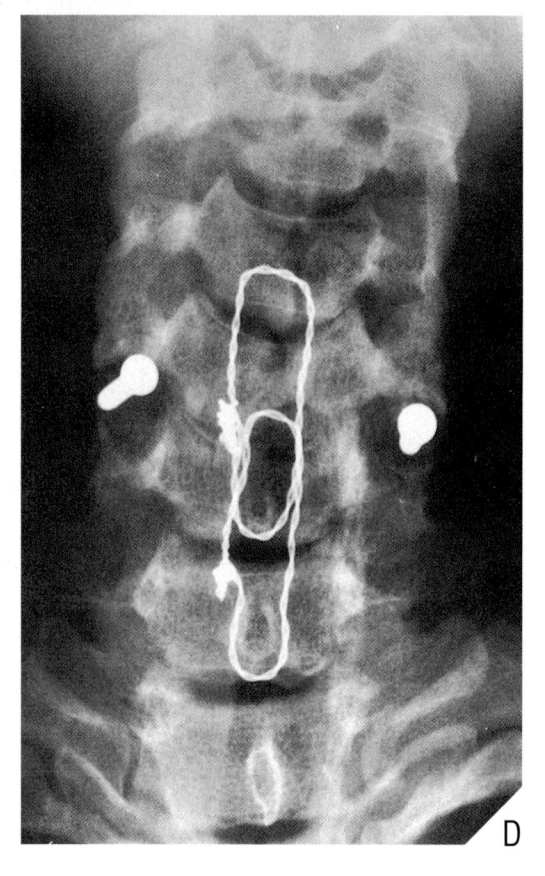

Imaging of the Spine in Clinical Practice

Clay-shoveler's Fracture

This oblique or vertical fracture of the spinous process of C6 or C7 is caused by an acute powerful flexion, such as that produced by shoveling. Deriving its name from its common occurrence in clay miners in Australia in the 1930s, clay-shoveler's fracture was simultaneously labeled with the same name in Germany, where it was seen among workers building the Autobahn. A direct blow to the cervical spine or indirect trauma to the neck in automobile accidents can result in similar injury.

Clay-shoveler's fracture is a stable injury, the posterior ligament complex remaining intact, and is therefore not associated with neurologic damage. The best radiographic projection for demonstrating this fracture is the lateral view of the cervical spine (Fig. 2.43A). If C7 cannot be visualized despite good positioning and technique (eg, because of a short, thick neck or wide shoulders), the swimmer's view should be obtained. This fracture can also be identified on the anteroposterior view by the so-called ghost sign (Fig. 2.43B), produced by displacement of the fractured spinous process. This is a stable injury that can be treated in a cervical orthosis for 8 to 12 weeks.

Simple Wedge (Compression) Fracture

Resulting from hyperflexion of the cervical spine, a simple wedge fracture generally occurs in the mid-cervical or lower cervical segment. There is anterior compression (wedging) of the vertebral body, and although the

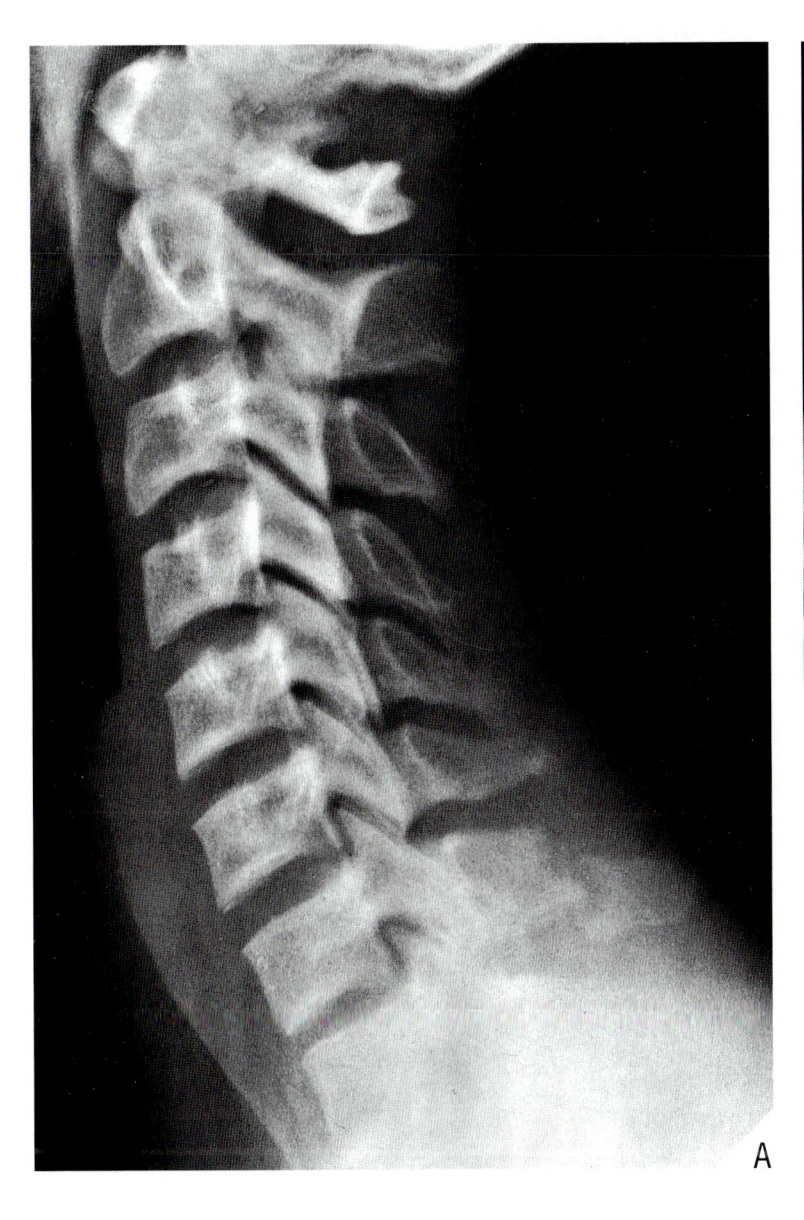

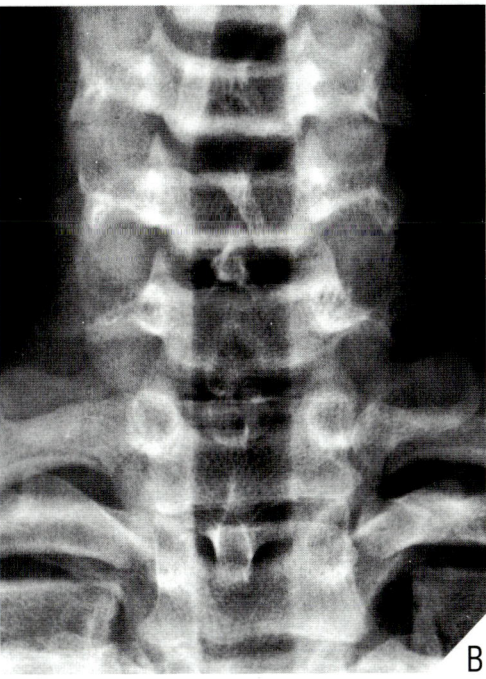

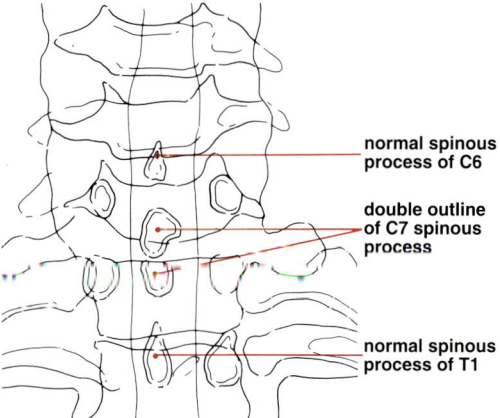

FIGURE 2.43 A 22-year-old man sustained a neck injury in an automobile accident. **(A)** Lateral view of the cervical spine shows a fracture of the spinous process of C7, identifying this injury as a clay-shoveler's fracture. **(B)** On the anteroposterior view, clay-shoveler's fracture can be identified by the appearance of a double spinous process for C7. This ghost sign is secondary to slight caudal displacement of the fractured tip of the spinous process.

Injury to the Cervical Spine

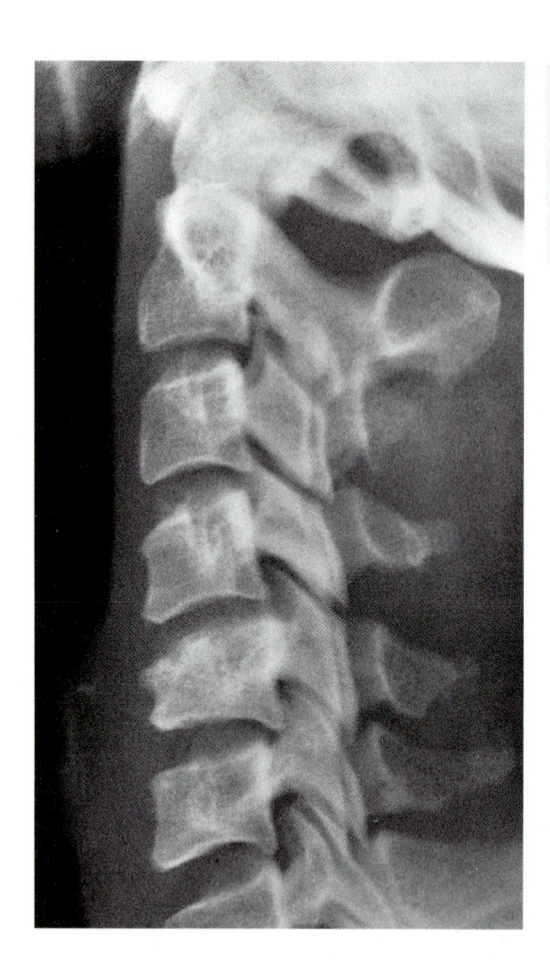

FIGURE 2.44 A 30-year-old woman sustained a neck injury in an automobile accident. Lateral view of the cervical spine demonstrates a simple wedge fracture of C5.

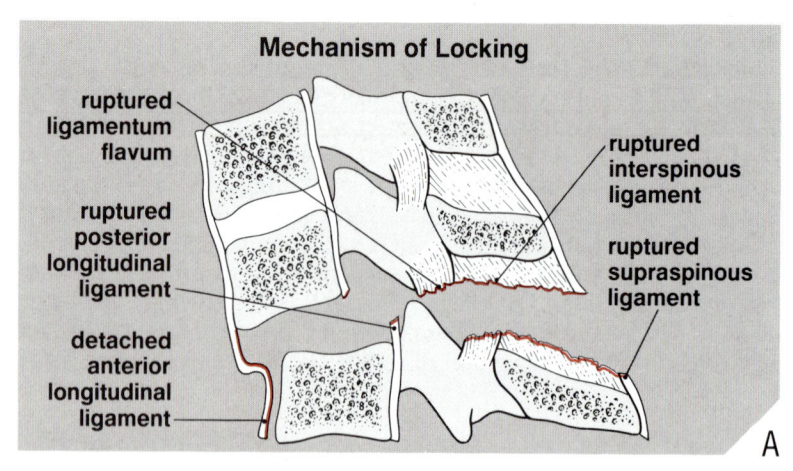

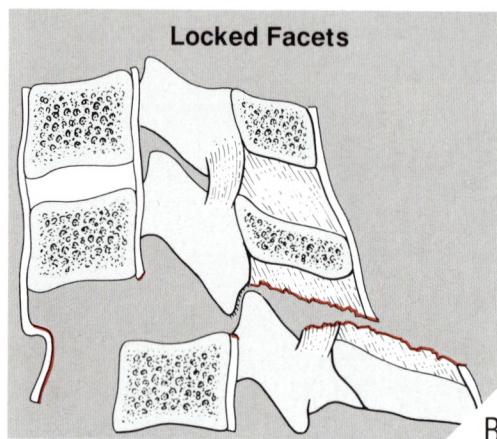

FIGURE 2.45 (A,B) Bilateral locked facets is a hyperflexion injury characterized by complete anterior dislocation of the affected vertebra. It is always associated with extension ligament disruption and carries a great risk of cervical spinal cord damage.

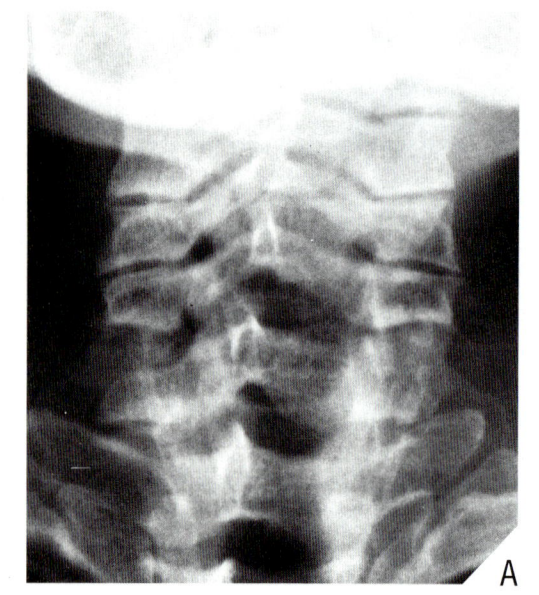

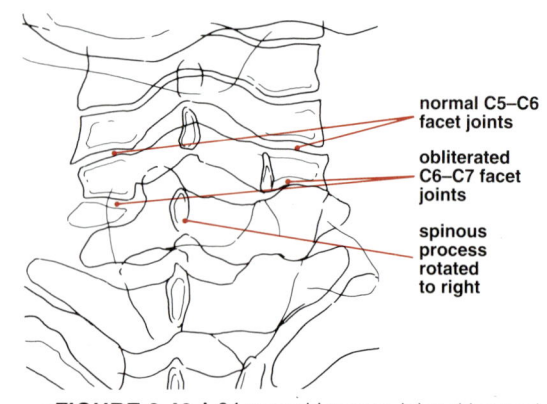

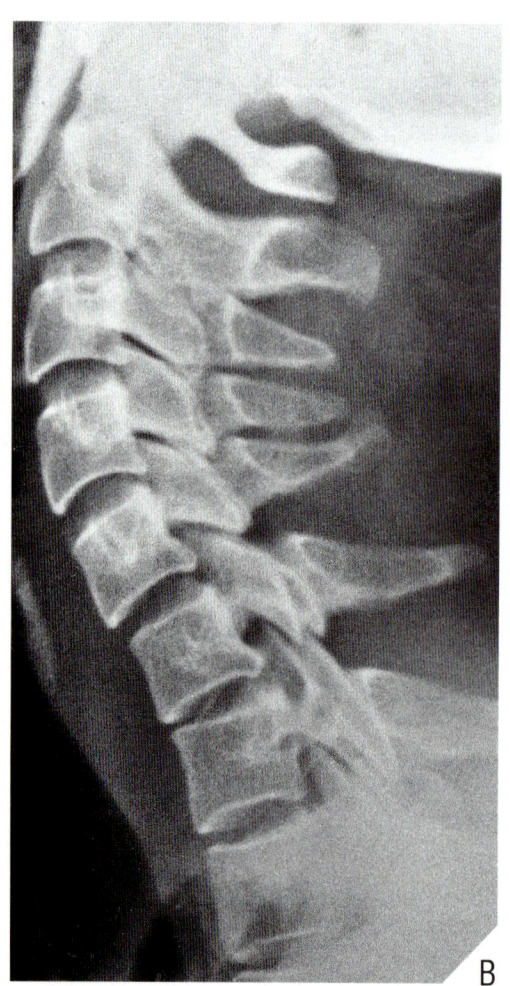

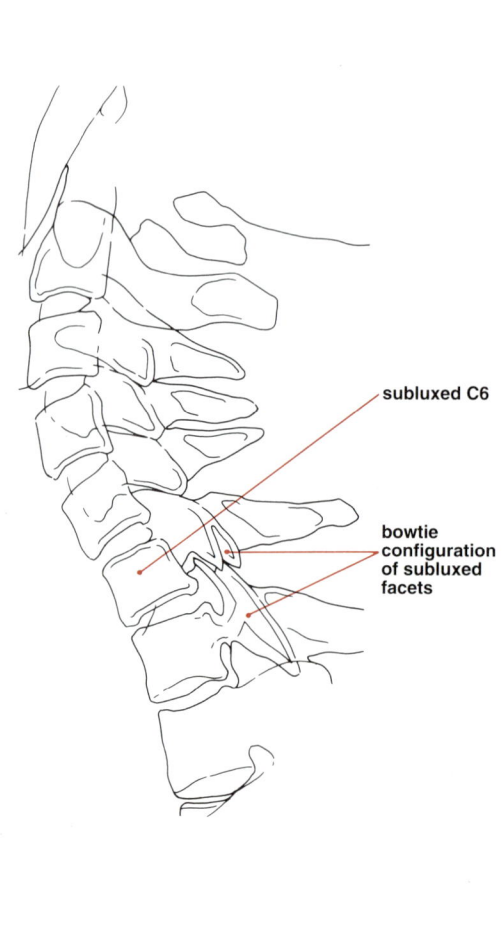

FIGURE 2.46 A 34-year-old woman injured her neck in a skiing accident. **(A)** Pillar view of the cervical spine demonstrates bilateral obliteration of the facet joints at the C6–C7 level. The joints above appear normal. Displacement of the spinous process to the right is the result of rotation. **(B)** Lateral view shows subluxation of C6 onto C7, as well as rotation, yielding the typical "bow tie" appearance of this injury.

2.34   *Imaging of the Spine in Clinical Practice*

posterior ligament complex is stretched it remains intact, making this a stable fracture. The lateral projection of the cervical spine adequately demonstrates this injury (Fig. 2.44). The treatment usually consists of cervical orthosis for 8 to 12 weeks.

Bilateral Locked Facets

Bilateral dislocation of the cervical spine in the facet joints is the result of extreme flexion of the head and neck; it is an unstable condition because it involves extensive disruption of the posterior ligament complex. Interlocking of the articular facets is initiated by the forward movement of the inferior articular facet of the underlying vertebra (Fig. 2.45). This causes the lamina and the spinous process of the two adjacent vertebrae to spread apart and the vertebral bodies to sublux. In the later stage of dislocation, the inferior articular facet of the upper vertebra locks in front of the superior articular facet of the lower vertebra, which results in complete anterior dislocation. The configuration of this injury leads to complete disruption of the posterior ligament complex, the posterior longitudinal ligament, the annulus fibrosus, and occasionally the anterior longitudinal ligament. It is also associated with a high incidence of damage to the cervical spinal cord.

The lateral projection of the cervical spine, preferably a cross-table lateral, is sufficient to demonstrate bilaterally locked facets. The key to the correct diagnosis is the presence of anterior displacement of 50% of the vertebral mid-sagittal diameter of the affected vertebra, evident from its oblique orientation, whereas the vertebrae below are seen in true lateral projection. This frequently results in a bow-tie or bat-wing appearance of the articular pillars of the dislocated vertebra (Fig. 2.46).

Treatment

In this injury, the capsules of both facet joints are disrupted; hence, although less stable, this injury is easier to reduce than unilateral facet dislocations. It usually results in severe neurologic damage. Bilateral facet dislocations require posterior cervical spine fusion (Fig. 2.47), occasion-

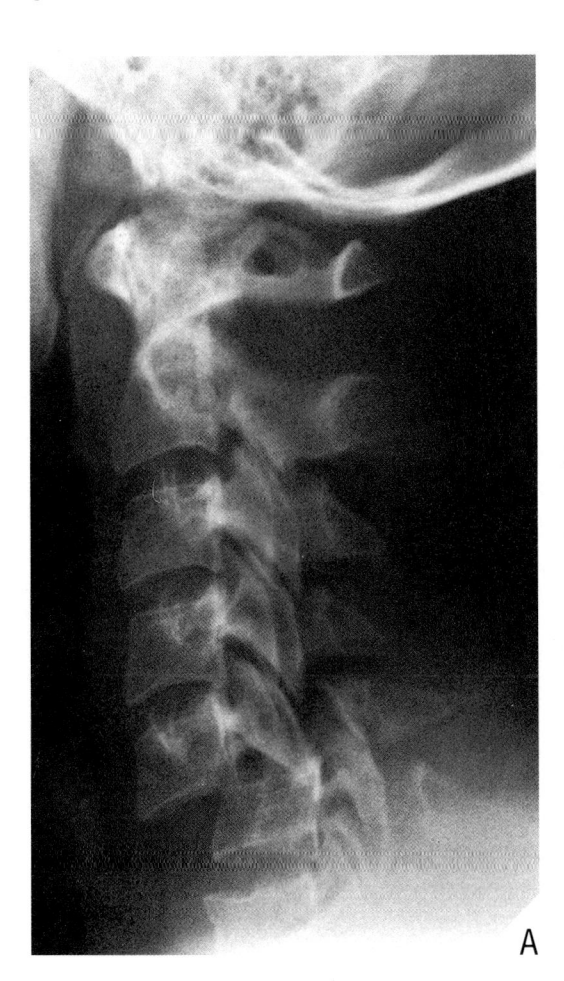

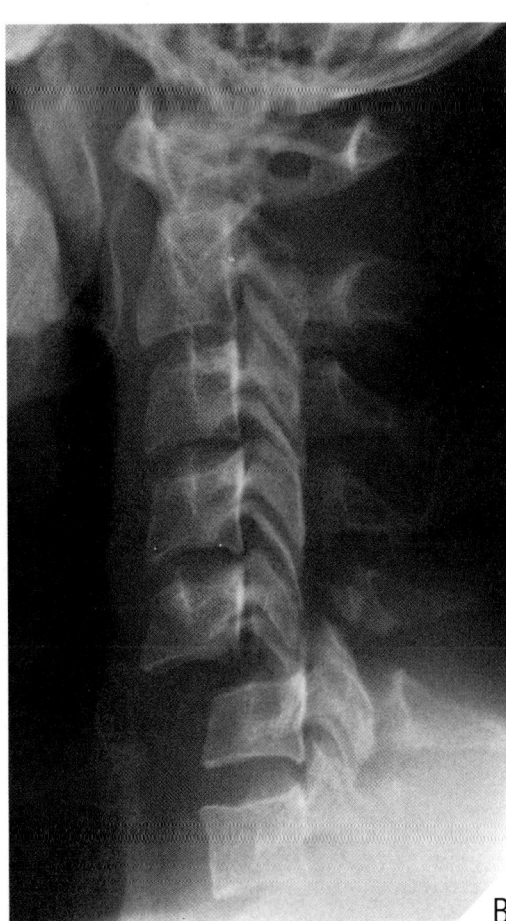

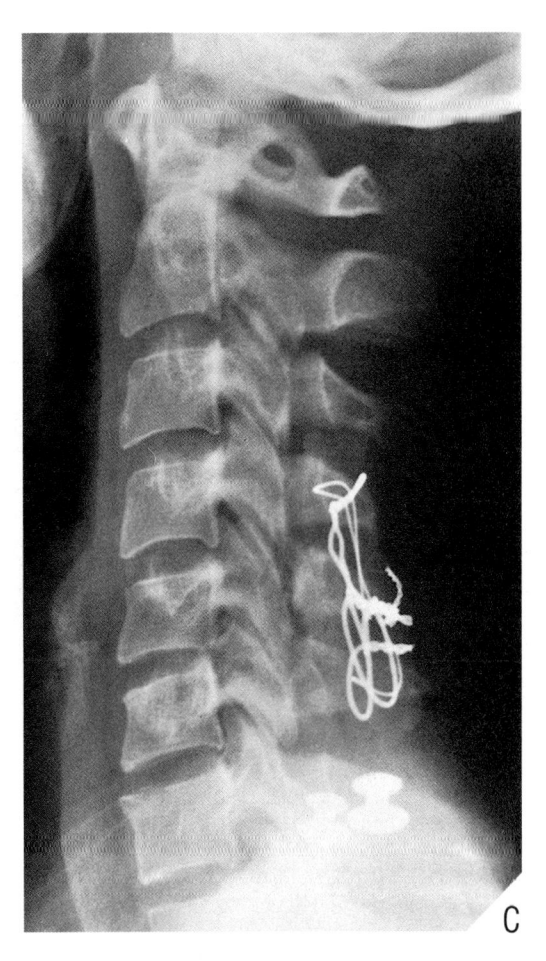

FIGURE 2.47 A 36-year-old man injured his neck in a motor vehicle accident that resulted in quadriplegia. **(A)** Lateral view of cervical spine demonstrates bilateral locked facets at C5–C6 level. **(B)** Cervical traction with application of up to 60 lbs of weight failed to "unlock" the joints. **(C)** Surgical procedure has been performed to reduce the dislocation and posterior fusion was done using bone graft and cerclage wire.

ally augmented by anterior interbody graft stabilization (Fig. 2.48). In patients who have only partial neurologic injury, or who are totally intact neurologically, CT myelogram or MRI should be performed before reduction to determine the location of the intervertebral disk. If the disk lies immediately posterior to the dislocated vertebral body, it may be inadvertently pulled into the spinal canal during reduction, producing complete and irreversible neurologic damage. If the disk is identified posteriorly to the dislocated vertebral body, anterior disk excision with tricortical interbody fusion should be performed. The patient should then be turned to the prone position for spinous process wiring and posterior cervical spine fusion. Alternate treatment consists of anterior plate fixation combined with anterior decompression and fusion.

Bilateral Perched Facets

This type of vertebral subluxation occurs as a result of a flexion injury. There is disruption of the posterior ligamentous complex. This injury, similarly to complete facet dislocation, is best diagnosed by lateral and oblique views of the spine or CT with sagittal and oblique reformation. Posterior spinous process wiring and fusion are indicated as the preferred method of treatment.

Unilateral Locked Facets

This type of injury is caused by flexion–rotation force, with subsequent tearing of the joint capsule of one facet and of the posterior ligamentous complex. Plain film examination reveals 25% anterior subluxation. These patients may sustain nerve root injury or, rarely, a Brown–Sequard type of spinal cord injury. Unilateral locked facets may be difficult to reduce in traction. One should begin with approximately 10 pounds and then gradually increase the weight until either reduction has been achieved or 40- to 60-pound traction (one third of body weight) has been attained. Complete radiologic and neurologic examination should be performed before each weight increase. If reduction is successful, the patient is placed in a halo jacket for 8 to 12 weeks. If reduction is unsuccessful, the treatment consists of posterior open reduction combined with posterior fixation and fusion.

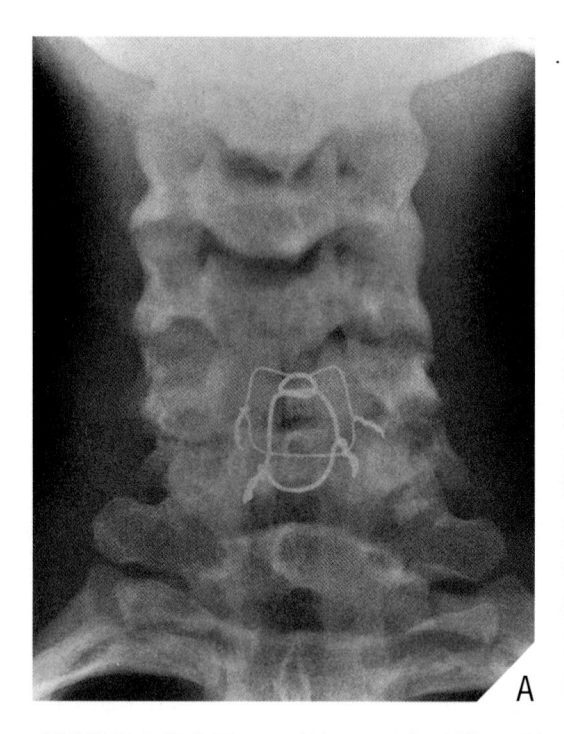

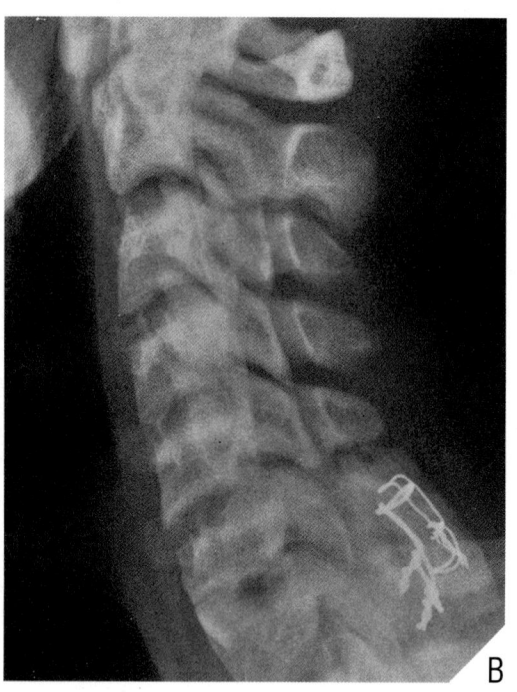

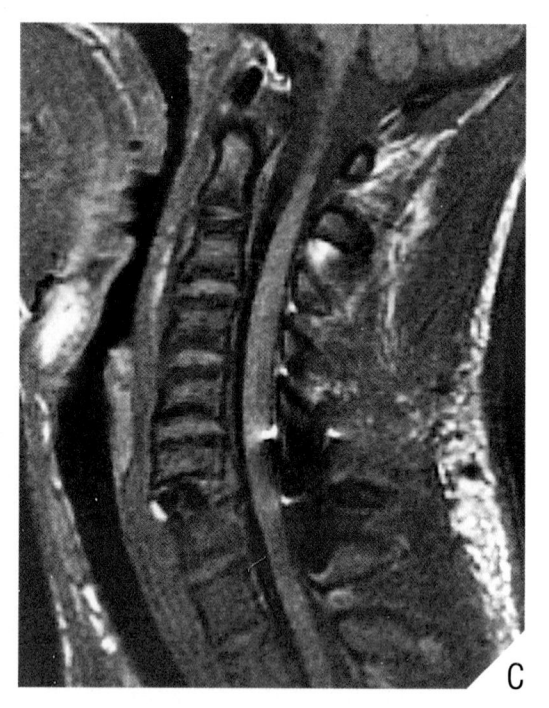

FIGURE 2.48 A 17-year-old boy sustained bilateral facet dislocation at C6–C7 level as a result of a pedestrian vs. automobile accident. He was neurologically intact. Anteroposterior **(A)** and lateral **(B)** radiographs demonstrate posterior fusion with bone graft and cerclage wire supplemented with anterior interbody fibular strut. **(C)** Postoperative sagittal MRI shows adequate alignment of the cervical spine and no encroachment on the spinal cord. Posterior and anterior grafts demonstrate low signal intensity.

Suggested Reading

Aebi M, Etter C, Coscia M: Fractures of the odontoid process: Treatment with anterior screw fixation. *Spine* 14:1065, 1989.

Aebi M, Mohler J, Zach GA, et al: Indication, surgical technique, and results of 100 surgically-treated fractures and fracture-dislocations of the cervical spine. *Clin Orthop* 203:244, 1986.

Amundsen P, Skalpe IO: Cervical myelography with a water soluble contrast medium (Metrizamide). *Neuroradiology* 8:209, 1975.

Anderson LD, D'Alonzo RT: Fractures of the odontoid process of the axis. *J Bone Joint Surg* 56A:1663, 1974.

Anderson PA, Montesano PX: Morphology and treatment of occipital condyle fractures. *Spine* 13:731, 1988.

Anderson PA, Montesano PX: Traumatic injuries to the occipital–cervical articulation. In Camins M, O'Leary P (eds): *Disorders of the Cervical Spine*. Baltimore, Williams & Wilkins, 1992.

Bohler J: Anterior stabilization for acute fractures and non-unions of the dens. *J Bone Joint Surg* 64A:18, 1985.

Borne GM, Bedou GL, Pinaudeau M, et al: Odontoid process fracture osteosynthesis with a direct screw fixation technique in nine consecutive cases. *J Neurosurg* 68:223, 1988.

Boyd WR, Gardiner A Jr: Metrizamide myelography. *Am J Roentgenol* 129:481, 1974.

Brant-Zawadzki M, Miller EM, Federle MP: T in the evaluation of spine trauma. *Am J Roentgenol* 136:369, 1981.

Brashear HR Jr, Venters G, Preston ET: Fractures of the neural arch of the axis: A report of twenty-nine cases. *J Bone Joint Surg* 57A:879, 1975.

Bucholz RW: Unstable hangman's fractures. *Clin Orthop* 154:119, 1981.

Burke JT, Harris JH: Acute injuries of the axis vertebra. *Skeletal Radiol* 18:335, 1989.

Cancelmo JJ: Clay shoveler's fracture. A helpful diagnostic sign. *Am J Roentgenol* 115:540, 1972.

Chance Q: Note on a type of flexion fracture of the spine. *Br J Radiol* 21:452, 1948.

Christenson P: The radiologic study of the normal spine: Cervical, thoracic, lumbar, and sacral. *Radiol Clin North Am* 15:133, 1977.

Clark R, White AA: Fractures of the dens. *J Bone Joint Surg* 67A:1340, 1985.

Clark WM, Gehweiler JA Jr, Laib R: Twelve significant signs of cervical spine trauma. *Skeletal Radiol* 3:201, 1979.

Daffner RH: "Fingerprints" of vertebral trauma—A unifying concept based on mechanism. *Skeletal Radiol* 15:518, 1986.

Daffner RH: *Imaging of Vertebral Trauma*. Rockville, MD, Aspen Publishers, 1988.

Dolan KD: Cervical spine injuries below the axis. *Radiol Clin North Am* 15:247, 1977.

Dovark J, Panjabi MM: Functional anatomy of the allyl ligaments. *Spine* 12:183, 1987.

Dunn ME, Seljeskog EL: Experience in the management of odontoid process injuries: An analysis of 128 cases. *Neurosurgery* 18:306, 1986.

Fuchs AW: Cervical vertebrae (Part 1). *Radiogr Clin Photogr* 16:2, 1940.

Fujii E, Kobayashi K, Hirabayashi K: Treatment in fractures of the odontoid process. *Spine* 13:604, 1988.

Geisler FH, Cheng C, Poka A, et al: Anterior screw fixation of posteriorly displaced type II odontoid fractures. *Neurosurgery* 25:30, 1989.

Gerlock AJ Jr, Kirchner SG, Heller RM, et al: *The Cervical Spine in Trauma*. Philadelphia, W B Saunders, 1978.

Gerlock AJ Jr, Mirfakhraee M: Computed tomography and hangman's fracture. *South Med J* 76:727, 1983.

Goldstein SJ, Woodring JH, Young AB: Occipital condyle fracture associated with cervical spine injury. *Surg Neurol* 17:350, 1982.

Hadley MN, Browner CM, Sonntag VKH: Axis fractures: A comprehensive review of management and treatment in 107 cases. *Neurosurgery* 17:281, 1985.

Han SY, Witten DM, Musselman JP: Jefferson fracture of the atlas: Report of six cases. *J Neurosurg* 44:368, 1976.

Hanssen AD, Cabanela ME: Fractures of the dens in adult patients. *J Trauma* 27:928, 1987.

Harding-Smith J, MacIntosh PK, Sherbon KJ: Fracture of the occipital condyle. *J Bone Joint Surg* 63A:1170, 1981.

Haughton VM: MR imaging of the spine. *Radiology* 166:297, 1988.

Hyman RA, Gorey MT: Imaging strategies for MR of the spine. *Radiol Clin N Am* 26:505, 1988.

Johansen JG, Orrison WW, Amundsen P: Lateral C1-2 puncture for cervical myelography. Part I: Report of a complication. *Radiology* 146:391, 1983.

Kim KS, Chen HH, Russell EJ, et al: Flexion teardrop fracture of the cervical spine: Radiographic characteristics. *AJR* 152:319, 1989.

Lesoin F, Autricque A, Franz K, et al: Transcervical approach and screw fixation for upper cervical spine pathology. *Surg Neurol* 27:928, 1987.

Levine AM, Edwards CC: The management of traumatic spondylolisthesis of the axis. *J Bone Joint Surg* 67A:217, 1985)

Lipson SJ: Fractures of the atlas associated with fractures of the odontoid process and transverse ligament ruptures. *J Bone Joint Surg* 59A:940, 1977.

McKim TH: Atlantoaxial injuries. *Semin Orthop* 2:110, 1987.

Mirvis SE, Geisler FH, Jelinek JJ, et al: Acute cervical spine trauma: Evaluation with 1.5T MR imaging. *Radiology* 166:807, 1988.

Mirvis SE, Young JWR, Lim C, et al: Hangman's fracture: Radiologic assessment in 27 cases. *Radiology* 163:713, 1987.

Montesano PX, Anderson PA, Schlehr F, et al: Odontoid fractures treated by anterior odontoid screw fixation. *Spine* 16:S33, 1991.

Montesano PX, Benson DR: The thoracolumbar spine. In Rockwood CA, Green DP, Bucholz RW (eds): *Rockwood and Green's Fractures in Adults*, 3rd ed. Philadelphia, J B Lippincott, 1991.

Nakanishi T, Sasaki T, Tokita N, et al: Internal fixation for the odontoid fracture. *Orthop Trans* 6:176, 1982.

Orrison WW, Eldevik OP, Sackett JF: Lateral C1–2 puncture for cervical myelography. Part III: Historical, anatomic and technical considerations. *Radiology* 146:401, 1983.

Pech P, Kilgore DP, Pojunas KW, et al: Cervical spinal fractures: T detection. *Radiology* 157:117, 1985.

Rogers LF: Cervical spine trauma. In Dalinka MK, Kaye JJ (eds): *Radiology in Emergency Room Medicine*. New York, Churchill Livingstone, 1984.

Russell EJ, D'Angelo M, Zimmerman RD, et al: Cervical disk herniation: CT demonstration after contrast enhancement. *Radiology* 152:703, 1984.

Schatzker J, Rorabeck H, Waddell JP: Non-union of the odontoid process. *Clin Orthop* 108:1975.

Scher AT: Unilateral locked facet in cervical spine injuries. *Am J Roentgenol* 129:45, 1977.

Schneider R, Livingston KE, Cave AJE, et al: "Hangman's fracture" of the cervical spine. *J Neurosurg* 22:141, 1965.

Spence KF, Decker S, Sell KW: Bursting atlantal fracture associated with rupture of the transverse ligament. *J Bone Joint Surg* 52A:543, 1970.

Spencer JA, Yeakley JW, Kaufman HH: Fracture of the occipital condyle. *Neurosurgery* 15:101, 1984.

Traynelis VC, Marano GD, Dunker RO, et al: Traumatic atlanto-occipital dislocation. *J Neurosurg* 65:863, 1988.

Wang GJ, Mabie KN, Whitehill R, et al: The nonsurgical management of odontoid fractures in adults. *Spine* 9:229, 1984.

Whittley JE, Forsythe HF: Classification of cervical spine injuries. *Am J Roentgenol* 83:633, 1958.

Zanca P, Lodmell EA: Fracture of spinous process: New sign for recognition of fractures of cervical and upper dorsal spinous processes. *Radiology* 56:427, 1951.

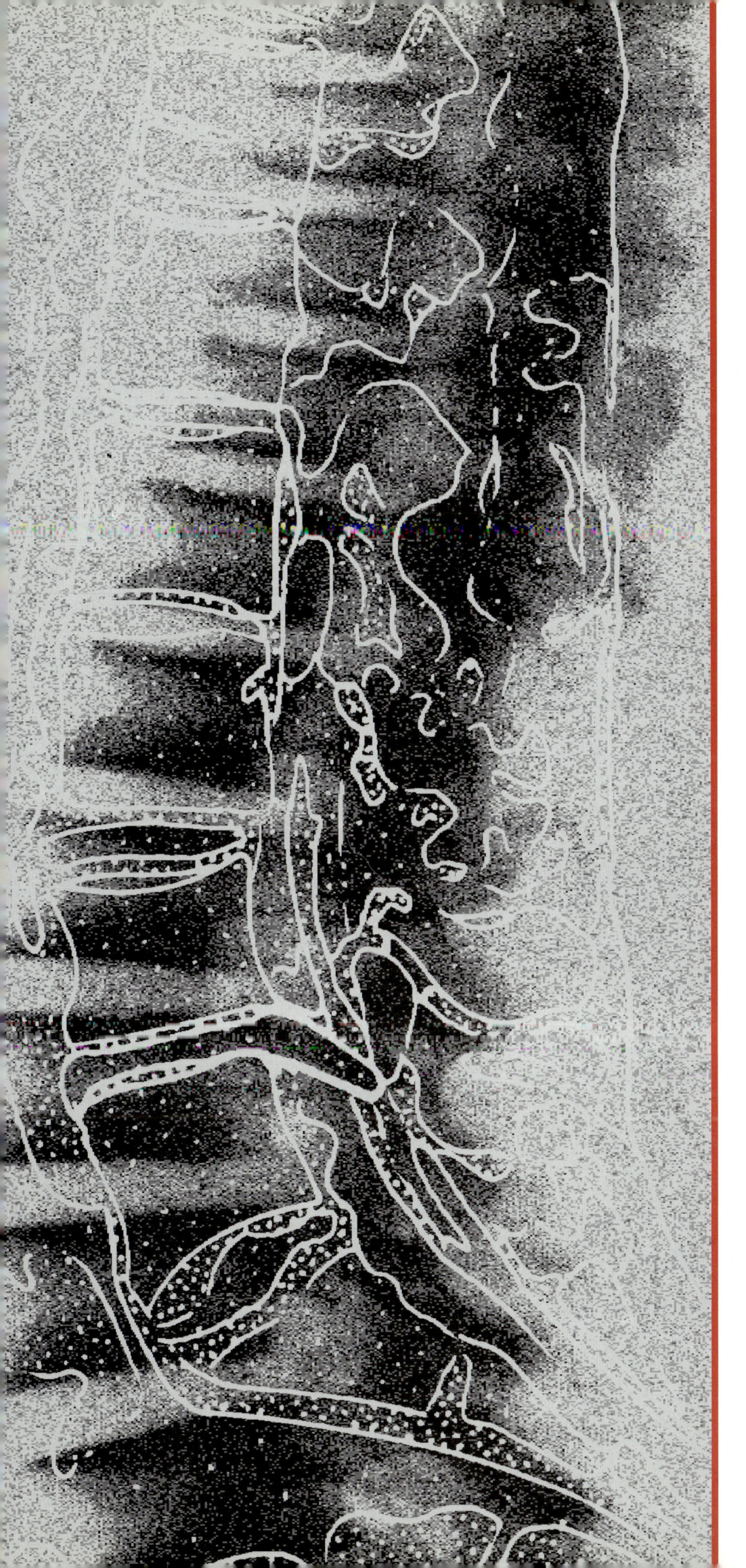

Injury to the Thoracolumbar Spine

3

ANATOMIC AND RADIOLOGIC CONSIDERATIONS

The standard radiographic projections for evaluating an injury to the *thoracic spine* are the anteroposterior (Fig. 3.1) and lateral (Fig. 3.2) views. The lateral projection is obtained using a technique called autotomography, which requires shallow breathing by the patient to blur the structures involved in respiratory motion and thus provide a clear view of the thoracic vertebral column.

As in cervical spine injuries, conventional tomography, CT, and MRI play leading roles in the evaluation of fractures of the thoracic spine, particularly in defining the extent of injury. Conventional tomography offers the possibility of obtaining direct coronal and sagittal sections of spine, but its disadvantages include the inability to obtain axial sections and exposure of the patient to a relatively high dose of radiation. Axial images can be obtained by CT, which also provides an excellent means of evaluating soft tissue injuries and exposes the patient to a relatively low dose of radiation. Unless reformation images are obtained, however, axially oriented fracture lines can be missed on axial CT sections. MR images are ideal to evaluate concomitant soft tissue injury, as well as injury to the spinal cord and thecal sac.

The standard radiographic examination for evaluating injuries of the *lumbar spine* includes the anteroposterior, lateral, and oblique projections, supplemented by coned-down lateral spot films of the lumbosacral junction (L5–S1). The anteroposterior view is usually sufficient for evaluating traumatic conditions involving the vertebral bodies and transverse processes; the intervertebral disk spaces are well demonstrated, except for the lowest (L5–S1) (Fig 3.3). However, the spinous processes, seen as "teardrops," and the articular facets are not well demonstrated on this projection. A characteristic configuration of the endplates of the L2–L5 vertebral bodies can be observed on the anteroposterior projection. Normally, the inferior aspects of these vertebrae form a "Cupid's bow" contour (Fig. 3.4), which is lost in cases of compression fractures affecting this part of the spine.

On the lateral view of the lumbar spine, the vertebral bodies are seen in profile, and the superior and inferior endplates are well demonstrated (Fig. 3.5). Fractures of the spinous processes can be adequately evaluated on this projection, as can abnormalities involving the intervertebral disk spaces, including L5–S1. As in the cervical spine, an oblique projection of the lumbar spine can be obtained from either the anterior or posterior aspect, although the posteroanterior oblique projection is preferable (Fig. 3.6). This view is particularly effective in demonstrating the facet joints (articular facets) and reveals a configuration of the elements of adjoining vertebrae, known as the "Scotty dog" formation (Fig. 3.7).

Ancillary imaging techniques are frequently used in the evaluation of traumatic conditions of the lumbar spine. As with cervical and thoracic injuries, conventional tomography and CT provide useful information; CT

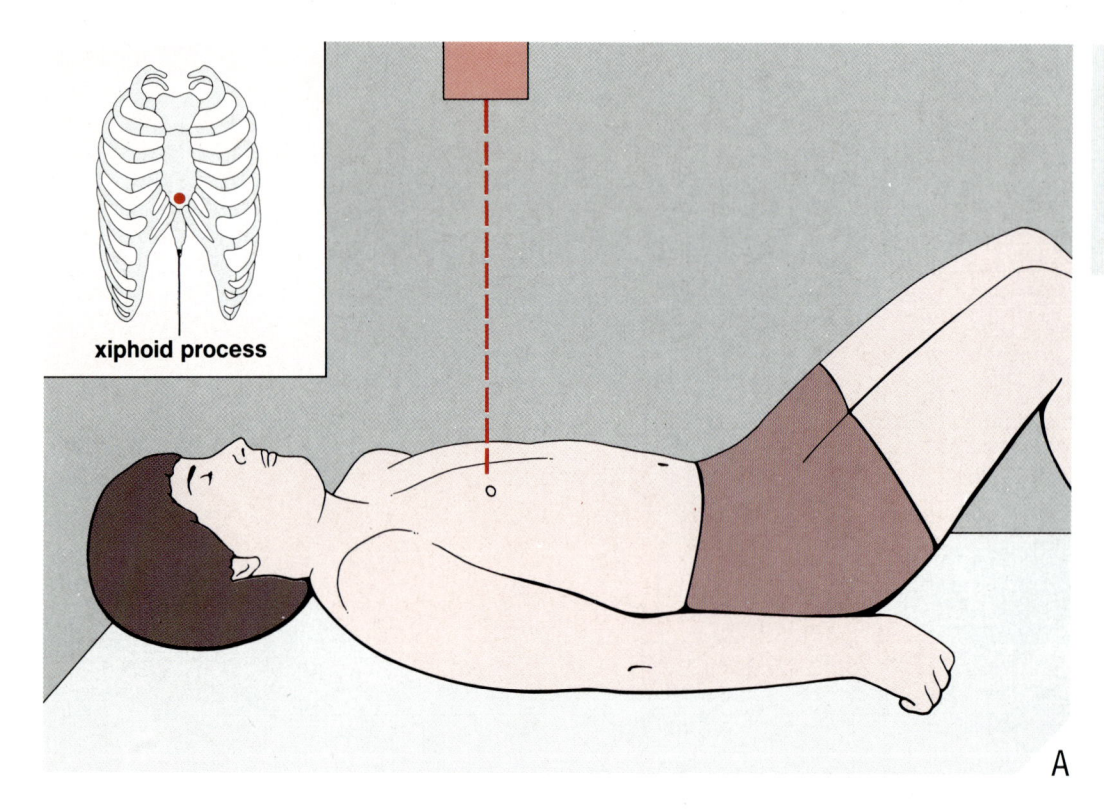

FIGURE 3.1 (A) For the anteroposterior view of the thoracic spine, the patient is supine on the table, with the knees flexed to correct the normal thoracic kyphosis. The central beam is directed vertically about 3 cm above the xiphoid process. **(B)** On the film in this projection, the vertebral endplates and pedicles and the intervertebral disk spaces are seen. The height of the vertebrae can be determined, and changes in the paraspinal line can be evaluated.

FIGURE 3.1 (cont.)

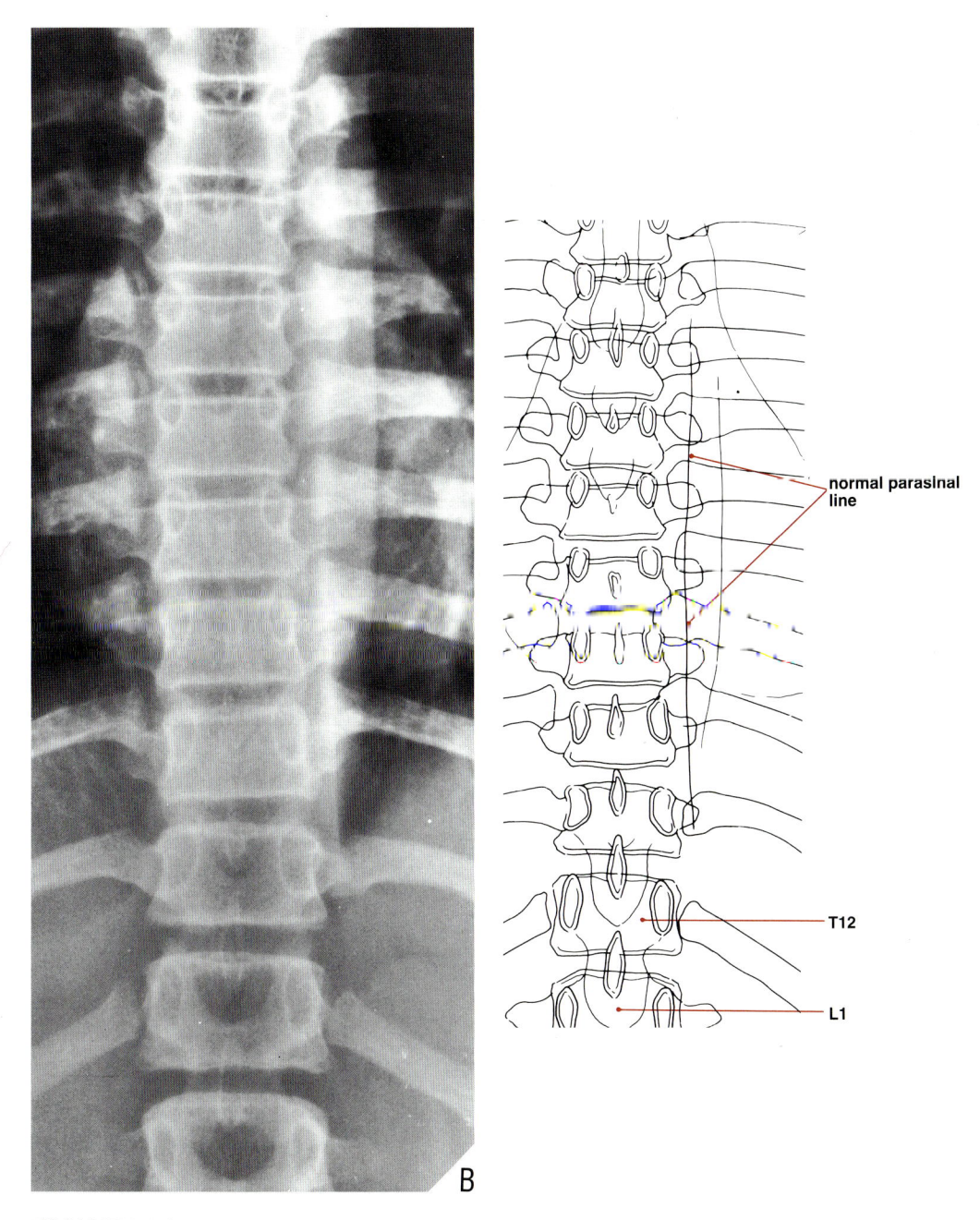

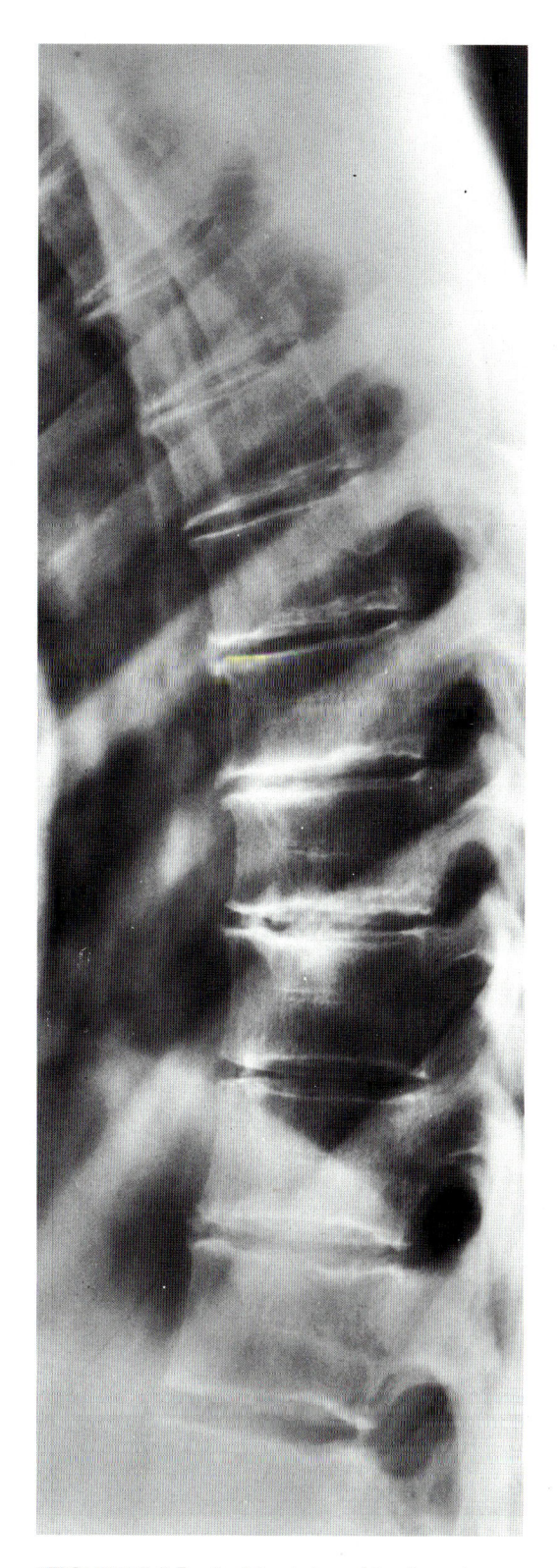

FIGURE 3.2 For the lateral view of the thoracic spine, the patient is erect with the arms elevated. To eliminate structures that would obscure the bony elements of the thoracic spine, the patient is instructed to breathe shallowly during the exposure. The central beam is directed horizontally to the level of the T6 vertebra with about 10° cephalad angulation. The film in this projection demonstrates a lateral image of the vertebral bodies and intervertebral disk spaces.

Injury to the Thoracolumbar Spine

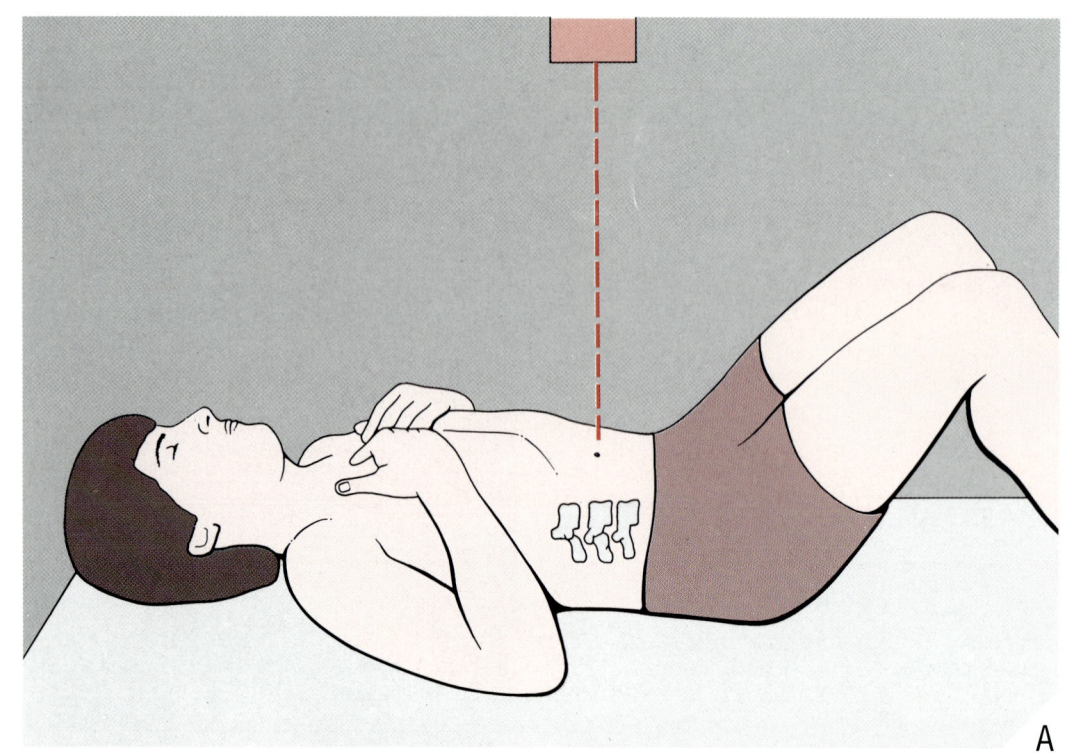

FIGURE 3.3 (A) For the anteroposterior projection of the lumbar spine, the patient is supine on the table, with the knees flexed to eliminate the normal physiologic lumbar lordosis. The central beam is directed vertically to the center of the abdomen at the level of the iliac crests. **(B)** The radiograph in this projection demonstrates the vertebral bodies, vertebral endplates, and the transverse processes; the intervertebral disk spaces are also well delineated. The spinous processes are seen en face, appearing as teardrops; and the pedicles, also visualized en face, project as oval densities on either side of the bodies.

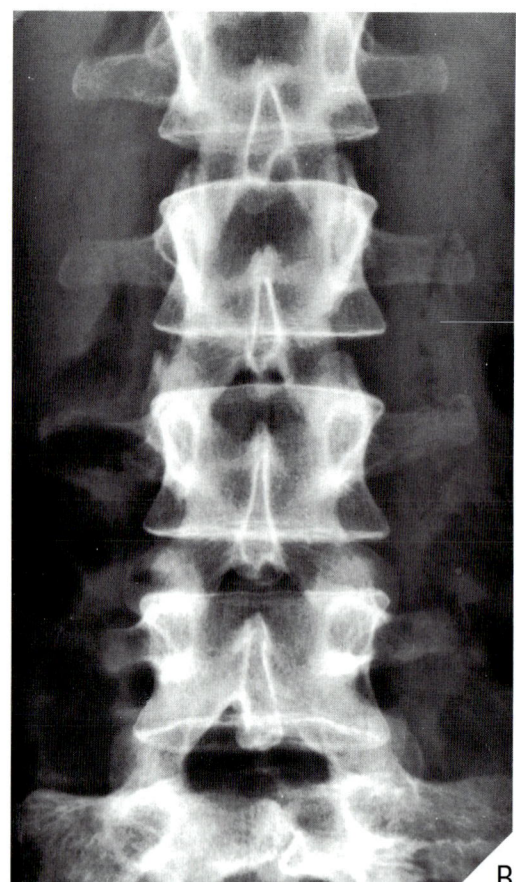

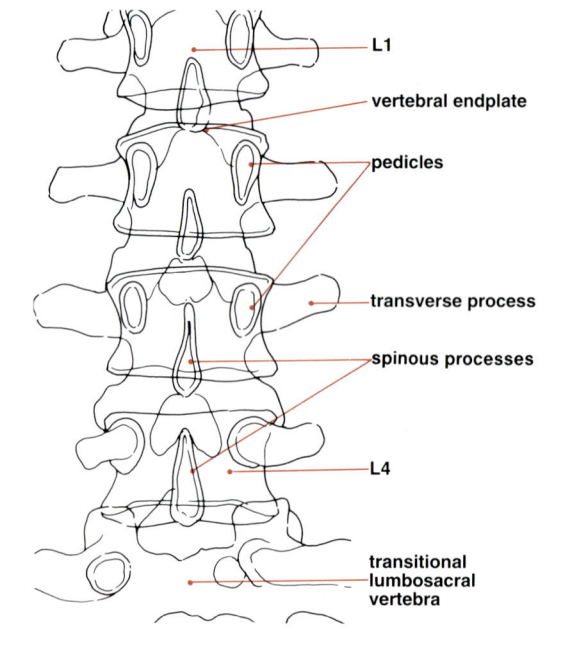

Imaging of the Spine in Clinical Practice

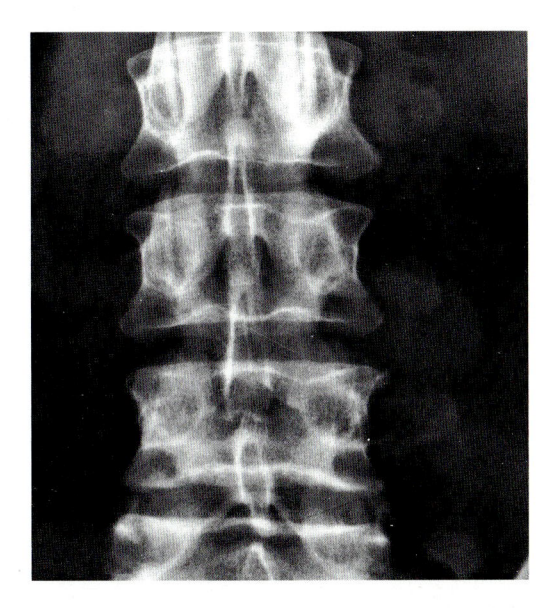

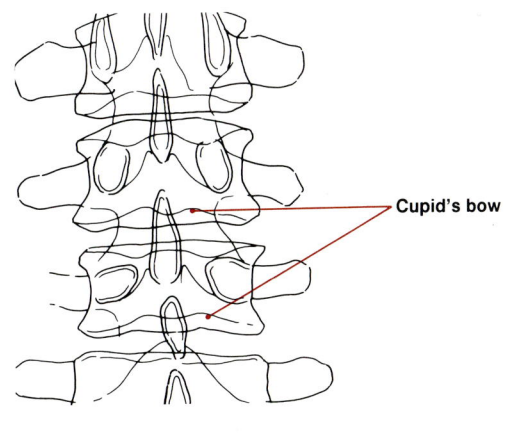

FIGURE 3.4 Anteroposterior coned-down view of the lumbar spine demonstrates a characteristic configuration of the lower aspects of L3 and L4. This "Cupid's bow" contour is lost in cases of compression fracture.

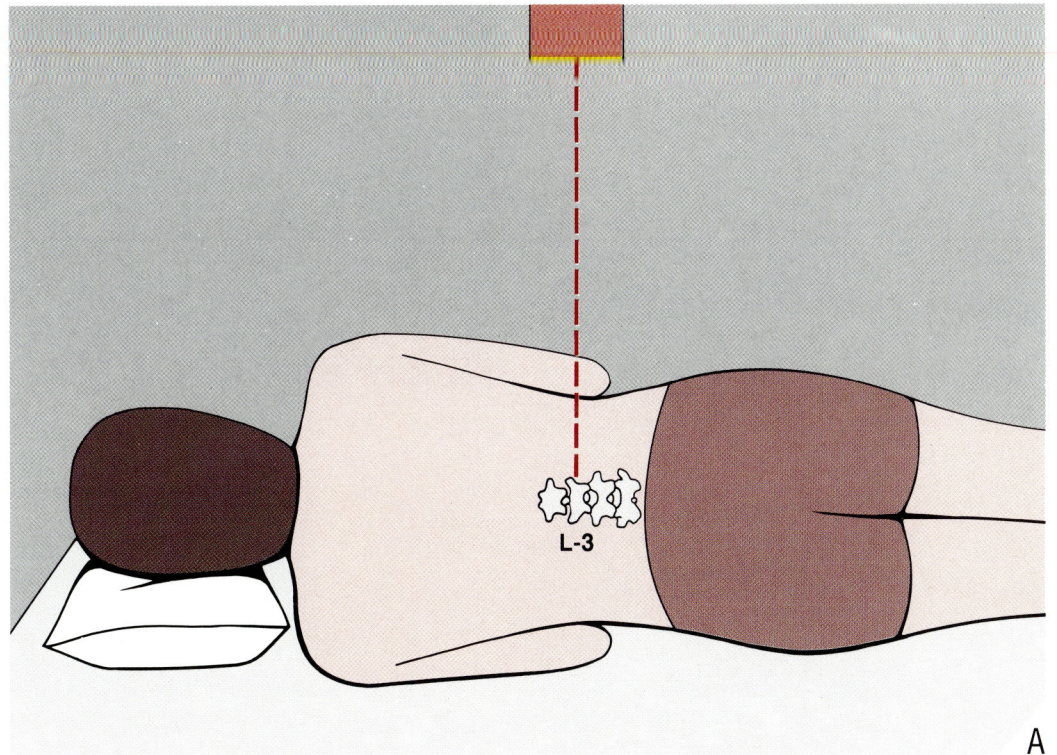

FIGURE 3.5 (A) For the lateral projection of the lumbar spine, the patient is recumbent on the radiographic table on either the left or right side; the knees and hips are flexed to eliminate the lordotic curve. The central beam is directed vertically to the center of the body of L3, at the level of the patient's waist. **(B)** The lateral film of the lumbar spine allows adequate demonstration of the vertebral bodies, pedicles, and spinous processes, as well as the intervertebral foramina and disk spaces.

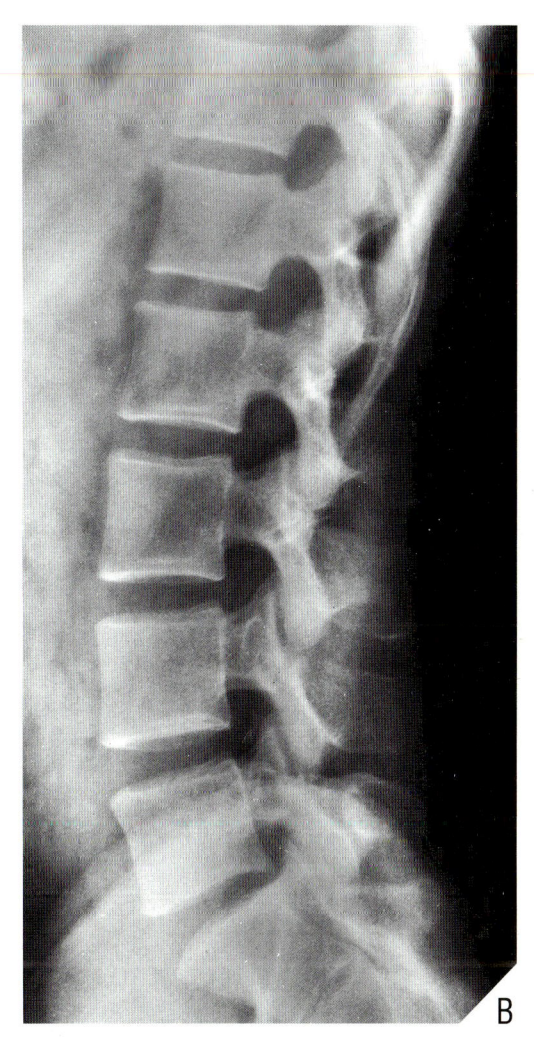

Injury to the Thoracolumbar Spine

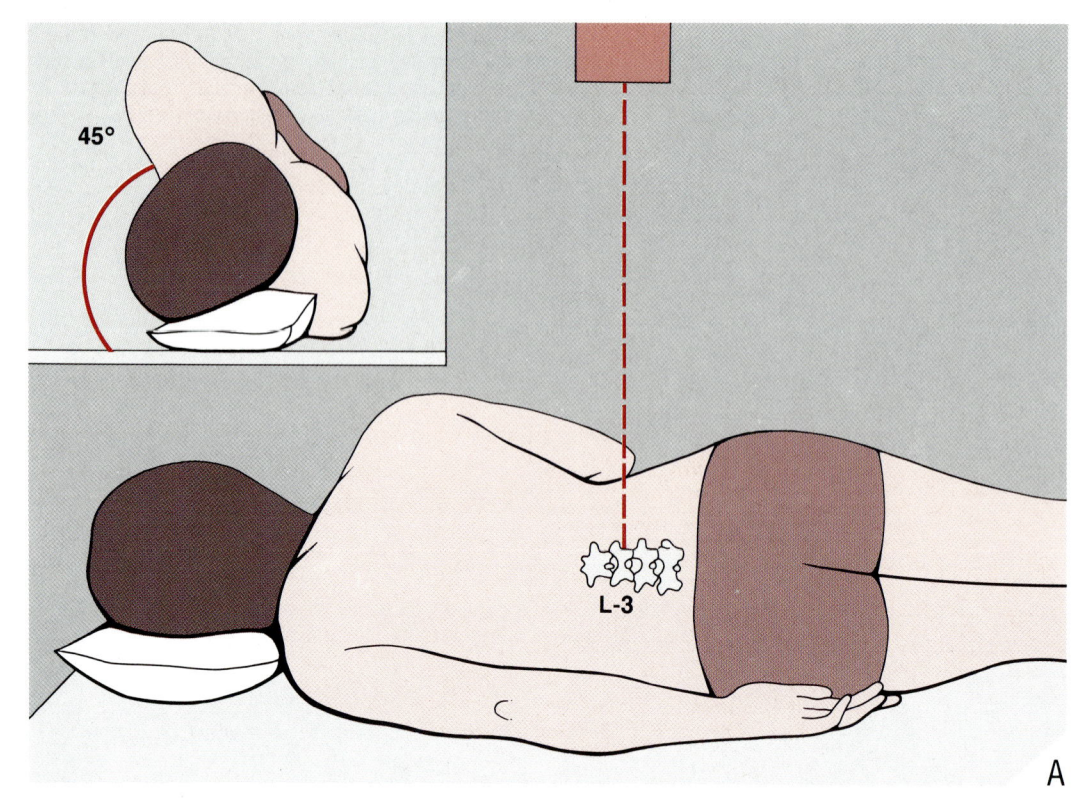

FIGURE 3.6 (A) For the posteroanterior oblique projection of the lumbar spine, the patient is recumbent on the table, with the right side rotated 45° to demonstrate the right-sided articular facets. (Elevation of the left side allows demonstration of the left-sided articular facets.) The central beam is directed vertically toward the center of L3. **(B)** The posteroanterior oblique film demonstrates the facet joints, the superior and inferior articular processes, the pedicles, and the pars interarticularis.

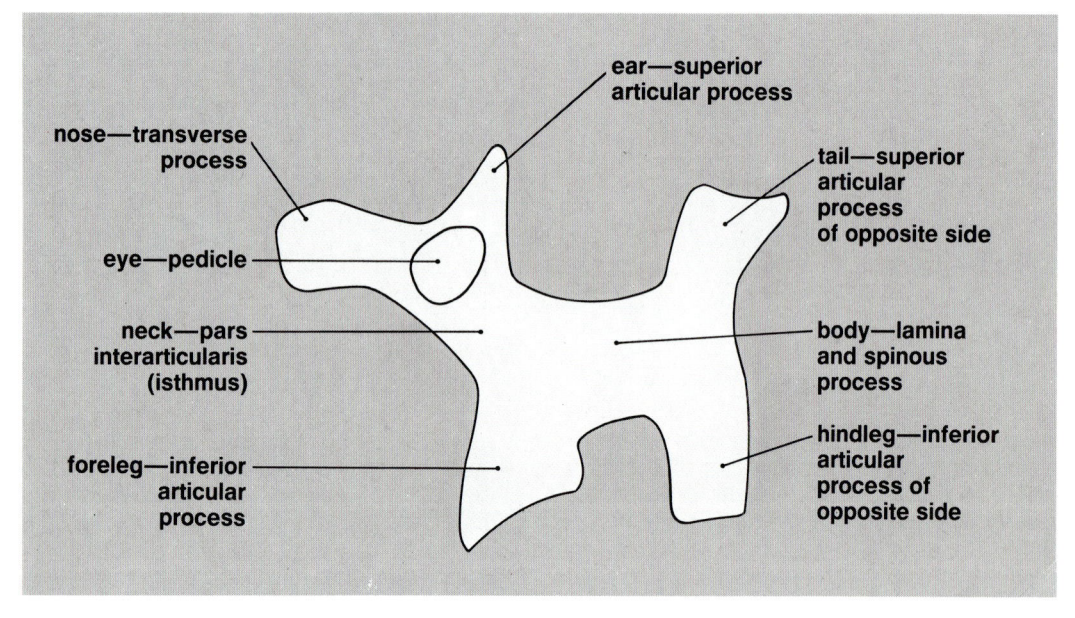

FIGURE 3.7 The oblique film also demonstrates a characteristic configuration of the elements of adjacent lumbar vertebrae known as the "Scotty dog" (see Fig. 3.6).

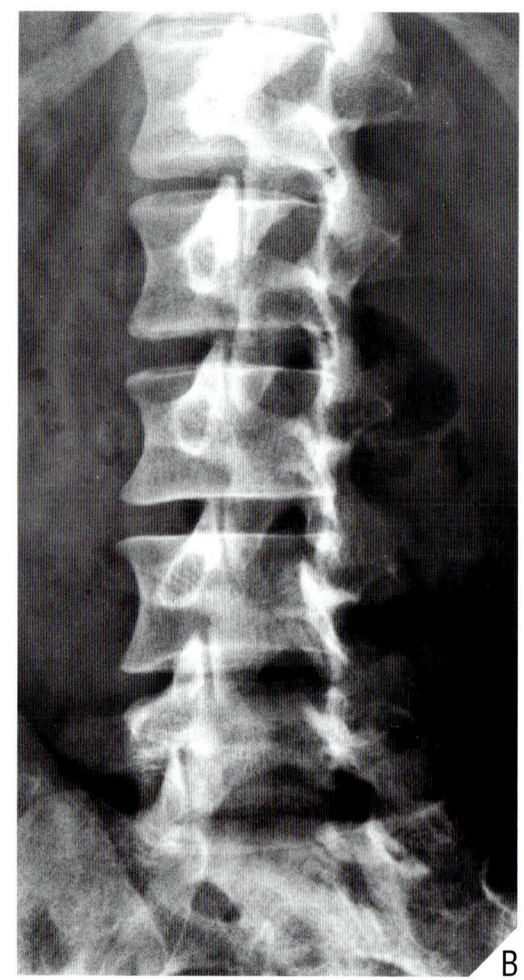

Imaging of the Spine in Clinical Practice

is often used to assess the extent of damage in vertebral body fractures and abnormalities involving the intervertebral disks (Fig. 3.8). Moreover, myelography (Fig. 3.9) and diskography (Fig. 3.10A) are occasionally required but as a rule are performed in conjunction with CT examination (Figs. 3.10B, 3.11).

MR imaging is now commonly used in the evaluation of injury to the thoracic and lumbar spine. In general, these images are obtained using a planar surface coil with its long axis oriented parallel to the spine. The slice thickness used to image thoracic and lumbar spine in both sagittal and axial planes is usually 5.0 mm, with a 1-mm gap between slices to reduce the artifactual signal from adjacent slices ("cross talk"). Sagittal images of the thoracic and lumbar spine are usually obtained with T1 and T2 weighting. In the axial plane, T1- and T2*-gradient (MPGR) or gradient-recalled acquisition (GRASS) sequences are most often obtained. On the sagittal images in T1 weighting, CSF is visualized with low signal intensity in contrast to intermediate signal intensity of the spinal cord.

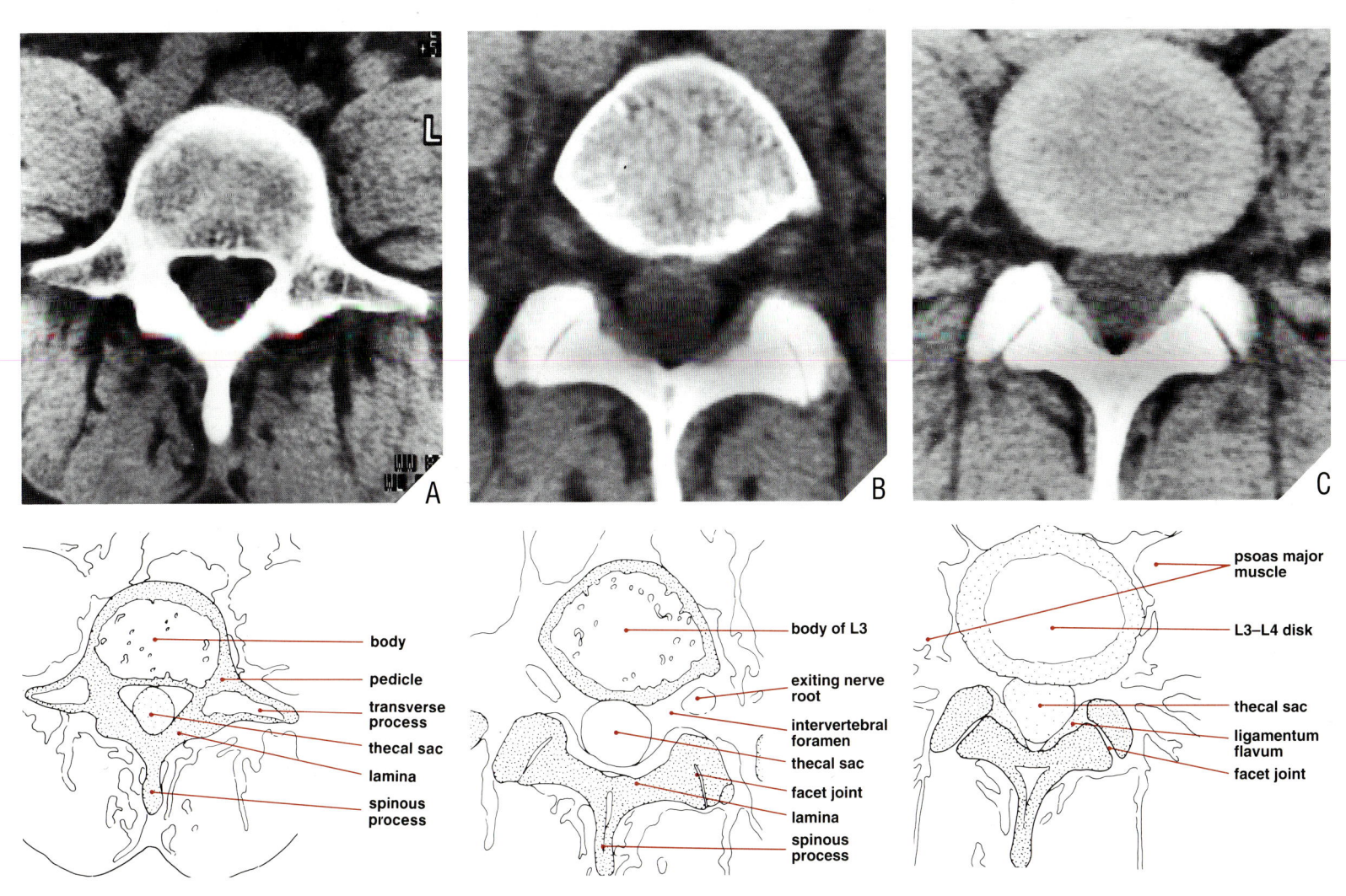

FIGURE 3.8 (A) CT section through the body of L3 demonstrates an axial view of the pedicles, transverse processes, and laminae, as well as a cross section of the thecal sac and the superior part of the spinous process. **(B)** In a section through the base of the intervertebral foramina, the caudal part of the body and spinous process are seen. Note the L3–L4 facet joints. **(C)** At the L3–L4 disk space, the facet joints are shown in full view, and the spinous process and laminae of L4 can now be seen. Note the appearance of the ligamentum flavum.

Injury to the Thoracolumbar Spine

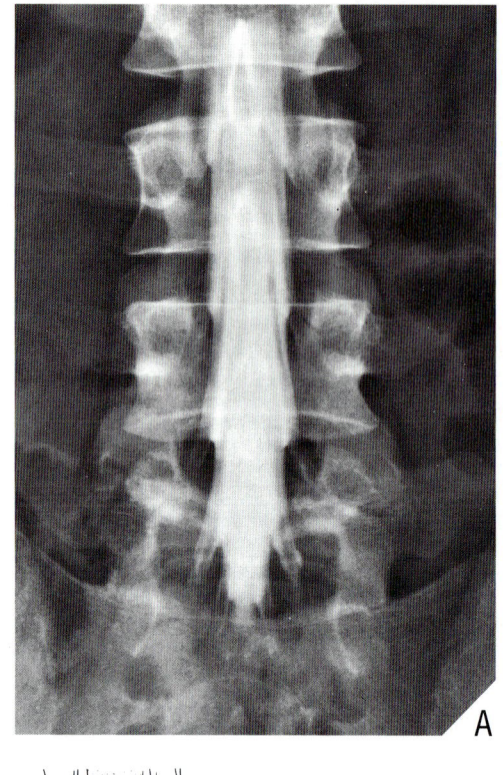

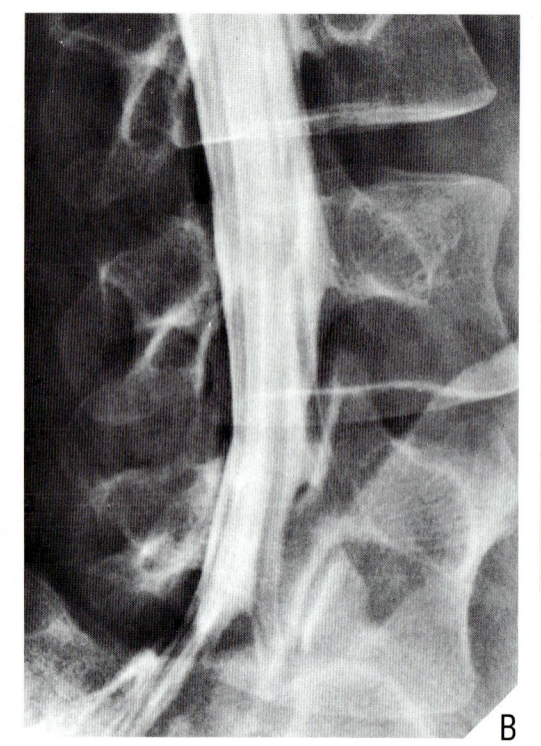

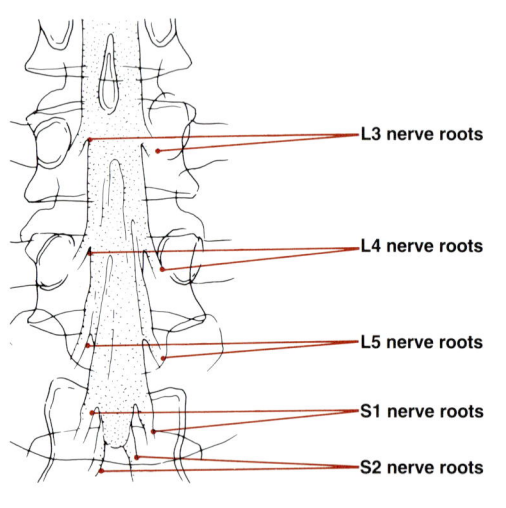

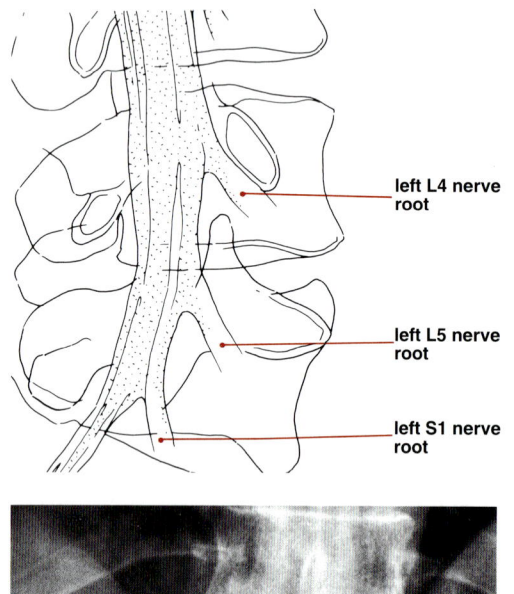

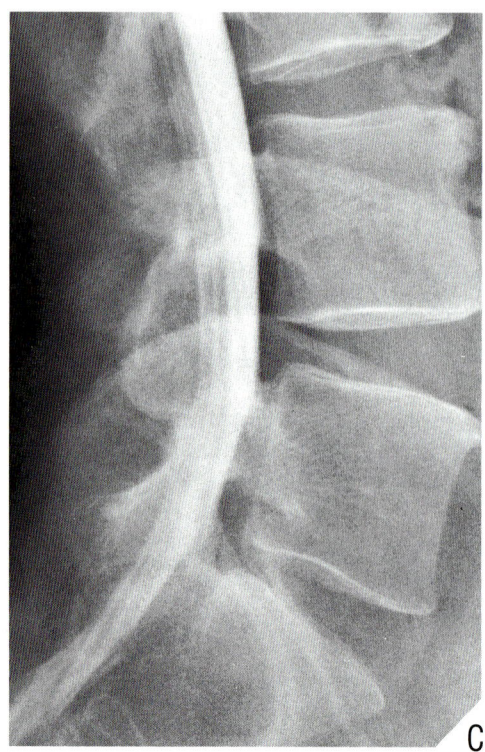

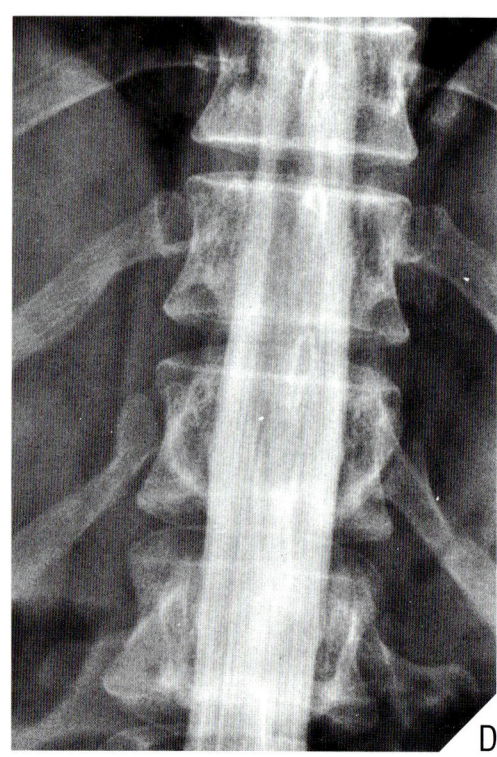

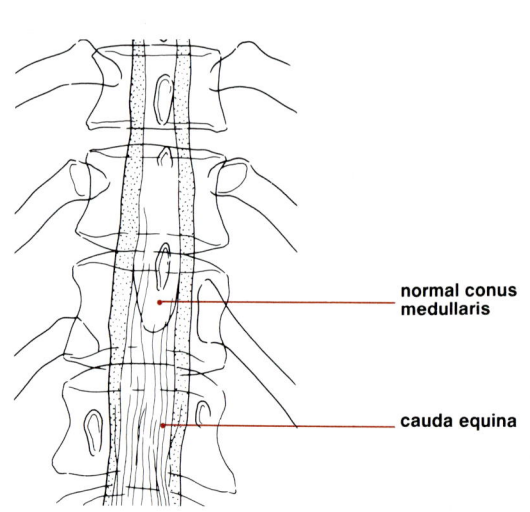

FIGURE 3.9 For myelographic examination of the lumbar spine, the patient is prone on the table. The puncture site, usually at the L3–L4 or L2–L3 level, is marked under fluoroscopic control. A 22-gauge needle is inserted into the subarachnoid space, and free flow of spinal fluid indicates proper placement. Fifteen milliliters of Iohexol in a concentration of 180 mg iodine/ml is slowly injected, and films are obtained in the posteroanterior **(A)**, left and right oblique **(B)**, and cross-table lateral **(C)** projections. In these normal studies, contrast is seen outlining the subarachnoid spaces of the thecal sac, as well as the cul-de-sac or most caudal part of the subarachnoid space. The nerve roots appear symmetric on both sides of the contrast column. A linear filling defect represents a nerve root in its contrast-filled sleeve. The length of the root pocket may vary from one patient to another, but in each patient all roots are approximately equal in length. It is imperative during myelographic examination of the lumbar segment to obtain one spot film of the thoracic segment at the level T10–T12 **(D)**, since tumors localized in the conus medullaris may mimic the clinical symptoms of a herniated lumbar disk.

3.8   *Imaging of the Spine in Clinical Practice*

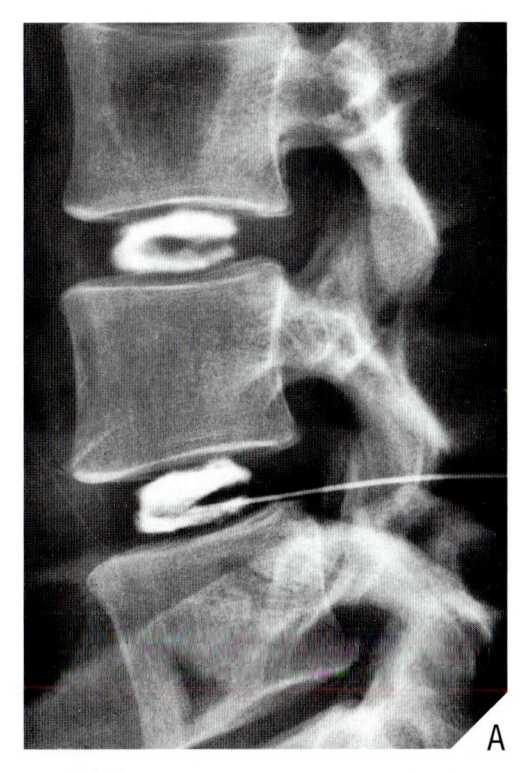

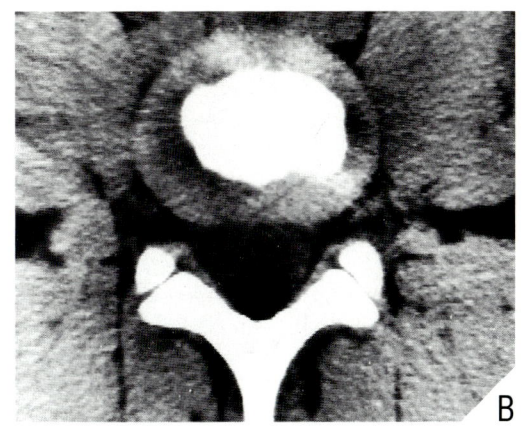

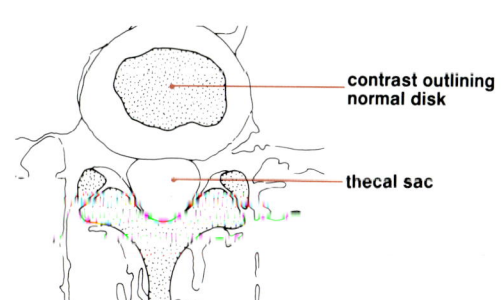

FIGURE 3.10 For diskographic examination of the lumbar spine, the patient is prone on the table, and the level of the injection, depending on the indication, is marked. The needle is inserted into the center of the nucleus pulposus, and about 2 to 3 ml of metrizamide is injected. **(A)** Lateral view of a normal diskogram shows a concentration of contrast medium while the needle is in place. **(B)** CT section through the L3–L4 disk space following diskography shows the normal appearance of this structure.

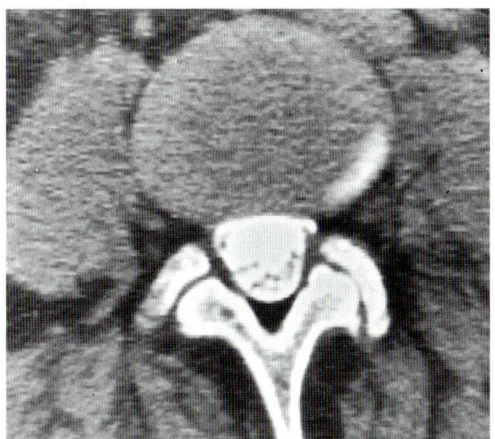

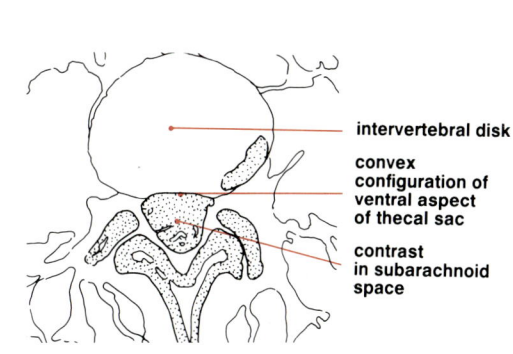

FIGURE 3.11 CT section obtained following myelography shows the normal appearance of contrast medium in the subarachnoid space. Note that the disk does not encroach on the ventral aspect of the thecal sac.

Injury to the Thoracolumbar Spine   **3.9**

The marrow within the vertebral bodies is imaged with an intermediate to high signal intensity, in contrast to slightly lower signal intensity of the intervertebral disks (Fig. 3.12A).

On T2-weighted images, the thoracic cord is visualized as a intermediate signal intensity structure in contrast to high signal intensity of the CSF. The intervertebral disks demonstrate high signal intensity on both T2 and T2*(MPGR and GRASS)-weighted images. The vertebral body marrow demonstrate intermediate signal intensity on T2-weighted images and low signal intensity on T2*-weighted images (Fig. 3.12B).

Axial images are effective to demonstrate the relation of intervertebral disks space to the thecal sac. The vertebral body, pedicles, laminae, and the transverse and spinous processes show high signal intensity. On axial T1-weighted images, the nucleus pulposus yields intermediate signal intensity, in contrast to peripheral low signal intensity of the annulus fibrosus. The nerve roots demonstrate low signal intensity and are in contrast with the high signal intensity of the surrounding fat (Fig. 3.12C). On T2-weighted images, the nucleus pulposus is imaged with high signal intensity in contrast to the low signal intensity of the annulus fibrosus. The nerve roots are imaged as low signal intensity structures (Fig. 3.12D).

For a summary of the preceding discussion in tabular form, see Figures 2.17, 2.19 and 3.13.

TRAUMA TO THE THORACOLUMBAR SPINE

Fractures of the Thoracolumbar Spine

Fractures of the thoracolumbar segment of the spine may involve the vertebral body and arch, as well as the transverse, spinous, and articular processes. In general, they can be grouped by mechanism of injury as compression fractures, burst fractures, distraction fractures (Chance and other seat-belt injuries), and fracture dislocations.

Because different classifications of thoracolumbar spine fractures have been used in the past by many authors, reports concerning the stability or lack of stability of a particular fracture pattern have varied. In 1983, Denis introduced the concept of the three-column spine classification of acute injuries to the thoracic and lumbar segments (Fig. 3.14). The significance of this system is its usefulness in determining the stability of various fractures, based on the site of injury in one or more of the spinal columns or elements.

The *anterior column* comprises the anterior two thirds of the annulus fibrosus and vertebral body, and the anterior longitudinal ligament. The *middle column* includes the posterior longitudinal ligament, and the posterior third of the annulus fibrosus and vertebral body. The *posterior column* consists of the posterior ligament complex, which has been defined by Holdsworth to include the supraspinous and infraspinous ligaments, the capsule of the intervertebral joints, and the ligamentum flavum (or interlaminar ligament), as well as the posterior portion of the neural arch. In general, one-column fractures are stable whereas three-column fractures are unstable; two-column fractures may be stable or unstable, depending on the extent of injury (Fig. 3.15).

COMPRESSION FRACTURES

Usually resulting from anterior or lateral flexion, compression fracture represents a failure of the anterior column under compression forces; the middle column remains intact, acting as a hinge, even in severe cases where there may also be partial failure of the posterior column. The standard radiographic examination of the thoracic and lumbar segments is usually sufficient to demonstrate this injury, although conventional tomography or CT may be required to delineate the extent of the fracture or to demonstrate obscure features. The anteroposterior view reveals buckling of the lateral cortices of the body close to the involved endplate, together with a decrease in the height of the body. In lateral flexion injuries, compression forces may cause a wedge-shaped deformity of the body. In subtle cases, a clue to the diagnosis may be seen in a localized

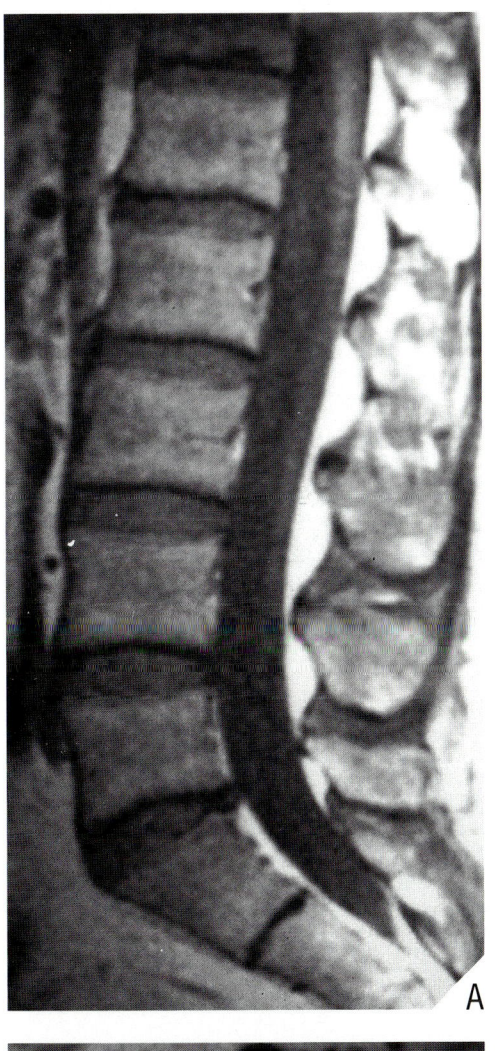

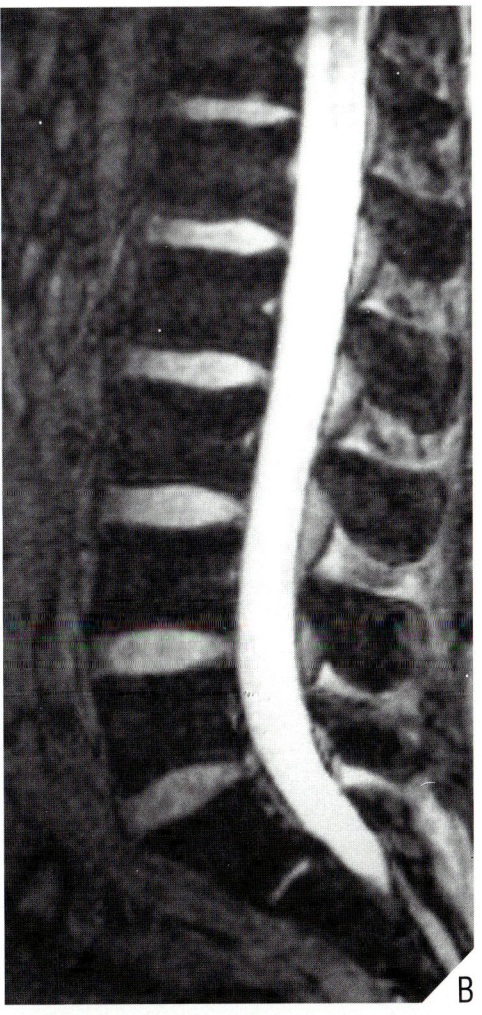

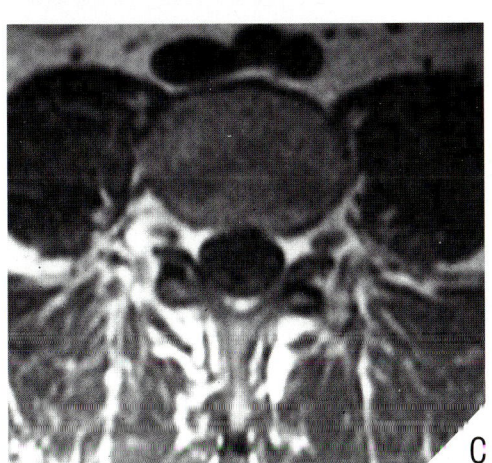

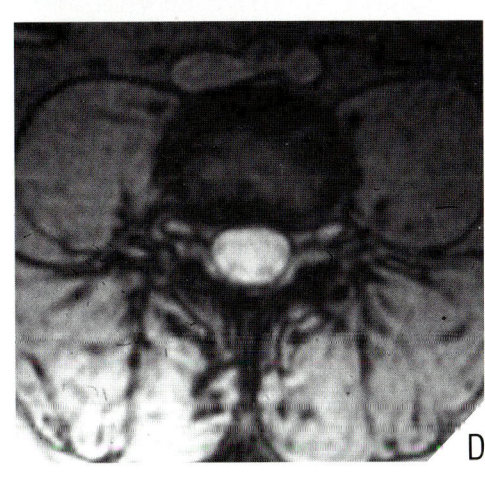

FIGURE 3.12 MRI appearance of a normal lumbar spine. **(A)** On this spin-echo T1-weighted sagittal midline section (TR 800/TE 20) the tip of the conus medullaris is identified at T12–L1 level, surrounded by low signal intensity cerebrospinal fluid. Epidural fat is of a very high signal intensity. It is most clearly seen posteriorly but some fat is also present anteriorly at the lumbosacral junction. Intervertebral disks are of a somewhat low signal intensity due to their high water content. The low signal intensity lines along the ventral and dorsal aspects of the vertebral body are related to the anterior and posterior longitudinal ligaments and cortical bone of the vertebral bodies. These ligaments also span and cover the anterior and posterior portions of the disks. The thin black line along the inferior endplate and the bright line at the superior portion of each vertebral body are due to a chemical shift artifact. **(B)** Gradient-echo T2-weighted sagittal midline section (TR 1000/TE 12, flip angle 22.5°) provides an image with an appearance similar to that of the myelographic technique, due to its very high gray-scale contrast. There is clear delineation of the thecal sac filled with high signal intensity cerebrospinal fluid. The posterior longitudinal ligament and dura are silhouetted against the high water signal of the cerebrospinal fluid and the intervertebral disks. The epidural fat is of intermediate to low signal intensity and the vertebral bodies are of a very low signal intensity. A high signal intensity midposterior cleft in the vertebral bodies is related to the basivertebral veins. **(C)** On the spin-echo T1-weighted axial section (TR 800/TE 20), the nerve roots are surrounded by high signal intensity fat in the neural foramen. The ventral margin of the thecal sac at the disk level is convex outward and the canal is ample in size. The facet joints are well demonstrated as the two low signal intensity arcs of the cortical bone. **(D)** Gradient-echo T2-weighted axial section (TR 1000/TE 12, flip angle 22.5°) demonstrates low signal nerve roots of the cauda equina surrounded by high signal intensity cerebrospinal fluid. The anterior margin of the thecal sac is well delineated. The individual nerve-root sheaths in the foramen also appear at a somewhat higher signal intensity. Some signal is visible from the disk interspace. (Reproduced with permission from Beltran J: *MRI: Musculoskeletal Sytem.* New York, Gower, 1990)

FIGURE 3.13 STANDARD AND SPECIAL RADIOGRAPHIC PROJECTIONS FOR EVALUATING INJURY TO THE THORACIC AND LUMBAR SPINE

PROJECTION	DEMONSTRATION
Anteroposterior	Fractures of
	Vertebral bodies
	Vertebral endplates
	Pedicles
	Transverse processes
	Fractures–dislocations
	Abnormalities of
	intervertebral disk spaces
	Paraspinal bulge
	Inverted "Napoleon's hat" sign
Lateral	Fractures of
	Vertebral bodies
	Vertebral endplates
	Pedicles
	Spinous processes
	Chance fracture
	(seat-belt fractures)
	Abnormalities of
	Intervertebral foramina
	Intervertebral disk spaces
	Limbus vertebra
	Schmorl's node
	Spondylolisthesis
	Spinous-process sign
Oblique	Abnormalities of
	Articular facets
	Pars interarticularis
	Spondylolysis
	"Scotty dog" configuration

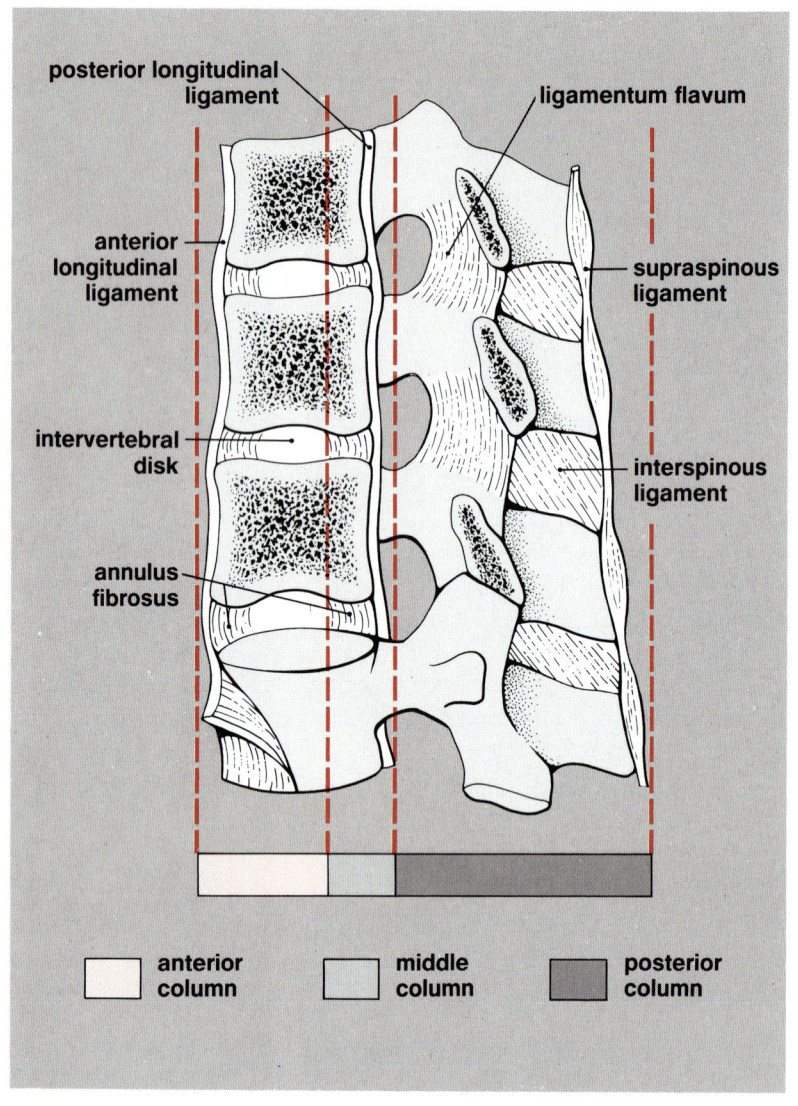

FIGURE 3.14 The three-column concept in viewing the thoracolumbar spine is helpful in determining the stability of various injuries. Fractures involving all three columns are unstable and those affecting one column are stable. (Adapted from Denis F: The three column spine and its significance in the classification of acute thoracolumbar spine injuries. *Spine* 8:817, 1983)

FIGURE 3.15 THE BASIC TYPES OF SPINAL FRACTURES AND THE COLUMNS INVOLVED IN EACH

COLUMN INVOLVEMENT

TYPE OF FRACTURE	Anterior	Middle	Posterior
Compression	Compression	None	None or distraction (in severe fractures)
Burst	Compression	Compression	None or distraction
Seat-belt	None or compression	Distraction	Distraction
Fracture–dislocation	Compression and/or rotation, shear	Distraction and/or rotation, shear	Distraction and/or rotation, shear

(Reproduced with permission from Montesano PX, Benson DR: The thoracolumbar spine. In Rockwood CA, Green DP, Bucholz RW (eds): *Rockwood and Green's Fracture in Adults*, 3rd ed. Philadelphia, J B Lippincott, 1991)

Imaging of the Spine in Clinical Practice

bulge of the paraspinal line secondary to hemorrhage and edema. However, it should be kept in mind that this finding may also represent a pathologic fracture secondary to metastasis to the vertebral body. On the lateral projection, a simple vertebral compression fracture can be identified by a decrease in the height of the anterior part of the body, while the height of the posterior part and posterior cortex is maintained (Fig. 3.16).

Treatment

Compression fractures are usually stable and rarely involve neurologic compromise. For the most part, they are treated symptomatically. Early ambulation is encouraged in a hyperextension orthosis. However, when there is a loss of more than 50% of vertebral body height, angulation of greater than 20°, or multiple adjacent compression fractures, the injury is considered to be potentially unstable. This usually requires treatment in a hyperextension cast, or possibly an open reduction and internal fixation using posterior instrumentation and fusion, depending on the severity.

BURST FRACTURES

A burst fracture results from a failure of the anterior and middle columns secondary to axial compression forces or a combination of axial compression with rotation or anterior or lateral flexion. Five subtypes of burst fractures have been described, depending on whether one or both endplates are fractured and the amount of rotation or lateral flexion observed (Fig. 3.17).

Anteroposterior and lateral projections of the thoracic and lumbar spine are usually adequate to demonstrate these fractures. The anteroposterior view characteristically reveals an increase in the interpedicular distance and splaying of the posterior facet joints (Fig. 3.18A). On the lateral view, fracture of the posterior part of the vertebral body is seen as a decrease in the height of this portion of the bone. Comminution is often present (Fig. 3.18B), and fragments are retropulsed into the spinal canal, leading to compression of the thecal sac. For this reason, CT is essential in the evaluation of burst fractures (Figs. 3.18C, 3.19A), and myelography (Fig. 3.19B) or MRI (Fig. 3.19C) may be required to localize the site and demonstrate the degree of compression of the thecal sac.

Treatment

In the absence of neurologic compromise, stable burst fractures can be treated in a hyperextension cast. However, when neurologic injury is present or there is loss of vertebral body height of more than 50%, angulation of greater than 20°, or canal compromise of more than 30%, early posterior stabilization is advocated to restore sagittal plane alignment. A distraction system is recommended because reduction by forceful distraction may lead to decompression of the retropulsed vertebral body fragment (Fig. 3.20). When distractive instrumentation is used, intraoperative radiographs should be obtained to confirm that sagittal plane alignment has been restored. This also allows evaluation for possible overdistraction, which is a particular risk when there is evidence of three column failure. A repeat CT is performed the day after surgery to determine the adequacy of canal decompression. In the event that residual canal compromise is greater than 25% to 30% (in a patient with an incomplete neurologic injury), a secondary anterior retroperitoneal decompression is performed (Fig. 3.21). (Residual canal compression is ignored in a neurologically

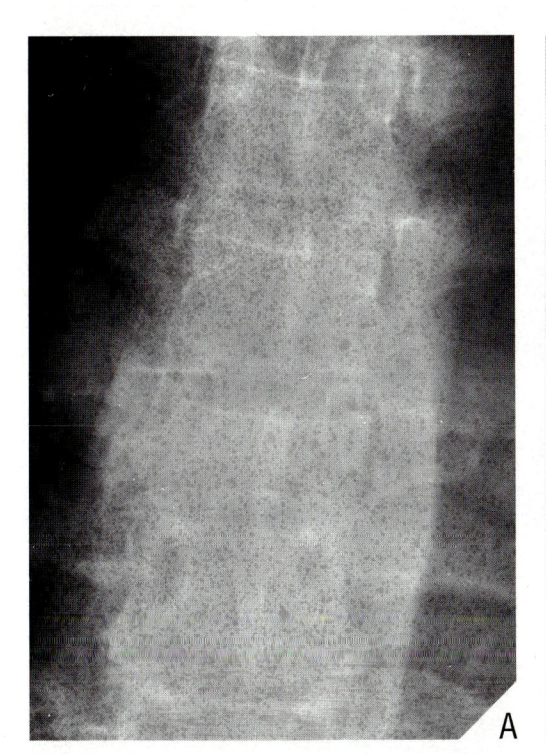

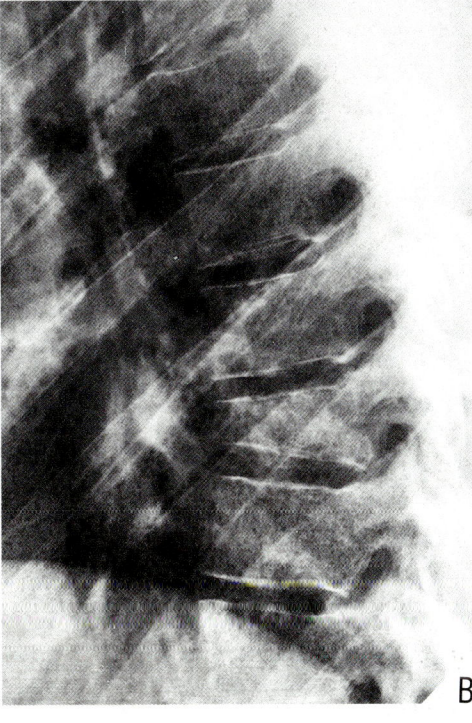

FIGURE 3.16 A 48-year-old woman fell from a ladder and hurt her back. **(A)** Anteroposterior view of the thoracic spine demonstrates a decrease in the height of the vertebral body of T8, secondary to compression fracture. Note the localized widening of the paraspinal line secondary to hemorrhage and edema. **(B)** The lateral view demonstrates anterior wedging. Note the intact posterior vertebral body line. These are the features of simple compression fracture affecting only the anterior column.

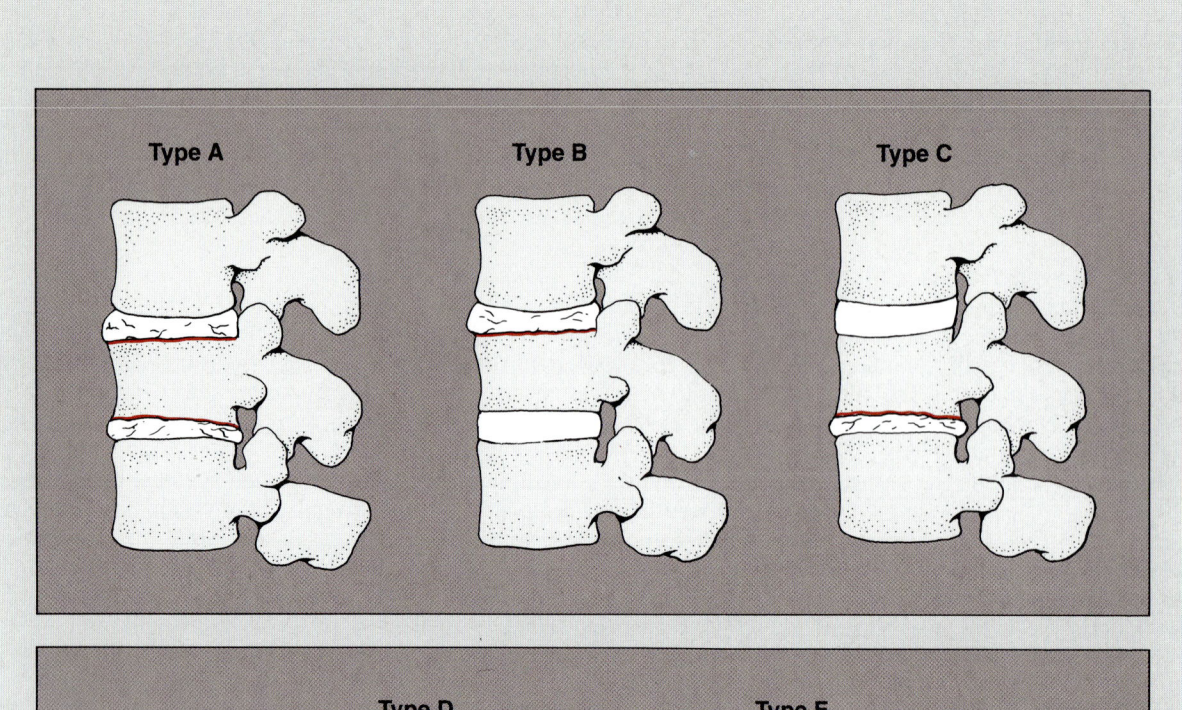

FIGURE 3.17 The five basic types of burst fractures, according to Denis. **(A)** Type A burst fracture involves both endplates. **(B)** Type B involves only the superior endplate. **(C)** Type C is a fracture of only the inferior endplate. **(D)** Type D involves rotation. **(E)** Type E fracture is characterized by lateral wedging of the vertebral body.

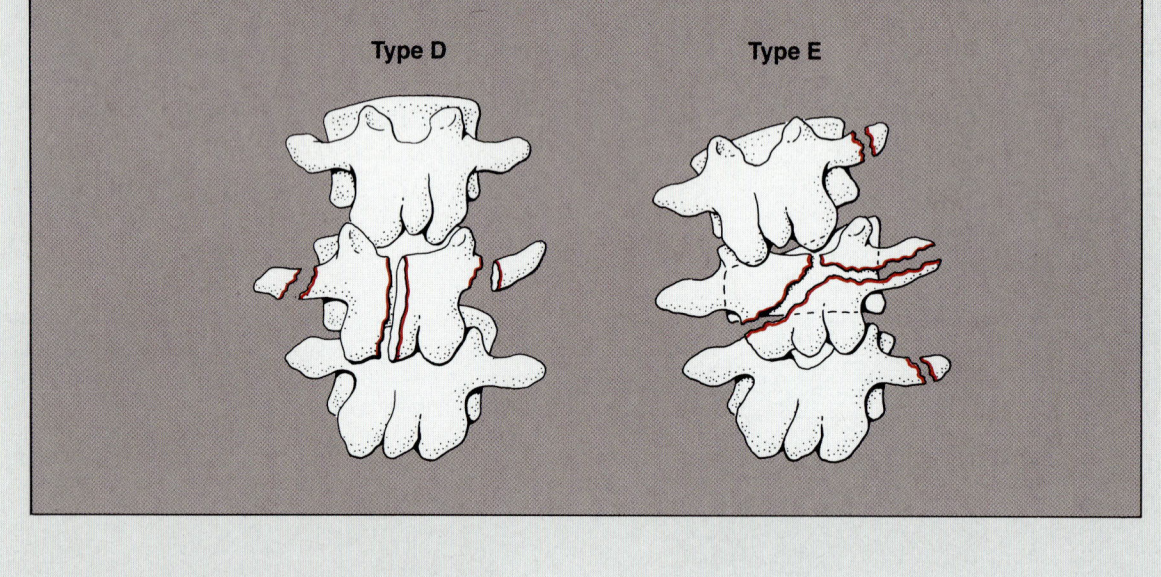

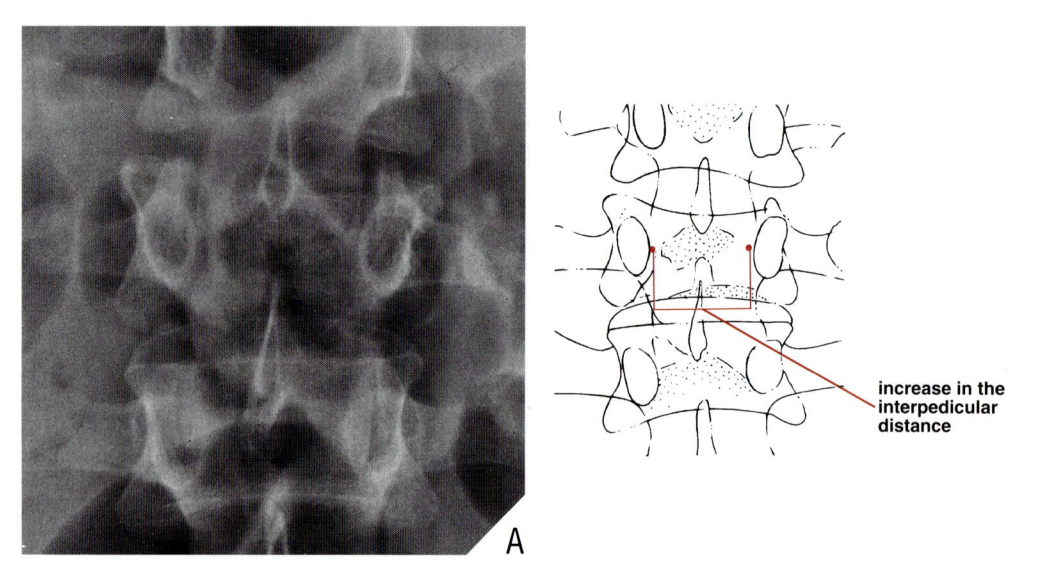

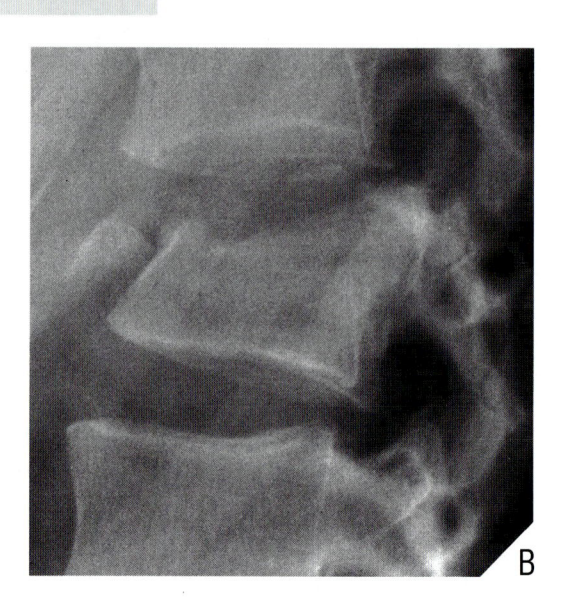

FIGURE 3.18 (A) Anteroposterior film shows an increase in the interpedicular distance of vertebra, indicative of a burst fracture. **(B)** Lateral radiograph demonstrates comminution of the posterior aspect of the vertebral body with retrograde displacement.

3.14 *Imaging of the Spine in Clinical Practice*

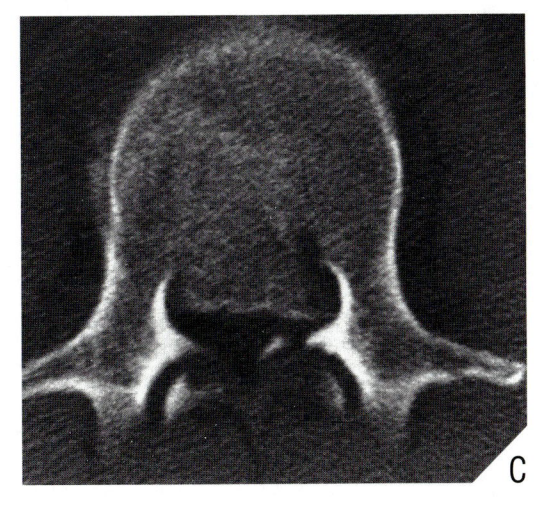

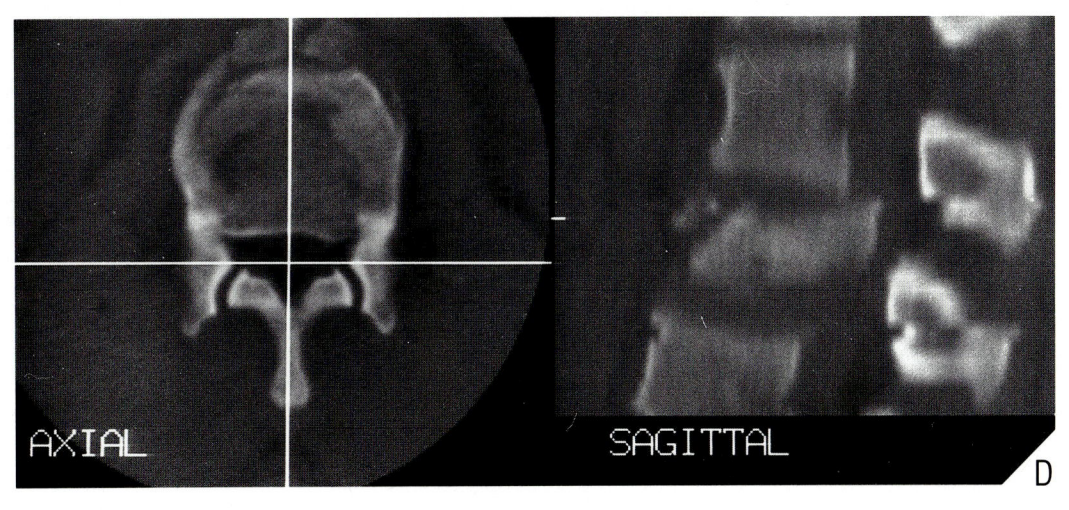

FIGURE 3.18 (cont.) **(C)** CT axial section clearly shows compromise of the spinal canal by posteriorly displaced fragment. **(D)** Sagittal CT reformation demonstrates this complication more dramatically, in addition allowing to obtain precise measurements of the width of compromised canal.

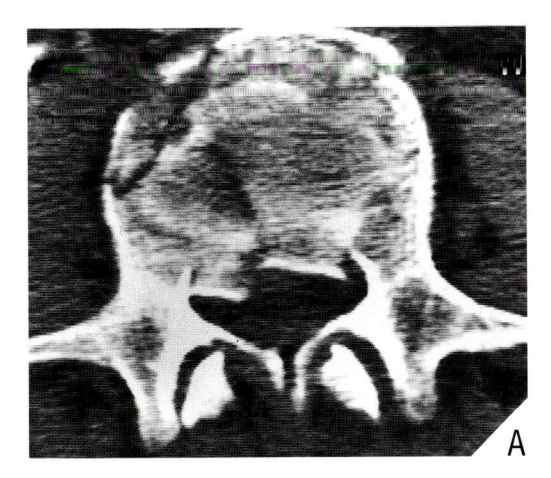

FIGURE 3.19 A 56-year-old merchant seaman fell from a 60-foot ladder on a ship. Anteroposterior and lateral films of the lumbar spine showed a burst fracture of the body of L3. The severity of the injury, however, is better appreciated on a CT section **(A)** through the body of L3. There is communinution of the vertebral fracture and displacement of two bony fragments into the spinal canal, with compression of the thecal sac, indicating involvement of anterior and middle columns. **(B)** Lateral view as part of a myelogram of another patient shows complete obstruction of the flow of contrast at the level of fracture of L1 due to a small bony fragment impinging on the thecal sac. **(C)** In yet another patient with a burst fracture of L3, sagittal MR image (SE, TR 800/TE 20) shows posterior displacement of the middle column with compression of the thecal sac. (C reproduced with permission from Beltran J: *MRI: Musculoskeleton System*. New York, Gower, 1990).

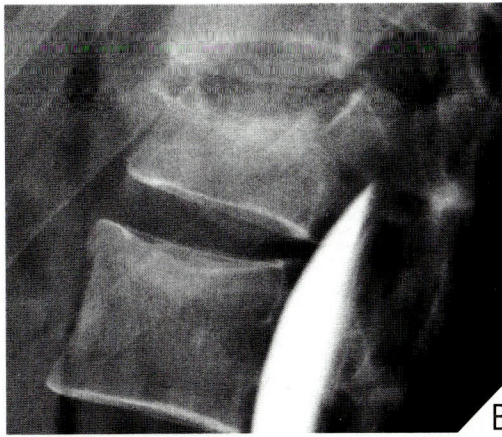

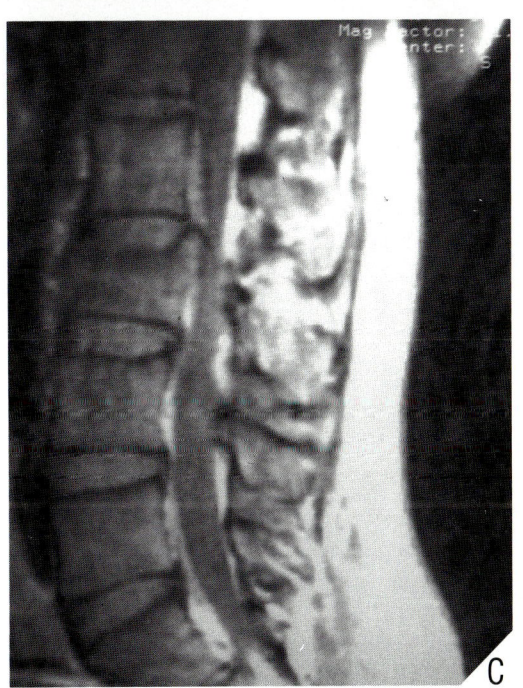

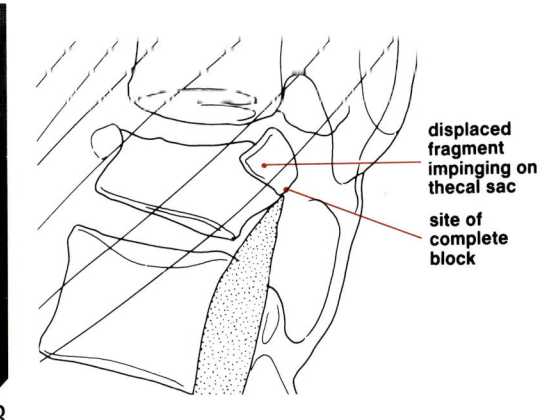

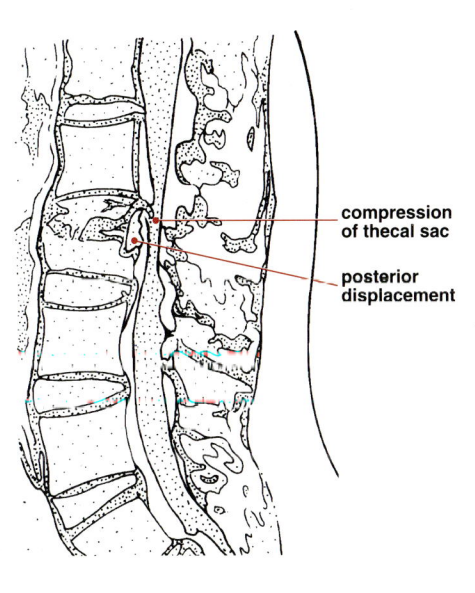

Injury to the Thoracolumbar Spine   3.15

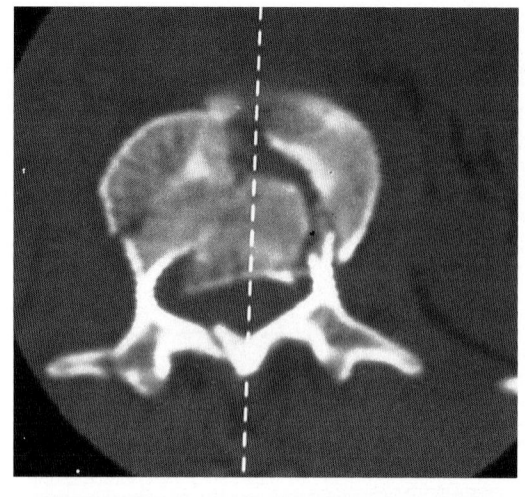

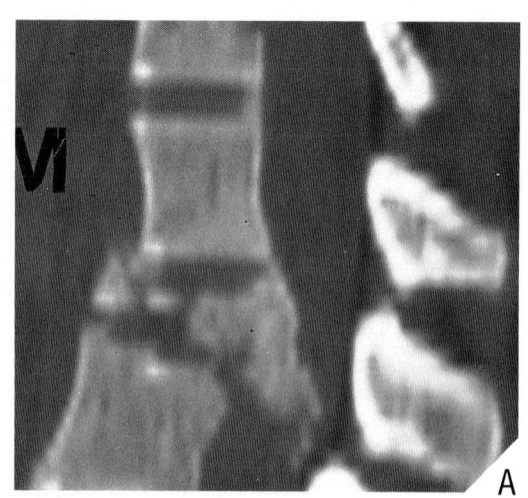

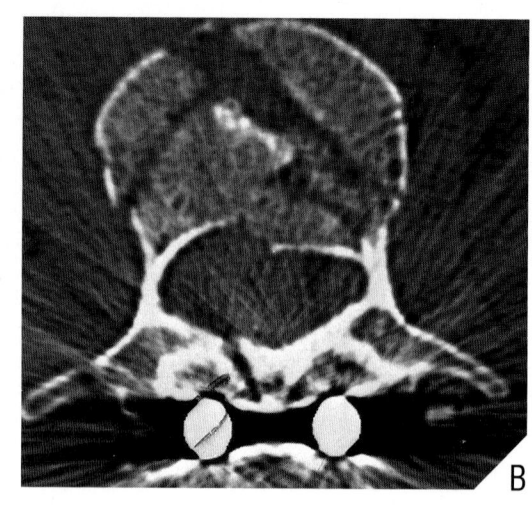

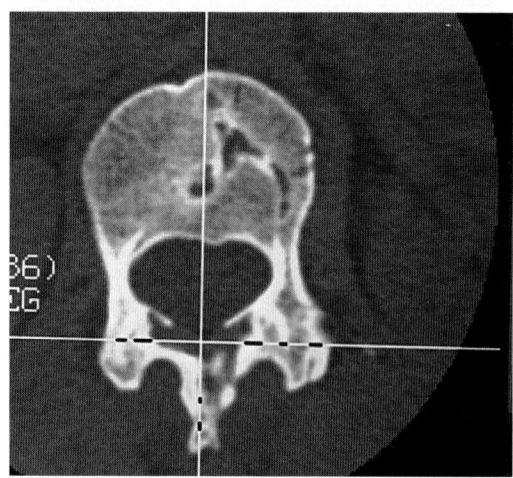

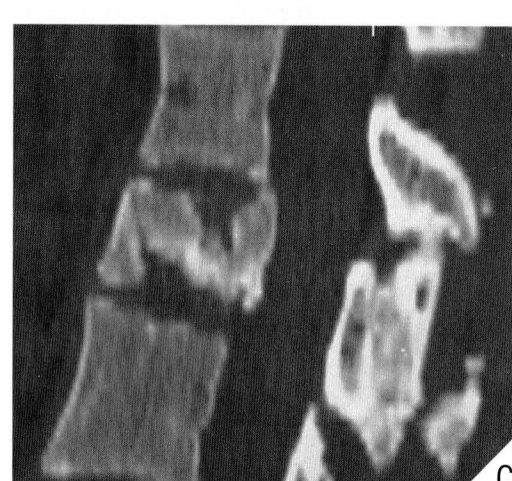

FIGURE 3.20 A 19-year-old woman sustained Denis type-A burst fracture of L1 in a motor vehicle accident. She presented with neurologically incomplete lesion with major weakness of both lower extremities. **(A)** Axial CT section and sagittal reformation show approximately 60% spinal canal compromise. **(B)** The patient was treated with the locking-hook spinal rod to reestablish sagittal plane alignment, and with judicious distraction to reconstitute vertebral body height. Postoperatively, near-complete restoration of the spinal canal was achieved. **(C)** Axial CT and sagittal reformation obtained one year after rod removal shows good fracture healing and almost normal width of the spinal canal. (Reprinted with permission from Montesano PX, Benson DR: The thoracolumbar spine. In Rockwood CA, Green DP, Bucholz RW (eds): *Rockwood and Green's Fractures in Adults*, 3rd ed, vol. 2. New York, J B Lippincott, 1991)

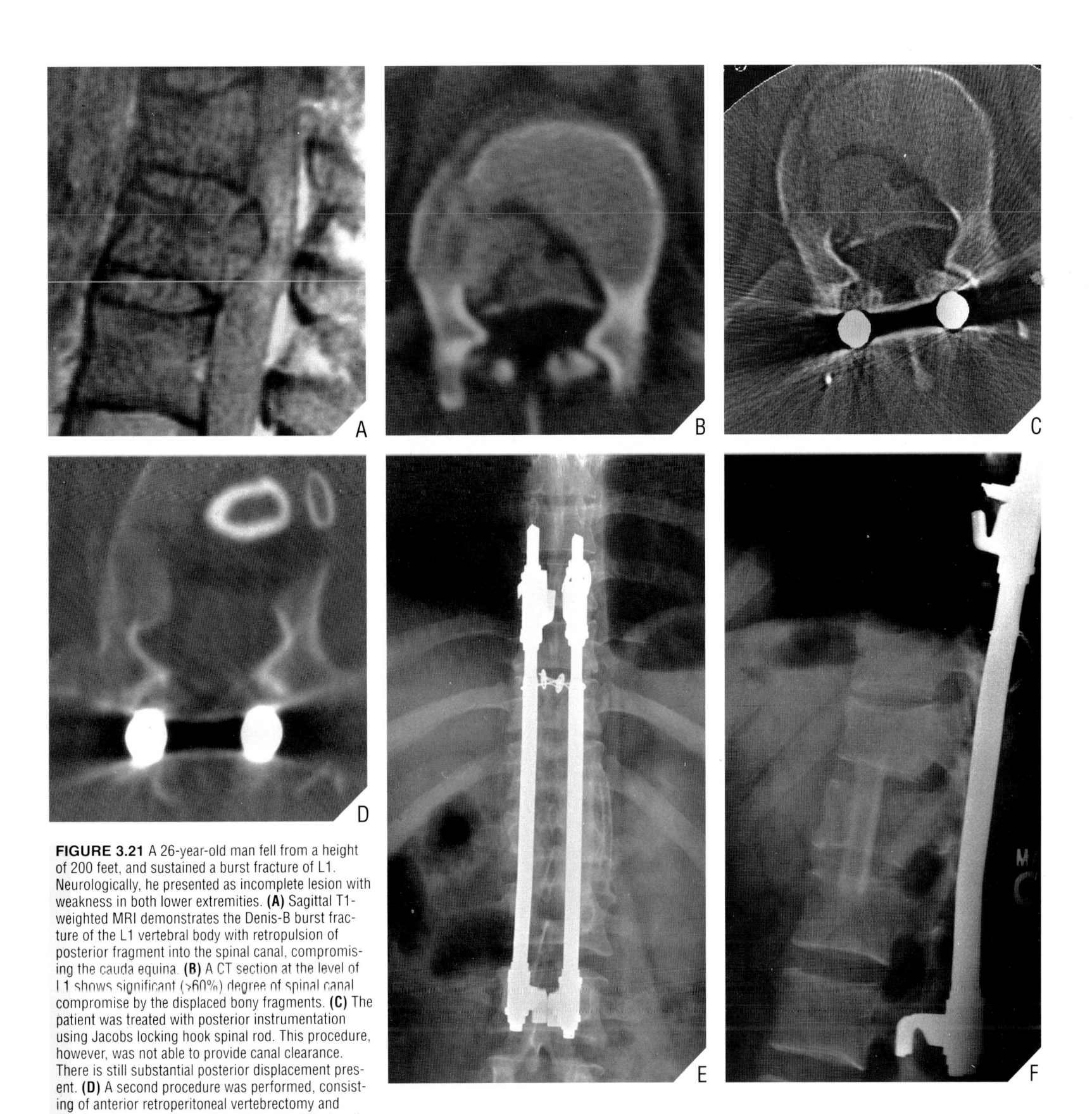

FIGURE 3.21 A 26-year-old man fell from a height of 200 feet, and sustained a burst fracture of L1. Neurologically, he presented as incomplete lesion with weakness in both lower extremities. **(A)** Sagittal T1-weighted MRI demonstrates the Denis-B burst fracture of the L1 vertebral body with retropulsion of posterior fragment into the spinal canal, compromising the cauda equina. **(B)** A CT section at the level of L1 shows significant (>60%) degree of spinal canal compromise by the displaced bony fragments. **(C)** The patient was treated with posterior instrumentation using Jacobs locking hook spinal rod. This procedure, however, was not able to provide canal clearance. There is still substantial posterior displacement present. **(D)** A second procedure was performed, consisting of anterior retroperitoneal vertebrectomy and anterior decompression of L1. A tricortical fibular allograft was used to provide anterior stability, at the same time serving as a template for anterior fusion. This resulted in excellent reduction and opening of the spinal canal. **(E,F)** Anteroposterior and lateral radiographs demonstrate the spinal reconstruction with the Jacobs locking hook spinal rod. Note the restoration of sagittal vertebral alignment and the position of the fibular allograft.

Injury to the Thoracolumbar Spine **3.17**

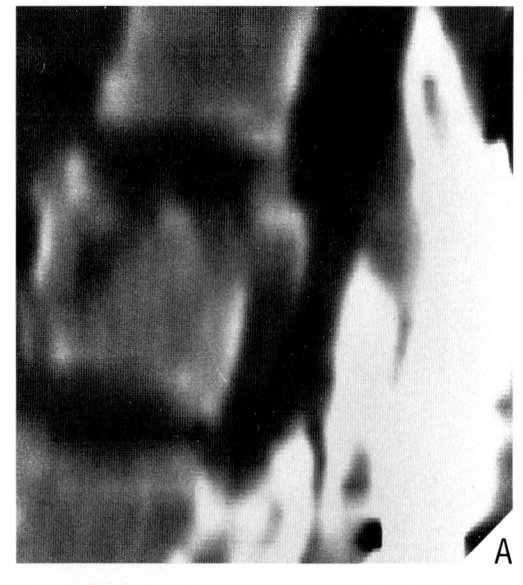

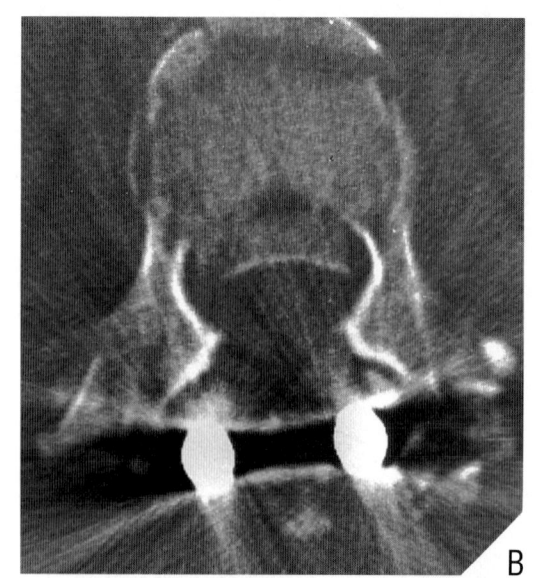

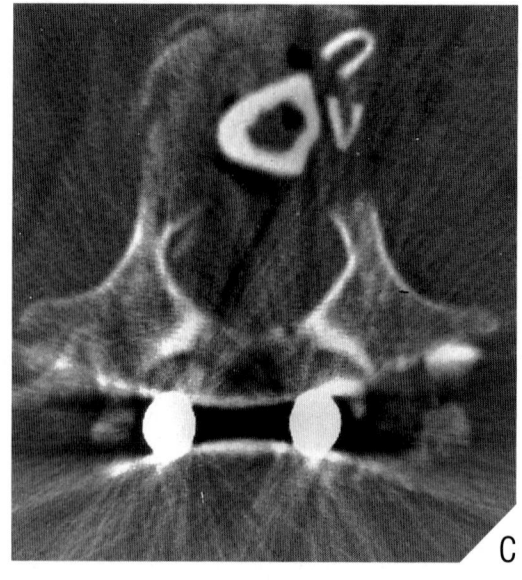

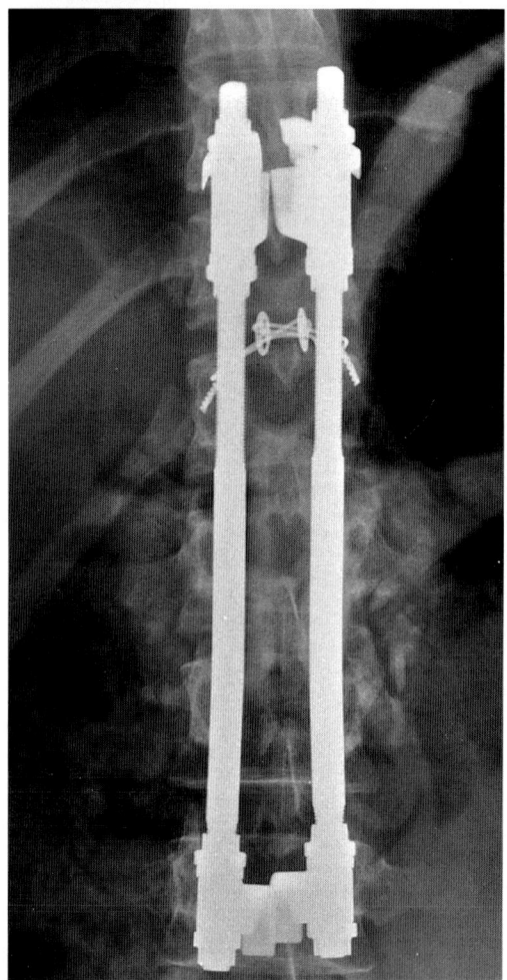

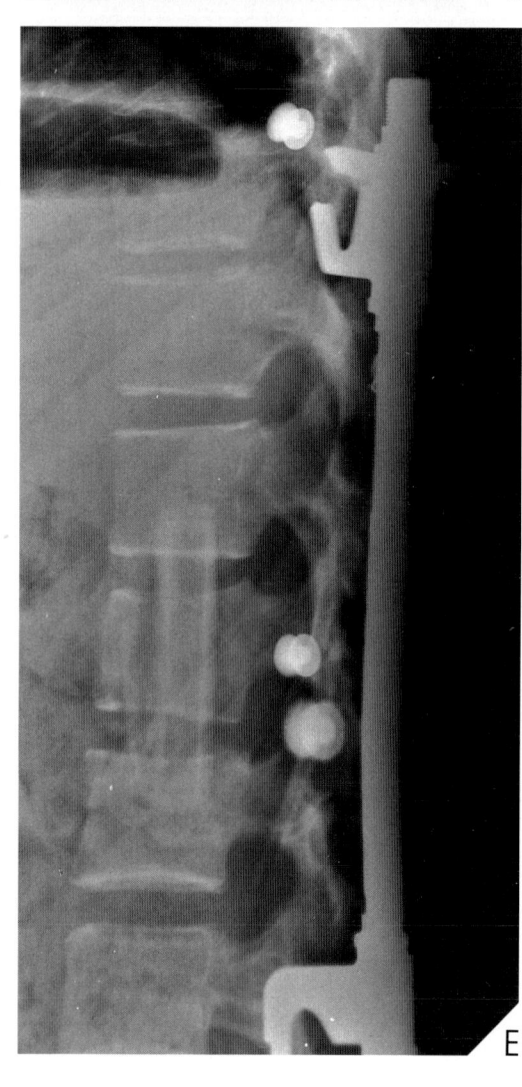

FIGURE 3.22 A 36-year-old woman was involved in a motor vehicle accident and sustained a burst fracture of L1. She presented with neurologically incomplete lesion resulting in weakness of both lower extremities. **(A)** Sagittal reformation CT image shows a Denis-B type of burst fracture. Note the retropulsion of fragments into the spinal canal. **(B)** Post-instrumentation axial CT section demonstrates that adequate canal decompression was not achieved as evidenced by the residual retropulsed bony fragment. **(C)** After anterior retroperitoneal decompression and fusion using fibular allograft and 12th rib autograft, there is an adequate width of spinal canal. **(D,E)** Postoperative radiographs in the anteroposterior and lateral projections demonstrate good spinal alignment and the proper position of the anterior allograft and autograft used in reconstruction procedure.

Imaging of the Spine in Clinical Practice

intact patient, because canal remodeling will result in decompression within 1 year.) On the other hand, when it can be predicted preoperatively that postoperative residual canal compromise will be more than 25% to 30% and the patient has a neurologically incomplete lesion, a simultaneous anterior and posterior approach is advocated. It has been determined that Denis Type A burst fractures can be reduced 80%, whereas Denis Type B burst fractures can be reduced 50% by distraction reduction alone. Therefore, Denis Type A may be reduced by posterior instrumentation alone (see Fig. 3.20) while Denis Type B with greater than 60% canal compromise in neurologically incomplete patients should undergo a simultaneous anterior and posterior approach, because the best that can be hoped for is a reduction to 30% canal compromise (Fig. 3.22).

An alternative to the simultaneous approach is combination of anterior internal fixation with anterior decompression and fusion. Anterior fixation can be achieved with either the Armstrong or the Yuan anterior spinal plate (Fig. 3.23). However, anterior rod screw systems such as the Kaneda device are also available which enable the surgeon to apply compressive or distraction forces.

Chance Fractures

Originally described by G.Q. Chance, this type of distraction injury of the lumbar spine is also called a "seat-belt" fracture because of its frequent occurrence in individuals wearing only lap seat belts during automobile accidents. Acute forward flexion of the spine across a restraining lap seat

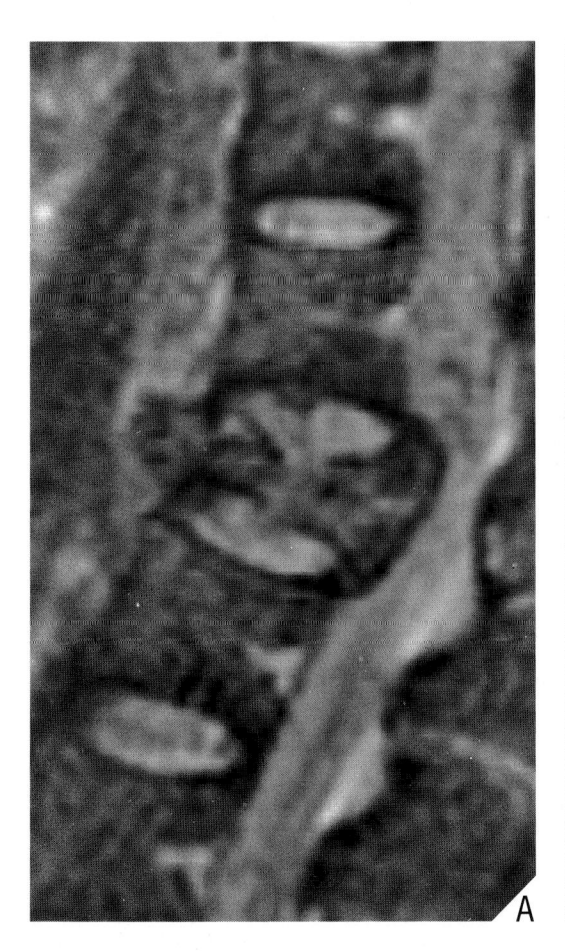

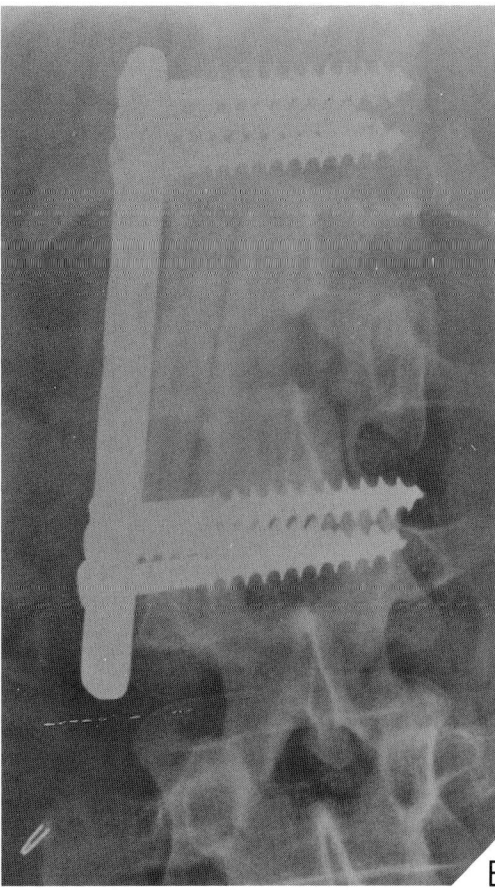

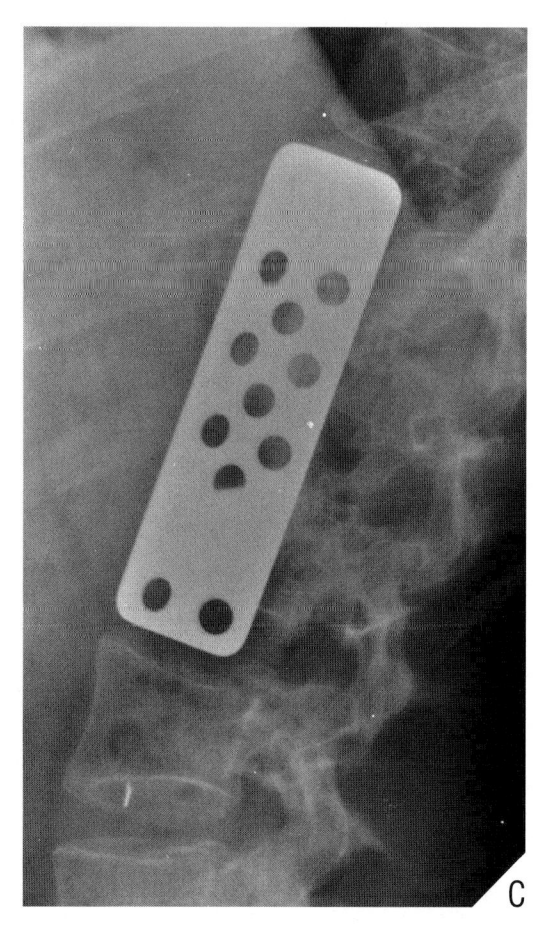

FIGURE 3.23 A 30-year-old man sustained a Denis-B burst fracture of L1 in a fall from the roof. He presented as an incomplete neurologic injury with weakness of both lower extremities. **(A)** Sagittal T2-weighted MRI shows the comminution of the L1 vertebra with compromise of 50% of the width of spinal canal. There is retropulsion of bone into the spinal canal resulting in compressure of the cauda equina. **(B,C)** Because of the significant amount of retropulsion it was elected to perform a primary anterior retroperitoneal vertebrectomy decompression of the spinal canal with anterior fusion, using a combination of a fibular allograft and 12th rib autograft. This was stabilized by application of the Armstrong plate.

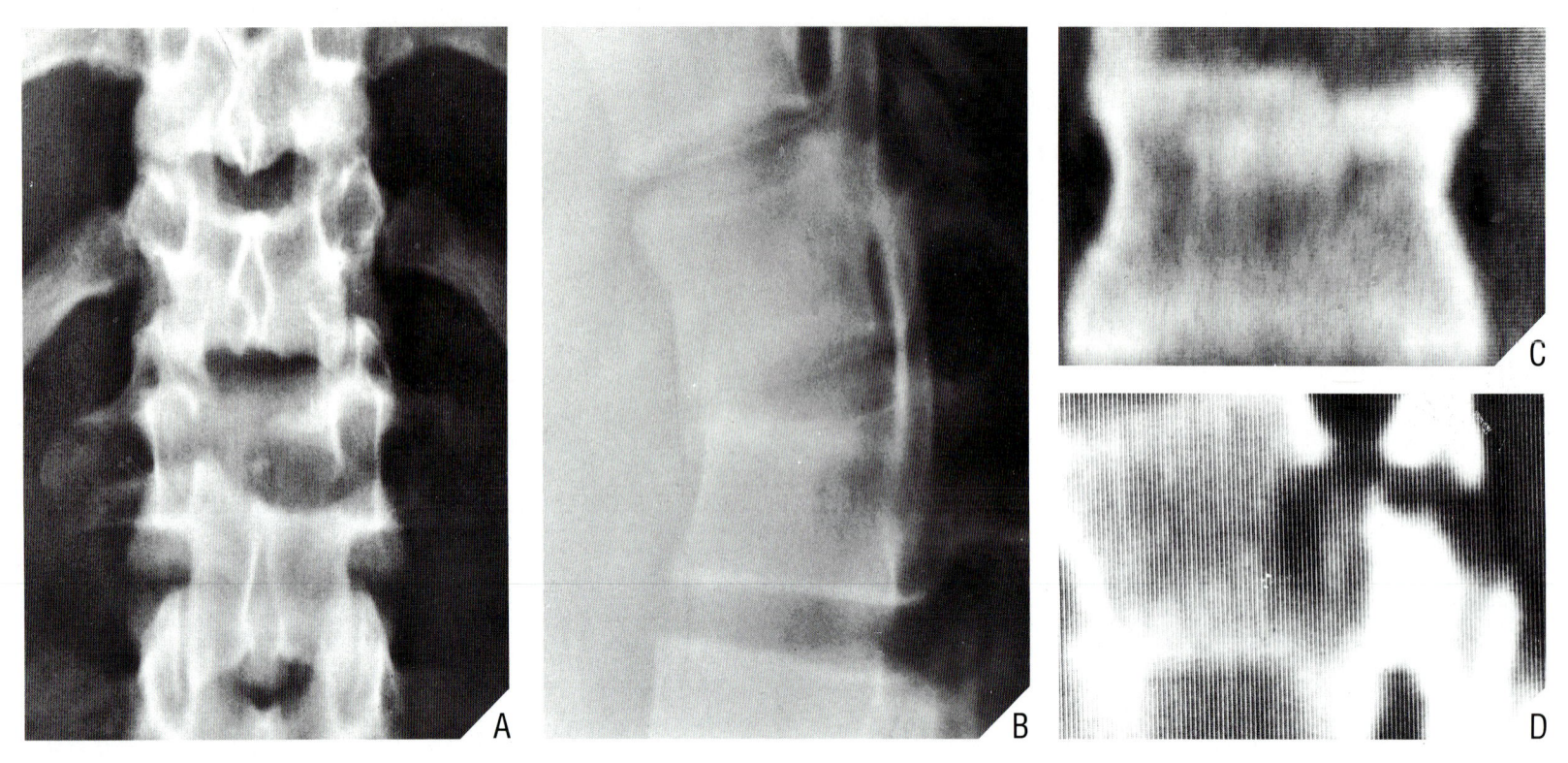

FIGURE 3.24 A 30-year-old woman sustained an injury to the lower back in a car collision; she had been wearing a lap seat belt. Anteroposterior **(A)** and lateral **(B)** tomograms of the lumbar spine show a fracture of the vertebral body of L1 extending into the lamina and spinous process. Coronal **(C)** and sagittal **(D)** CT reformation images confirm the conventional tomographic findings. (Courtesy of David Faegenburg, MD, Mineola, NY)

SPECTRUM OF SEAT-BELT INJURIES

One-Level

- Chance fracture—horizontal splitting of vertebra; no ligament disruption
  - posterior longitudinal ligament
  - interspinous ligament
  - anterior longitudinal ligament
  - supraspinous ligament
- rupture of ligaments and intervertebral disk

Two-Level

- fracture of posterior column; rupture of ligaments and intervertebral disk
- fracture of posterior and middle columns; rupture of ligaments and intervertebral disk

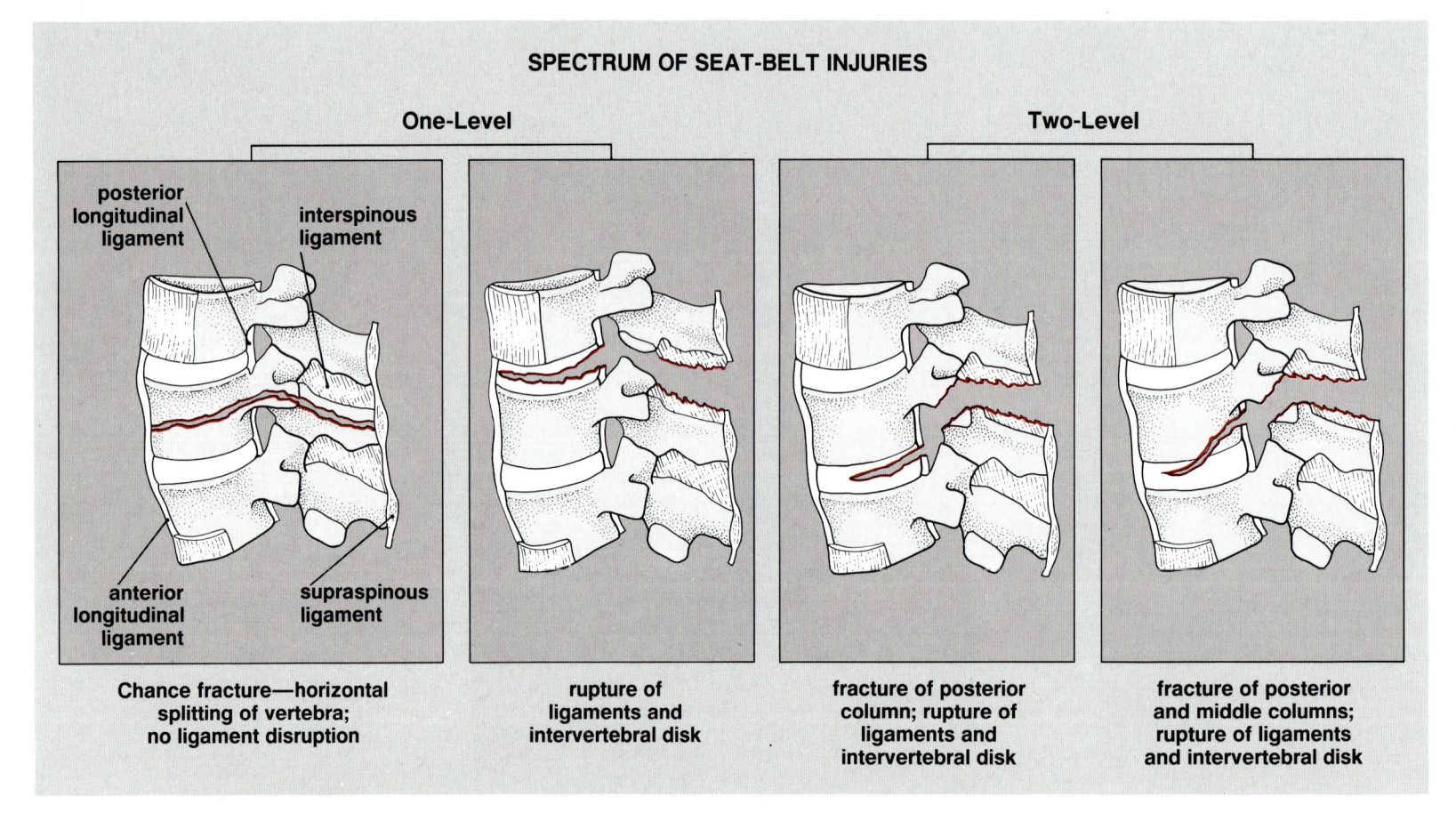

FIGURE 3.25 The spectrum of seat-belt injuries involving the lumbar spine.

Imaging of the Spine in Clinical Practice

belt with sudden deceleration causes the spine above the belt to be pushed forward and to be distracted from the lower, fixed part of the spine. The classic Chance fracture involves a horizontal splitting of the vertebra, beginning in the spinous process or lamina and extending through the pedicles and the vertebral body without damage to ligament structures. Its constant feature is a transverse fracture without dislocation or subluxation (Fig. 3.24). The transverse process may be horizontally fractured as well, and at times there is compression of the anterior aspect of the vertebral body. A Chance fracture tends to be stable, because the upper half of the neural arch remains firmly attached to the vertebra above and the lower half to the vertebra below. Since the original description of this fracture, three more types of seat-belt fractures have been reported, which involve various degrees of ligament and intervertebral disk disruption (Figs. 3.25, 3.26). According to Denis' three-column concept of thoracolumbar spine injuries, these latter types of fracture are essentially the result of failure of the posterior and middle columns, with the intact anterior element acting as a hinge. These injuries can be stable or unstable, depending on their extent and severity.

Treatment

When these injuries occur entirely through bone, treatment is a hyperextension cast. When the posterior and middle columns fail because of ligamentous disruption, translaminar facet screw fixation (Fig. 3.27) or posterior spinal fusion with a compression system (Fig. 3.28) is advocated. However, it is important to determine that the middle column is capable of load-bearing. If this is not the case, the use of a compression system could lead to retropulsion of bone and disk fragments into the canal.

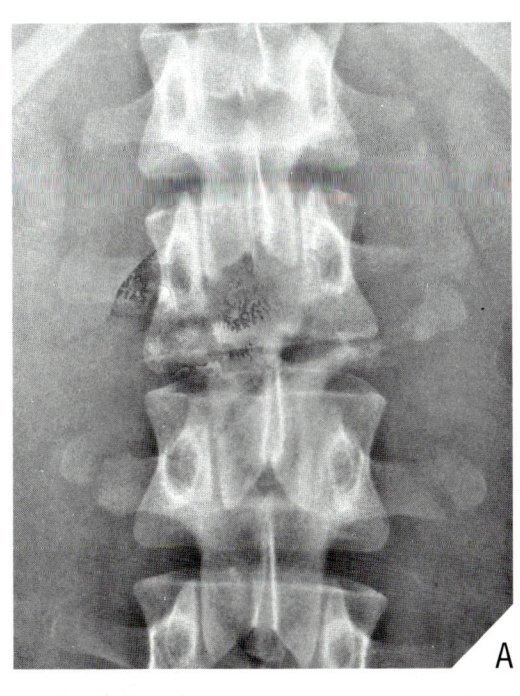

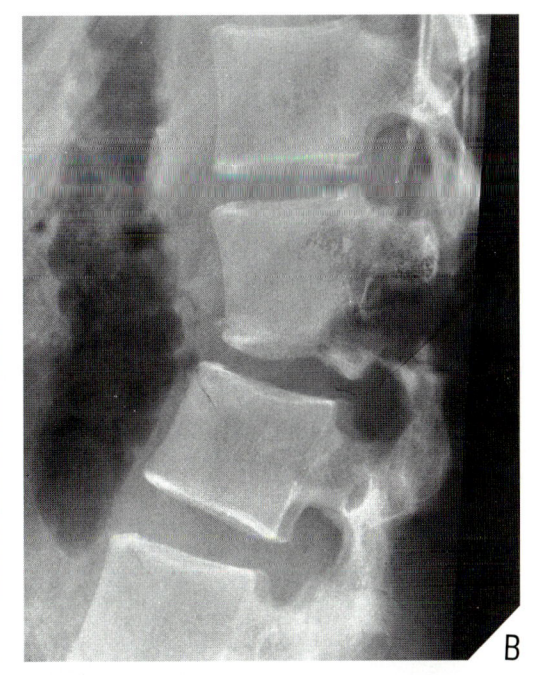

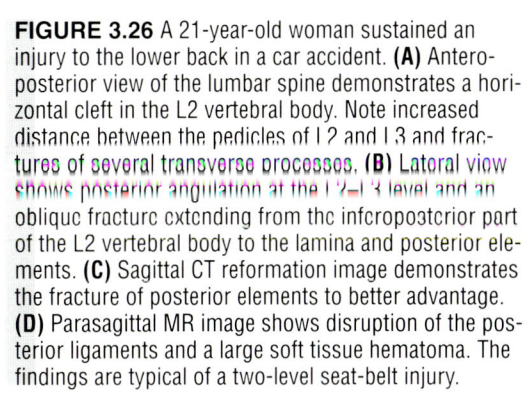

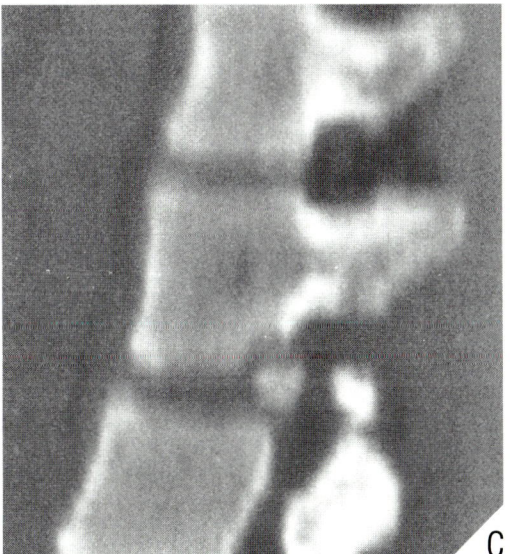

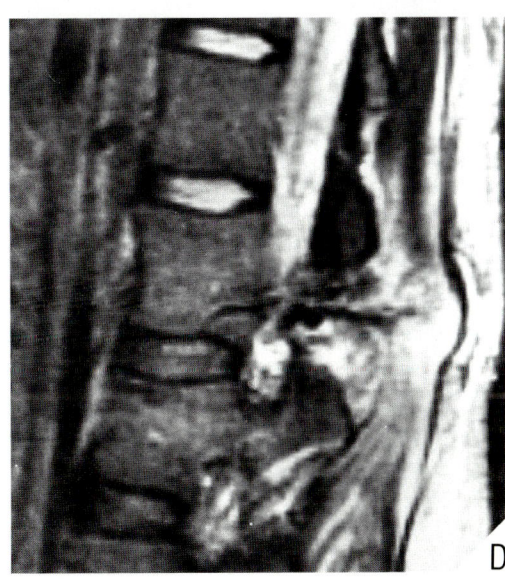

FIGURE 3.26 A 21-year-old woman sustained an injury to the lower back in a car accident. **(A)** Anteroposterior view of the lumbar spine demonstrates a horizontal cleft in the L2 vertebral body. Note increased distance between the pedicles of L2 and L3 and fractures of several transverse processes. **(B)** Lateral view shows posterior angulation at the L2–L3 level and an oblique fracture extending from the inferoposterior part of the L2 vertebral body to the lamina and posterior elements. **(C)** Sagittal CT reformation image demonstrates the fracture of posterior elements to better advantage. **(D)** Parasagittal MR image shows disruption of the posterior ligaments and a large soft tissue hematoma. The findings are typical of a two-level seat-belt injury.

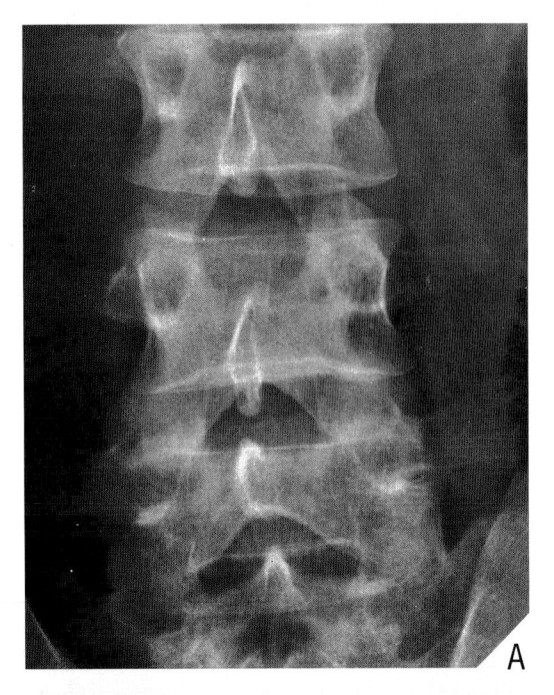

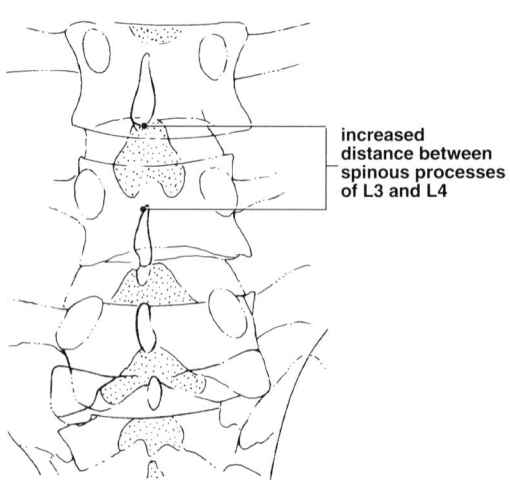

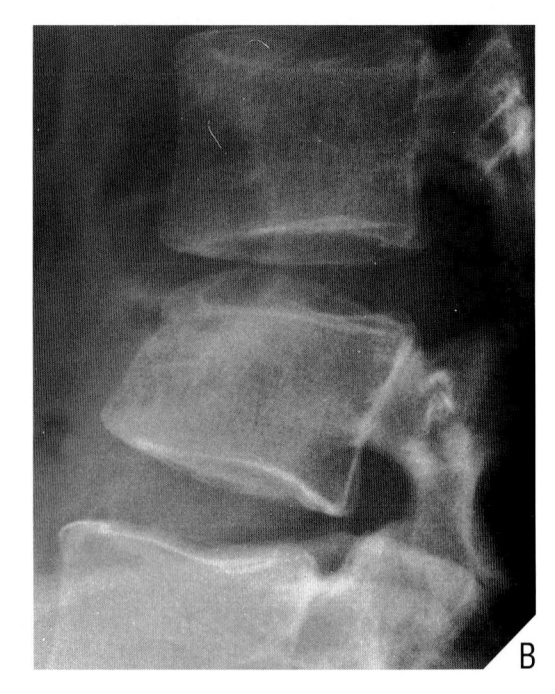

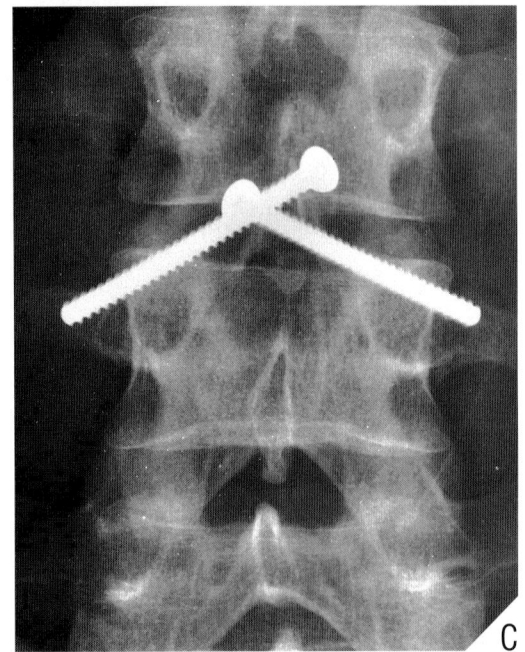

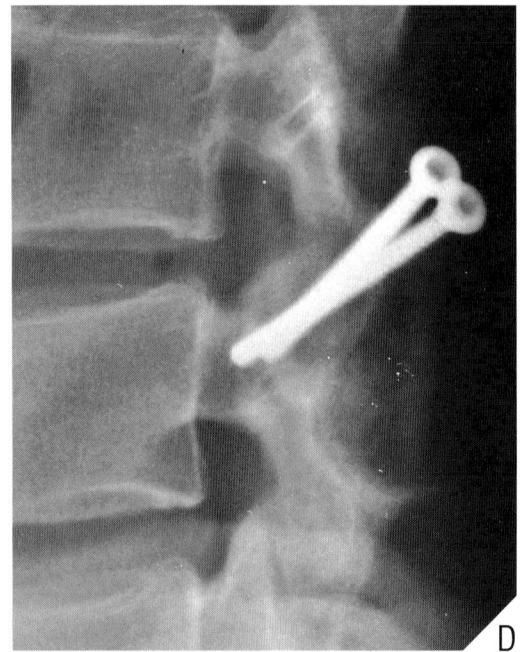

FIGURE 3.27 A 23-year-old man, a restrained passenger in a motor vehicle accident, sustained a flexion–distraction type of seat-belt injury at L3–L4. He was neurologically intact. **(A)** Anteroposterior radiograph of lumbar spine shows increased distance between spinous processes of L3 and L4, indicative of distraction injury. **(B)** Lateral film shows the kyphotic deformity at the level of L3–L4 and slight compression of the superior endplate of L4, as well as opening of the facets posteriorly, resulting from the severe ligamentous injury. **(C,D)** The patient was treated with translaminar facet screws which are stabilizing the posterior column. Normal interspinous processes distance and sagittal plane alignment have been restored.

3.22 *Imaging of the Spine in Clinical Practice*

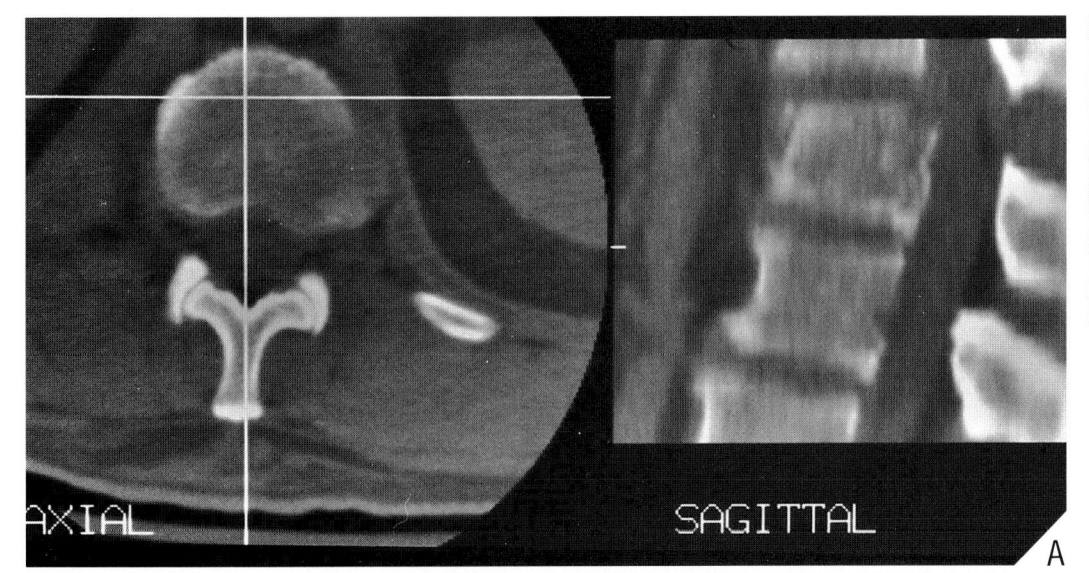

FIGURE 3.28 A 46-year-old man was involved in a motor vehicle accident and sustained a flexion–distraction injury at the level of T11–T12. He was neurologically intact. **(A)** Axial CT section and sagittal reformation, supplemented with **(B)** parasagittal reformation show mild compression of superior part of vertebral body T12 and widening of the interspinous distance T11–T12. **(C,D)** The postoperative radiographs in anteroposterior and lateral projections show the use of a modified Synthes compression system which has restored alignment of the spine in the sagittal plane.

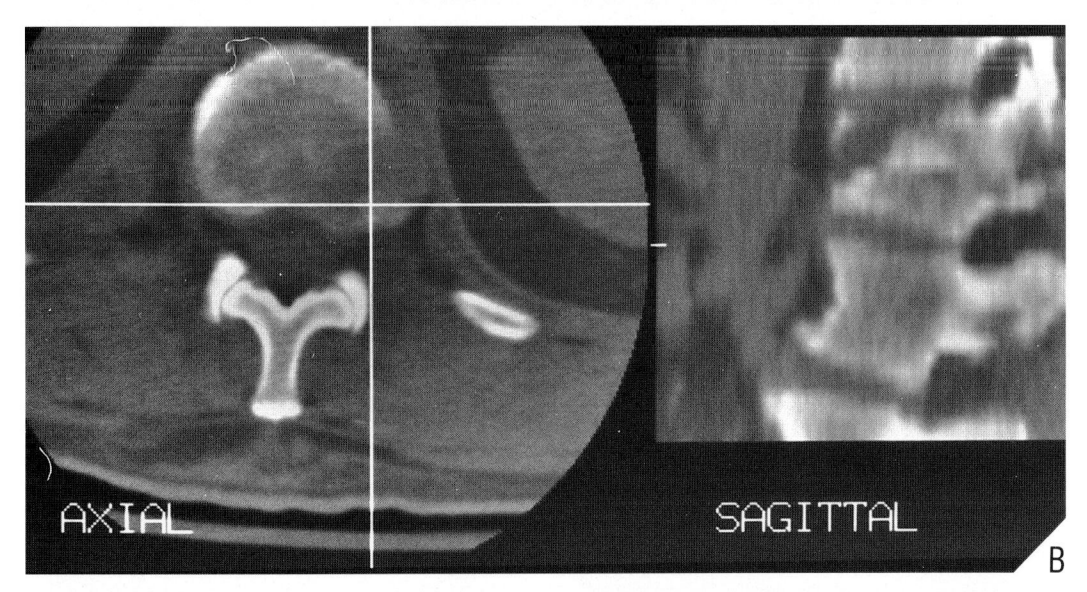

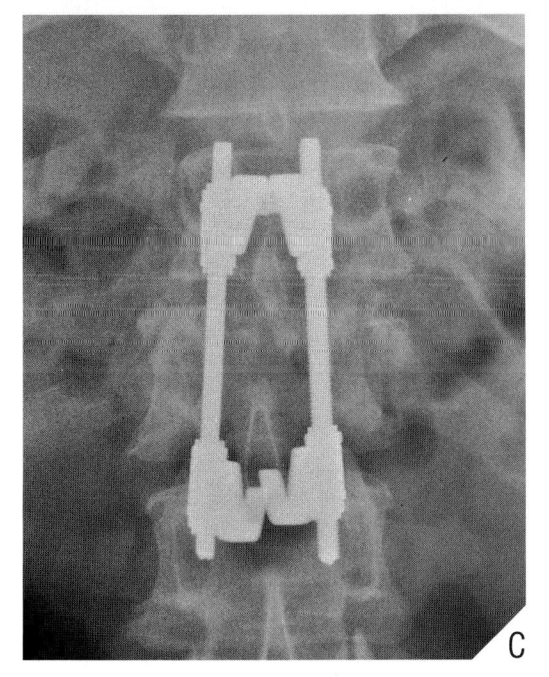

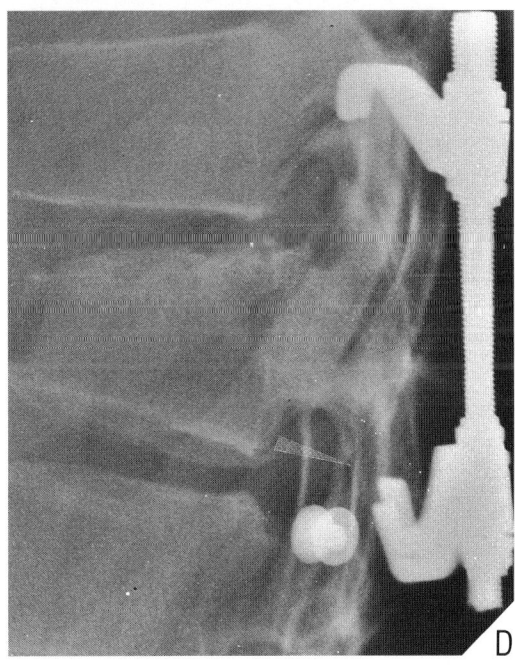

Injury to the Thoracolumbar Spine

Fracture Dislocations

Resulting from various forces—flexion, rotation, distraction, or anteroposterior or posteroanterior shear—acting on the thoracolumbar segment either alone or in combination, fracture dislocations lead to failure of all three columns of the spine; such injuries are therefore unstable and are usually associated with severe neurological complications.

In the *flexion–rotation* type of injury (Fig. 3.29), the posterior and middle columns are completely disrupted, and the anterior column may show anterior wedging of the vertebral body (Fig. 3.30). The lateral film also demonstrates subluxation or dislocation, together with an increase in the interspinous distance. The posterior wall of the vertebral body may remain intact if the dislocation occurs at the level of the intervertebral disk. Although the anteroposterior projection is not always diagnostic, occasionally it reveals a displaced fracture of the superior articular process on one side, representing failure of the posterior column secondary to rotational forces (see Fig. 3.30A).

In the *shear* types of fracture dislocation, all three columns are disrupted, including the anterior longitudinal ligament. The *posteroanterior shear* variant is characterized by forward displacement of the spinal segment onto the vertebra below at the point of shear (Fig. 3.31); the vertebral bodies are intact, without any decrease in their anterior or posterior height. However, the posterior elements of the dislocated vertebral segment, including the laminae, articular facets, and the spinous processes, are usually fractured at several levels. In *anteroposterior shear*, the spinal segment above the point of shear is dislocated posterior to the segment below (Fig. 3.32). It may be accompanied by a fracture of the spinous process. Fracture dislocation of the *flexion–distraction* type resembles a seat-belt injury involving failure of the posterior and middle columns.

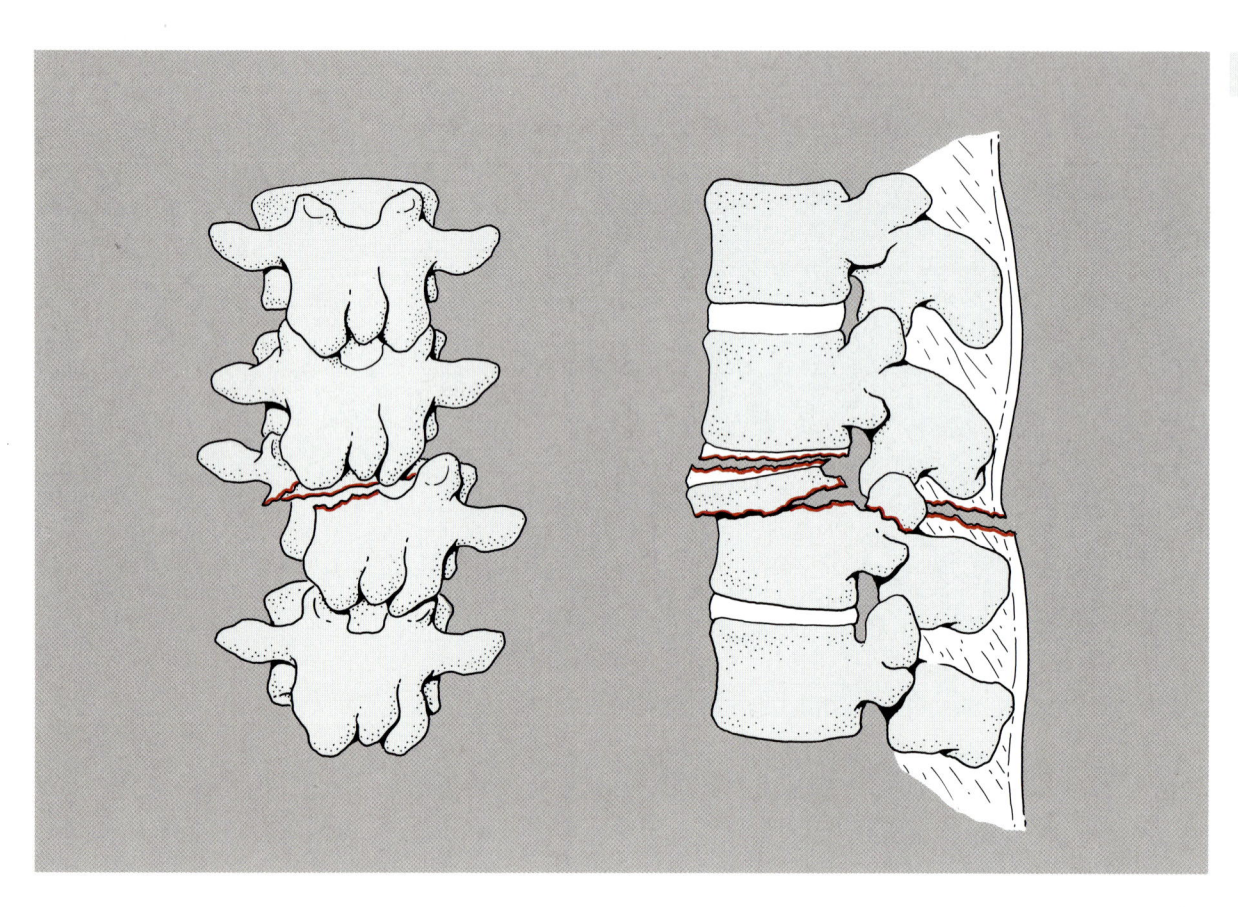

FIGURE 3.29 The flexion–rotation type of fracture dislocation.

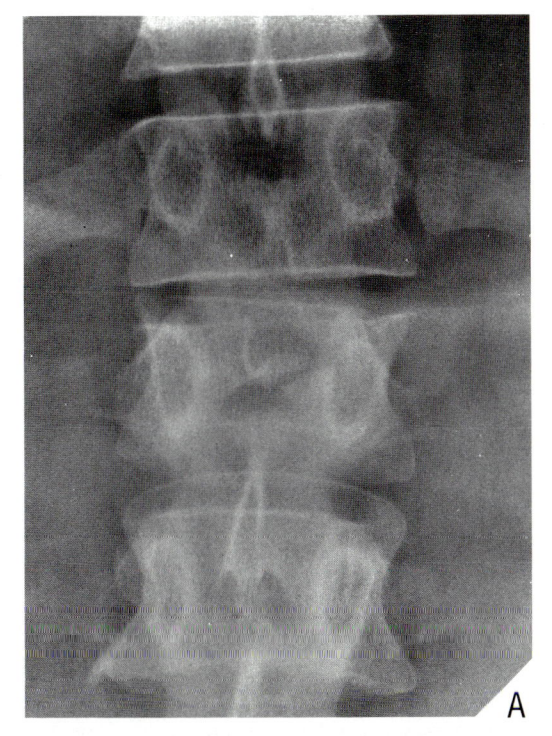

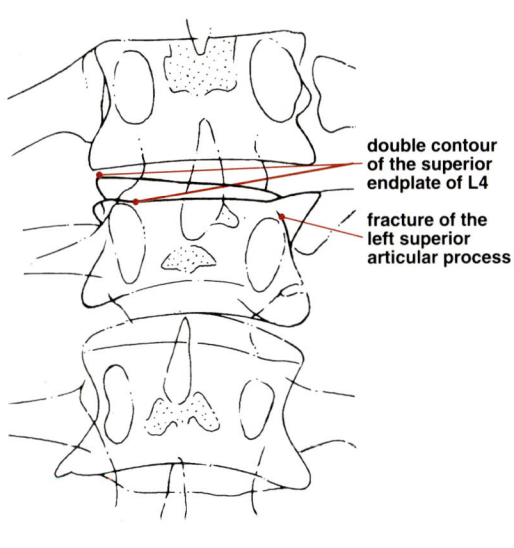

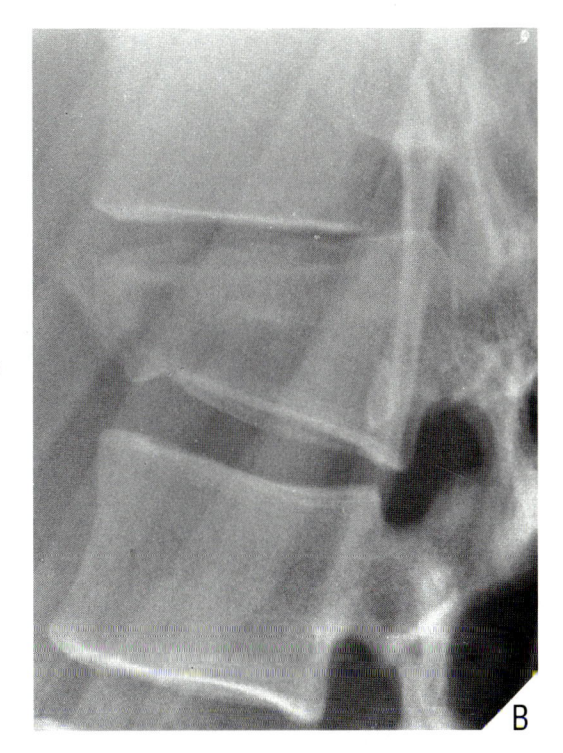

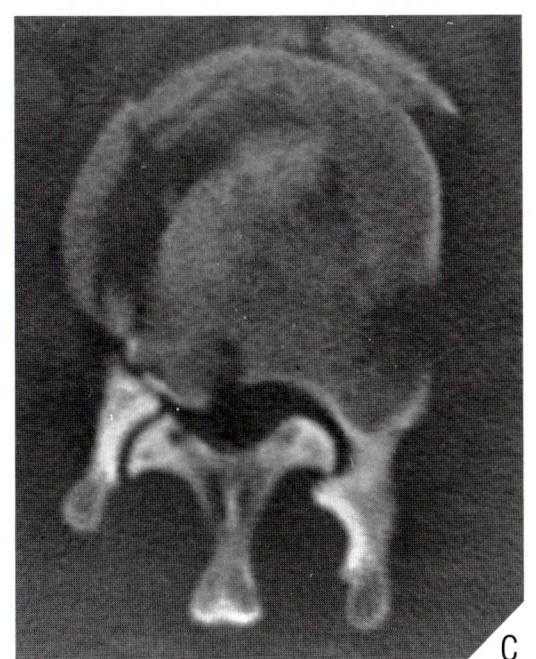

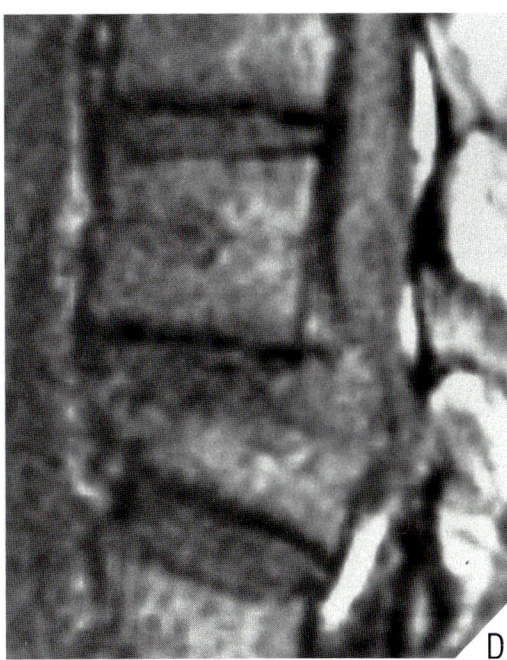

FIGURE 3.30 A 27-year-old man was involved in a motorcycle accident and sustained flexion–rotation fracture–dislocation at T12–L1 level. **(A)** Antero-posterior film shows double contour of the superior endplate of L1 due to compression fracture, and fracture of the left superior articular process. **(B)** Lateral radiograph shows anterior wedging of the body of L1 together with disruption of the middle column and malaligment of vertebrae T12 and L1. **(C)** CT section through the vertebra L1 shows fracture of the middle column with retropulsion of the fractured fragment into the spinal canal, similar to that present in the burst fractures. The spinal canal is compromised more than 80%. **(D)** Sagittal T2-weighted MRI, in addition, shows disruption of the posterior column and compression of the thecal sac.

Injury to the Thoracolumbar Spine **3.25**

FIGURE 3.31 A posteroanterior shear-type fracture dislocation.

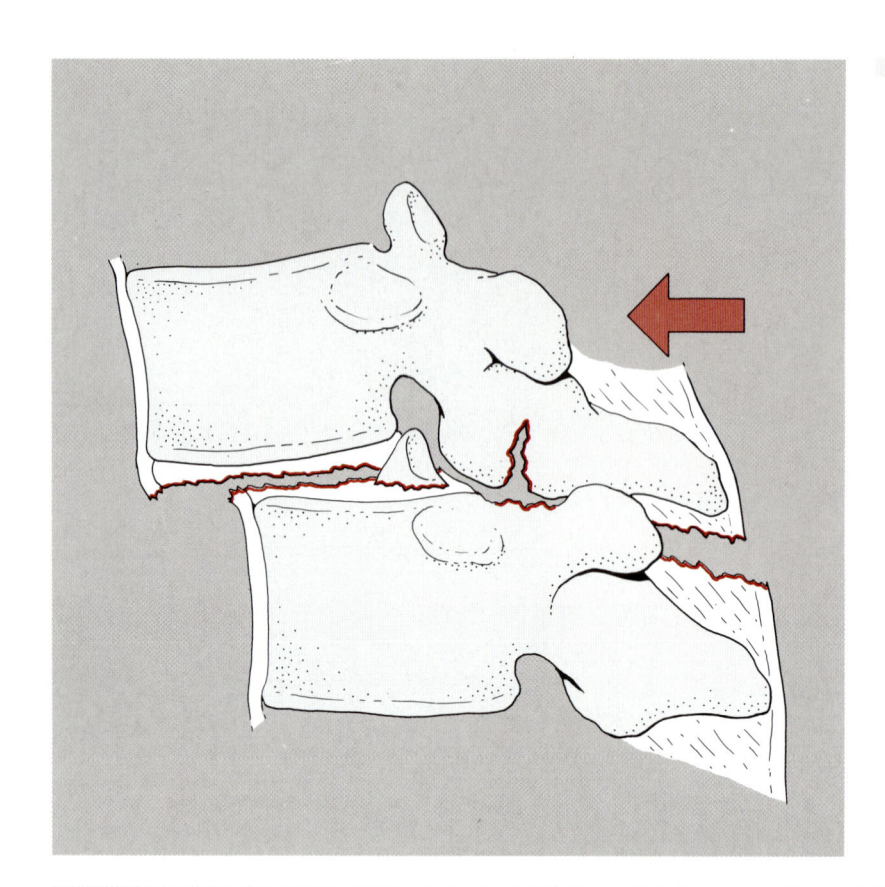

FIGURE 3.32 An anteroposterior shear-type fracture dislocation.

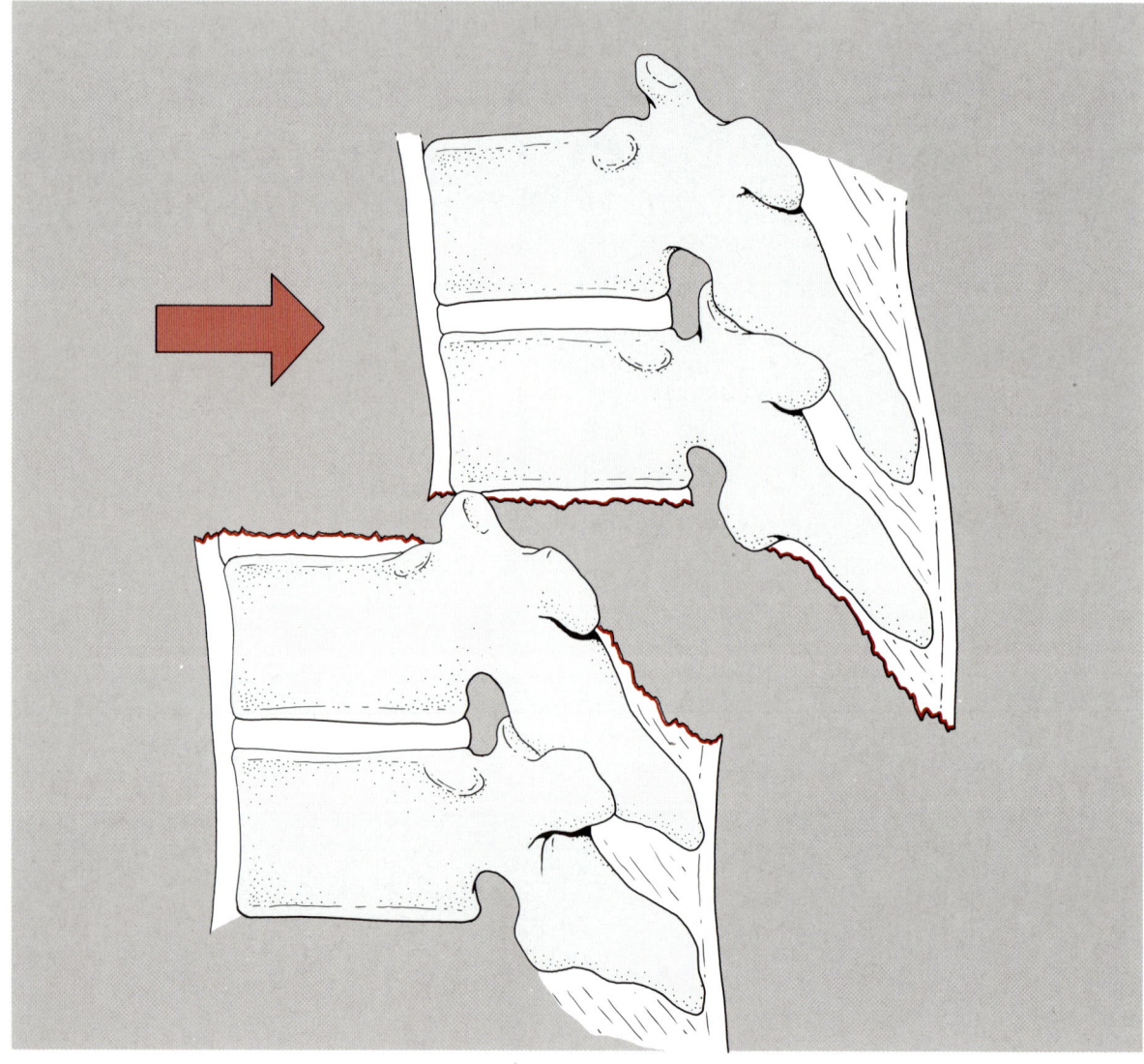

However, unlike seat-belt injuries, the entire annulus fibrosus is torn, allowing the vertebra above to dislocate or sublux onto the affected vertebra (Fig. 3.33). The latter is best documented on lateral radiography. Unlike the seat-belt injury, the flexion–distraction fracture dislocation is often associated with neurologic loss and intra-abdominal injury.

Treatment

The goal of treatment is to realign the spinal column and provide adequate posterior stabilization so as to allow early mobilization (Figs. 3.34–3.36). Early mobilization has been shown to decrease morbidity and mortality while enhancing the patient's ability to return to a productive lifestyle.

SPONDYLOLYSIS AND SPONDYLOLISTHESIS

Spondylolysis, a defect in the pars interarticularis (neck of the "Scotty dog") of a vertebra may be an acquired abnormality secondary to an acute fracture or, more commonly, may result from chronic stress (stress fracture). Rarely is it seen as a result of a congenital defect in the isthmus.

Spondylolisthesis is defined as ventral slipping or gliding of all or part of one vertebra over a stationary vertebra beneath it. These abnormalities occur predominantly in the lumbar spine (90% of cases) and most commonly at the L4–L5 and L5–S1 levels.

It is important to distinguish spondylolisthesis associated with spondylolysis from spondylolisthesis occurring without an associated defect in the pars interarticularis (Fig. 3.37). As a rule this latter form, designated "pseudospondylolisthesis" by Junghanns (1931), is associated with degenerative disk disease and degeneration and subluxation in the apophyseal joints; it is often referred to as *degenerative spondylolisthesis*. Although the defect in the pars interarticularis cannot always be demonstrated on conventional radiography—particularly if oblique views are not obtained—true spondylolisthesis can be differentiated from pseudospondylolisthesis by the spinous process sign introduced by Bryk and Rosenkranz (1969) (Fig. 3.38). The sign is a logical outgrowth of the different processes at work in the two conditions. In true spondylolisthesis, a bilateral defect in the pars interarticularis leads to forward (ventrad) slippage of the body, pedicles, and superior articular process of the involved vertebra, while the spinous process, laminae, and inferior articular process remain in normal position. Therefore, study of the most dorsal aspects of the spinous processes reveals a step-off at the interspace above the level of the slip (Fig.

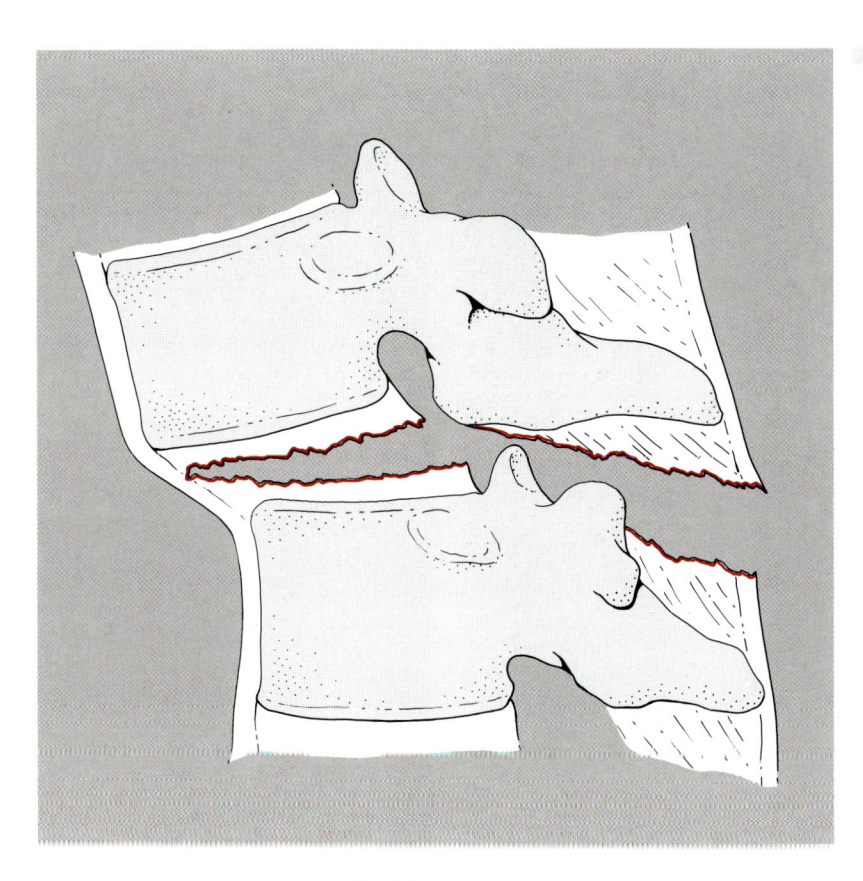

FIGURE 3.33 A flexion–distraction type of dislocation.

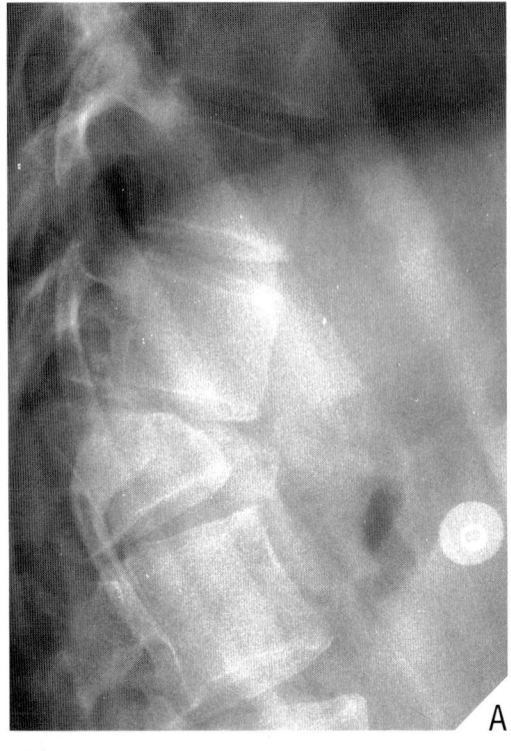

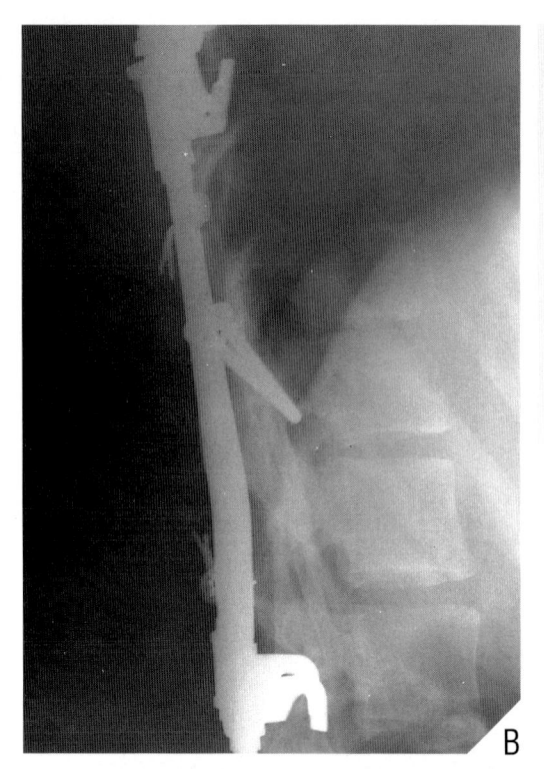

FIGURE 3.34 An 18-year-old woman sustained a fracture-dislocation at the level of T11–T12 when she was involved in a motor vehicle accident. Neurologically, she presented with a complete injury with no function below the level of T11. **(A)** Lateral radiograph demonstrates fracture–dislocation at T11–T12 level. **(B)** The postoperative lateral views show the spinal reconstruction using the Synthes Jacobs lock and hook spinal rod. Translaminar facet screws were used to stabilize the posterior column and prevent overdistraction at the level of injury. Note the reconstruction of normal sagittal alignment. (Reproduced with permission from Montesano PX, Benson DR: The thoracolumbar spine. In Rockwood CA, Green DP, Bucholz RW (eds): *Rockwood and Green's Fractures in Adults*. 3rd ed. vol 2. New York, J B Lippincott, 1991)

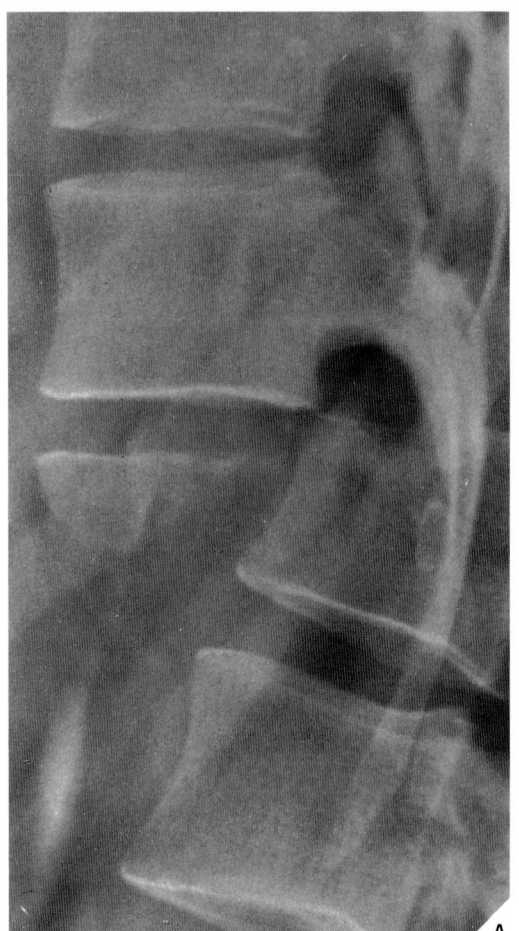

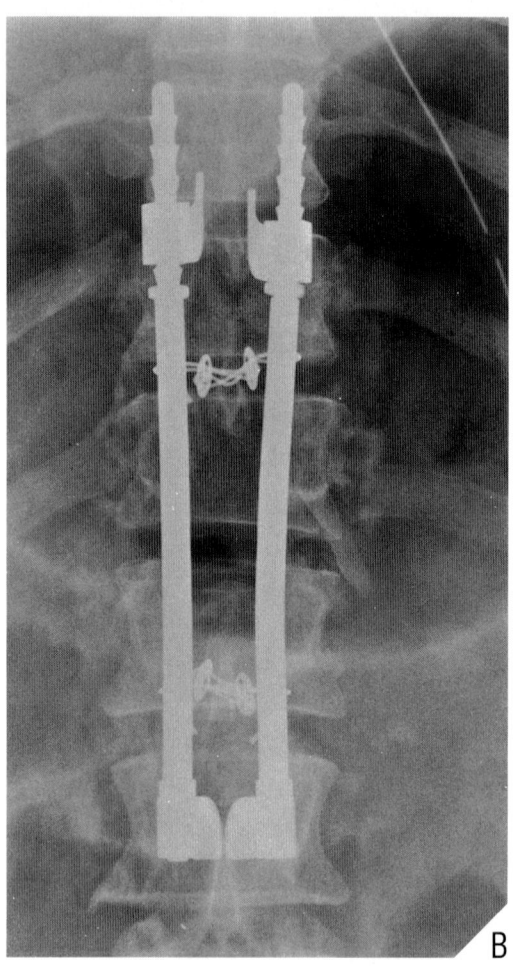

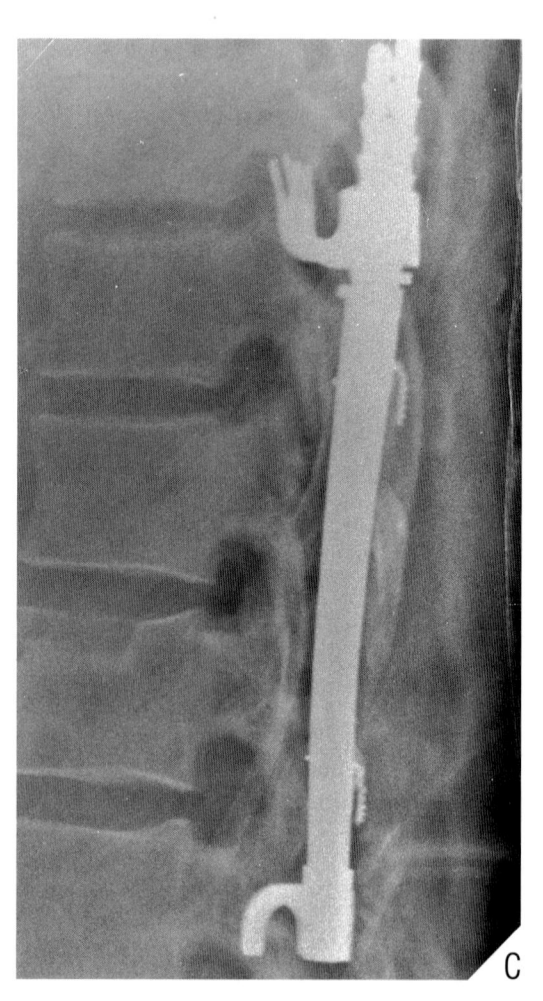

FIGURE 3.35 A 25 year-old man was found unconscious on the side of the road after being hit by a car. Physical examination revealed a completely neurological lrsion. **(A)** Lateral radiograph shows a posteroanterior sheer fracture dislocation. **(B,C)** The treatment of application of the Harrington distraction system using Cotrel pedicle hooks and Drummond spinous process wires through the bases of the spinous processes to supplement the internal fixation. Note the re-establishing of the normal spinal alignment. This type of treatment allows for early mobilization of the patient.

Imaging of the Spine in Clinical Practice

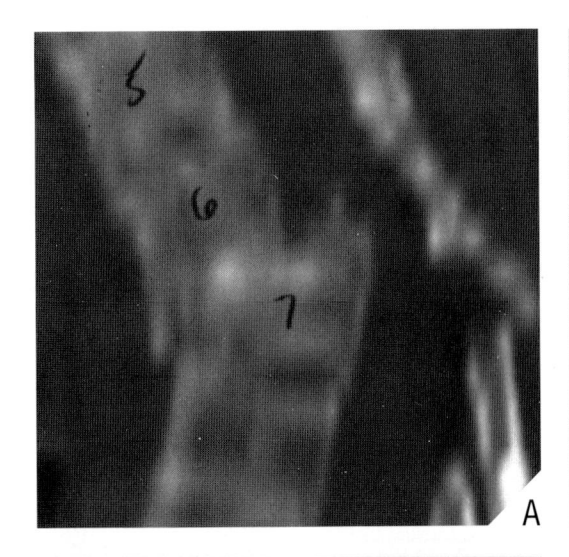

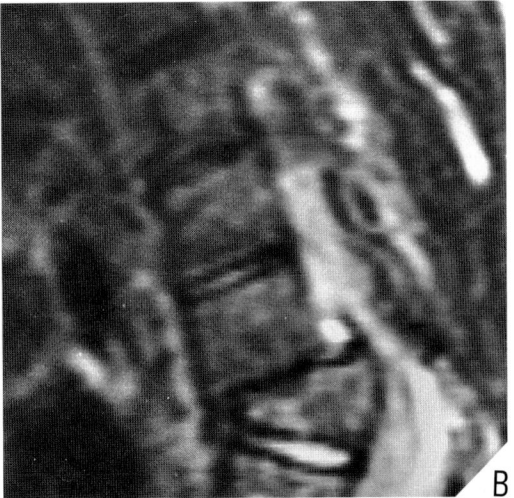

FIGURE 3.36 A 17-year-old man was involved in a motor vehicle accident and sustained a flexion–distraction fracture dislocation at T6–T7 with complete paralysis below the level of this injury. **(A)** CT sagittal reformation image shows significant degree of spinal canal compromise. **(B)** Sagittal T2-weighted MRI demonstrate the transection of the cord at T6–T7 level. **(C,D)** The treatment consisted of a transthoracic T7 vertebrectomy and fusion using autograft rib and simultaneous posterior instrumentation and fusion using the Cotrel–Dubousset instrumentation system in compression. Note that the pedicle hook at T9 has slipped out from underneath the pedicle and is in a lateral position. Despite this complication, postoperative stabilization was maintained and the patient went on to a solid fusion.

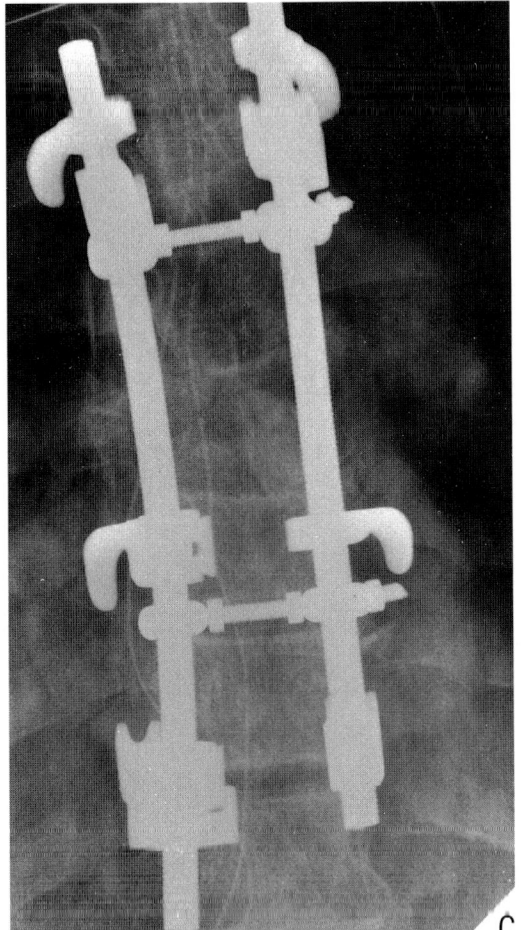

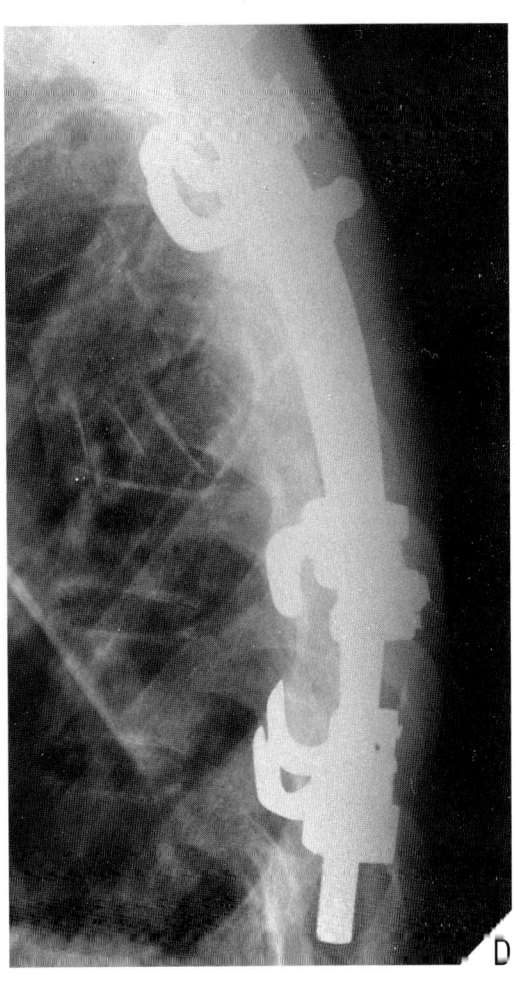

Injury to the Thoracolumbar Spine

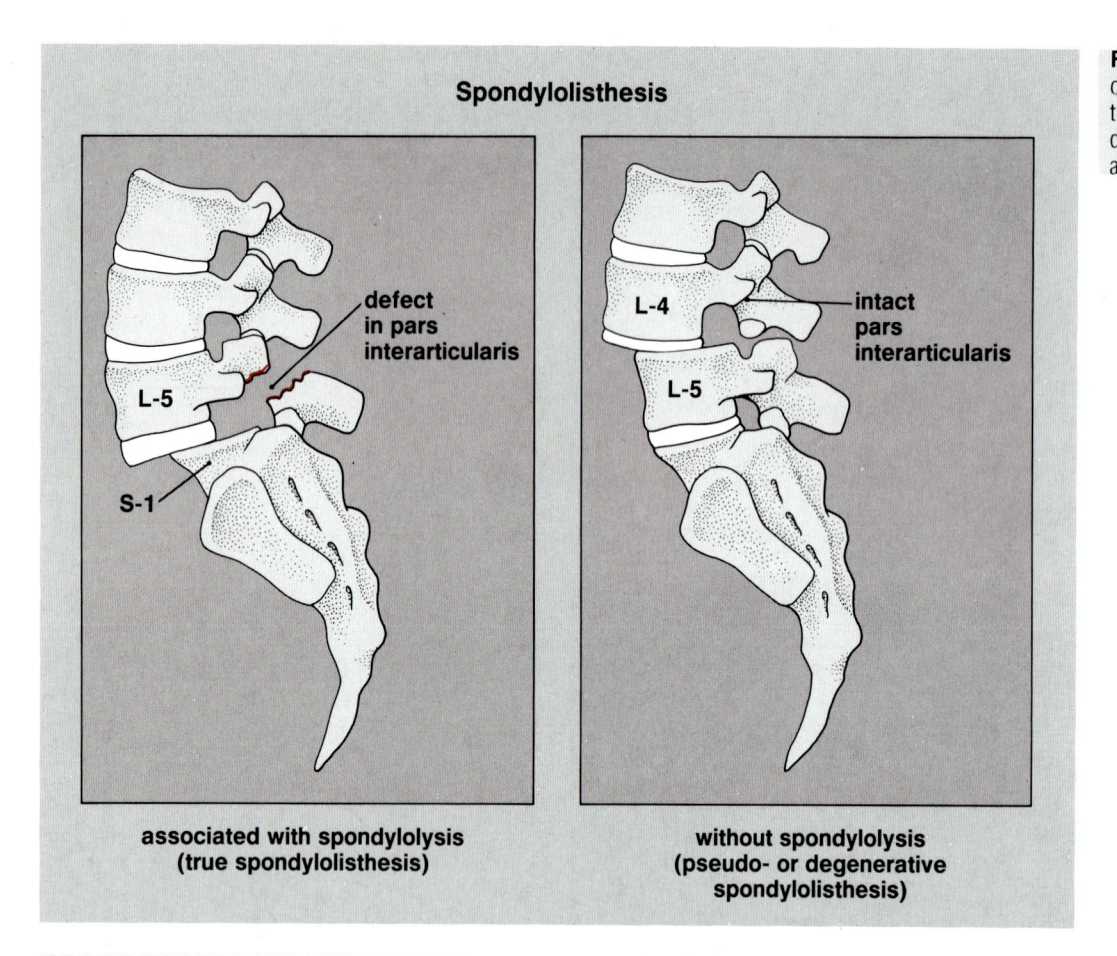

FIGURE 3.37 Spondylolisthesis may occur in association with spondylolysis resulting from a defect in the pars interarticularis or secondary to degenerative disk disease and osteoarthritis and subluxation of the apophyseal joints (pseudospondylolisthesis).

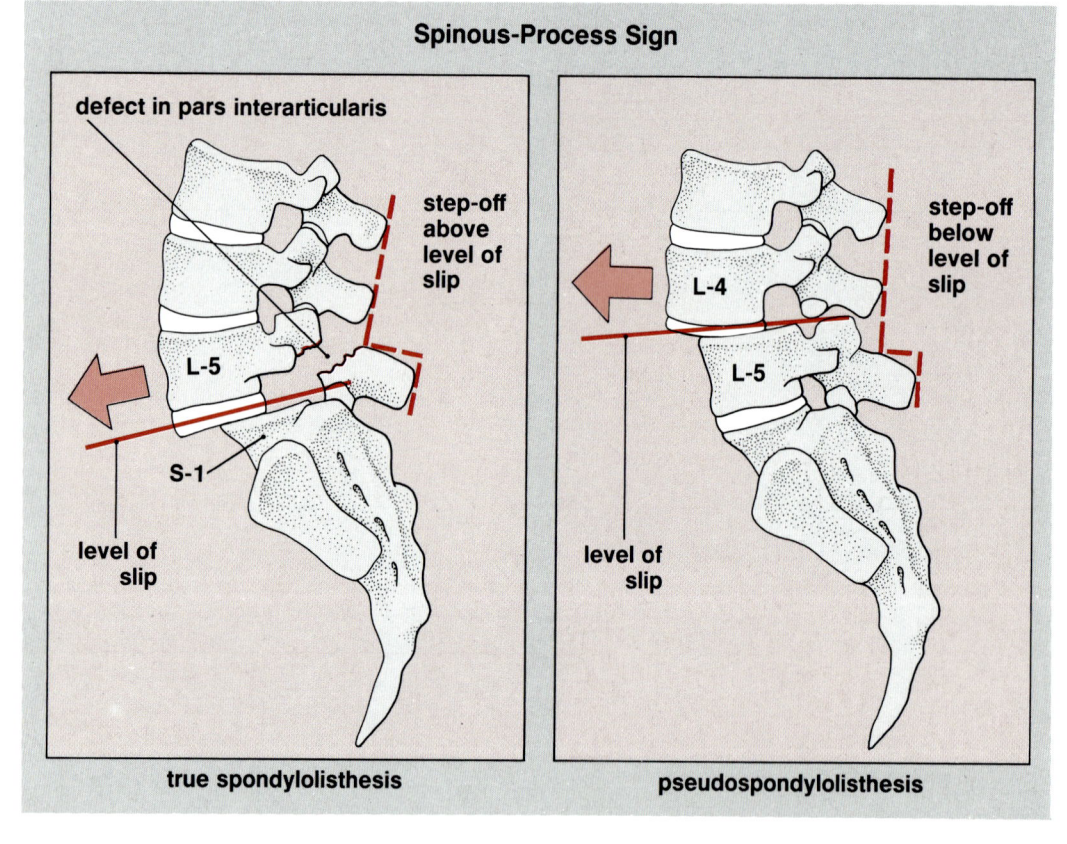

FIGURE 3.38 The spinous-process sign can help differentiate true spondylolisthesis from pseudospondylolisthesis by the appearance of a step-off in the spinous processes above the level of vertebral slip in the former and below that level in the latter.

3.30 Imaging of the Spine in Clinical Practice

3.39 A,B). In pseudospondylolisthesis, on the other hand, the entire vertebra, including the spinous process, moves forward, and the most dorsal aspects of the spinous processes exhibit a step-off at the interspace below the level of the slipped vertebra (see Figs. 3.39 A,B). Application of this sign enables the correct diagnosis to be made on a single lateral film; oblique projections are not necessary. In obtaining the films, however, it is important to avoid overexposure, which may obscure the posterior margins of the spinous processes.

The pars interarticularis defect that precipitates spondylolisthesis can be demonstrated on the standard oblique projection of the lumbar spine (Fig. 3.39C), which may need to be supplemented by conventional tomography (Fig. 3.39D) or CT (Fig. 3.39E); myelography on the lateral view may show an extradural defect on the ventral aspect of the thecal sac, similar to that created by disk herniation (Fig. 3.39F). A severe degree of spondylolisthesis at the L5–S1 level can be identified on the anteroposterior view by the ventrocaudal displacement of L5 over the sacrum. This configuration creates curvilinear densities which form the "inverted Napoleon's hat" sign (Fig. 3.40). The simple grading of spondylolisthesis proposed by Meyerding is based on the amount of forward slippage (Fig. 3.41). The other important measurement is ventral rotation in sagittal plane (also known as *degree of lumbosacral kyphosis* or *slip angle*), which is the angular relationship between the bodies of L5 and S1 (Fig. 3.42.)

Treatment

Spondylolysis usually presents as a back-pain syndrome; however, there may be an element of radiculopathy usually secondary to accumulation of fibrocartilage at the site of defect in pars interarticularis. The treatment for spondylolysis is rest and avoidance of stressful activity. If patients do not respond to a prolonged course of conservative management, then surgical intervention may be necessary, usually in the form of a one-level posterolateral fusion.

When treating spondylolisthesis it is important to take into account the patient's age, the grade of list, the slipped angle, and the predominate symptoms (ie, back pain, radiculopathy). For patients who fail to respond to conservative measures—rest, avoidance of stressful activity, anti-inflammatory medication, low-impact aerobic activity—surgical intervention may be indicated. We believe it is the slip angle rather than the grade that is the most important determinate in choosing which operation to perform (anterior fusion, posterior fusion or combined). In those patients with a grade 1 to 2 slippage, we prefer to perform a posterolateral one-level fusion without instrumentation. As the percent of slippage increases beyond the second degree, we believe that the treatment is more dependent on the slip angle or the amount of L5–S1 kyphosis. If the slip angle is extreme, fusion of L4 to the sacrum combined with an anterior L5–S1 arthrodesis is preferred. We have not chosen to attempt to obtain intraoperative reduction, but are glad to accept any amount of reduction that occurs secondary to positioning. Our reluctance to attempt intraoperative reduction is secondary to the high rate of neurologic complications that has been reported in the literature.

In those cases that are associated with radiculopathy unrelieved by rest, we suggest a limited laminotomy—a resection of fibrocartilage build-up around the pars defect, as well as a foraminal nerve root exploration.

Injury to the Diskovertebral Junction

One of the most common conditions affecting the diskovertebral junction is herniation of an intervertebral disk. The chief structural unit between adjacent vertebral bodies, the intervertebral disk comprises a soft central portion, the *nucleus pulposus*, composed of collagen fibrils and mucoprotein gel, lying eccentrically and somewhat posteriorly, and a firm, fibrocartilaginous ring, the *annulus fibrosus*, surrounding the nucleus pulposus and reinforced by the anterior and posterior longitudinal ligaments (Fig. 3.43). Injury to the intervertebral disk and the diskovertebral junction can result from acute trauma or from subtle subclinical, often endogenous, injury. Depending on the direction of herniation of disk material, a spectrum of injuries of the intervertebral disk and adjacent vertebrae may be seen (Fig. 3.44).

Anterior Disk Herniation

When the normal attachments of the annulus fibrosus to the vertebral rim by Sharpey fibers and those to the anterior longitudinal ligament loosen, disk material (nucleus pulposus) herniates anteriorly. Elevation of the anterior longitudinal ligament by herniating material stimulates the formation of peripheral osteophytes, leading to a degenerative condition known as spondylosis deformans, which can be demonstrated on the lateral view of the lumbar spine (Fig. 3.45A). Anterior herniation can also be demonstrated by diskography (Fig. 3.45B).

Intravertebral Disk Herniation

Ventrocaudal disk herniation, as well as the much less common, ventrocephalad herniation, produces an abnormality known as *limbus vertebra*. Herniation of disk material into a vertebral body at the site of attachment of the annulus fibrosus to the body's rim separates a small, triangular fragment of bone, which is commonly mistaken for an acute fracture or infectious spondylitis. Reactive bone sclerosis adjacent to the defect, however, indicates a chronic process. The adjacent disk space is invariably narrowed, and a radiolucent cleft known as the *vacuum phenomenon* may be seen in the disk space, representing degeneration of the disk (Fig. 3.46).

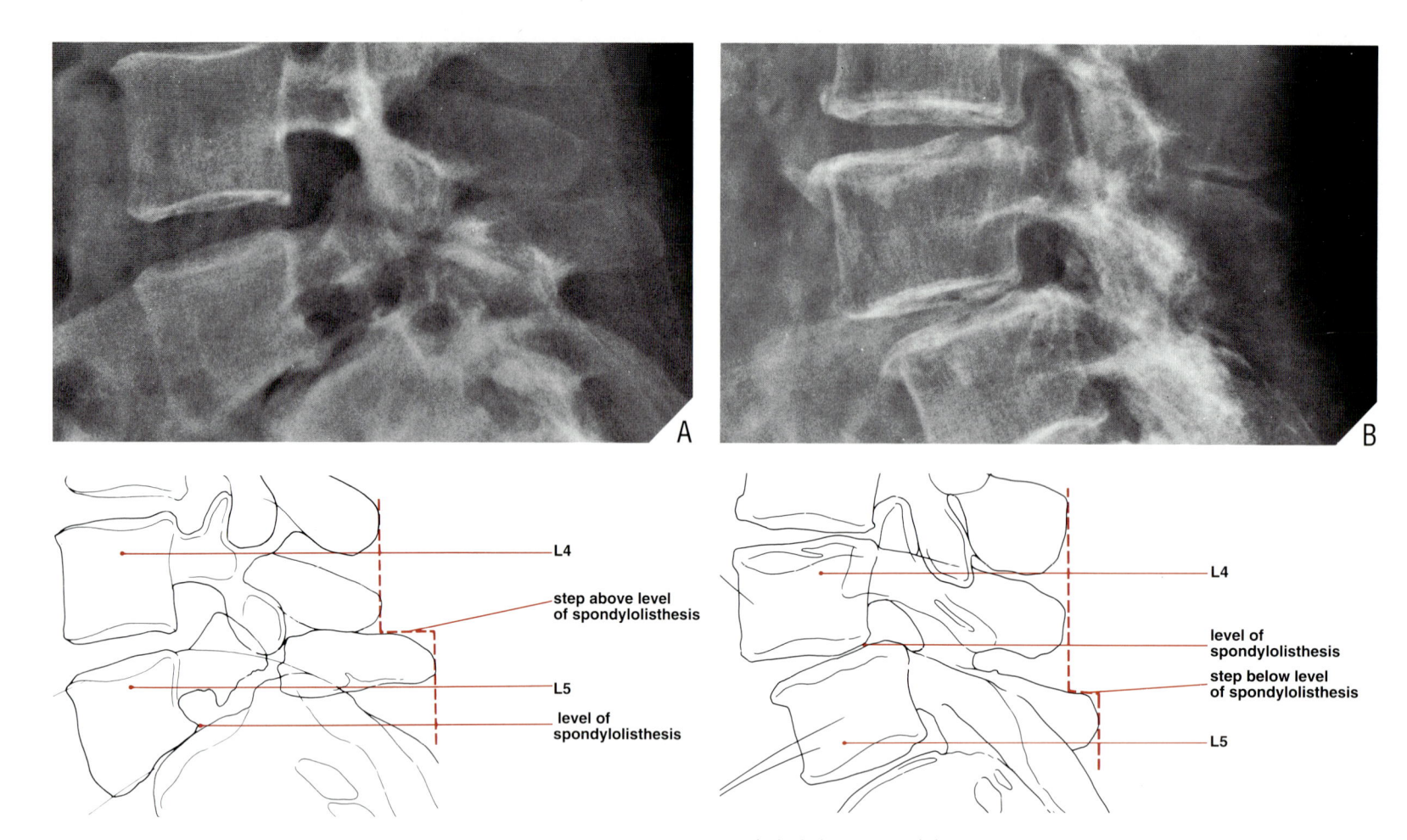

FIGURE 3.39 (A) Lateral view of the lumbar spine demonstrates the typical appearance of spondylolisthesis secondary to a defect in the pars interarticularis. Note that the most dorsal aspect of the spinous process of L5 forms a step with that of L4 above the level of slippage of L5. **(B)** In spondylolisthesis without spondylolysis (degenerative spondylolisthesis), a step-off in the spinous processes below the level of vertebral slippage is an identifying feature. Oblique plain film **(C)** and trispiral tomogram **(D)** of the lumbar spine in a 28-year-old man show a defect in the pars inarticularis (neck of the "Scotty dog") of L4 typical of spondylolysis. **(E)** CT section through the body clearly demonstrates defects in the left and right pars interarticularis. **(F)** Lateral spot film obtained during myelography shows an extradural defect, similar to that of disk herniation, on the ventral aspect of the thecal sac due to grade 2 spondylolisthesis at L4–L5.

FIGURE 3.39 (cont.)

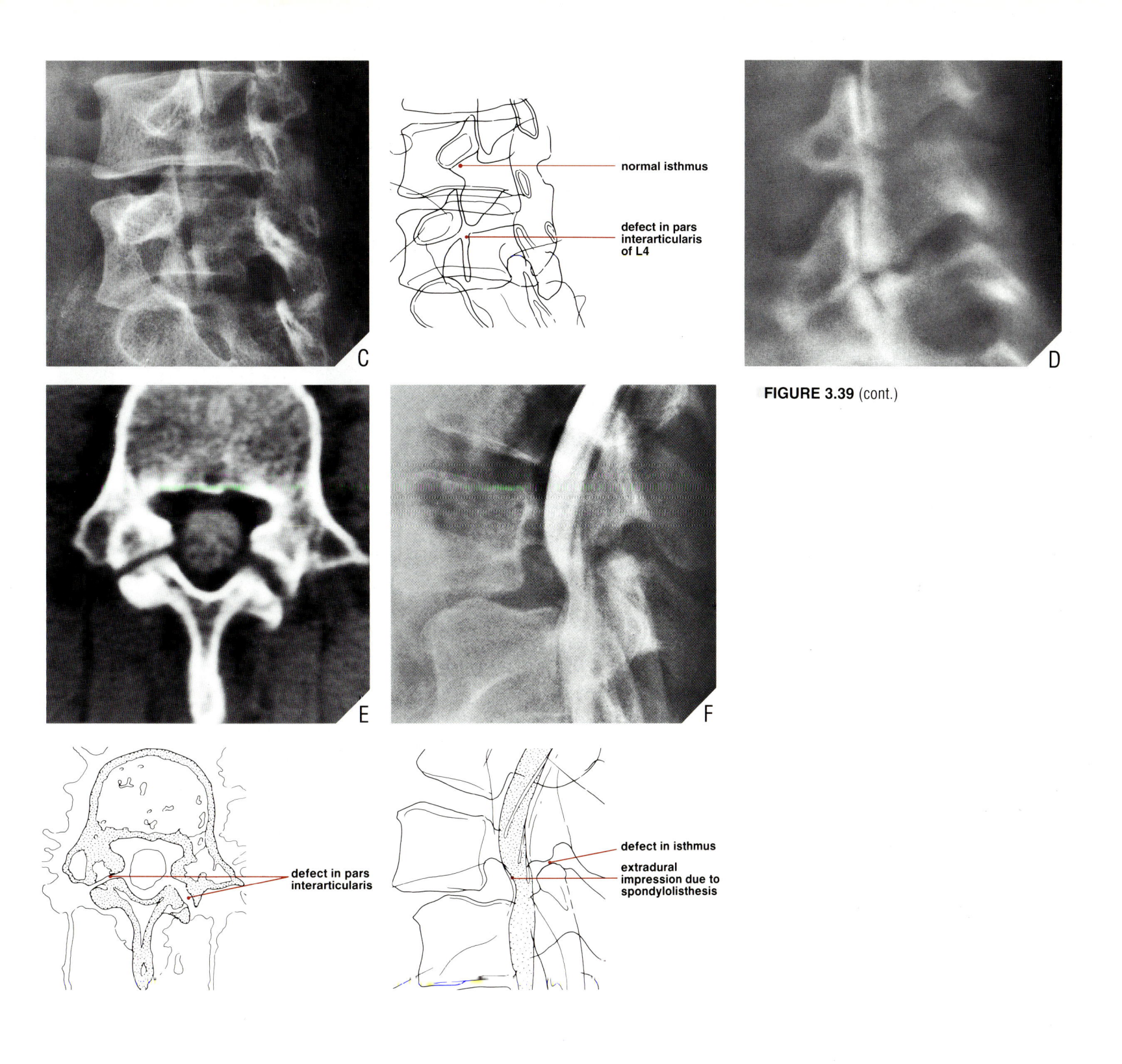

Injury to the Thoracolumbar Spine **3.33**

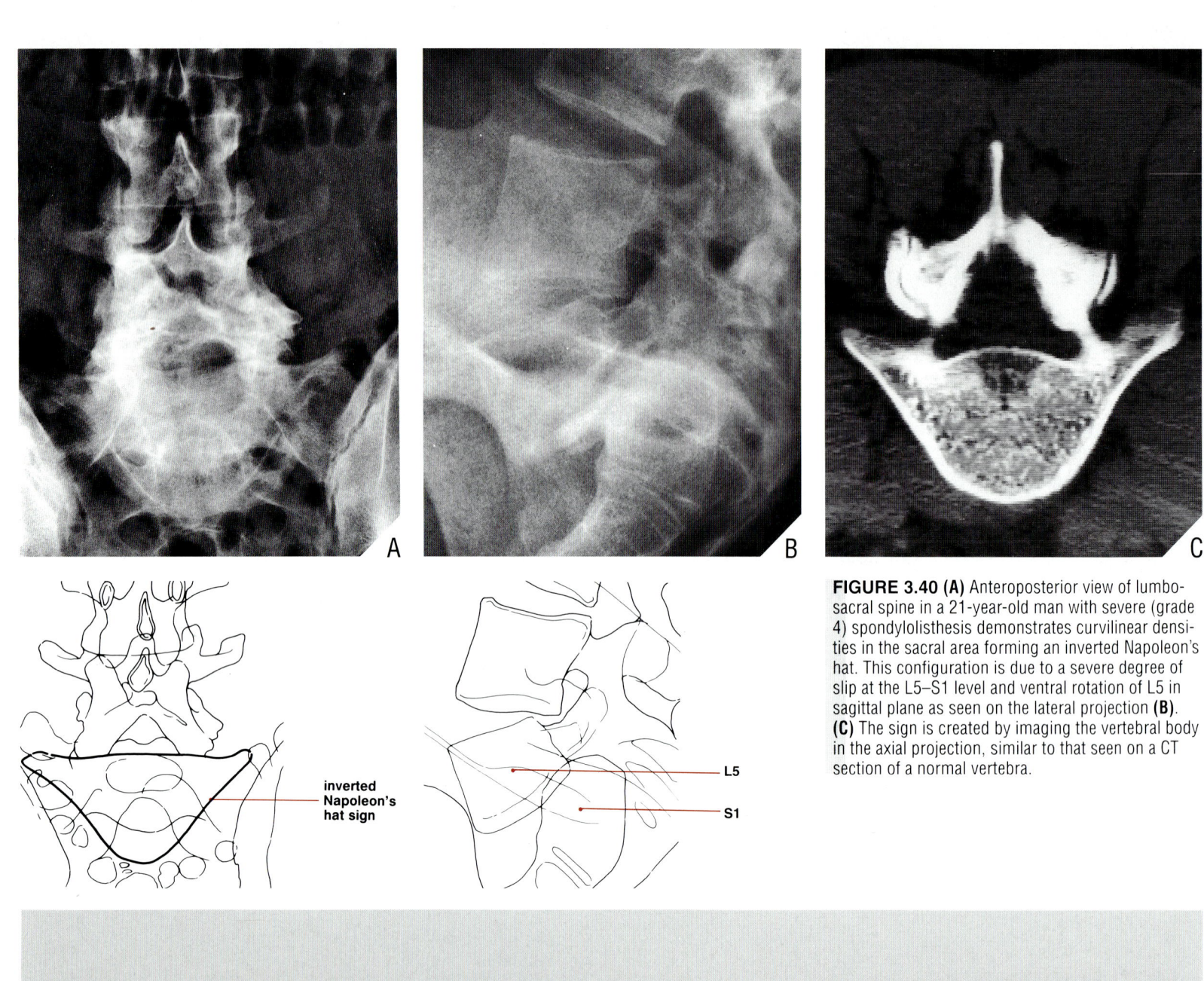

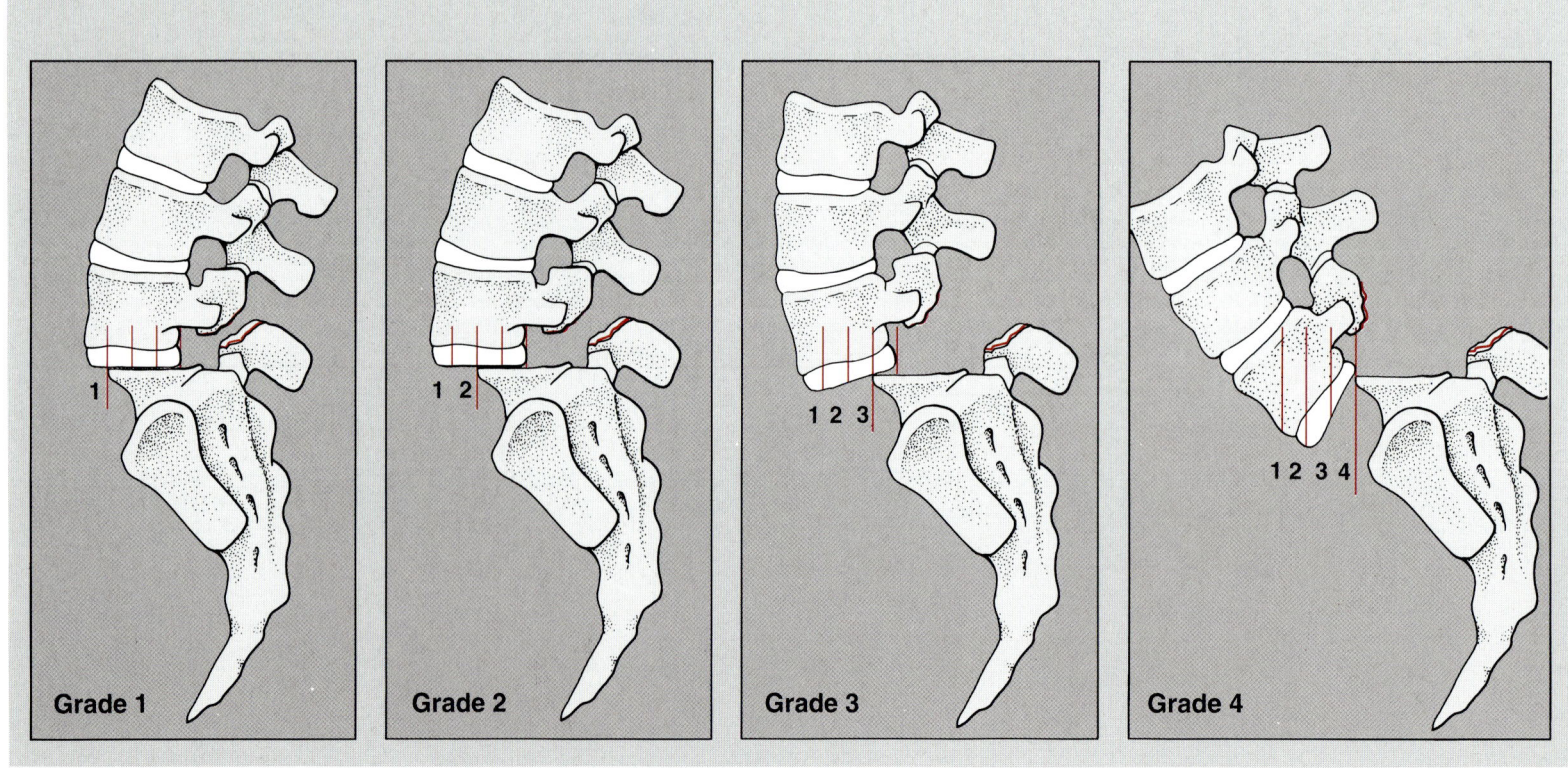

FIGURE 3.40 (A) Anteroposterior view of lumbosacral spine in a 21-year-old man with severe (grade 4) spondylolisthesis demonstrates curvilinear densities in the sacral area forming an inverted Napoleon's hat. This configuration is due to a severe degree of slip at the L5–S1 level and ventral rotation of L5 in sagittal plane as seen on the lateral projection **(B)**. **(C)** The sign is created by imaging the vertebral body in the axial projection, similar to that seen on a CT section of a normal vertebra.

FIGURE 3.41 The grading of spondylolisthesis, as proposed by Meyerding, is based on the amount of forward displacement of L5 on S1.

Imaging of the Spine in Clinical Practice

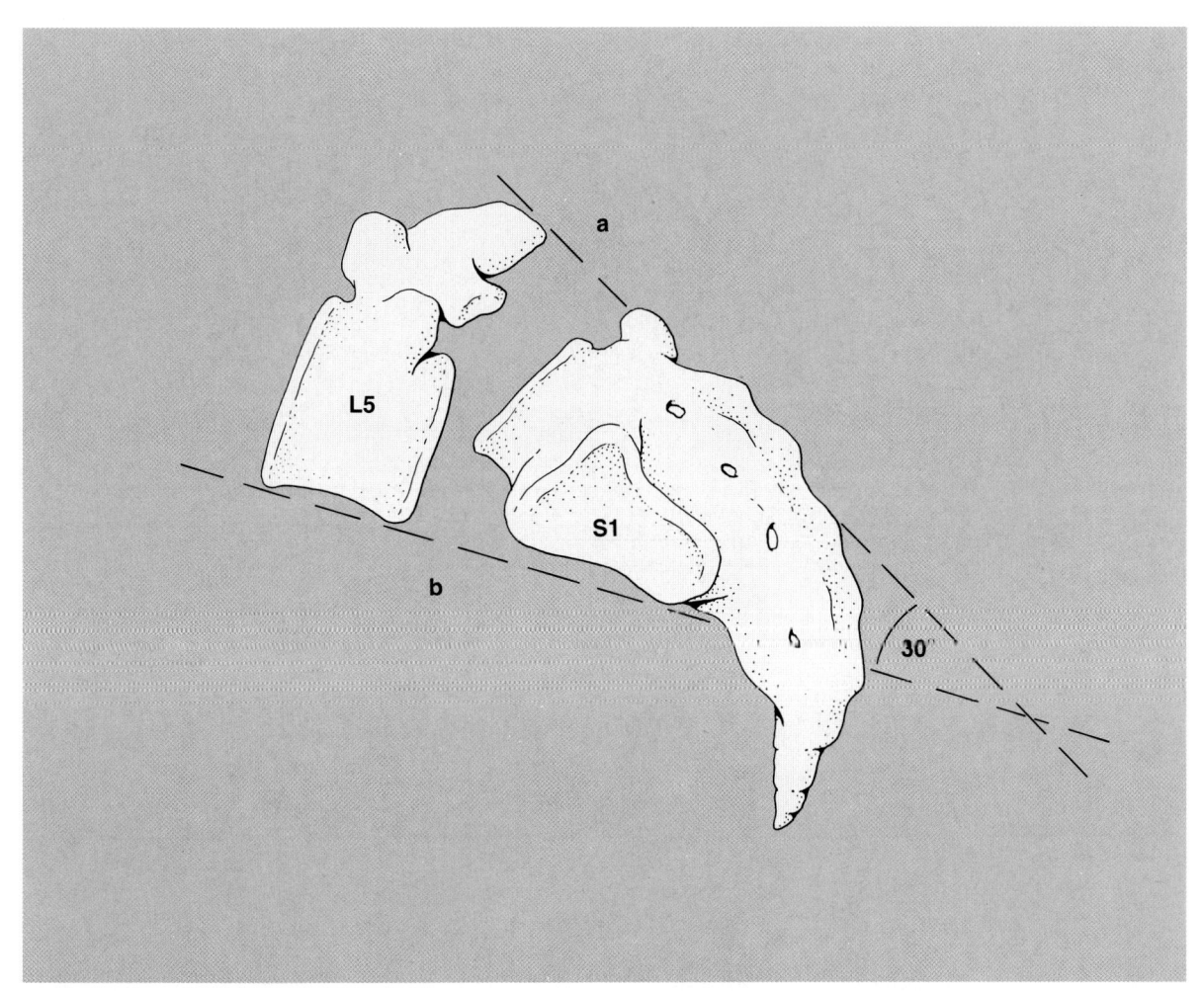

FIGURE 3.42 Ventral rotation of L5 in sagittal plane is determined by the angular relationship between L5 and S1. It is measured by extending a line along the posterior aspect of the body of S1 (a) and another line along the anterior aspect of L5 (b). The intersection of these two lines form an angle of rotation (or "slip angle"). (Modified from Wiltse LL, Winter RB: Terminology and measurement of spondylolisthesis. *J Bone Joint Surg* 65A:768, 1983)

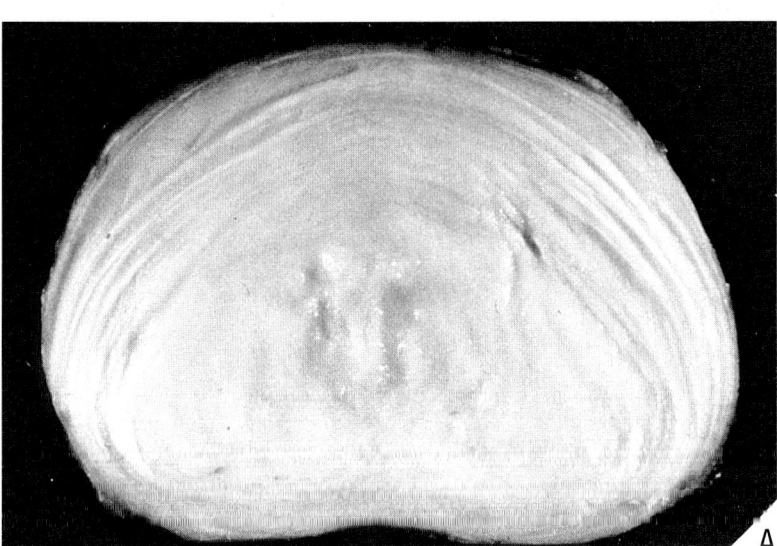

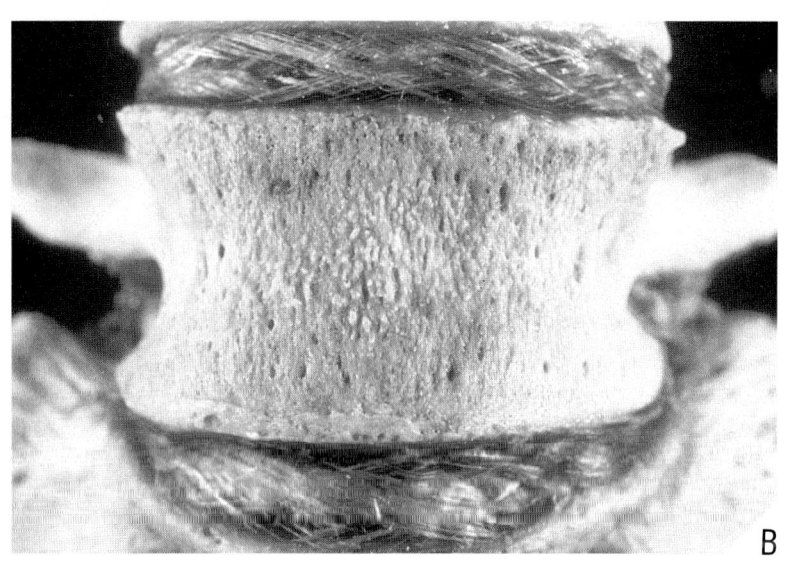

FIGURE 3.43 (A) Intervertebral disk seen from above. Note the layers of circumferential fibers that make up the annulus fibrosus in comparison to the bulging central mass of the nucleus pulposus. **(B)** Frontal view of L5 with the adjacent intervertebral disks. Note the oblique disposition of the collagen fibers of the annulus fibrosus in this macerated specimen. (Reproduced with permission from Bullough PG, Boachie-Adjei O: *Atlas of Spinal Diseases*. New York, Gower, 1988)

Injury to the Thoracolumbar Spine **3.35**

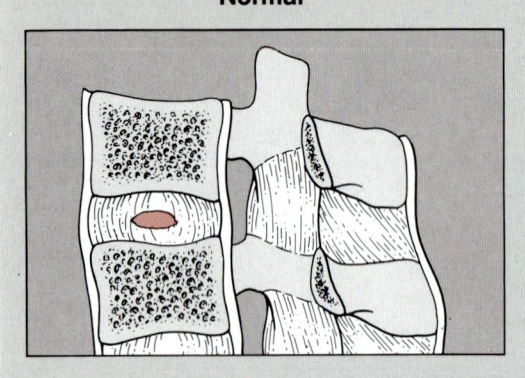

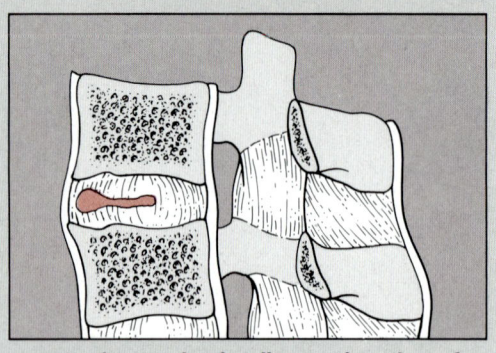

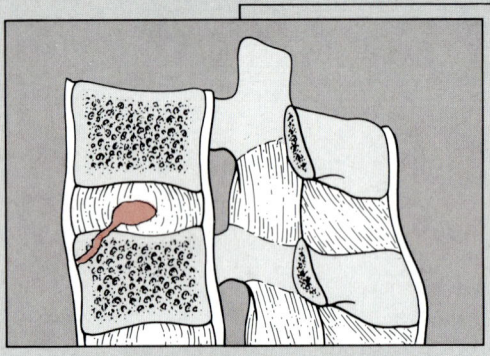

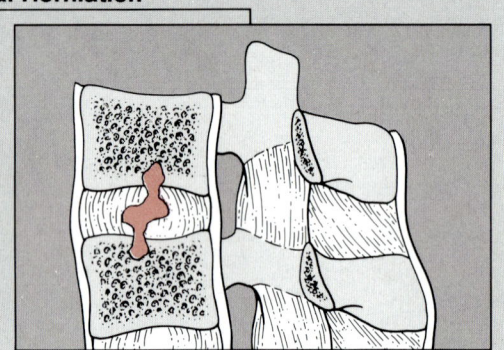

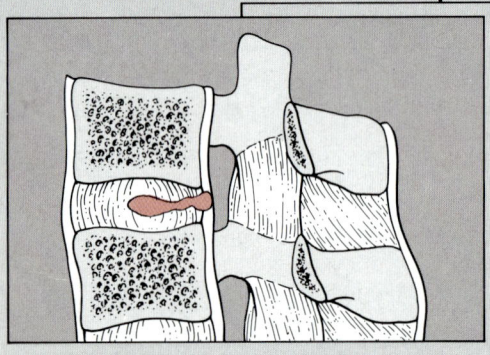

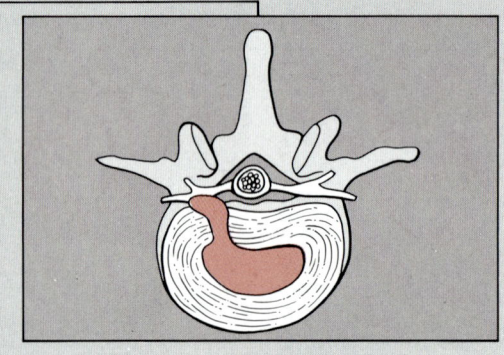

FIGURE 3.44 The spectrum of intervertebral disk herniation.

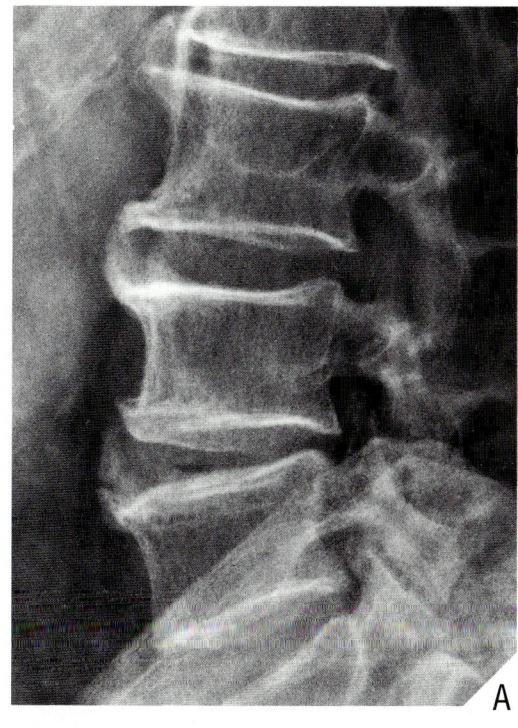

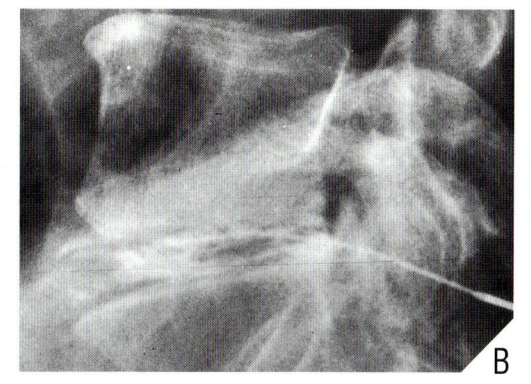

FIGURE 3.45 (A) Lateral view of the lumbar spine shows a late stage of spondylosis deformans at the L2–L3, L3–L4, and L4–L5 levels characterized by large osteophytes on the anterior aspects of adjacent vertebral bodies as a result of anterior disk herniation. **(B)** Anterior disk herniation can also be identified on diskography by contrast outlining the extruded material, as seen here at the L5–S1 level.

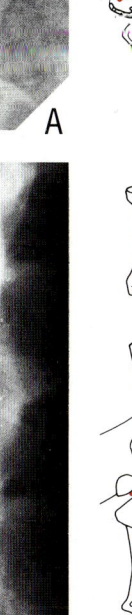

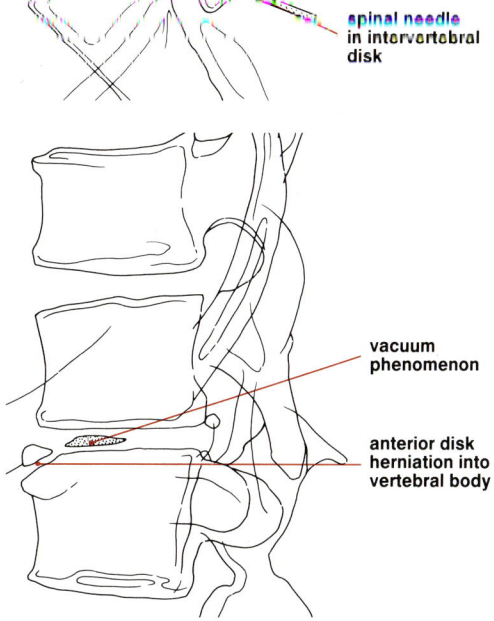

FIGURE 3.46 Lateral view of the lumbar spine in a 55-year-old woman with breast cancer who underwent radiographic examination to exclude bone metastases shows anterior disk herniation into the body of L2 (limbus vertebra). Note the vacuum phenomenon indicating disk degeneration.

Injury to the Thoracolumbar Spine

This abnormality is invariably asymptomatic because it is the product of chronic, endogenous trauma. The characteristic radiographic changes are best seen on the lateral projection of the lumbar spine; only rarely is conventional tomography (Fig. 3.47A) or CT (Fig. 3.47B) necessary to exclude a true vertebral fracture. Occasionally, more than one vertebra is affected, and although limbus vertebra is usually seen in the lumbar spine it may also be present in a thoracic vertebra.

Limbus vertebra should not be confused with the secondary ossification centers of the vertebral ring apophysis that are commonly seen in the growing skeleton (Fig. 3.48); at skeletal maturity, these centers become fully united with the vertebral body.

Intravertebral disk herniation may also occur when the nucleus pulposus breaks through the vertebral endplate, extruding into a vertebra. This abnormality may be the result of acute trauma, as in a burst fracture, but much more commonly it is secondary to weakening of the vertebral body, as in osteoporosis. In the latter condition the lesion is known as a *Schmorl node*. It may be large and diffuse (often referred to as *ballooned disk*, Fig. 3.49) or small and localized.

Involvement of more than three consecutive thoracic vertebrae by Schmorl nodes is frequently seen in *Scheuermann disease*. This condition, which usually affects adolescent boys and young adults, is characterized by anterior wedging of the vertebral bodies and a kyphotic curve of

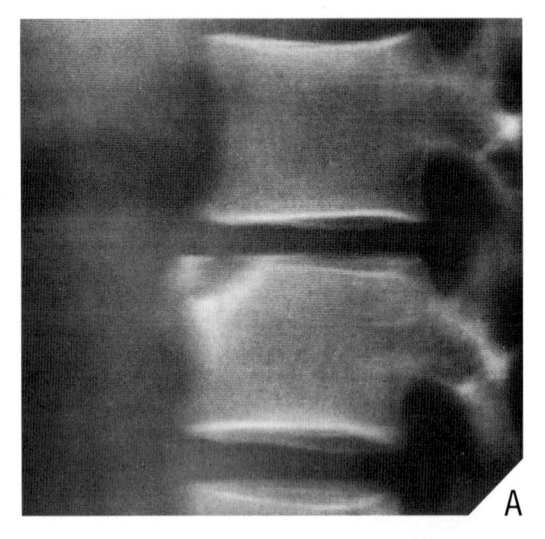

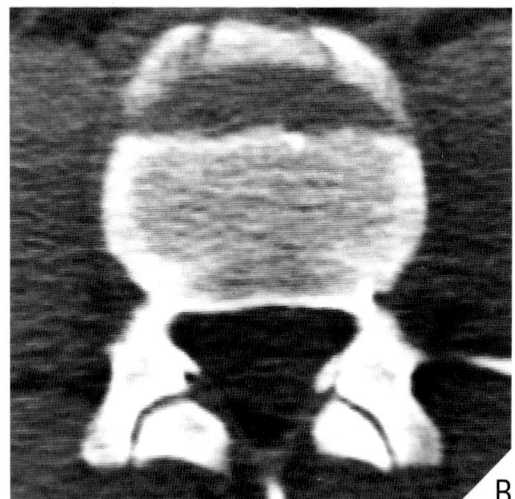

FIGURE 3.47 An 18-year-old male injured his lumbar spine in an automobile accident. The standard radiographic examination was equivocal regarding fracture. **(A)** Lateral tomogram shows the typical appearance of a limbus vertebrae secondary to anterior herniation of the nucleus pulposus. The small triangular segment is separated from the body of L4 by a rim of reactive sclerosis, indicating a chronic process. Note the characteristic disk space narrowing. **(B)** CT examination was performed to investigate the possibility of concomitant posterior disk herniation into the spinal canal. The examination was negative for posterior herniation but confirmed the anterior herniation into the vertebral body, as seen in this more cephalad section.

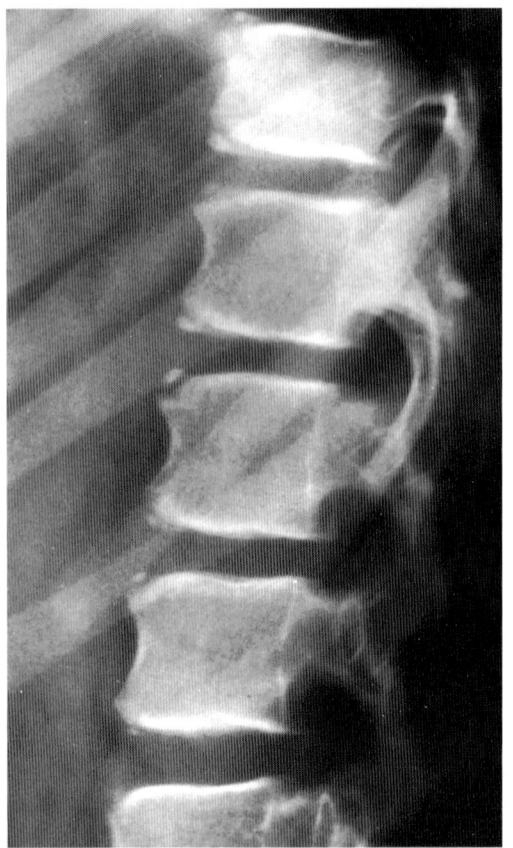

FIGURE 3.48 The secondary ossification centers of the vertebral ring apophysis in the growing skeleton, as seen here in a 5-year-old girl, should not be mistaken for limbus vertebrae.

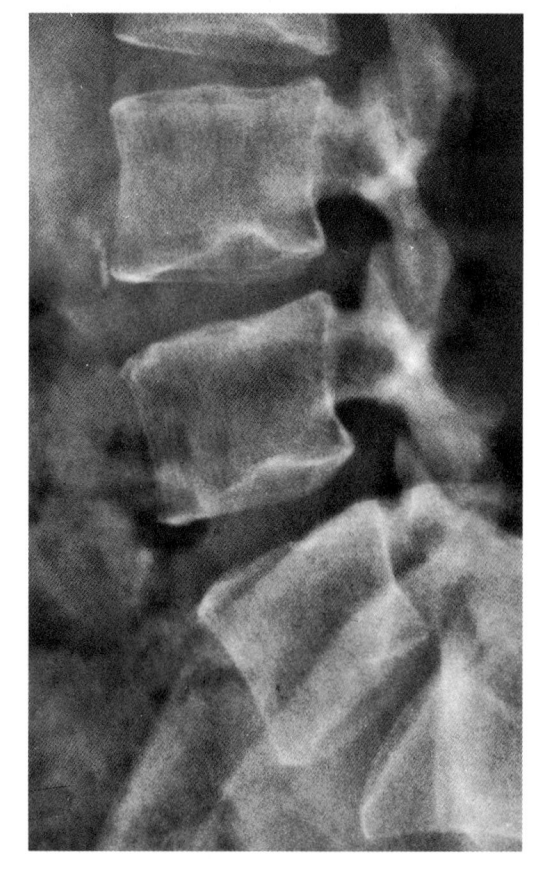

FIGURE 3.49 Lateral radiograph of the lumbar spine in an asymptomatic 77-year-old woman with osteoporosis of the spine shows multiple indentations, particularly of the inferior endplates of the L2 to L5 vertebrae, representing Schmorl nodes, secondary to intravertebral disk herniation due to weakening of the vertebral endplates.

the thoracic spine ("juvenile thoracic kyphosis"), in addition to a wavy outline of the vertebral endplates (Fig. 3.50A). The treatment of this condition usually involves intravertebral bone grafting and posterior instrumentation with Cotrel–Dubousset rods (Figs. 3.50B,C).

Posterior and Posterolateral Disk Herniation

Intraspinal herniation or "herniated disk" is the most serious of the three variants of diskovertebral junction injury. It is most commonly observed in the lumbar spine, particularly at L4–L5 and L5–S1, although it is occasionally seen in the cervical and even in the thoracic region. It is usually associated with clinical symptoms such as sciatica and weakening of the ipsilateral lower extremity, especially when herniation in the lumbar segment causes compression on an exiting nerve root or the thecal sac. A predisposing factor in some patients may be a loss of elasticity of the annulus fibrosus caused by degenerative changes, with subsequent rupture of the annulus or even the posterior longitudinal ligament and retropulsion of the nucleus pulposus into the spinal canal. Typically, the patient is a young adult man, who gives a history of straining his back by lifting a heavy object. The subsequent pain in the lumbar region radiates

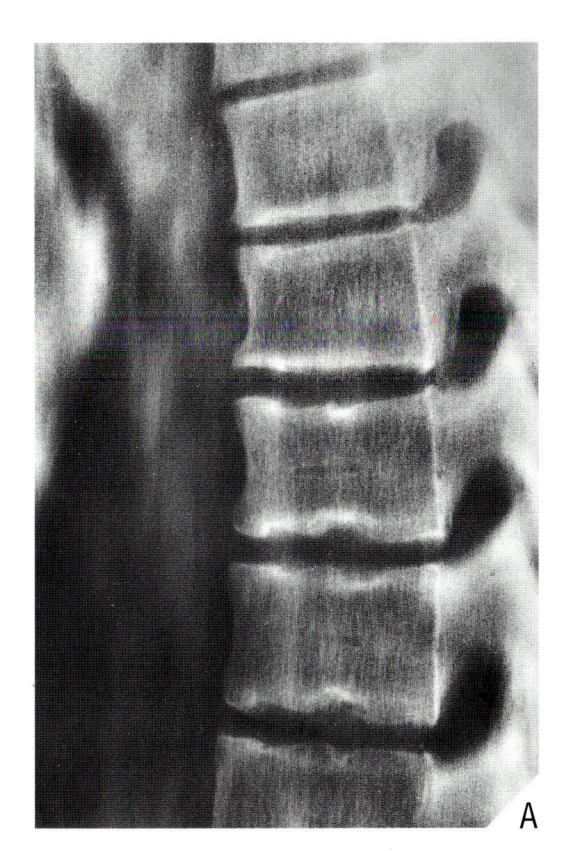

FIGURE 3.50 (A) Lateral tomogram of the thoracic spine in a 23-year-old man demonstrates several Schmorl nodes in T5 to T8 and slight anterior wedging of the bodies. Involvement of multiple thoracic vertebrae by Schmorl nodes is seen in Scheuermann disease, an abnormality called *juvenile thoracic kyphosis*. Note the wavy outline of the superior and inferior endplates and the mild kyphotic curve of the thoracic spine in this patient. **(B,C)** Another patient with Scheuermann juvenile kyphosis has been treated with intervertebral bony grafts and posterior instrumentation using Cotrel–Dubousset hardware and pedical screws. This type of treatment prevents the progression of kyphotic deformity.

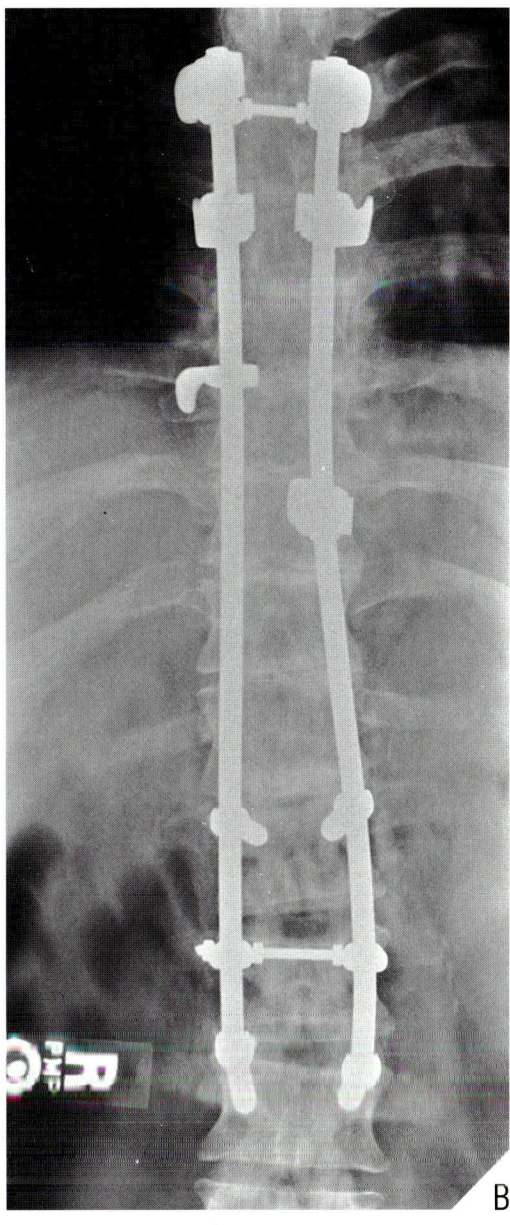

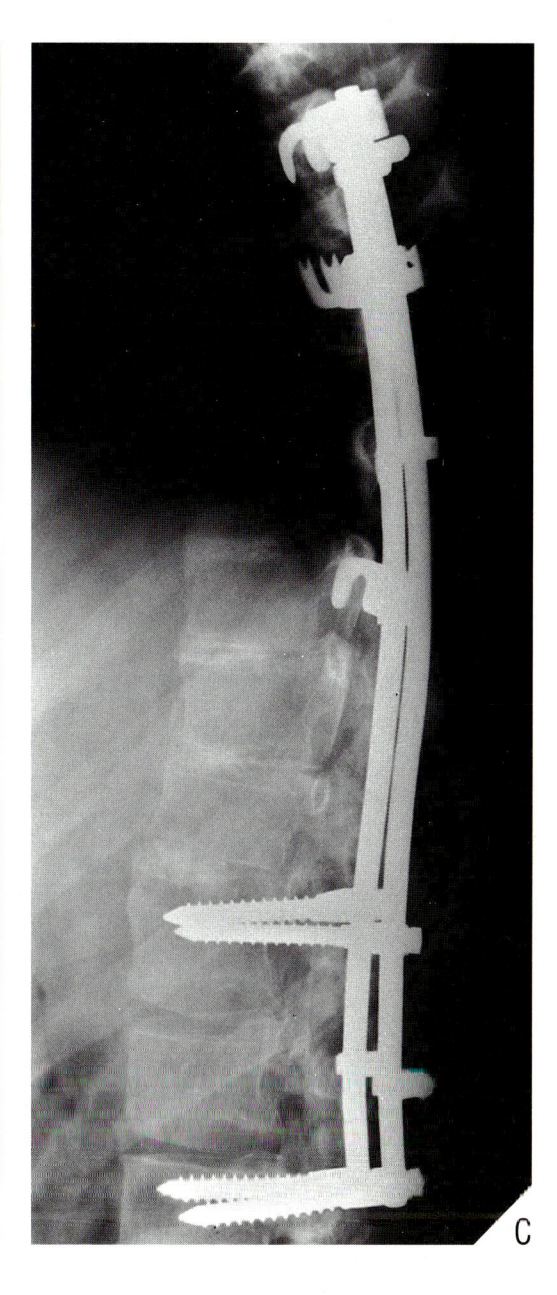

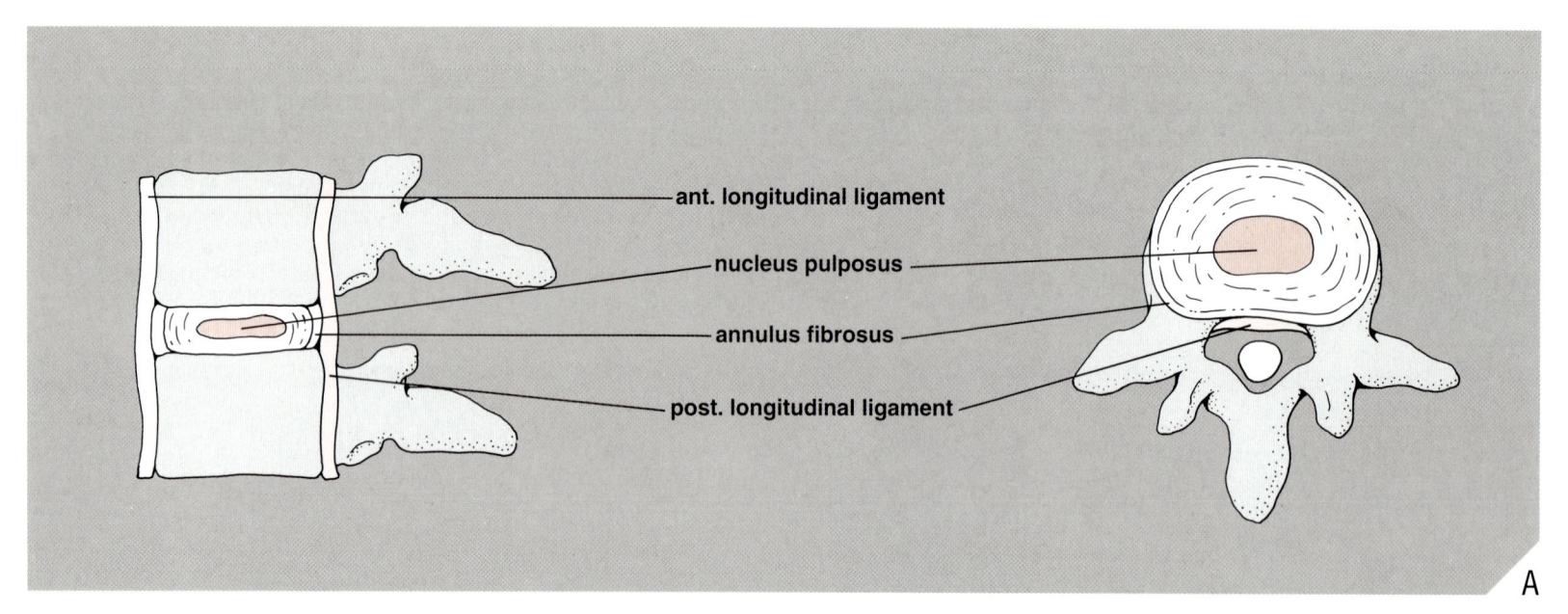

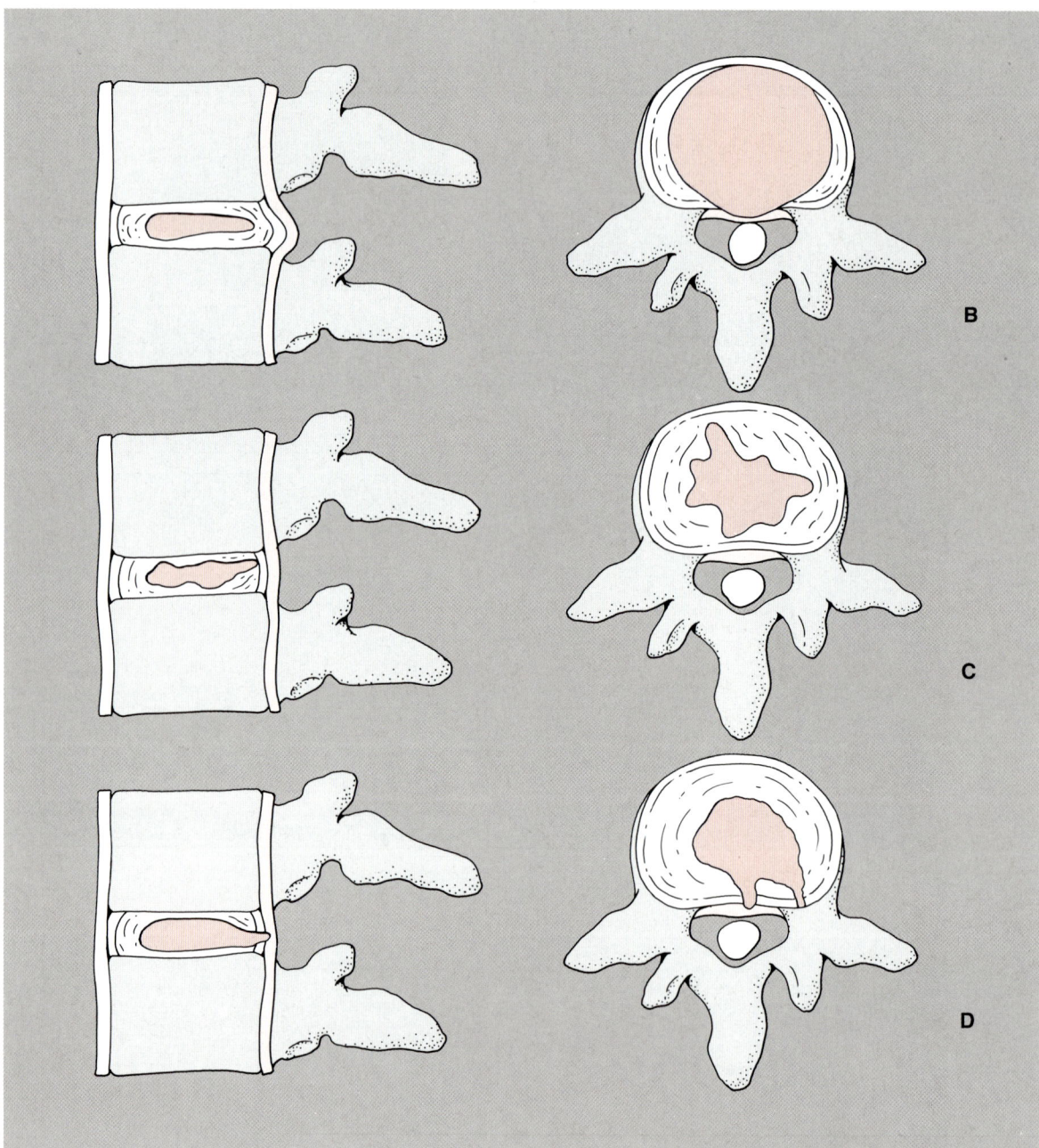

FIGURE 3.51 Staging of disk abnormalities. (A) Stage 0 = normal disk. (B) Stage 1 = bulging disk. (C) Stage 2 = degenerative disk. (D) Stage 3 = annular tear. (E) Stage 4 = herniated disk: (E1) substage 4A = protrusion (intact annulus and PLL); (E2) substage 4B = extrusion (either rupture of annulus and intact PLL, or rupture of both the annulus and PLL); (E3) substage 4C = sequestration of disk fragment in spinal canal (rupture of both annulus and PLL). (Modified from Greenspan A: CT-diskography vs. MRI in the evaluation of intervertebral disk herniation. *Appl Radiol*, in press)

Imaging of the Spine in Clinical Practice

to the posterior aspect of the thigh and buttock and the lateral aspect of the leg, and is aggravated by coughing and sneezing; sometimes there is associated paresthesia or numbness in the foot. Physical examination reveals muscular spasm, limitation of forward bending, and restriction of straight-leg raising on the affected side. Various other symptoms and physical findings may be pres-ent, depending on the level and degree of injury.

The standard radiographic examination in herniated disks is usually normal. Therefore, ancillary radiologic techniques, including myelography and CT either alone or in conjunction with one another, as well as diskography and MRI, are required to make a diagnosis. The staging of disk abnormalities modified by the authors is based on classification scheme proposed by Modic (1989): stage 0, normal disk; stage 1, bulging disk; stage 2, degenerative disk; stage 3, annular tear with no herniation; and stage 4, herniated disk. Stage 4 is further subdivided: substage 4A, protrusion with an intact annulus; substage 4B, extrusion with either rupture of annulus and intact posterior longitudinal ligament, or rupture of both the annulus and the posterior longitudinal ligament; and substage 4C, rupture of the annulus and the posterior longitudinal ligament with sequestration of a disk fragment in spinal canal (Fig. 3.51). The myelographic findings in disk herniation may be very subtle, such as absent

FIGURE 3.51 (cont.)

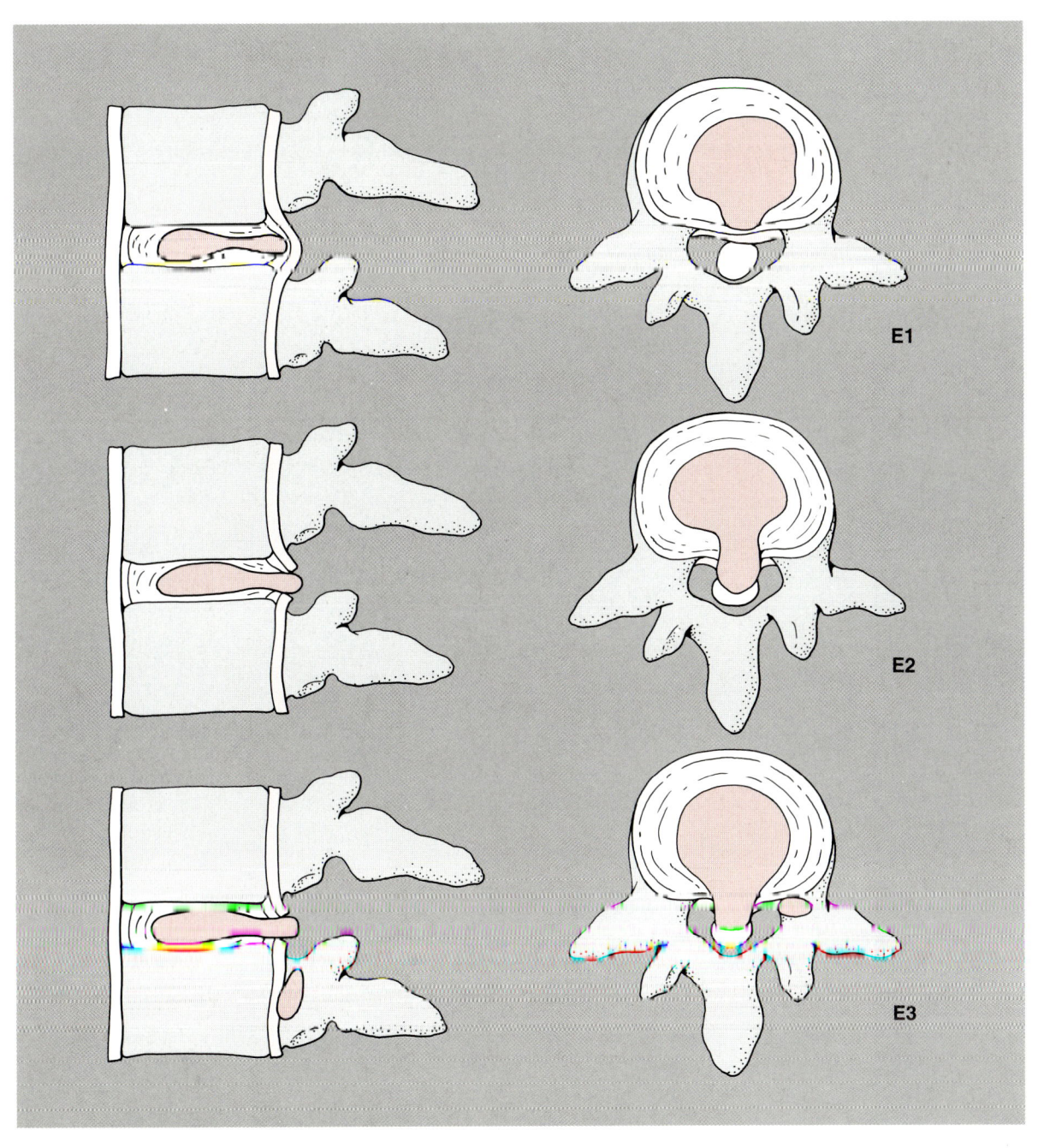

opacification of a nerve sheath (Fig. 3.52), or more obvious, such as an extradural pressure defect in the contrast-filled thecal sac (Fig. 3.53). Disk herniation can also be diagnosed on plain CT examination (Fig. 3.54), on CT sections obtained following myelography (Fig. 3.55) or diskography (Fig. 3.56), and on MRI examination (Fig. 3.57).

MRI is being used increasingly for the diagnosis of conditions that cause acute low back pain and sciatica. The sensitivity of MRI in the diagnosis of herniated disk and spinal stenosis is equivalent to or better than that of CT, even when the latter is combined with myelography. Radicular symptoms represent one of the most common reasons for patient referral for MRI of

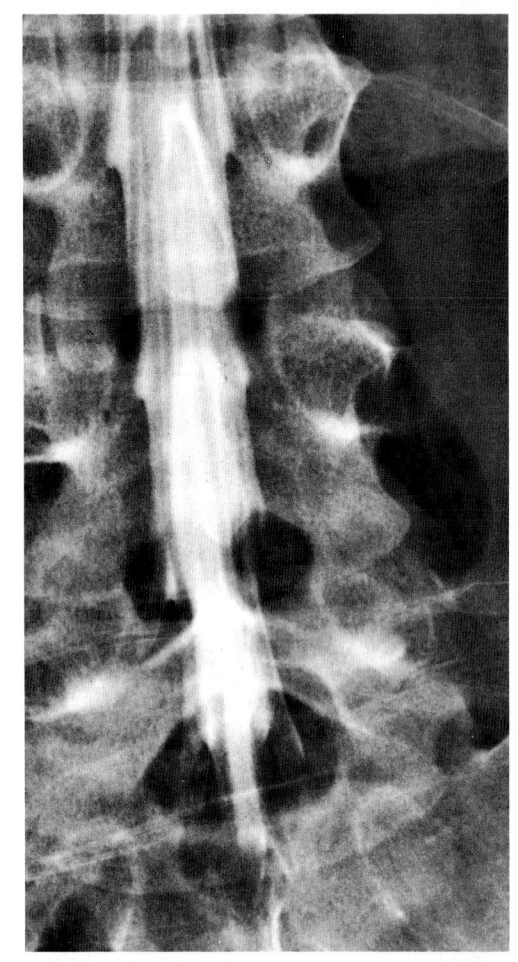

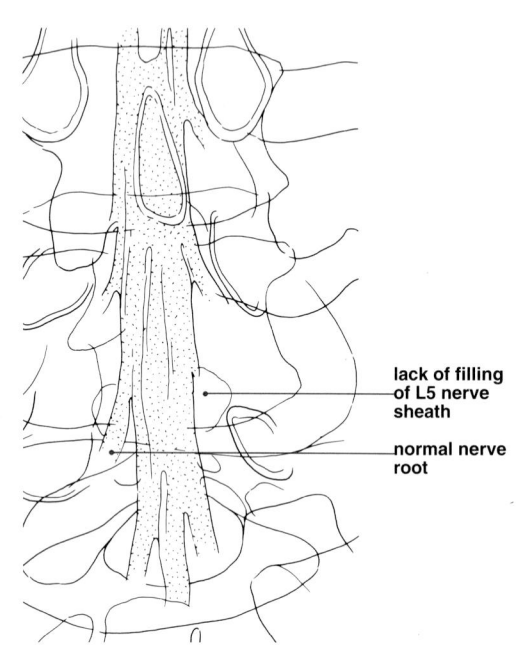

FIGURE 3.52 In lifting a heavy object, a 27-year-old man felt sudden, sharp pain in the lower back radiating to the left lower extremity. The standard radiographs of the lumbosacral spine were normal. Myelogram shows a subtle lack of filling of the left L5 nerve sheath, which at surgery was found to be compressed by a lateral herniation of the L4–L5 disk.

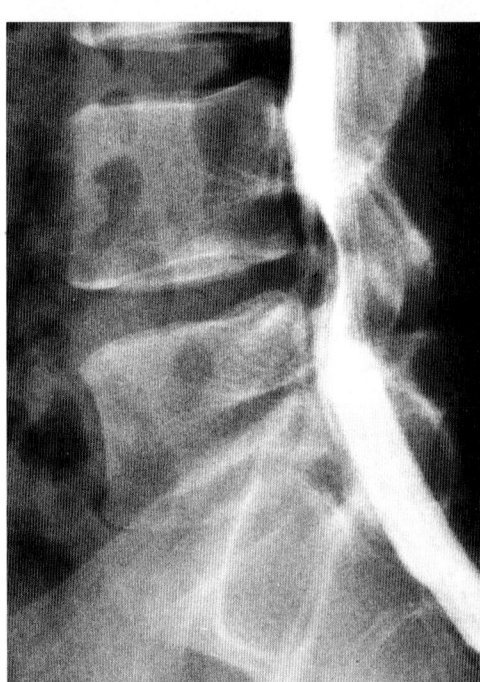

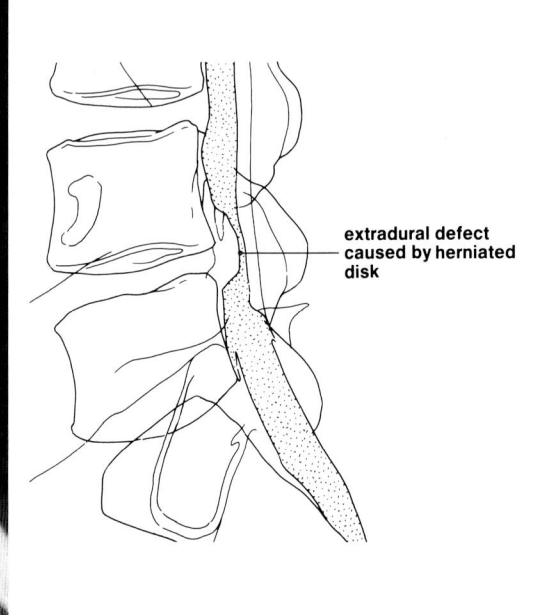

FIGURE 3.53 Lateral spot film obtained during myelography in a 38-year-old man demonstrates a large posterior herniation of the intervertebral disk at L4–L5.

Imaging of the Spine in Clinical Practice

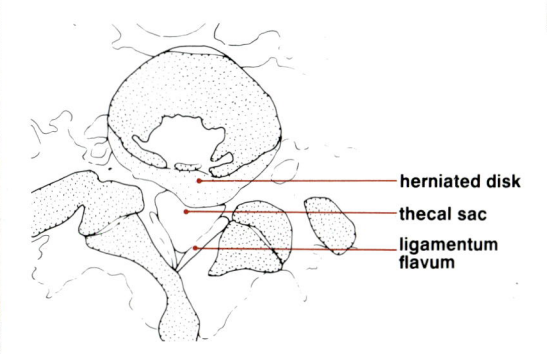

FIGURE 3.54 CT section of the lumbar spine at the L5–S1 level shows a large centrolateral disk herniation encroaching on the left neural foramen.

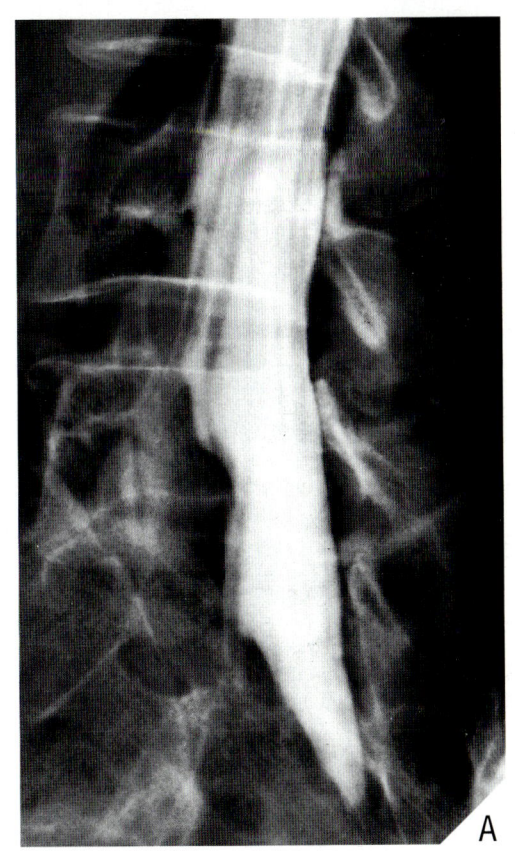

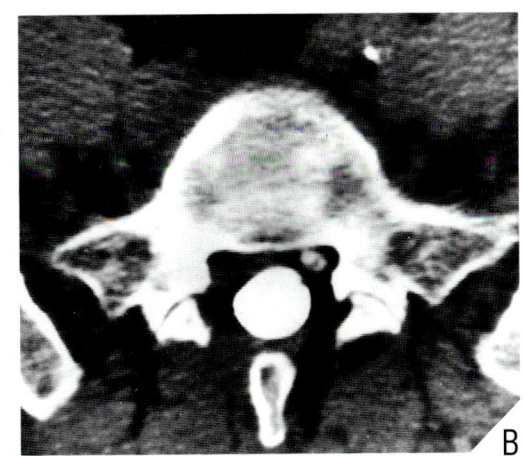

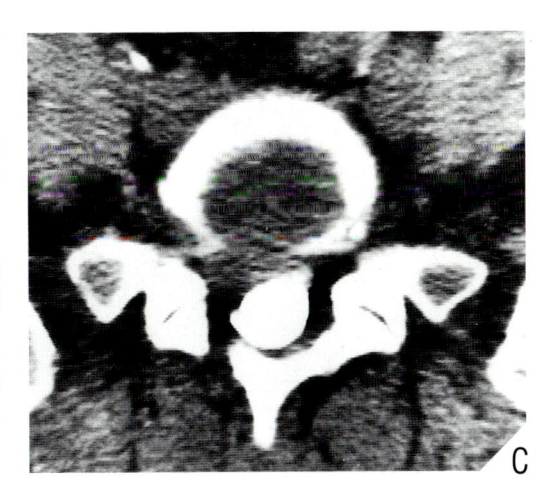

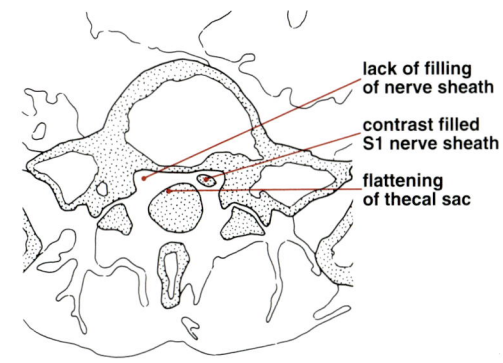

FIGURE 3.55 A 47-year-old man presented with severe back pain radiating to the right buttock and leg. **(A)** Spot film in the oblique projection obtained during myelography shows an extradural defect on the right side of the thecal sac at the L5–S1 disk space involving the right S1 nerve root. The L5 and S2 nerve roots are normally outlined. **(B,C)** Postmyelography CT sections demonstrate the lack of opacification of the S1 nerve root on the right side and a large herniation of the L5–S1 disk compressing the thecal sac.

Injury to the Thoracolumbar Spine   **3.43**

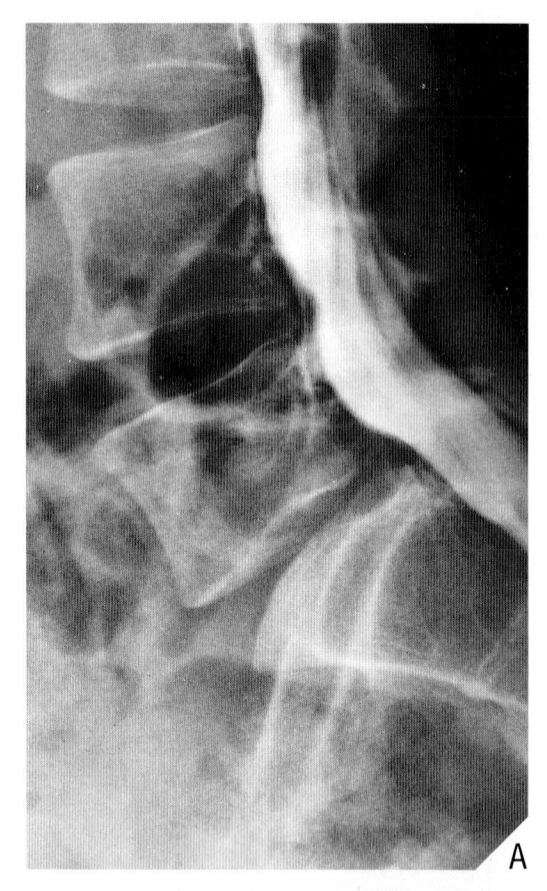

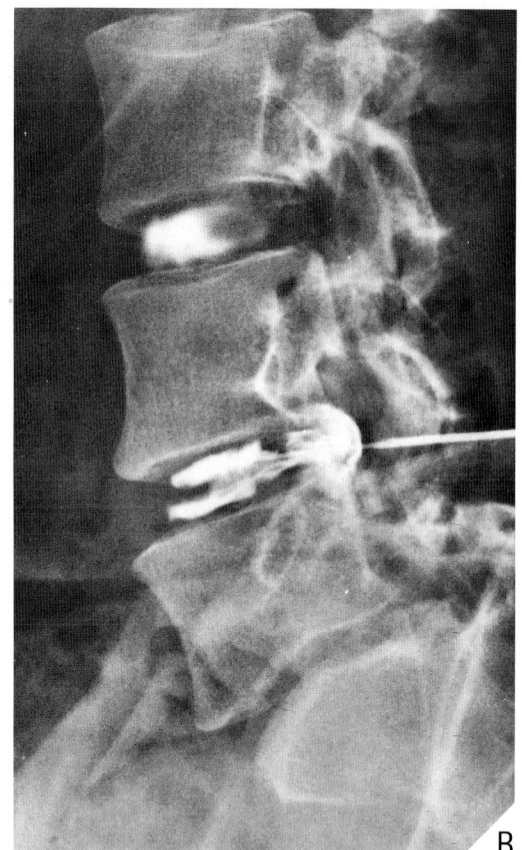

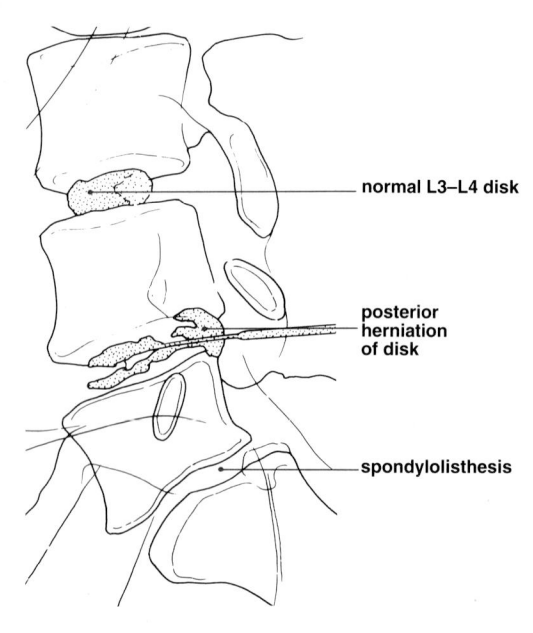

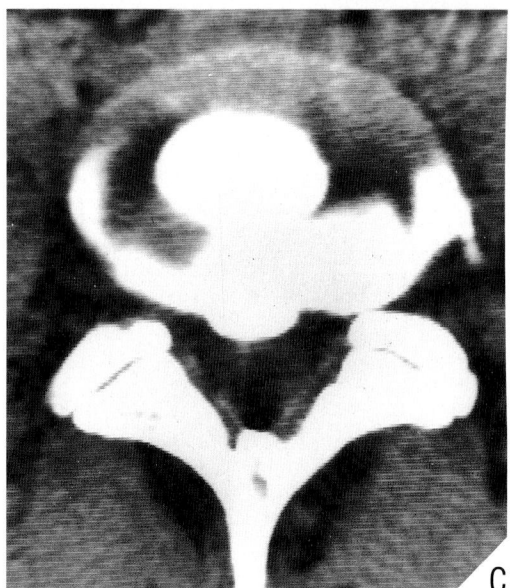

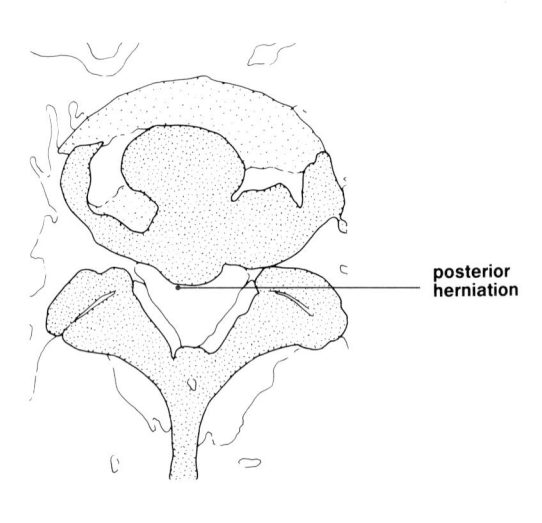

FIGURE 3.56 A 30-year-old male construction worker strained his lower back at work and was admitted to the hospital with severe sciatica. **(A)** Lateral view of the lumbar spine during myelographic examination reveals a slight separation of the ventral aspect of the dural sac from the dorsal aspect of L5 due to grade-1 spondylolisthesis. In addition, there is an extradural pressure defect on the ventral aspect of the thecal sac at the L4–L5 level and a much smaller defect at the L3–L4 disk space. **(B)** A diskogram using metrizamide was performed at the L3–L4 and L4–L5 levels, the latter demonstrating posterior herniation. **(C)** CT scan at the L4–L5 level following diskography shows posterior protrusion of the opacified disk material.

Imaging of the Spine in Clinical Practice

the spine. MRI is a particularly sensitive modality for detection and characterization of disk herniation, because it allows direct evaluation of the internal morphology of the disk. The sagittal imaging plane is very effective for identifying disk impingement on the thecal sac, and for demonstration of extruded fragments and their relationship to the vertebral bodies and intervertebral disk spaces (see Fig. 3.57A). The axial imaging plane can demonstrate the effect of the herniated disk on the exiting nerve roots and thecal sac (see Fig. 3.57B). Axial images are also important in evaluating neural foramina and nerve root effacement in cases of lateral and posterolateral disk herniation. Free disk fragments can be easily identified.

Use of T1-weighted images in the axial plane provides excellent contrast between high signal of fat and low signal of thecal sac, nerve roots, and disk fragments. Fast-scan techniques provide increased signal of CSF and allow increased contrast between herniated fragments and CSF. Some advantages of MRI in comparison with myelography and CT of lumbar disk degeneration are evident. MRI is sensitive to the water content of the nucleus pulposus. As the water content of this structure decreases with aging or degeneration, decreased signal is particularly notable on T2-weighted images. In addition, the myelographic effect that is provided by heavily T2-weighted images and fast-scan techniques allows the visualization of nerve roots within the thecal sac. Anomalies such as conjoint nerve roots, which may simulate herniated nucleus pulposus on CT studies, can be visualized directly with MRI. It must be stressed, however, that the evaluation of patients with radiculopathy and herniated disk is an area in which both MRI and CT can be complementary. When an extradural defect is identified by MRI yet it may be difficult to ascertain whether the lesion represents a herniated nucleus pulposus or an osteophyte, CT can make the distinction easily by identifying the increased mineralization within the osteophyte. When the herniated fragment is clearly in continuity with the intervertebral disk and of the same signal intensity, the diagnosis of disk herniation is suggested by MRI alone.

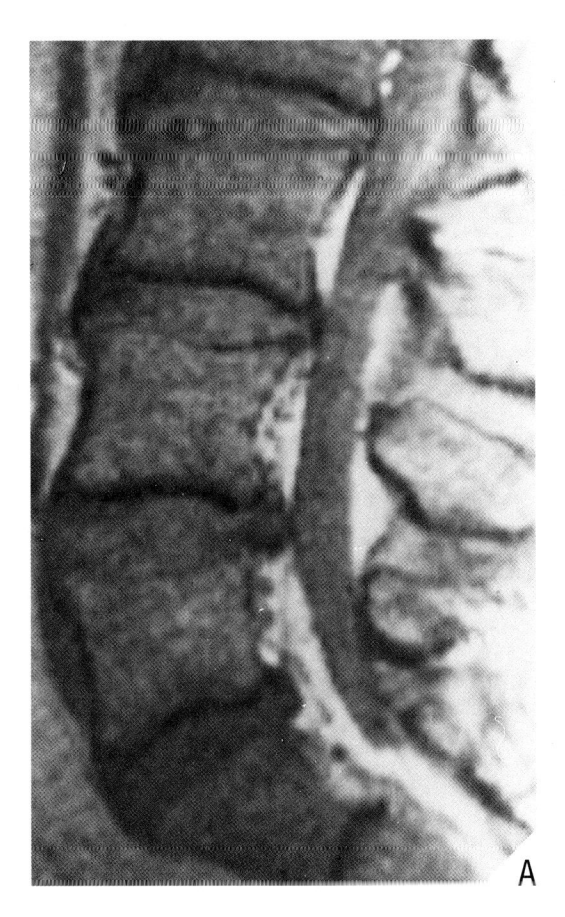

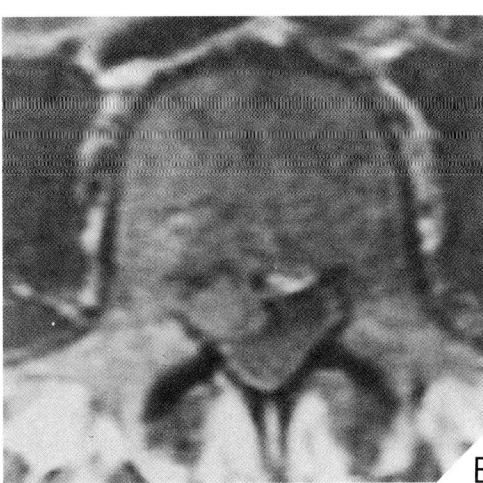

FIGURE 3.57 A 44-year-old man presented with sciatic pain radiating to the right buttock and thigh. **(A)** Sagittal MRI (SE, TR 1500/TE 20) demonstrates a posterior herniation of the disk L4-L5 and a bulging disk at L5-S1. **(B)** Axial MRI (SE, TR 1500/TE 30) clearly shows posterolateral disk herniation with marked compression of the thecal sac.

Suggested Reading

Amato M, Toffy WG, Gilula LA: Spondylolysis of the lumbar spine: Demonstration of defects and laminal fragmentation. *Radiology* 153:627, 1984.

Anand AK, Lee BP: Plain and metrizamide CT of lumbar disk disease: Comparison with myelography. *Am J Nucl Radiol* 3:567, 1982.

Boden SD, Davis DO, Dina TS, et al: Abnormal magnetic-resonance scans of the lumbar spine in asymptomatic subjects. *J Bone Joint Surg* 72A:403, 1990.

Brodsky AE, Binder WF: Lumbar discography—Its value in diagnosis and treatment of lumbar disc lesions. *Spine* 4:110, 1979.

Brown R, Evans ET: What causes the "eye in the Scotty dog" in the oblique projection of the lumbar spine? *Am J Roentgenol* 118:435, 1973.

Bryk D, Rosenkranz W: True spondylolisthesis and pseudospondylolisthesis—The spinous process sign. *J Can Assoc Radiol* 20:53, 1969.

Collins JS Jr, Gardner WJ: Lumbar discography: An analysis of one thousand cases. *J Neurosurg* 19:452, 1962.

Daffner RH: Injuries of the thoracolumbar vertebral column. In Dalinka MK, Kaye JJ (eds): *Radiology in Emergency Room Medicine*. New York, Churchill Livingstone, 1984.

Denis F: Spinal instability as defined by the three-column spine concept in acute spinal trauma. *Clin Orthop* 189:65, 1984.

Denis F: The three column spine and its significance in the classification of acute thoracolumbar spine injuries. *Spine* 8:817, 1983.

Dietz GW, Christensen EE: Normal "Cupid's bow" contour of the lower lumbar vertebrae. *Radiology* 121:577, 1976.

Dortwarth RH, DeGroot J, Sauerland EK, et al: Computed tomography of the lumbosacral spine: Normal anatomy, anatomic variants and pathologic anatomy. *RadioGraphics* 2:459, 1982.

Dublin AB, McGahan JP, Reid MH: The value of computed tomographic metrizamide myelography in the neuroradiological evaluation of the spine. *Radiology* 146:79, 1983.

Epstein BS, Epstein JA, Jones MD: Lumbar spondylolisthesis with isthmic defect. *Radiol Clin North Am* 15:261, 1977.

Ferguson RL, Allen BL Jr: A mechanistic classification of thoracolumbar spine fractures. *Clin Orthop* 189:77, 1984.

Firooznia H, Benjamin V, Kricheff II, et al: CT of lumbar spine disc herniation: Correlation with surgical findings. *Am J Roentgenol* 142:587, 1984.

Gehweiler JA, Osborn RL, Becker FG: *The Radiology of Vertebral Trauma*. Philadelphia, W B Saunders, 1980.

Glickstein MF, Burke DL, Kressel HY: Magnetic resonance demonstration of hyperintense herniated discs and extruded disc fragments. *Skeletal Radiol* 18:527, 1989.

Greenspan A: CT-diskography vs. MRI in the evaluation of intervertebral disk herniation. *Appl Radiol* (in press).

Guerra J Jr, Garfin SR, Resnick D: Vertebral burst fractures: CT analysis of the retropulsed fragment. *Radiology* 153:769, 1984.

Gumley G, Taylor TKF, Ryan MD: Distraction fractures of the lumbar spine. *J Bone Joint Surg* 64B:520, 1982.

Harrington PR, Tullos HS: Spondylolisthesis in children: Observations and surgical treatment. *Clin Orthop* 79:75, 1971.

Hartman JT, Kendrick I, Lorman P: Discography as an aid in evaluation for lumbar and lumbosacral fusion. *Clin Orthop* 81:77, 1971.

Haughton VM: MR imaging of the spine. *Radiology* 166:297, 1988.

Haughton VM, Eldevik OP, Magnacs B, et al: A prospective comparison of computed tomography and myelography in the diagnosis of herniated lumbar disks. *Radiology* 142:103, 1982.

Hayes W, Conway WF, Walsh JW, et al: Seat belt injuries: Radiologic findings and clinical correlation. *RadioGraphics* 11:23, 1991.

Holdsworth F, Chir M: Fractures, dislocations, and fracture dislocations of the spine. *J Bone Joint Surg* 52A:1534, 1970.

Holt EP: The question of lumbar discography. *J Bone Joint Surg* 50A:720, 1968.

Irstan L: Lumbar myelography with Amipaque. *Spine* 3:70, 1978.

Kassel EE, Cooper PW, Rubenstein JD: Radiology of spinal trauma: Practice experience in a trauma unit. *J Can Assoc Radiol* 34:189, 1983.

Keene JS, Goletz TH, Lilleas F, et al: Diagnosis of vertebral fractures: A comparison of conventional radiography, conventional tomography, and computed axial tomography. *J Bone Joint Surg* 64A:585, 1982.

Kornberg M: Discography and magnetic resonance imaging of the diagnosis of lumbar disc disruption. *Spine* 14:1368, 1989.

Martel W, Seeger JF, Wicks JD, et al: Traumatic lesions of the discovertebral junction in the lumbar spine. *Am J Roentgenol* 127:457, 1976.

Meyer GA, Haughton VM, Williams AL: Diagnosis of herniated lumbar disk with computed tomography. *N Engl J Med* 301:1166, 1979.

Modic MT: Degenerative disorders of the spine. In: Modic MT, Masaryk TJ, Ross JS (eds): *Magnetic Resonance Imaging of the Spine*. Chicago, Year Book Medical Publishing, 1989.

Modic MT: Magnetic resonance imaging of the spine. In Modic MT, Masangle TJ, Ross JS (eds): *Magnetic Resonance Imaging of the Spine*. Chicago, Year Book Medical Publishers, 1989.

Montesano PX, Benson DR: The thoracolumbar spine. In Rockwood CA, Green DP, Bucholz RW (eds): *Rockwood and Green's Fractures in Adults*, 3rd ed. Philadelphia, JB Lippincott, 1991.

Myerding HW: Spondylolisthesis. *Surg Gynecol Obstet* 34:371, 1932.

Newman PH: The etiology of spondylolisthesis. *J Bone Joint Surg* 45B:39, 1963.

Raskin SP, Keating JW: Recognition of lumbar disk disease: Comparison of myelography and computed tomography. *Am J Nucl Radiol* 3:215, 1982.

Rogers LF: The roentgenographic appearance of transverse or Chance fractures of the spine: The seat belt fracture. *Am J Roentgenol* 111:844, 1971.

Smith GR, Northrop H, Loop JW: Jumper's fractures: Patterns of thoracolumbar spine injuries associated with vertical plunges. A review of 38 cases. *Radiology* 122:657, 1977.

Turski PA, Sackett JF: Application of computed tomography in spinal trauma. *Appl Radiol* Sept–Oct 87, 1982.

Wiltse LL: Spondylolisthesis: Classification and etiology. In: *Symposium on the Spine. American Academy of Orthopedic Surgery*. St. Louis, CV Mosby, 1969.

Wiltse LL, Newman PH, McNab I: Classification of spondylolysis and spondylolisthesis. *Clin Orthop* 117:23, 1976.

Wiltse LL, Winter RB: Terminology and measurement of spondylolisthesis. *J Bone Joint Surg* 65A:768, 1983.

Yu S, Sether LA, Ho PSP, et al: Tears of the annulus fibrosus: Correlation between MR and pathologic findings in cadavers. *Am J Nucl Radiol* 9:367, 1988.

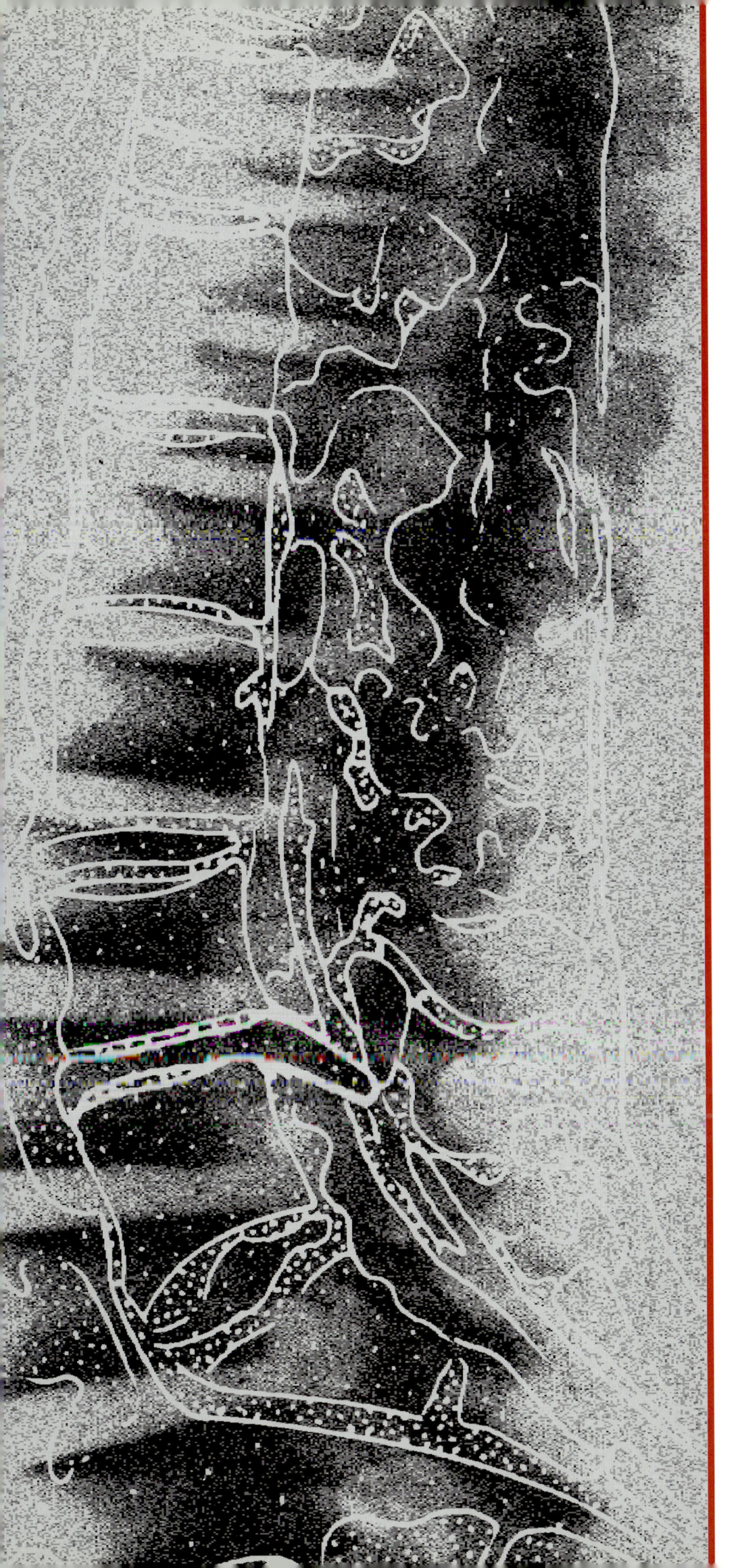

Radiologic Evaluation of the Arthritides Affecting the Spine

4

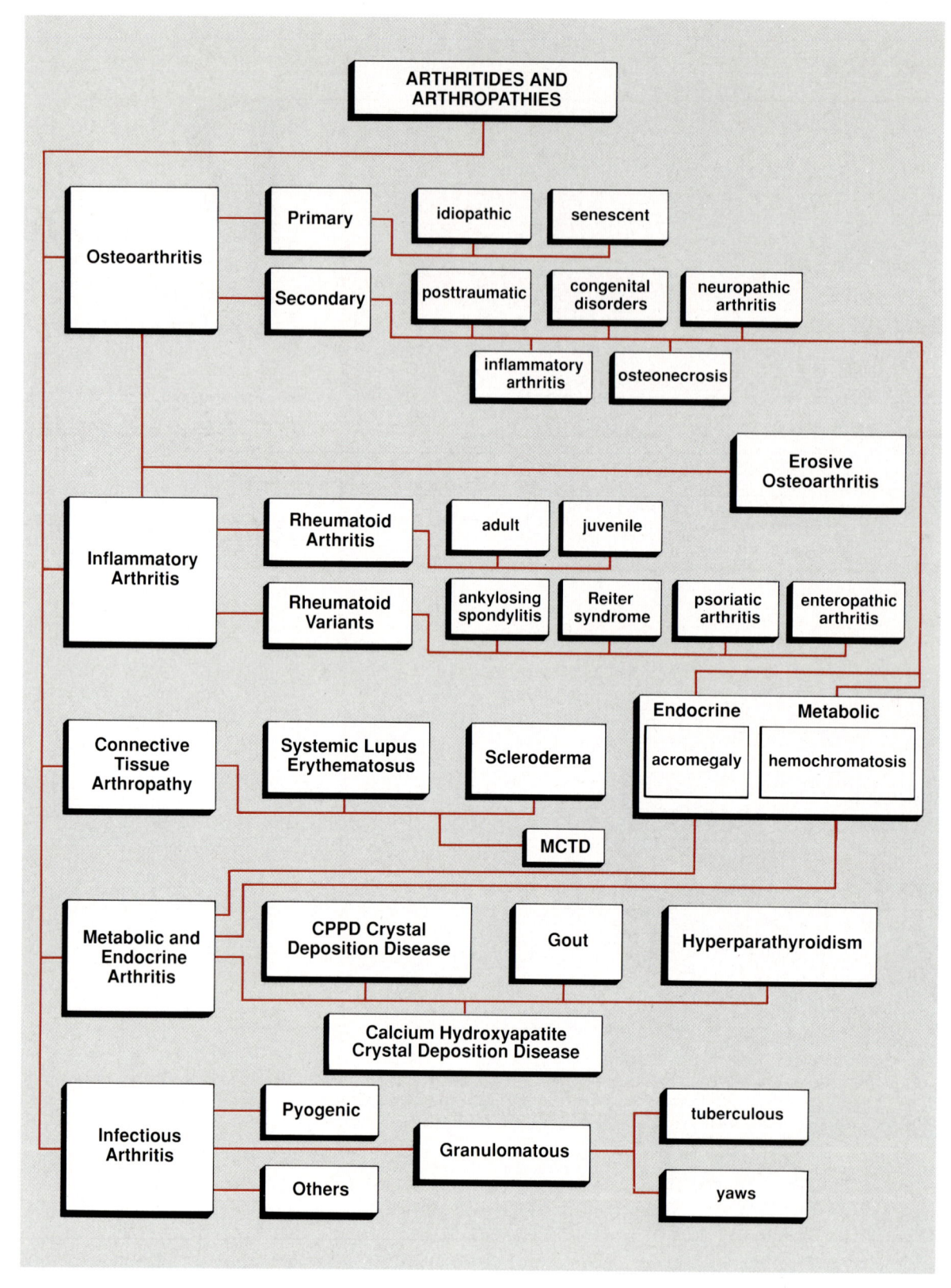

FIGURE 4.1 Classification of the arthritides.

In its general meaning, the term *arthritis* indicates an abnormality of the joint caused by a degenerative, inflammatory, infectious, or metabolic process, each giving the term applied to the various groups of arthritic disorders (Fig. 4.1). Also included among the arthritides are connective tissue arthropathies, such as those associated with systemic lupus erythematosus and scleroderma.

Clinical Findings

The clinical manifestations and laboratory data, in conjunction with the radiographic findings, are of significant help in making the diagnosis of a specific arthritic process. The various arthritides, for example, have different frequencies of occurrence between the sexes. Rheumatoid arthritis is much more common in females, and erosive osteoarthritis is seen almost exclusively in middle-aged women. Psoriatic arthritis, Reiter syndrome, and gouty arthritis, on the other hand, are more common in men. Clinical symptoms are of further assistance. Patients with Reiter syndrome, for example, usually present with urethritis, conjunctivitis, and mucocutaneous lesions, and those with psoriatic arthritis may present with swelling of a single finger, the so-called "sausage digit," as well as changes in the skin and fingernails. Patients with gouty arthritis may exhibit soft tissue masses on the dorsal aspect of the hands or feet, representing chronic tophi.

Laboratory data are also essential. Gouty arthritis, for example, is associated with elevated serum uric acid concentrations, and a synovial fluid examination reveals monosodium urate crystals in leukocytes in the fluid. The synovial fluid of patients with pseudogout (CPPD), on the other hand, contains calcium pyrophosphate crystals. The detection of auto-antibodies is another important aid in the diagnostic workup. A positive test for rheumatoid factor (RF) is a typical finding in rheumatoid arthritis. Patients who lack the specific antibodies represented by RF are said to have "seronegative" arthritis. Patients with lupus arthritis have a positive lupus erythematosus (LE) cell test. Lastly, identification of the antigens of the major histocompatibility complex (MHC), particularly human leukocyte-associated antigens HLA-B27 and HLA-DR4, has in recent years become a crucial test in the diagnosis of arthritic disease. It has been reported that 95% of patients with ankylosing spondylitis, 86% of patients with Reiter syndrome, and 60% of patients with psoriatic arthropathy test positively for antigen HLA-B27, while a great majority of those with rheumatoid arthritis exhibit the HLA-DR4 antigen. This is helpful in differentiating certain types of arthritides, as well as in distinguishing psoriatic arthritis from rheumatoid arthritis in patients whose radiographic findings are equivocal.

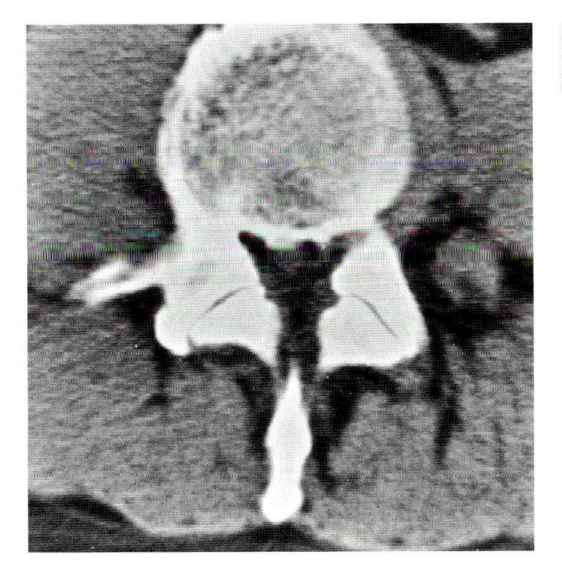

Radiologic Evaluation

Plain Film Radiography and Magnification Radiography

The radiologic modalities used to evaluate arthritic disorders of the spine are very similar to those employed in traumatic conditions involving the spine, although there are some modifications. The most important modality for the evaluation of arthritis is plain film radiography. As in the radiographic examination of traumatic conditions, standard films of the spine should be obtained in at least two projections at 90° angles to each other. Special projections are sometimes required to better demonstrate destructive changes in the spine to better advantage. Magnification radiography is used to diagnose the very early changes of arthritis, which are not well appreciated on standard projections. This technique involves a special screen–film system and geometric enlargement that yields magnified images of the bones and joints with greater sharpness and bone detail.

Conventional Tomography and Computed Tomography

Among the ancillary imaging techniques used to evaluate the arthritides, conventional tomography is rarely employed for the purpose of making a specific diagnosis, its major usefulness being in demonstrating to better advantage the degree of joint destruction. Except for its use in evaluating degenerative changes in the spine, particularly spinal stenosis (Fig. 4.2), computed tomography (CT) is less commonly used in arthritis than in trauma. In the assessment of spinal stenosis secondary to degenerative changes, CT examination may also be performed after myelography (Fig. 4.3), although myelography alone is often sufficient (Fig. 4.4). Arthrography has a very limited application in the evaluation of degenerative and inflammatory conditions of the facet joints.

FIGURE 4.2 CT scan in a 66-year-old patient with advanced osteoarthritis of the facet joints shows marked narrowing of the spinal canal secondary to degenerative changes. At 8 mm, the transverse diameter is well below normal.

Scintigraphy

Radionuclide bone scan is much more commonly used than the techniques discussed above, mainly for evaluating the distribution of arthritic lesion in the spine. The radiopharmaceuticals presently used in bone scanning include organic diphosphonates—ethylene diphosphonate (HEPD) and methylene diphosphonate (MDP)—labeled with ^{99m}Tc, a gamma emitter with a 6-hour half-life; MDP is more commonly used, typically in a dose that provides 15 mCi (555 MBq) of ^{99m}Tc. After intravenous injection of the radiopharmaceutical, approximately 50% of the dose localizes in bone, while the remainder circulates freely in the body and eventually is excreted by the kidneys. A gamma camera can then be used in a procedure known as a *three-phase isotope bone scan*.

Magnetic Resonance Imaging

Magnetic resonance imaging (MRI) of the spine provides excellent contrast between soft tissues and bone. Articular cartilage, fibrocartilage, intervertebral disk, cortex, and spongy bone can be readily distinguished from one another on the basis of their specific signal intensities (see Fig. 2.15).

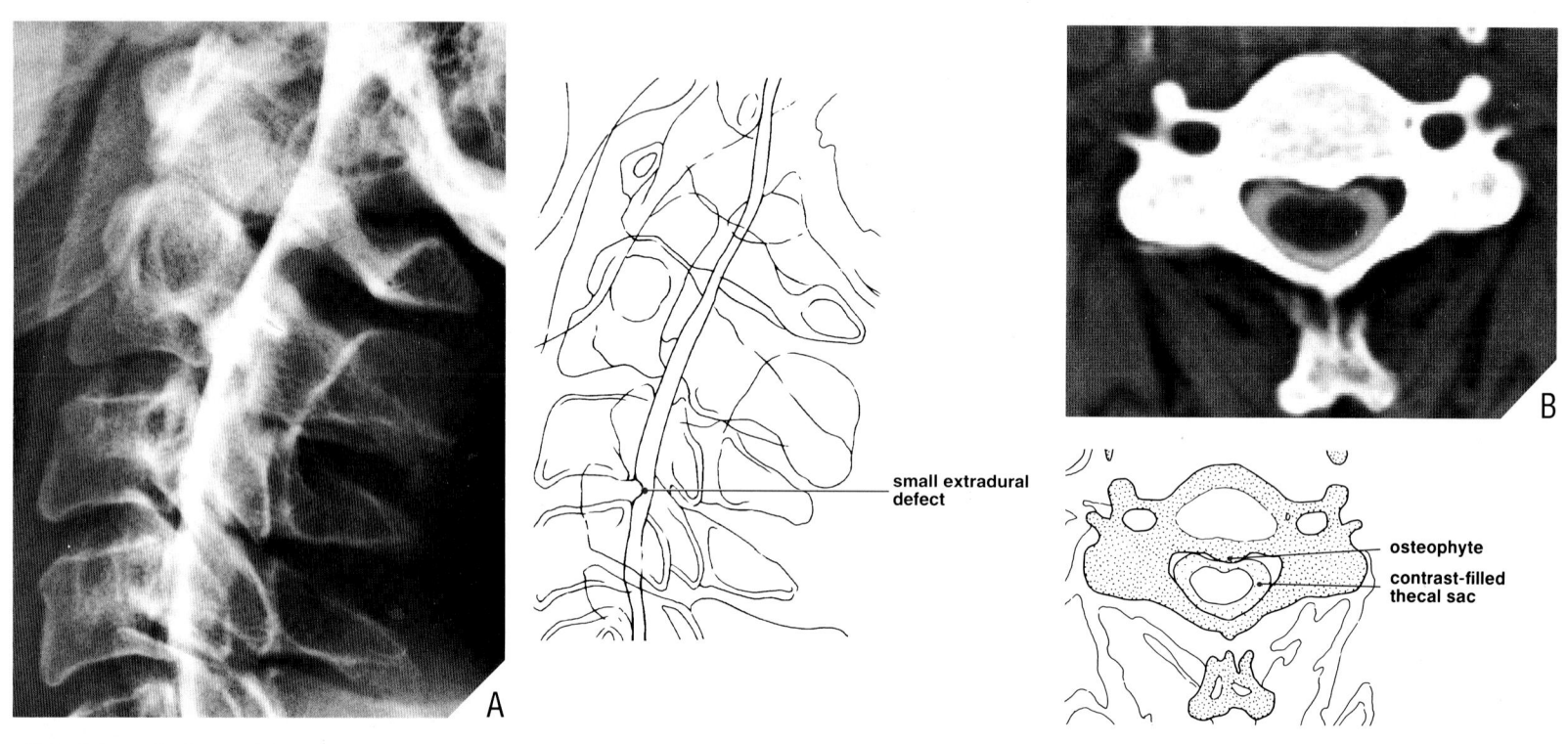

FIGURE 4.3 A 56-year-old man presented with neck pain radiating to the left arm; there was also associated weakness and numbness in the left hand. **(A)** Cervical myelogram in the lateral projection shows a small extradural defect on the ventral aspect of the thecal sac at C3–C4. **(B)** CT section obtained following myelography shows impingement of a posterior osteophyte on the thecal sac at the corresponding level.

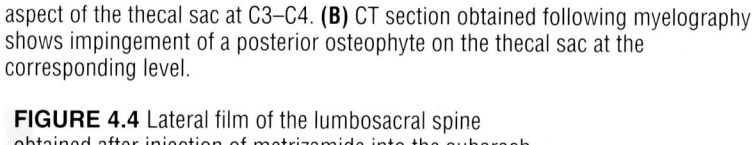

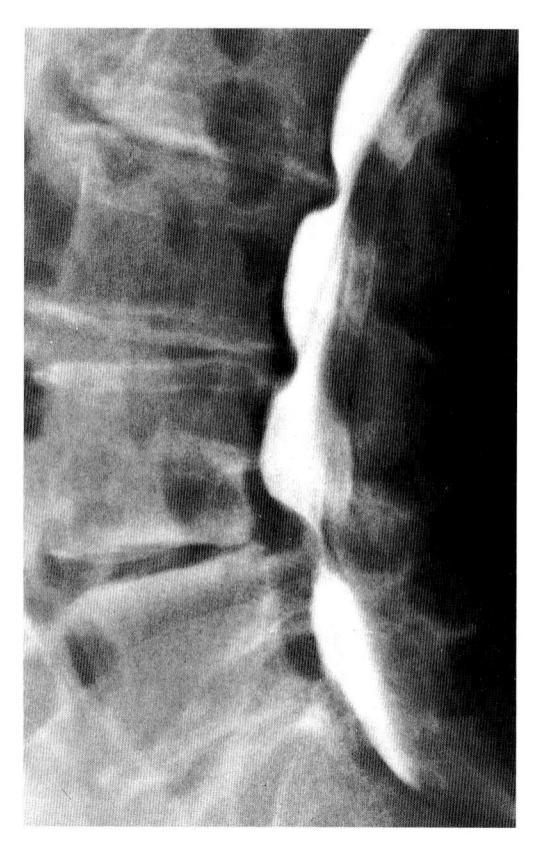

FIGURE 4.4 Lateral film of the lumbosacral spine obtained after injection of metrizamide into the subarachnoid space shows an "hourglass" configuration of the contrast medium in the thecal sac, a feature characteristic of spinal stenosis. This appearance results from concomitant hypertrophy of the facet joints and posterior bulging of the intervertebral disks.

MR images in the sagittal plane are useful to demonstrate hypertrophy of the ligamentum flavum or the vertebral facets, to grade the degree of foraminal stenosis, and to measure the diameter of the spinal cord. MR images in the axial plane facilitate detailed analysis of the facet joints and more accurate measurement of the thickness of the ligamentum flavum and spinal canal diameter.

The usefulness of MRI in evaluation of cervical spinal cord abnormalities in patients with rheumatoid arthritis (Fig. 4.5) and in evaluation of spinal stenosis in patients with advanced degenerative changes of the spine surpasses that of other modalities. MRI is particularly useful in examination of patients with pain related to disk disease, since it can differentiate normal, degenerated, and herniated disks noninvasively. In fact, the changes of disk degeneration can be identified by MRI long before they are detectable by conventional radiography or CT (Fig. 4.6).

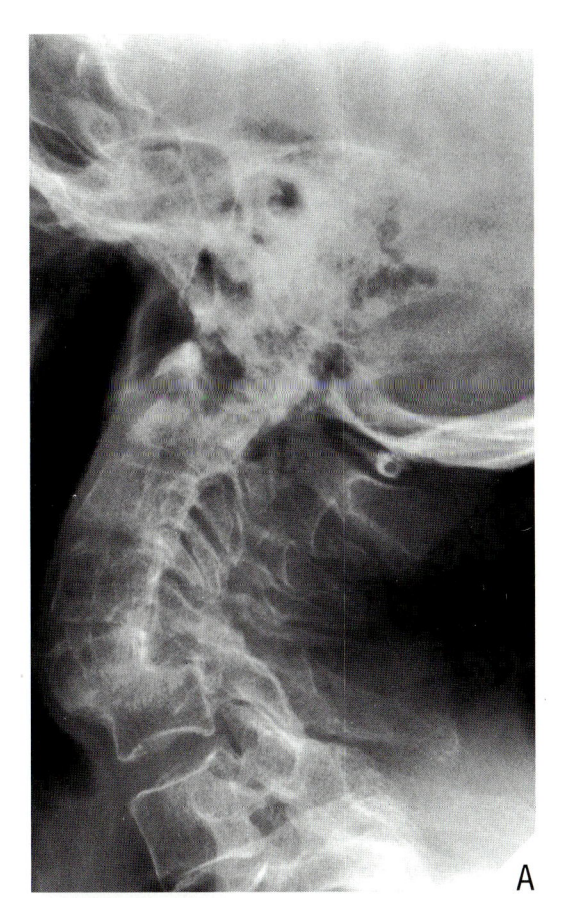

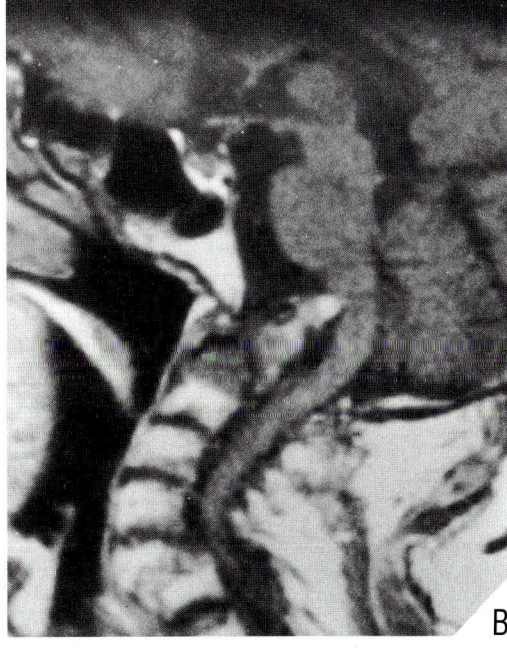

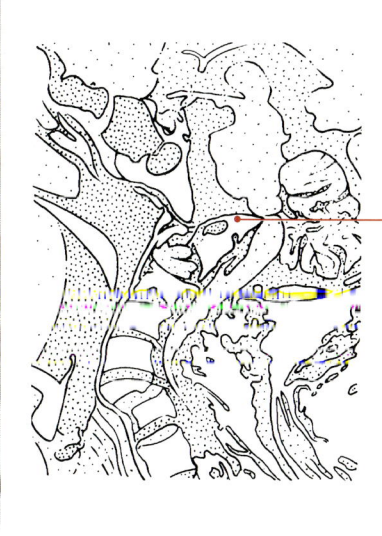

FIGURE 4.5 A 52-year-old woman with advanced rheumatoid arthritis presented with chronic neck pain, weakness of the upper limbs, numbness in both hands, and occasional dyspnea and cardiac arrythmia. **(A)** Plain radiograph demonstrates some of the abnormalities in the cervical spine: advanced osteopenia, erosive changes of the odontoid, diskovertebral junction, and apophyseal joints, as well as whittling of the spinous processes. **(B)** T1-weighted spin-echo sagittal MRI shows in addition the inflammatory pannus eroding odontoid, and cranial settling with superior migration of C2 impinging on medulla oblongata.

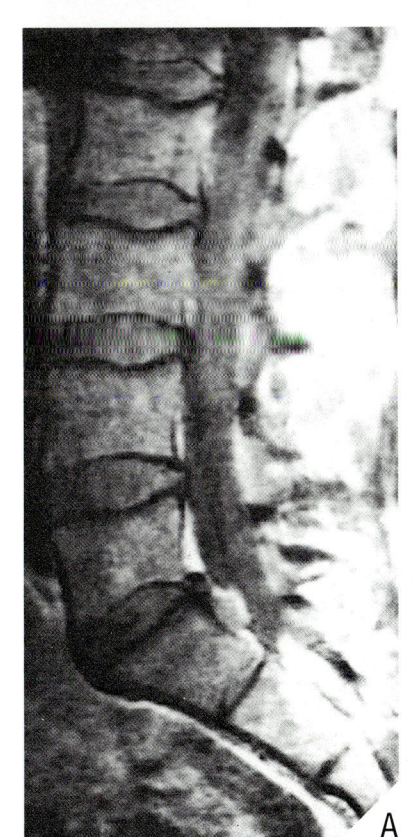

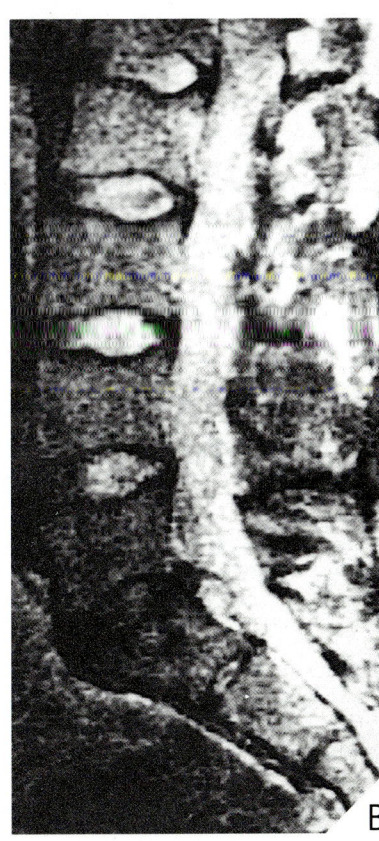

FIGURE 4.6 (A) Proton density-weighted sagittal MRI of lumbosacral spine shows mild bulging of annuli fibrosa at multiple levels. Central disk protrusion is present at L5–S1. **(B)** T2-weighted MRI demonstrates degenerative changes of disk L5–S1 by means of decrease in signal intensity of this structure. This change of signal is related to loss of water content by degenerative ("dry") disk.

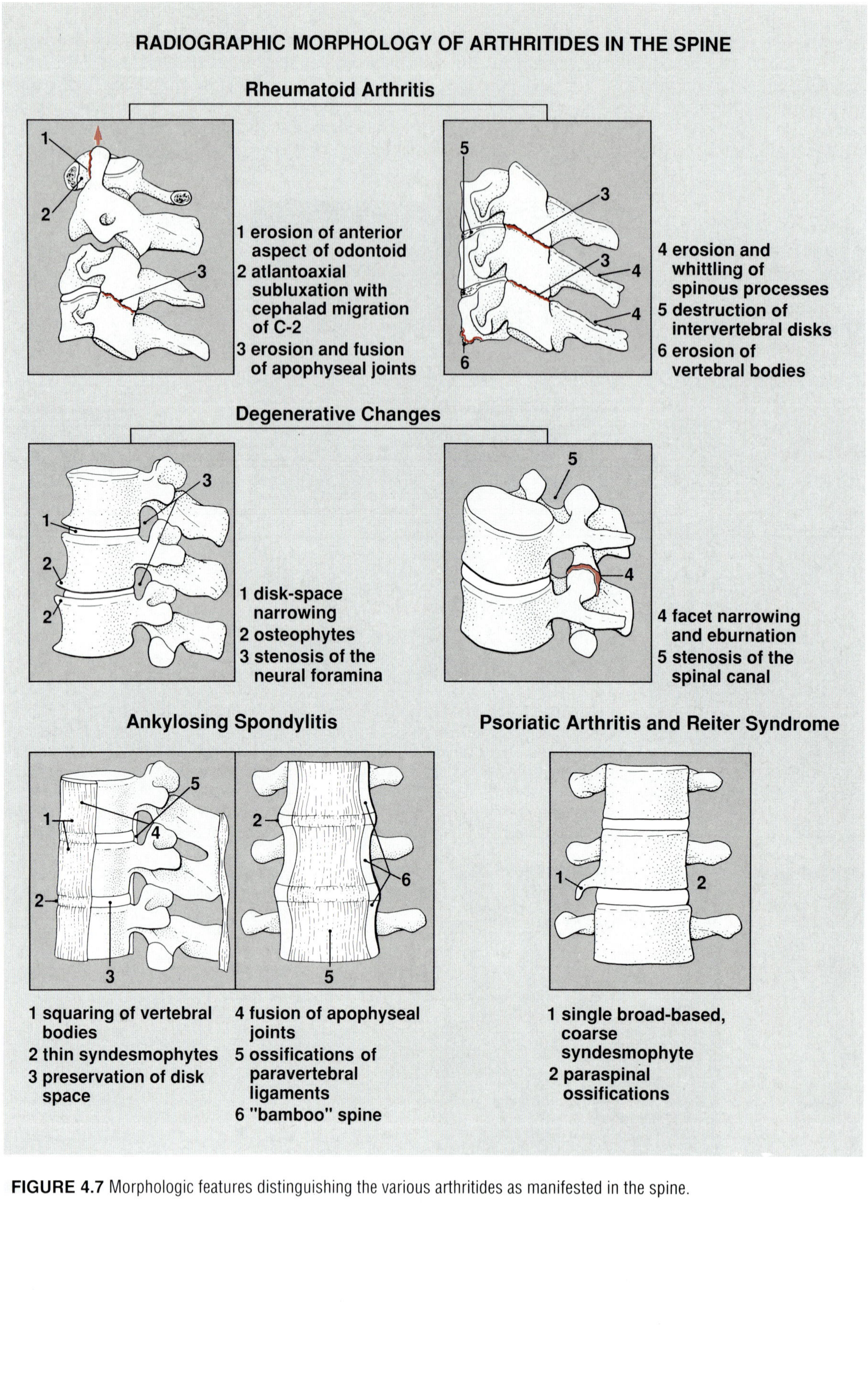

RADIOGRAPHIC MORPHOLOGY OF ARTHRITIDES IN THE SPINE

Rheumatoid Arthritis

1. erosion of anterior aspect of odontoid
2. atlantoaxial subluxation with cephalad migration of C-2
3. erosion and fusion of apophyseal joints
4. erosion and whittling of spinous processes
5. destruction of intervertebral disks
6. erosion of vertebral bodies

Degenerative Changes

1. disk-space narrowing
2. osteophytes
3. stenosis of the neural foramina
4. facet narrowing and eburnation
5. stenosis of the spinal canal

Ankylosing Spondylitis

1. squaring of vertebral bodies
2. thin syndesmophytes
3. preservation of disk space
4. fusion of apophyseal joints
5. ossifications of paravertebral ligaments
6. "bamboo" spine

Psoriatic Arthritis and Reiter Syndrome

1. single broad-based, coarse syndesmophyte
2. paraspinal ossifications

FIGURE 4.7 Morphologic features distinguishing the various arthritides as manifested in the spine.

Imaging of the Spine in Clinical Practice

Radiographic Features of the Arthritides

The true or diarthrodial joint consists of cartilage covering the articular ends of the bones that form the joint, the articular capsule, which is reinforced by ligamentous structures, and the joint space, which is lined with synovial membrane and filled with synovial fluid. In the spine the true synovial joints include atlanto–axial articulation, uncovertebral (Luschka) joints, apophyseal (facet) joints, costovertebral joints, and sacroiliac joints. Because of its physicochemical constitution, articular cartilage absorbs only a minimal amount of x-ray irradiation, and therefore appears radiolucent on radiographic film. The radiolucent articular cartilage, together with the joint cavity filled with synovial fluid, creates the so-called radiographic joint space. The abnormality of the joint in arthritis usually consists of destruction of the articular cartilage, which appears on the film as a narrowing of the radiographic joint space, usually accompanied by subchondral erosion; narrowing of the joint is the cardinal sign of arthritis.

Morphology of the Articular Lesion

The various arthritides exhibit morphologically distinct features, as observed radiographically in the large and small joints. In the degenerative form of the disease (osteoarthritis), thinning of the articular cartilage results in localized narrowing of the joint space; there is also subchondral sclerosis and osteophyte and cyst formation, but osteoporosis is usually absent. Inflammatory arthritides, such as rheumatoid arthritis, are characterized by a diffuse, usually multicompartmental narrowing of the joint space associated with marginal or central erosions, periarticular osteoporosis, and by symmetric periarticular soft tissue swelling; subchondral sclerosis is minimal or absent, and formation of osteophytes is lacking. In a metabolic arthritis such as gout, well-defined bone erosions displaying a so-called overhanging edge are usually associated with preservation of part of the joint space and a localized, asymmetric soft tissue mass; osteophyte formation and osteoporosis are absent. Infectious arthritis is characterized by the complete destruction of the articular ends of the bones that form the joint; all communicating joint compartments are invariably involved, with diffuse osteoporosis, joint effusion, and periarticular soft tissue swelling. Neuropathic arthritis is marked by destruction of the articular surfaces, which releases bone debris, and a substantial joint effusion; osteoporosis is absent. Depending on the amount of destruction, various degrees of joint instability are present.

Analysis of the morphologic features of an arthritic lesion at certain sites other than the diarthrodial joints may be of further assistance in differentiating the various arthritides and reaching a correct diagnosis. Two such sites that are frequently affected are the heel and the spine.

The morphology of arthritic lesions in the spine offers important indications of the disease process at work (Fig. 4.7). Among the inflammatory arthritides, for example, rheumatoid arthritis causes a characteristic erosion of the odontoid process (Fig. 4.8). Moreover, as a result of inflammatory pannus and erosion of the transverse ligament between the anterior arch of the atlas and C2, there may be subluxation in the atlanto–axial joint. This is usually manifested by an increase to more than 3 mm in the

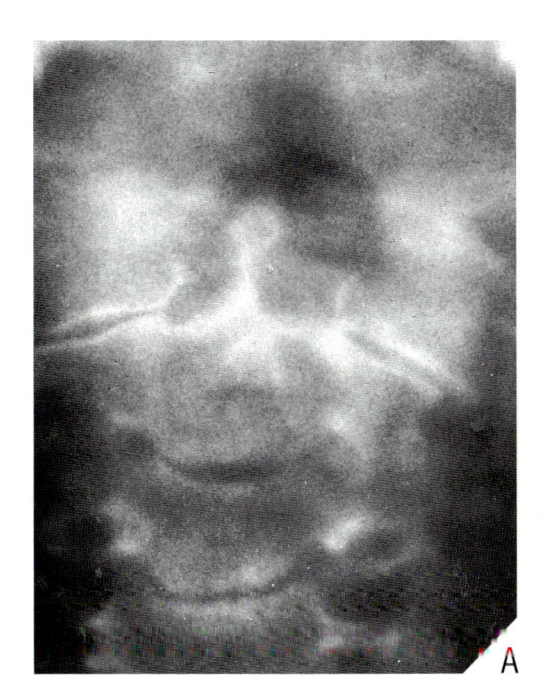

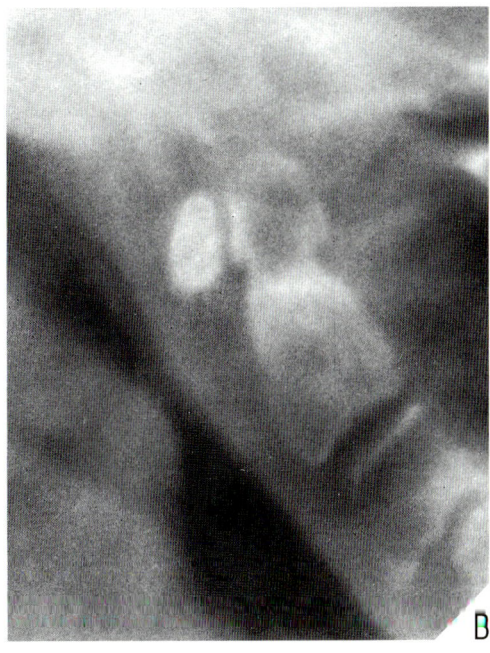

FIGURE 4.8 Anteroposterior (**A**) and lateral (**B**) trispiral tomograms of the cervical spine in a 55-year-old woman with a 15-year history of rheumatoid arthritis show erosion of the odontoid process typical for this condition.

distance between the arch of the atlas and the dens, as demonstrated on a lateral view of the cervical spine in flexion (Fig. 4.9). Erosion of the apophyseal joints of the cervical spine, sometimes leading to fusion, is frequently seen in juvenile rheumatoid arthritis (Fig. 4.10).

Arthritic lesions involving other segments of the spine also exhibit distinguishing features that assist in differentiating the disease process. Degenerative changes may manifest in the cervical, thoracic, or lumbar (Fig. 4.11) spine as the appearance of marginal osteophytes, narrowing and sclerosis of the apophyseal joints, and narrowing of the disk spaces. In ankylosing spondylitis, there is a characteristic "squaring" of the vertebral bodies, with the formation of delicate syndesmophytes (which differ morphologically from degenerative osteophytes) arising from the anterior aspects of the vertebral bodies. In the later stages of this condition, inflammation and fusion of the apophyseal joints lead to the appearance of the "bamboo" spine; the sacroiliac joints are also invariably affected (Fig. 4.12). In psoriasis and Reiter syndrome, one can occasionally see a single, coarse osteophyte in the lumbar spine, frequently bridging adjacent vertebral bodies, or paravertebral ossifications; there are also associated inflammatory changes in the sacroiliac joints (Fig. 4.13).

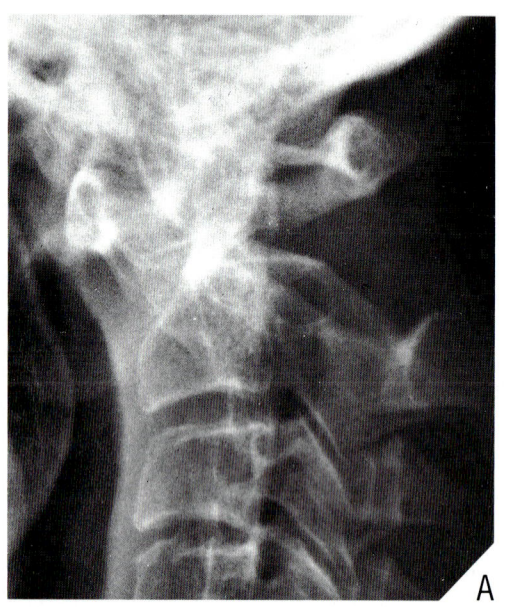

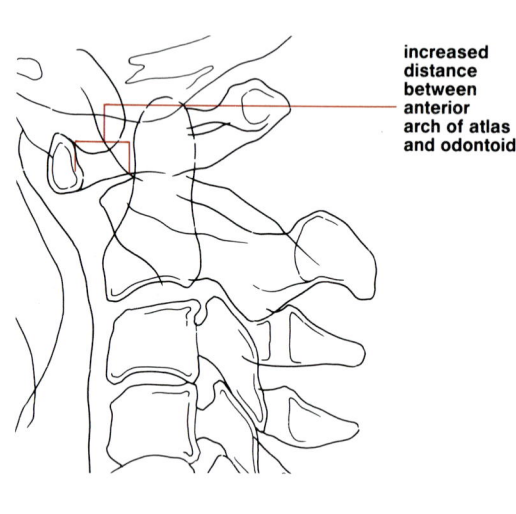

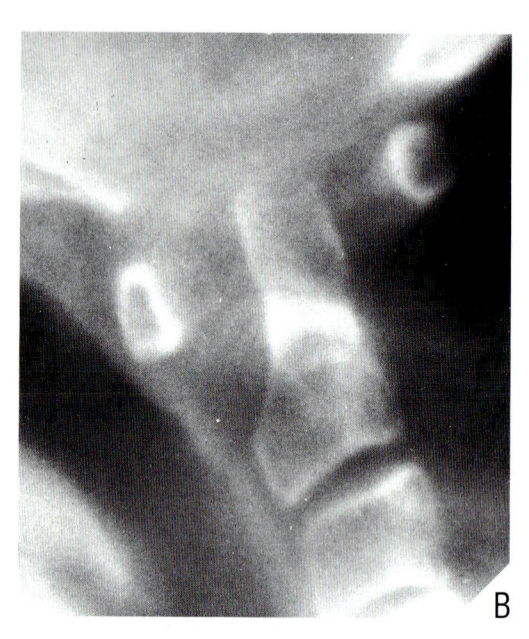

FIGURE 4.9 (A) Lateral film of the cervical spine in flexion in a 68-year-old woman with a long history of rheumatoid arthritis shows a marked increase in the distance between the anterior arch of the atlas and the odontoid process, measuring 10.2 mm; normally, it should not exceed 3 mm. **(B)** Trispiral tomogram demonstrates the antlantoaxial subluxation in detail.

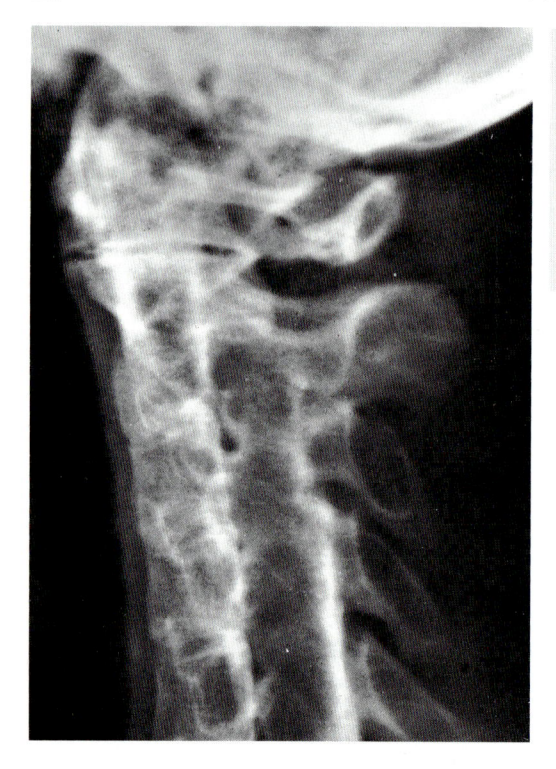

FIGURE 4.10 Lateral view of the cervical spine in a 34-year-old woman with juvenile rheumatoid arthritis since age 20 shows the typical involvement of the apophyseal joints. In this case, there is complete fusion of the joints.

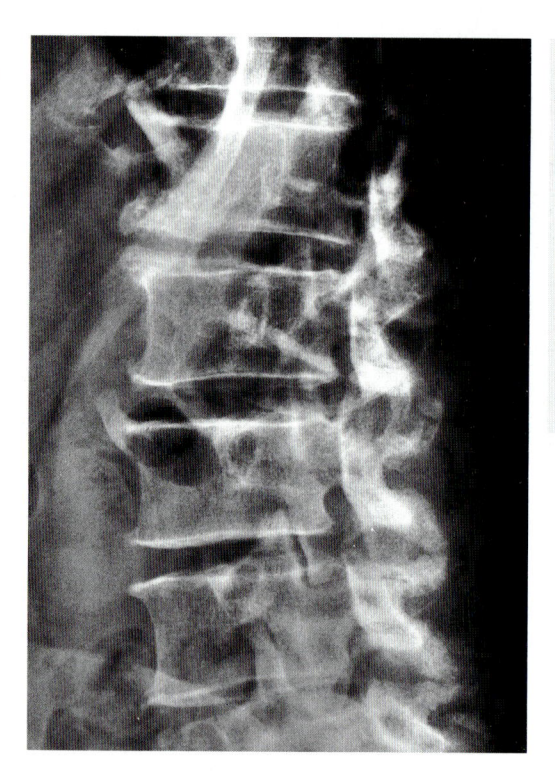

FIGURE 4.11 Oblique view of the lumbar spine in a 72-year-old woman shows narrowing and eburnation of the articular margins of the facet joints, osteophytosis, and narrowing of the intervertebral disk spaces—a combination of the effects of true facet joint arthritis, spondylosis deformans, and degenerative disk disease.

Imaging of the Spine in Clinical Practice

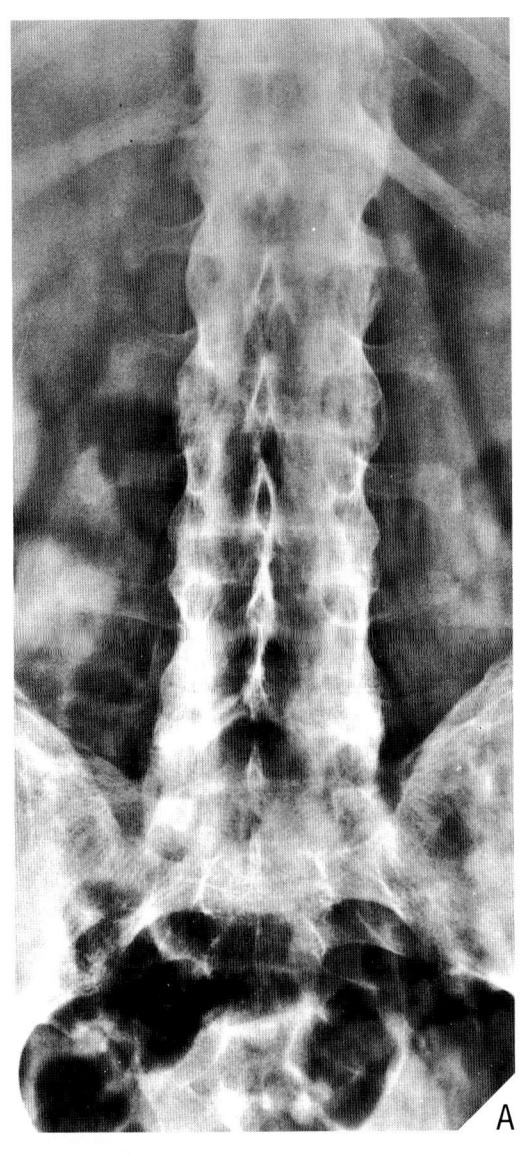

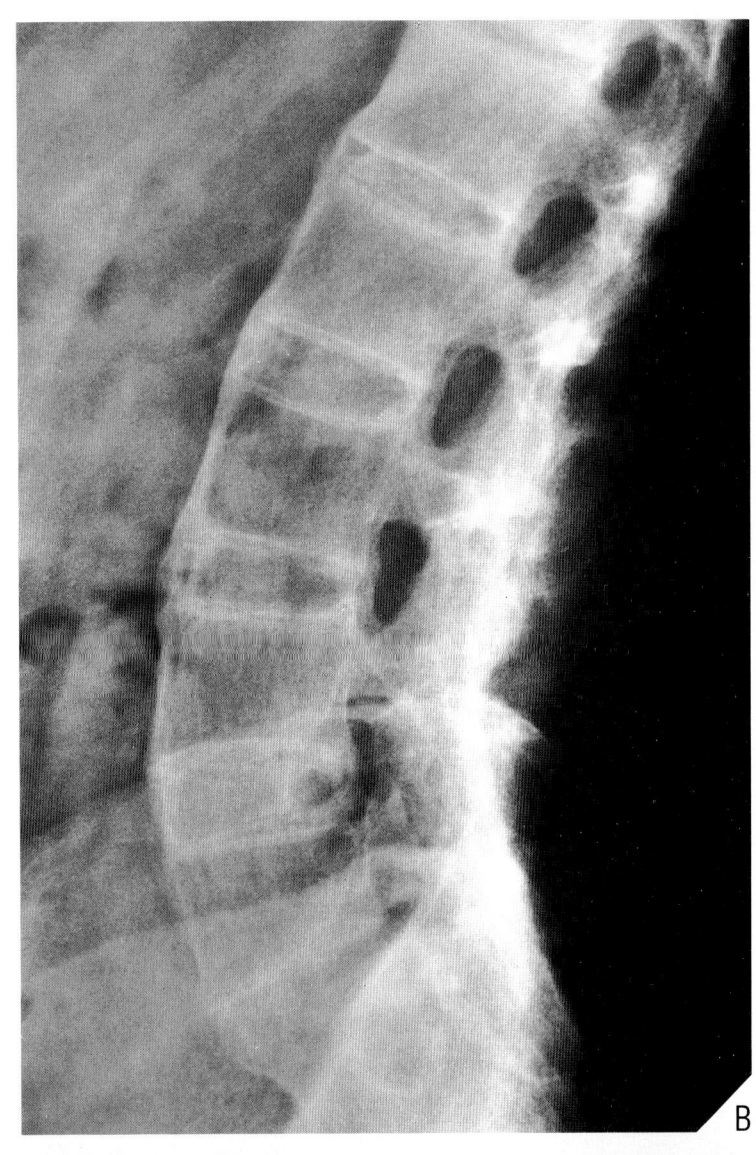

FIGURE 4.12 Anteroposterior **(A)** and lateral **(B)** radiographs of the lumbar spine in a 31-year-old man with advanced ankylosing spondylitis demonstrate the typical appearance of "bamboo" spine secondary to inflammation, ossification, and fusion of the apophyseal joints, associated with ossification of the anterior and posterior longitudinal ligaments, as well as the supraspinous and interspinous ligaments. Note also the fusion of the sacroiliac joints.

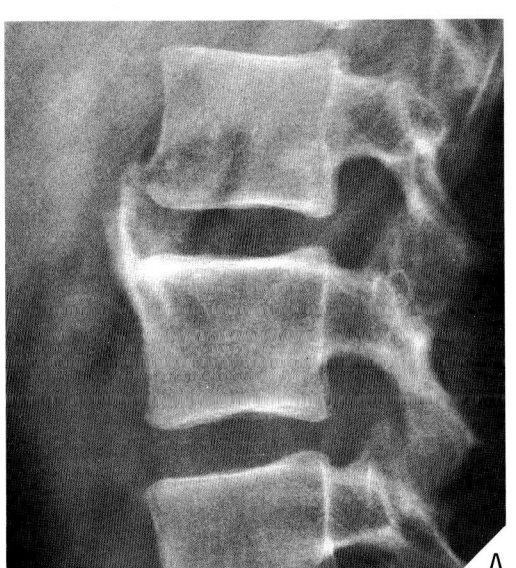

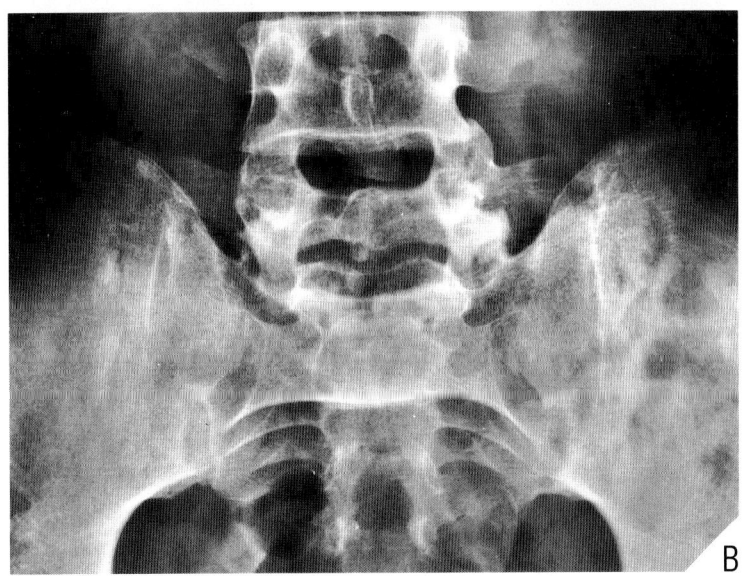

FIGURE 4.13 (A) Lateral view of the lumbar spine in a 27-year-old man with psoriasis shows a single, coarse osteophyte bridging the bodies of L1 and L2. **(B)** Anteroposterior view of the lumbosacral segment shows the effects of the inflammatory process on the sacroiliac joints.

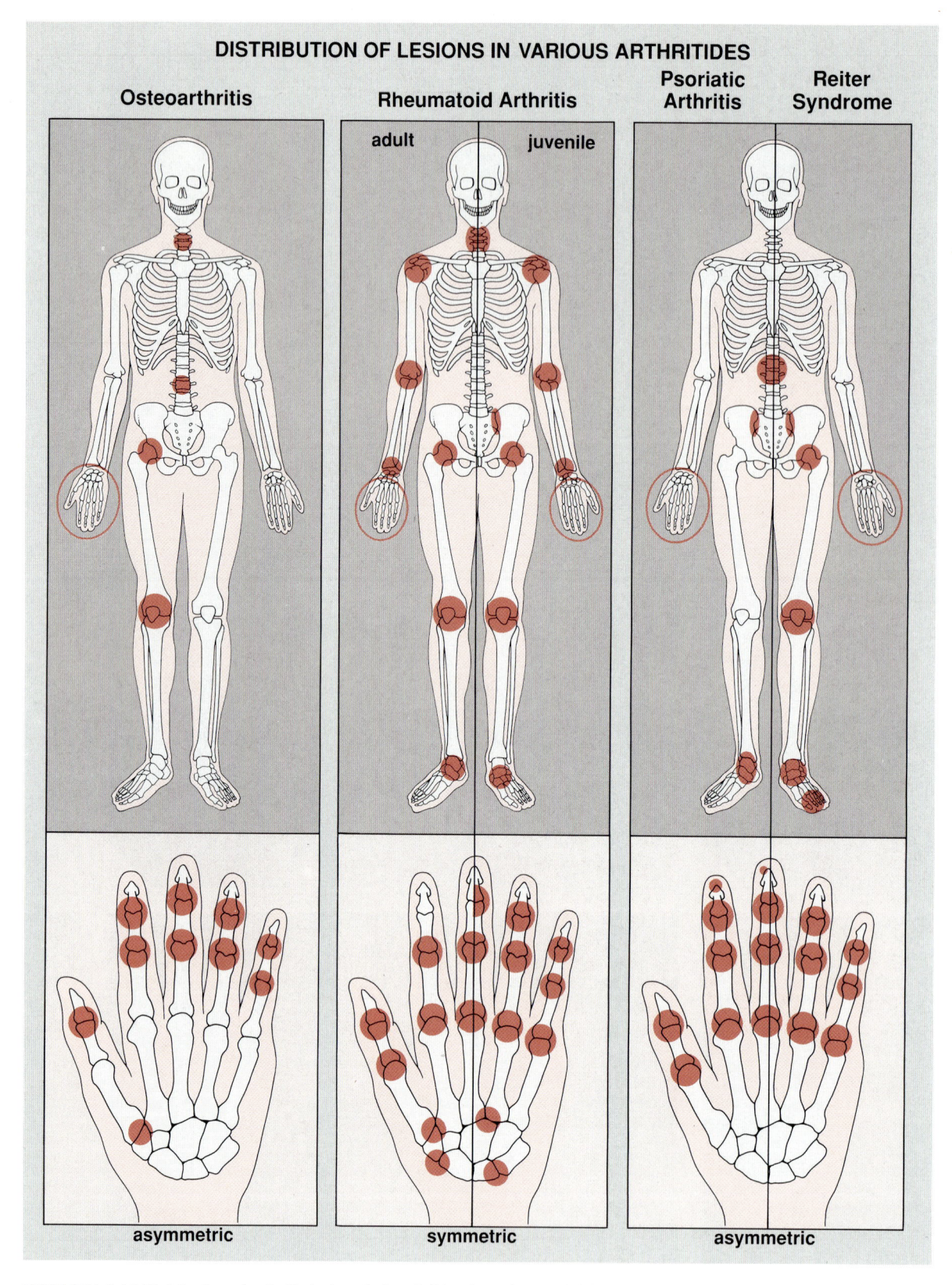

FIGURE 4.14 Distribution of arthritic lesions in the skeleton in various arthritides.

4.10 *Imaging of the Spine in Clinical Practice*

Distribution of the Articular Lesions

Osteoarthritis tends to have a characteristic distribution in the skeletal system. Typically, the large joints (eg, the hip, knee, small joints of the hand and wrist) are involved, whereas the shoulder, elbow, and ankle are spared (Fig. 4.14). In the spine, apophyseal joints and intervertebral disk spaces are affected. Inflammatory arthritides have different sites of predilection in the skeleton, depending on the specific variant of the disease. Rheumatoid arthritis, for example, involves most of the large joints such as the hips, knees, elbows, and shoulders. In the hand, it has a characteristic distribution that spares the distal interphalangeal joints, and in the cervical spine, the C1–C2 articulation and the apophyseal joints are frequently affected. Juvenile rheumatoid arthritis has a similar pattern of distribution, except that the distal interphalangeal joints of the hand may also be affected. Psoriatic arthritis, in contrast to rheumatoid arthritis, has a predilection for the distal interphalangeal joints and the sacroiliac joints, resembling Reiter syndrome. Erosive osteoarthritis, which some consider a variant of osteoarthritis, others a variant of rheumatoid arthritis, and still others a distinct form of arthritis, has a tendency to affect the proximal and distal interphalangeal joints. The spine may be affected by degenerative disease (facet and sacroiliac joints, intervertebral disks), rheumatoid arthritis (facet joints, particularly in the cervical segment, Luschka joints, atlanto–axial joint and dens, diskovertebral junction, and occasionally the costovertebral joints), ankylosing spondylitis (sacroiliac joints, diskovertebral junction, apophyseal joints, posterior ligamentous attachment), psoriatic arthritis (sacroiliac joints, costovertebral joints, paravertebral soft tissues), Reiter syndrome (sacroiliac joints, paravertebral soft tissues), and enteropathic arthropathies (sacroiliac joints, diskovertebral junction).

Suggested Reading

Alsen AM, Martel W, Ellis JE, et al: Cervical spine involvement in rheumatoid arthritis: MR imaging. *Radiology* 165:159, 1987.

Beltran J, Caudill JL, Herman LA, et al: Rheumatoid arthritis: MR imaging manifestations. *Radiology* 165:153, 1987.

Breedveld FC, Algra PR, Vielvoye CJ, et al: Magnetic resonance imaging in the evaluation of patients with rheumatoid arthritis and subluxations of the cervical spine. *Arthritis Rheum* 30:624, 1987.

Brower AC: *Arthritis in Black and White*. Philadelphia, W B Saunders, 1988.

Forrester DM, Brown JC: *The Radiology of Joint Diseases*, 3rd ed. Philadelphia, W B Saunders, 1987.

Larsson EM, Holtas S, Zygmunt S. Pre- and postoperative MR imaging of the craniocervical junction in rheumatoid arthritis. *AJR* 152:561, 1989.

McAfee JG: Update on radiopharmaceuticals for medical imaging. *Radiology* 171:593, 1989.

Steinbach L, Hallman D, Petri M, et al: Magnetic resonance imaging: A review of rheumatologic applications. *Semin Arthritis Rheum* 16:79, 1986.

Subramanian G, McAfee JG, Blair RJ, et al: Technetium 99m methylene diphosphonate—A superior agent for skeletal imaging. Comparison with other technetium complexes. *J Nucl Med* 16:744, 1975.

Weissman BN: Spondyloarthropathies. *Radiol Clin North Am* 25:1235, 1987.

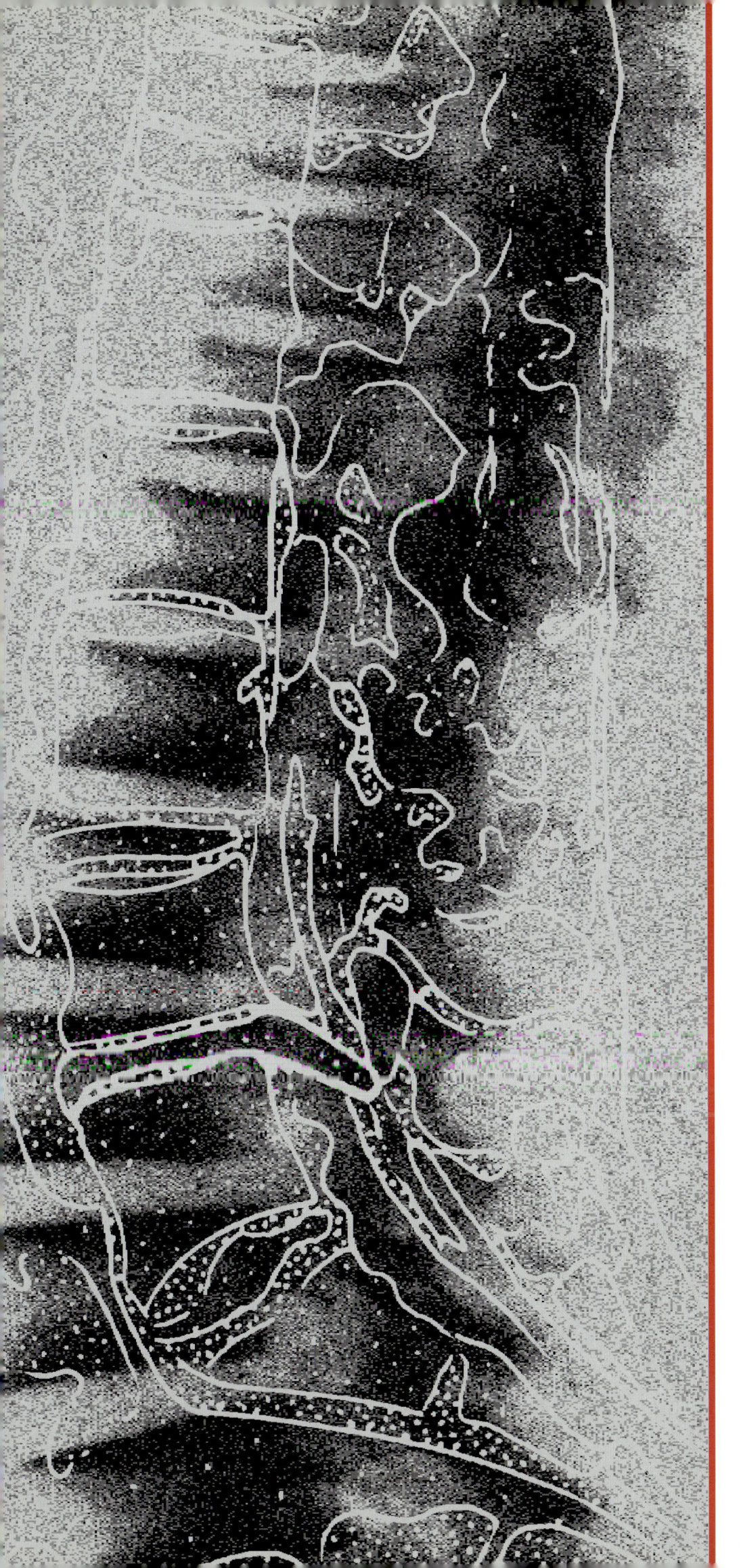

Degenerative Diseases of the Spine

5

Degenerative joint disease (osteoarthritis, osteoarthrosis) is the most common form of arthritis. In its primary (idiopathic) form, it affects individuals in their fifth decade and above; in its secondary form, however, osteoarthritis may be seen in a much younger age group. Patients in the latter group have clearly defined underlying conditions leading to the development of degenerative joint disease.

Some authorities postulate that there are two types of primary degenerative joint disease. The first form is apparently closely related to the aging process ("wear and tear") and represents not a true arthritis but a senescent process of the joint. It is characterized by limited destruction of the cartilage, slow progression, lack of significant joint deformity, and no restriction of joint function. This process is not affected by sex or race. The second type, a true osteoarthritis, is unrelated to the aging process, although it shows an increased prevalence with age. Marked by progressive destruction of the articular cartilage and reparative processes such as osteophyte formation and subchondral sclerosis, true osteoarthritis progresses rapidly, leading to significant joint deformity. This form may be related to genetic factors, as well as to sex, race, and obesity. Osteoarthritis

HIGHLIGHTS OF PRIMARY OSTEOARTHRITIS

Morphology

Large Joints

1 localized joint-space narrowing
2 subchondral sclerosis
3 osteophytes
4 cyst or pseudocyst

Small Joints

1 Heberden nodes
2 Bouchard nodes
3 joint-space narrowing
4 subchondral sclerosis

Spine

1 facet narrowing and eburnation
2 foraminal stenosis
3 stenosis of spinal canal

Distribution

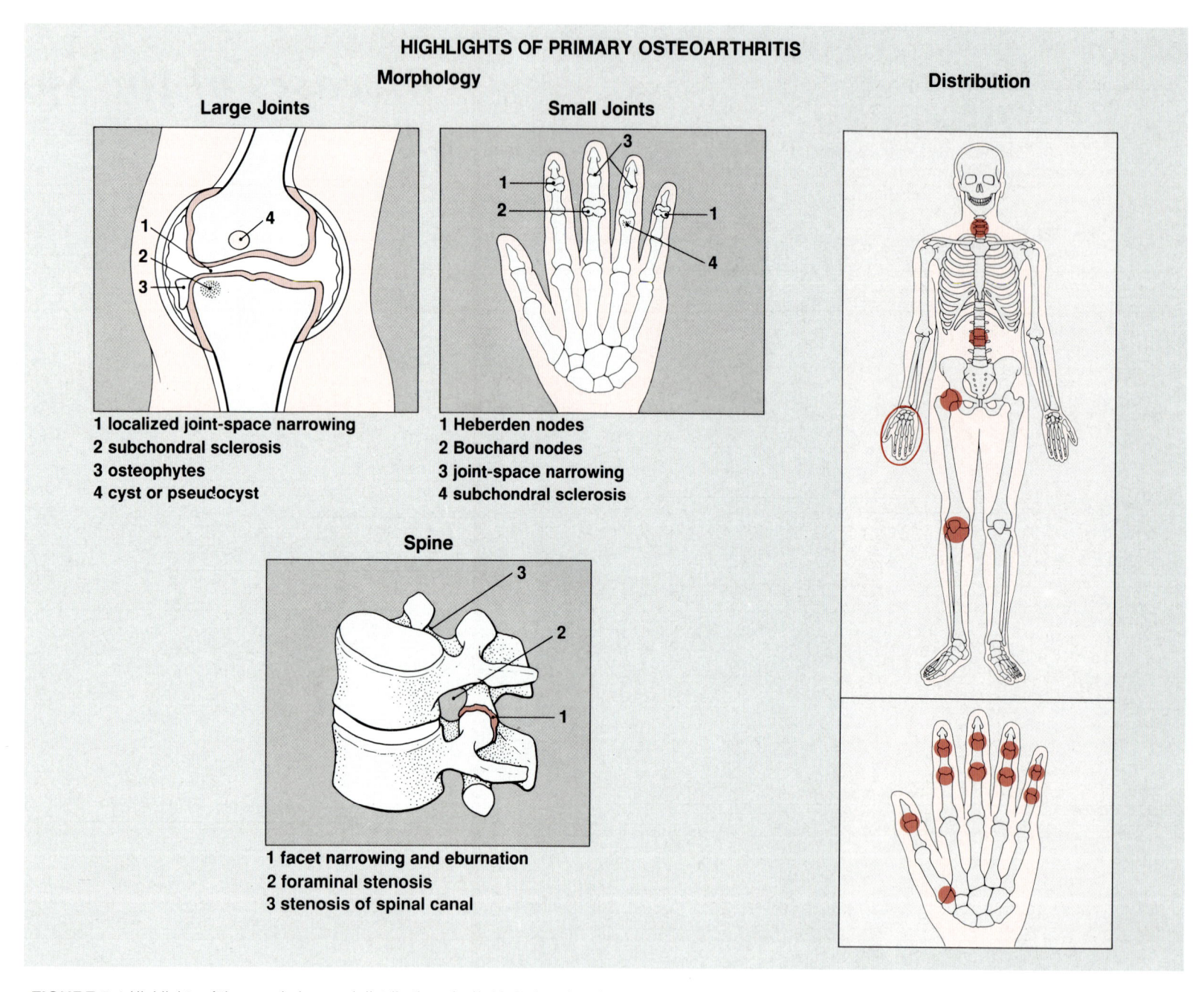

FIGURE 5.1 Highlights of the morphology and distribution of arthritic lesions in primary osteoarthritis.

Imaging of the Spine in Clinical Practice

tends to affect women more commonly than men, particularly in the proximal and distal interphalangeal joints and in the first carpometacarpal joints. In the population over age 65, osteoarthritis affects whites more frequently than blacks. Obesity is associated with a higher incidence of osteoarthritis in the knees, which may be related to an excessive weight-bearing load on these joints.

Generally speaking, osteoarthritis most often affects the large diarthrodial joints, such as the hip or knee, and the small joints, such as the interphalangeal joints of the hand. The spine, however, is just as frequently involved in the degenerative process (Fig. 5.1).

Degenerative Diseases of the Spine

Degenerative changes may involve the spine at the following sites:

1. The synovial joints—atlantoaxial, apophyseal, costovertebral, and sacroiliac—leading to *osteoarthritis* of these structures.
2. The intervertebral disks, leading to the condition known as *degenerative disk disease*.
3. The vertebral bodies and annulus fibrosus, resulting in the condition known as *spondylosis deformans*.
4. The fibrous articulations, ligaments, or sites of ligament attachment to the bone (entheses), leading to the condition known as *diffuse idiopathic skeletal hyperostosis* (DISH).

It is not uncommon for all four conditions to coexist in the same patient.

Osteoarthritis of the Synovial Joints

Degenerative changes of the vertebral facet joints are very common, particularly in the mid and lower cervical and the lower lumbar segments. As in the other synovial joints, the characteristic radiographic features include diminution of the joint space, eburnation of subchondral bone, and osteophyte formation, all of which are most easily demonstrated on the oblique projection of the spine (Fig. 5.2). In the cervical spine, osteophytes on the posterior aspect of a vertebral body may encroach on the neural foramina or the thecal sac, causing various neurologic symptoms. In addition to the standard oblique views (Fig. 5.3), conventional tomography or computed tomography (CT) is usually required to demonstrate these changes (Fig. 5.4). Anterior osteophytes, on the other hand, are usually asymptomatic unless they are unusually prominent. Involvement of the apophyseal joints may be accompanied by a "vacuum phenomenon" (Fig. 5.5), which in fact represents gas in the joint. This finding is almost pathognomonic for a degenerative process.

As in other diarthrodial joints, degenerative changes of the sacroiliac joints are manifested by narrowing of the joint space, subchondral sclerosis, and osteophytosis (Fig. 5.6). It is important to note in the evaluation of the sacroiliac joints that only the lower half of the radiographic sacroiliac joint space is lined by synovium; the upper portion is a syndesmotic joint (Fig. 5.7).

Degenerative Disk Disease

In degenerative disk disease, the vacuum phenomenon in the disk space is common. These radiolucent collections of gas (principally nitrogen)

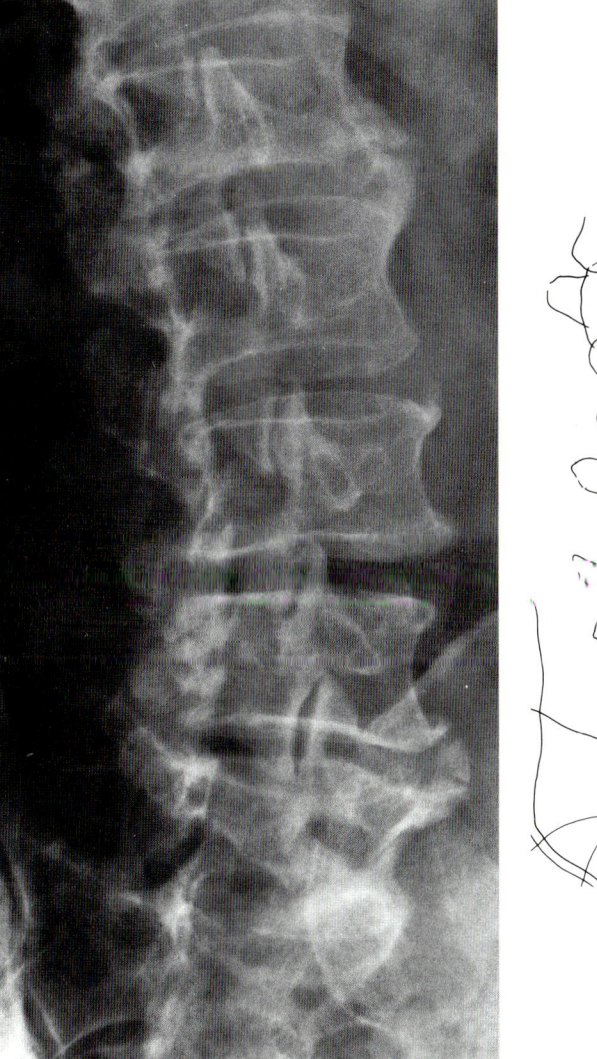

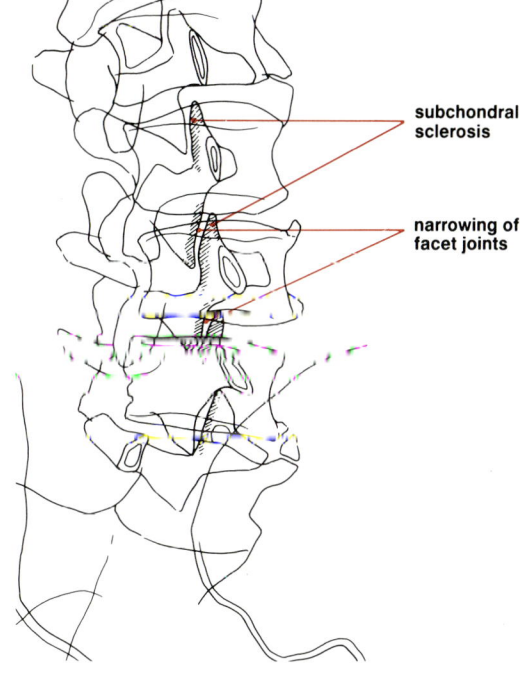

FIGURE 5.2 Oblique view of the lumbar spine in a 68-year-old man demonstrates advanced osteoarthritis of the facet joints. Narrowing of the joint spaces, eburnation of the articular margins, and small osteophytes are similar to the changes seen in osteoarthritis of the large synovial joints.

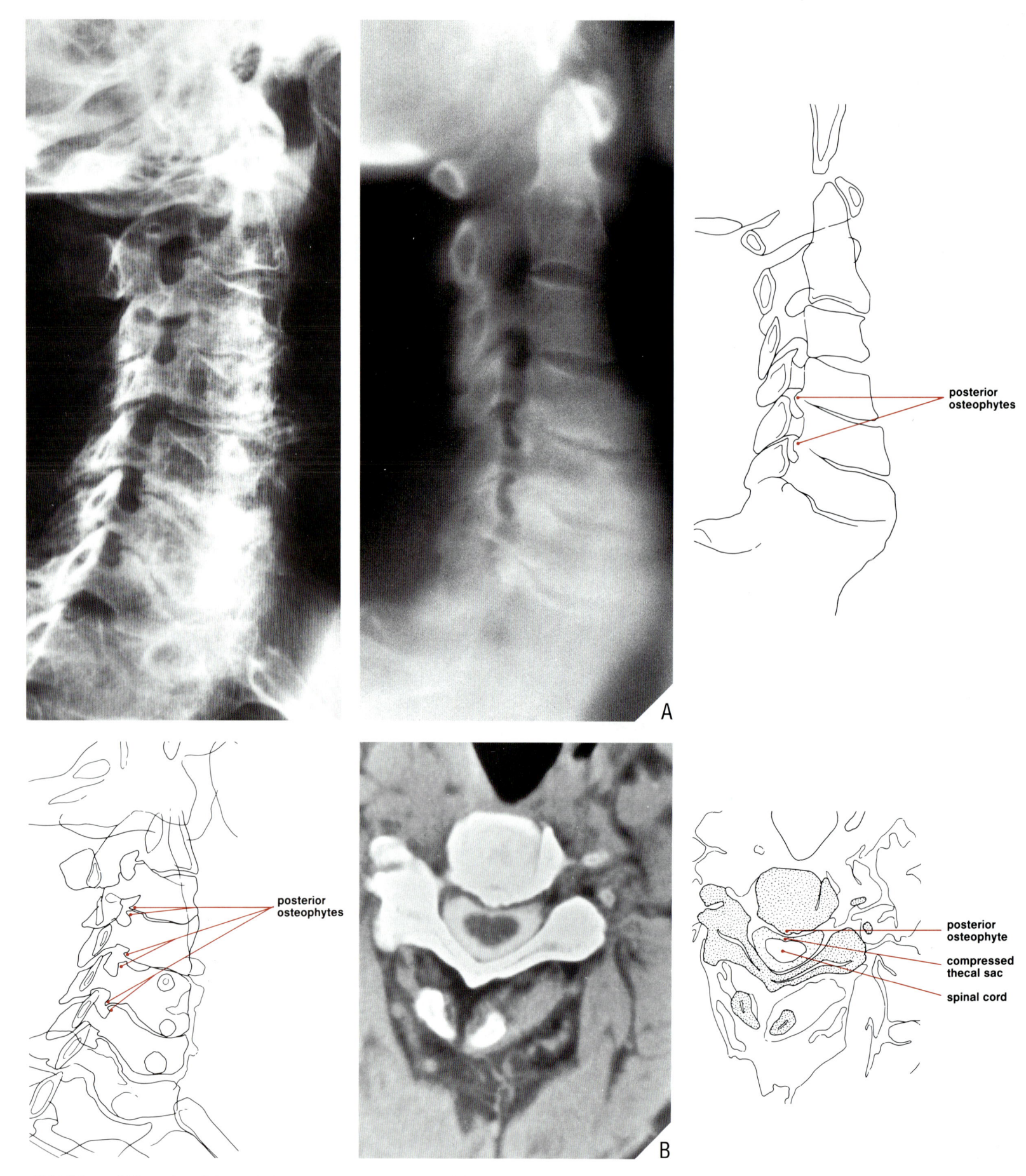

FIGURE 5.3 Oblique view of the cervical spine in a 72-year-old woman who complained of neck pain radiating to both shoulders reveals multiple posterior osteophytes encroaching on numerous neural foramina.

FIGURE 5.4 (A) Conventional lateral tomogram of the cervical spine in a 56-year-old man demonstrates encroachment of the neural foramina by posterior osteophytes. **(B)** CT section at the level of C3 obtained during myelography demonstrates a large posterior osteophyte impinging on the thecal sac and compressing the subarachnoid space filled with contrast medium.

5.4   Imaging of the Spine in Clinical Practice

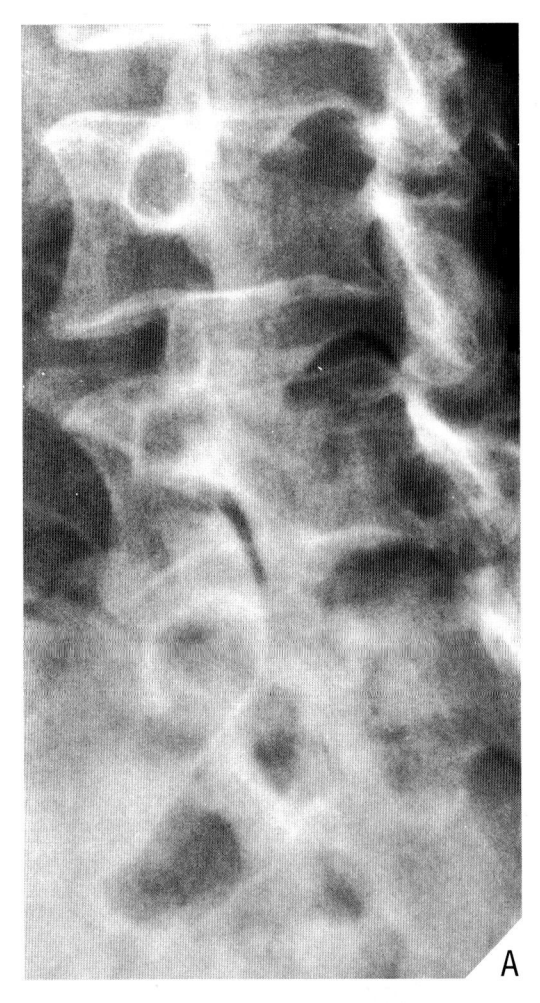

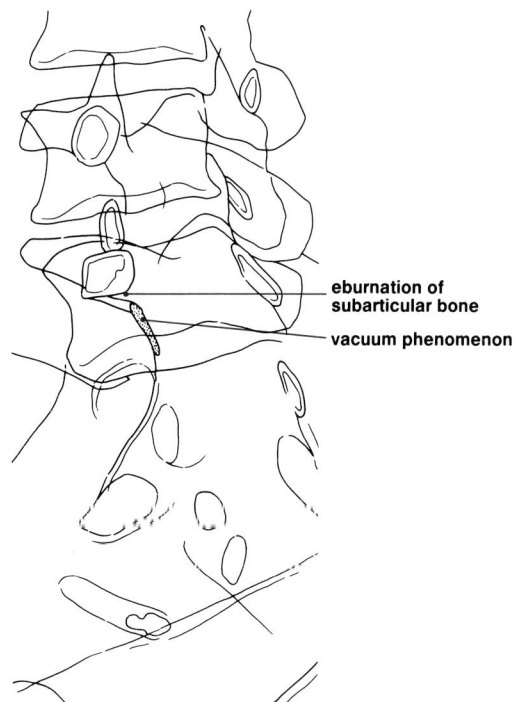

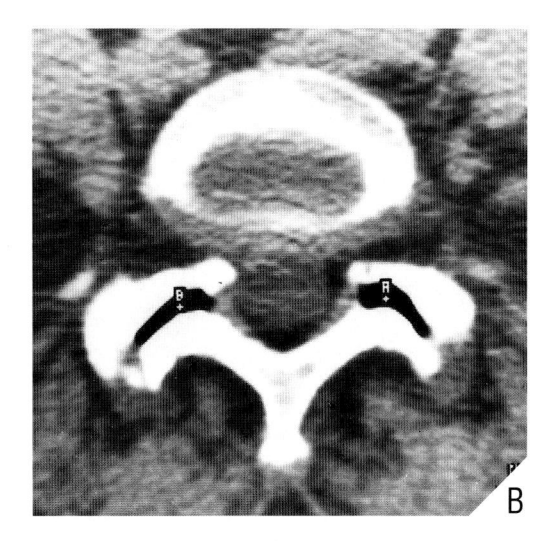

FIGURE 5.5 A 56-year-old man with osteoarthritis affecting the apophyseal joints of the lumbar spine. **(A)** Oblique view of the lumbosacral spine shows a vacuum phenomenon of the facet joint L5–S1 and eburnation of the subarticular bone. **(B)** CT section through both facets clearly demonstrates the presence of gas, as confirmed by the Hounsfield values. These units are related to the attenuation coefficient for various tissues in the body and represent absorption values directly related to tissue density. Note also the hypertrophic spur arising from the right facet and encroaching on the spinal canal.

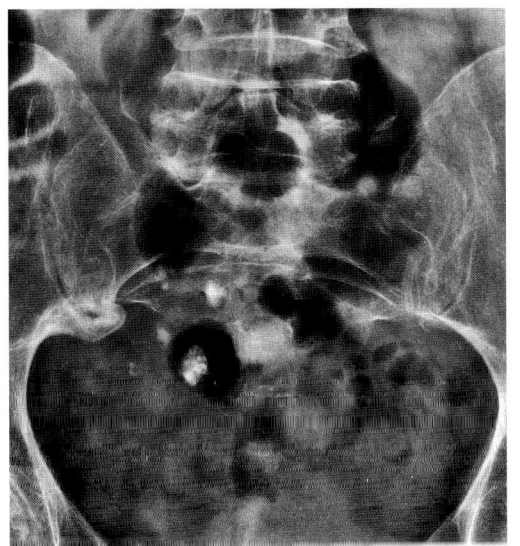

FIGURE 5.6 Degenerative changes in the sacroiliac joints, seen here affecting predominantly the right sacroiliac joint in an 82-year-old woman, are manifested by narrowing of the joint space and osteophytosis.

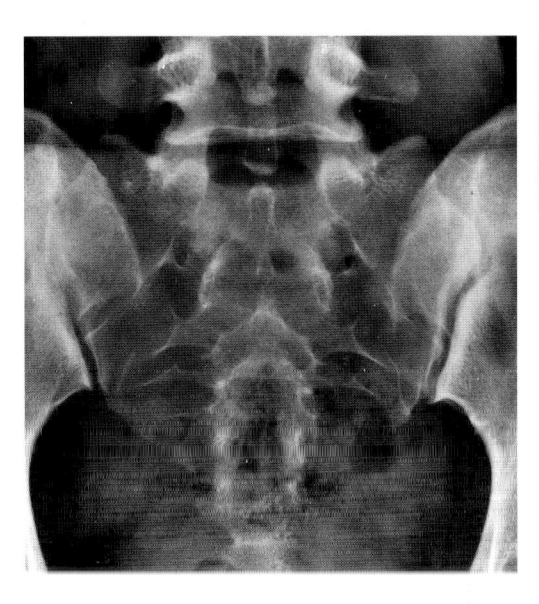

FIGURE 5.7 The true diarthrodial portion of the sacroiliac joint comprises only about 50% of the radiographic joint space. The upper part is a syndesmotic joint.

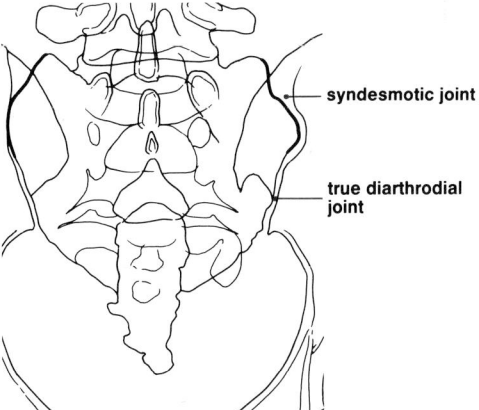

Degenerative Diseases of the Spine **5.5**

are related to the negative pressure created by abnormally altered disk spaces.

Other radiographic findings of degenerative disk disease include disk space narrowing and osteophytosis at the marginal borders of the adjacent vertebral bodies. Degenerative disk disease, in combination with degenerative changes in the apophyseal joints, may lead to degenerative spondylolisthesis (Fig. 5.8).

Spondylosis Deformans

Spondylosis deformans is a degenerative condition marked by the formation of anterior and lateral osteophytes as a result of anterior and anterolateral disk herniation (see Fig. 3.41A). As Schmorl (1971) and other investigators have pointed out, the initiating factors in the development of this condition are abnormalities in the peripheral fibers of the annulus fibrosus that result in weakening of the anchorage of the intervertebral disk to the vertebral body at the site of attachment of Sharpey fibers to the vertebral rim. Unlike degenerative disk disease, the intervertebral spaces in spondylosis deformans are relatively well preserved, the primary radiographic feature being extensive osteophytosis (Fig. 5.9). These osteophytes must be differentiated from the delicate syndesmophytes of ankylosing spondylitis, from the large, characteristically asymmetric bone excrescences that are seen in psoriatic arthritis and Reiter syndrome involving the lateral aspect of vertebral bodies, and from the flowing, usually anterior, hyperostosis of the DISH syndrome.

Diffuse Idiopathic Skeletal Hyperostosis (DISH)

DISH, originally described by Forestier and Rotes Querol (1950) and elaborated on by Resnick et al. (1975), is characterized by flowing ossification along the anterior aspect of the vertebral bodies extending across the disk spaces. It is also associated with hyperostosis at the sites of tendon and ligament attachment to the bone, ligament ossification, and osteophytosis involving the axial and appendicular skeleton. A lateral radiograph of the spine best demonstrates these changes. As in spondylosis deformans, the disk spaces, at least initially, are usually well preserved (Fig. 5.10). It is important to distinguish this condition from the apparently similar "bamboo spine" seen in ankylosing spondylitis (see Fig. 6.6).

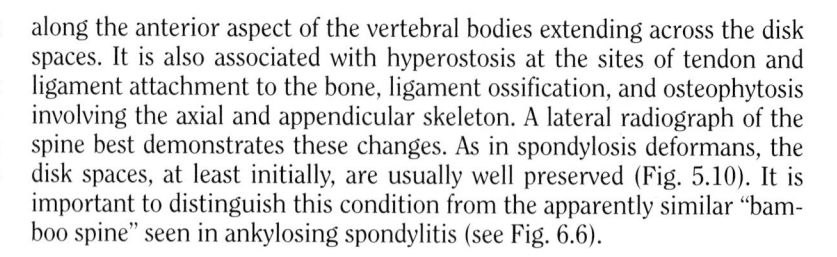

COMPLICATIONS OF DEGENERATIVE DISEASES OF THE SPINE

Degenerative Spondylolisthesis

One of the most common complications of degenerative disease of the spine, degenerative spondylolisthesis, results from degenerative changes in the disk and apophyseal joints. In this condition, there is anterior displacement of a vertebra onto the one below, which can usually be easily recognized on the lateral view of the spine by the spinous-process sign (Fig. 5.11; see also Fig. 3.38). MRI may also be useful in demonstrating this abnormality (Fig. 5.12). However, on occasion, the displacement may not be obvious on the standard lateral film, and radiographs must be obtained while the patient maximally extends and flexes the spine (Fig. 5.13). As Milgram (1986) pointed out, the stress applied by forward and backward motion of the spine discloses instability (spondylolisthesis) that might be overlooked on other projections.

Degenerative spondylolisthesis occurs in approximately 4% of patients with degenerative disk disease, affecting females more often than males. It has a predilection for the L4–L5 spinal level. This predilection has been

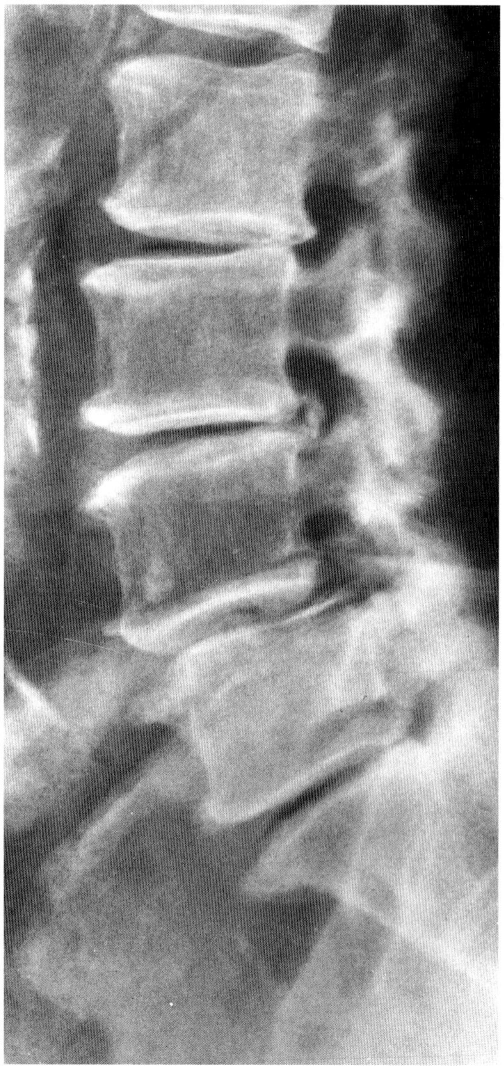

FIGURE 5.8 Lateral view of the lumbosacral spine in a 66-year-old woman demonstrates advanced degenerative disk disease at multiple levels. Note the radiolucent collections of gas in several disks (the vacuum phenomenon) as well as the narrowing of the disk spaces and marginal osteophytes. Grade 1 degenerative spondylolisthesis is seen at the L4–L5 level.

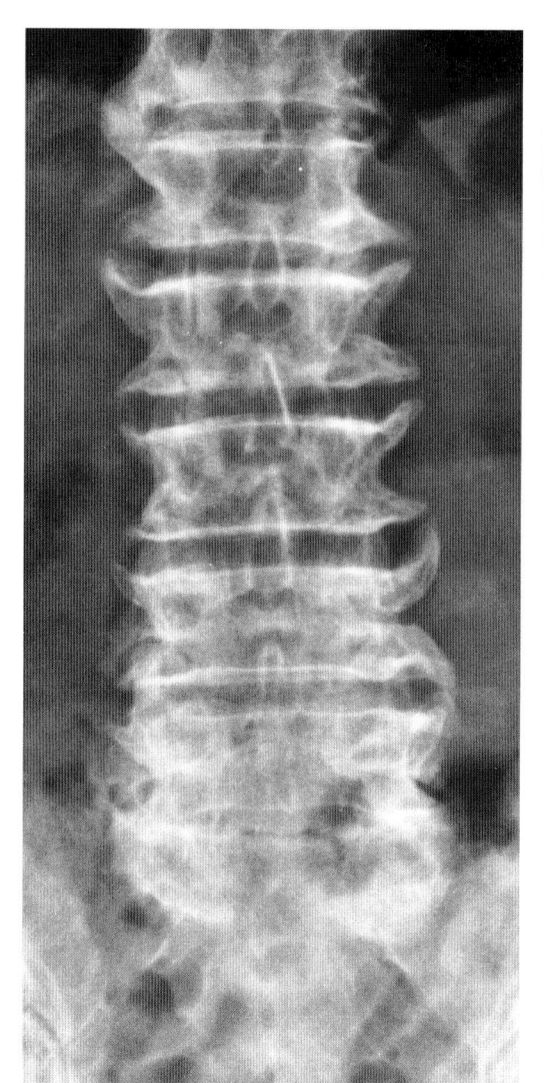

FIGURE 5.9 Anteroposterior projection of the lumbosacral spine in a 68-year-old woman demonstrates the typical changes of spondylosis deformans. Note the extensive osteophytosis and relatively well preserved intervertebral disk spaces.

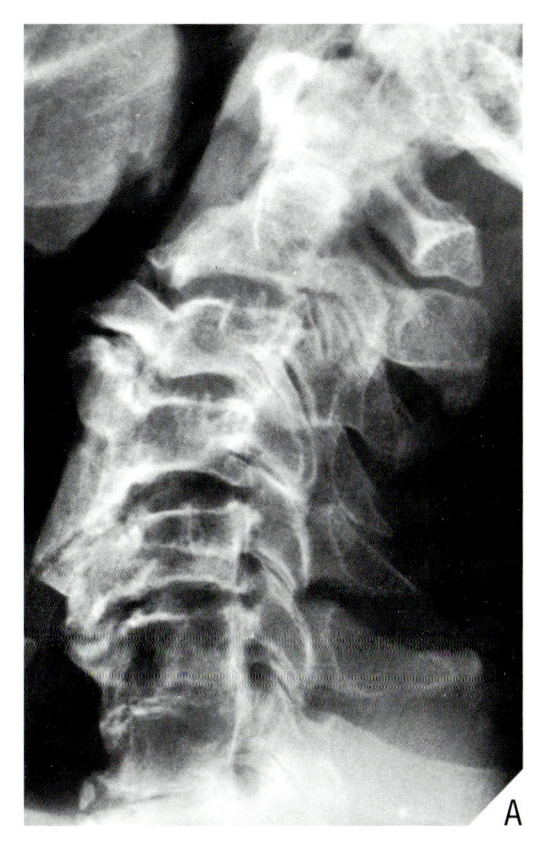

FIGURE 5.10 Lateral views of the cervical **(A)**, thoracic **(B)**, and lumbar **(C)** spine in a 72-year-old man with Forestier disease (DISH) show the characteristic flowing hyperostosis extending across the vertebral disk spaces, which are relatively well preserved.

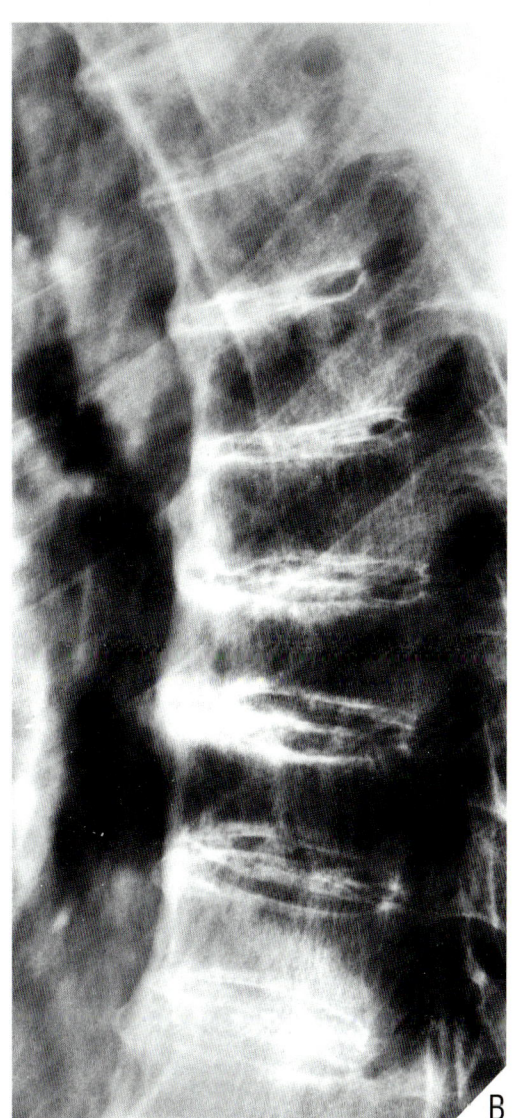

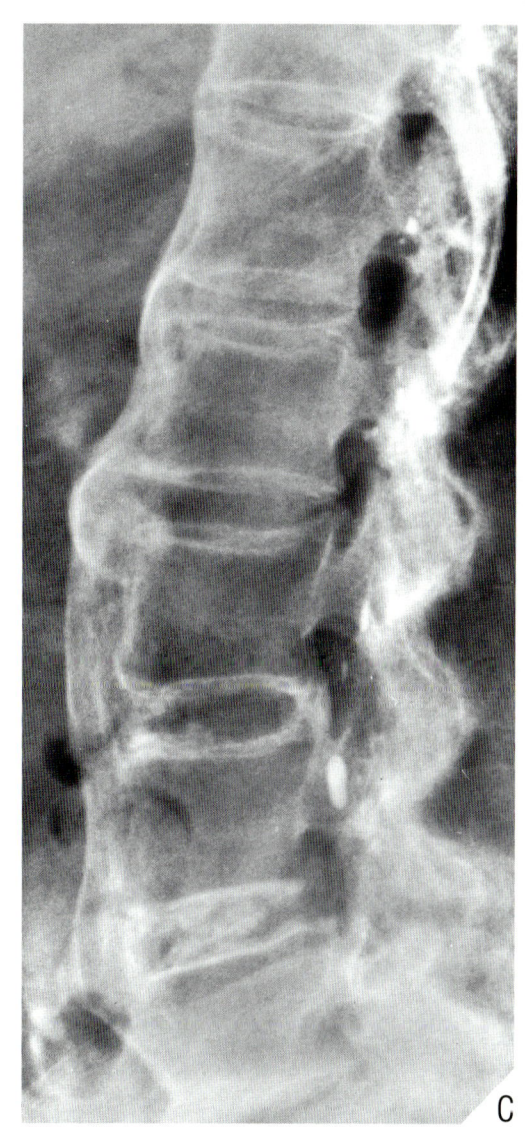

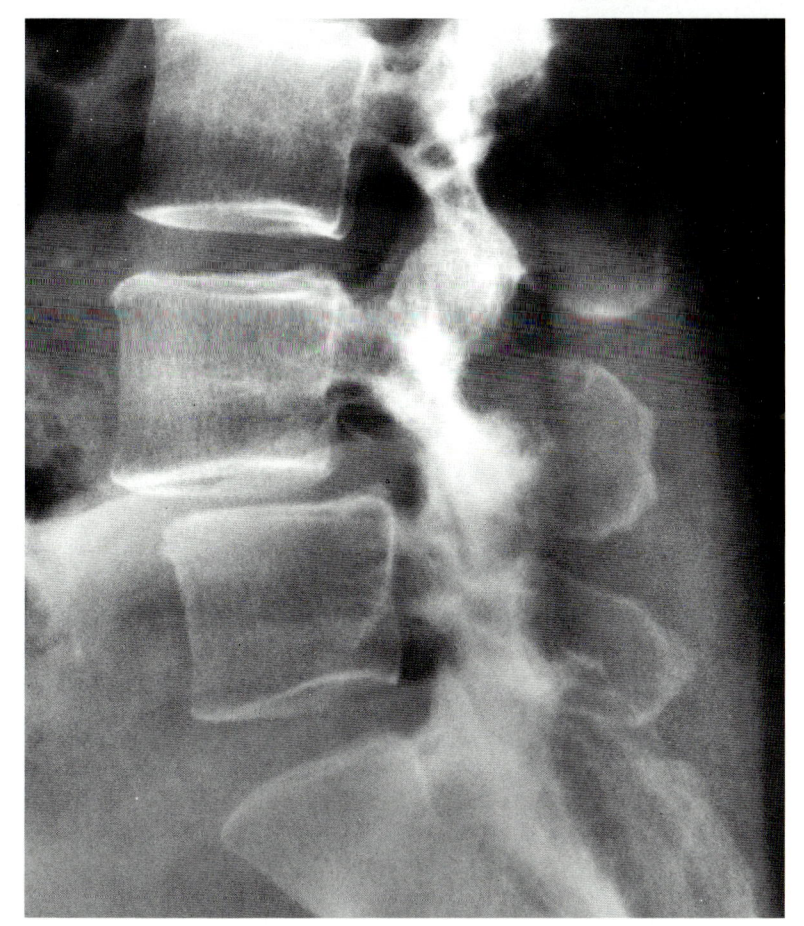

FIGURE 5.11 A 55-year-old woman with degenerative disk disease at L4–L5 and degenerative facet arthritis developed spondylolisthesis, a common complication of this condition. Lateral view of the lumbosacral spine is sufficient to differentiate this condition from spondylolisthesis associated with spondylolysis by the appearance of a step-off of the spinous process at the vertebra below the involved intervertebral space.

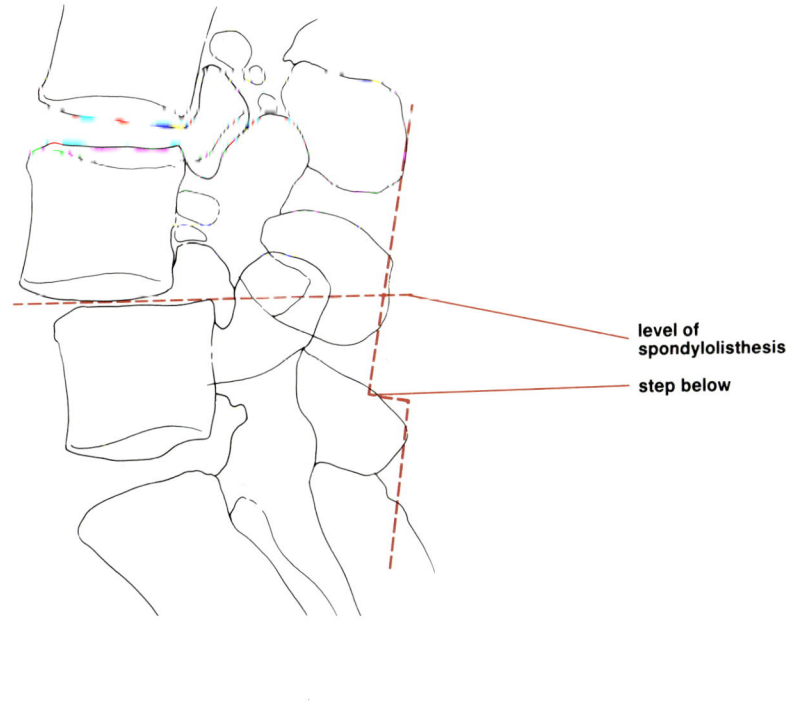

level of spondylolisthesis

step below

Degenerative Diseases of the Spine **5.7**

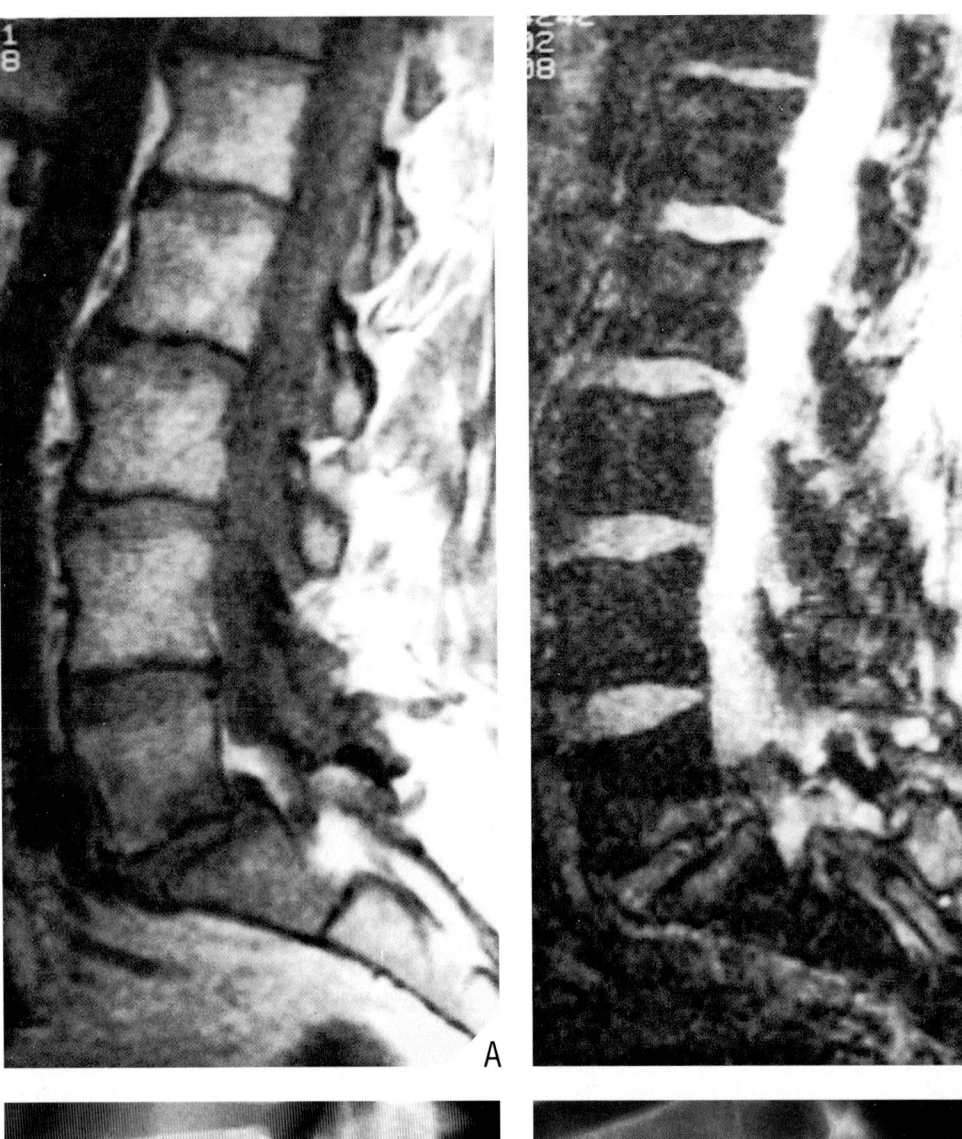

FIGURE 5.12 (A) Sagittal T1-weighted MRI [SE, TR 800/TE 20] demonstrates slight anterior spondylolisthesis of the fifth lumbar vertebral body on the first sacral body due to both degeneration of the intervertebral disk and facet disease. The lumbosacral disk space is narrowed and shows decreased signal intensity. The juxtaposed endplates show lower signal intensity than the remaining fatty marrow spaces secondary to bony sclerosis. **(B)** Sagittal gradient-echo section [GRASS, TR 1000/TE 12, flip angle 22.5°] shows normal high signal from disk interspaces. The lumbosacral intervertebral disk is imaged clearly lower in signal intensity than in the other disks, which is consistent with degeneration. (Reproduced with permission from Beltran J: *MRI: Musculoskeletal System.* New York, Gower, 1990)

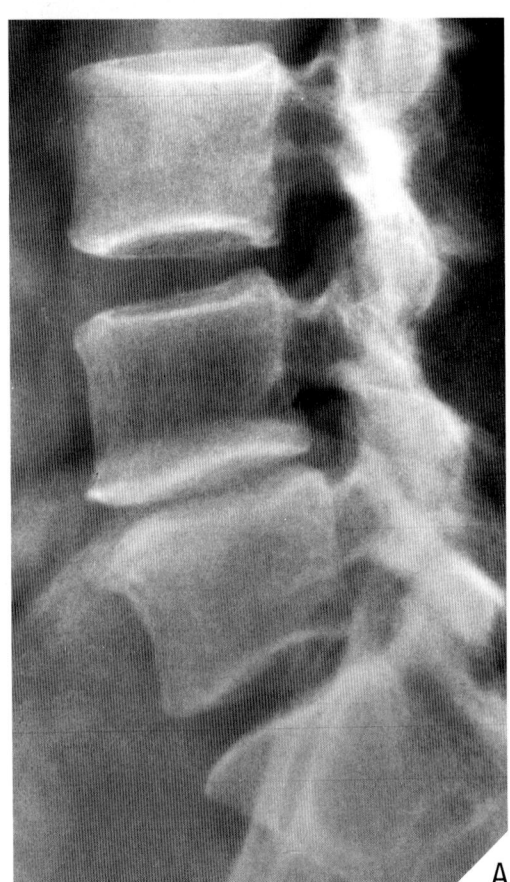

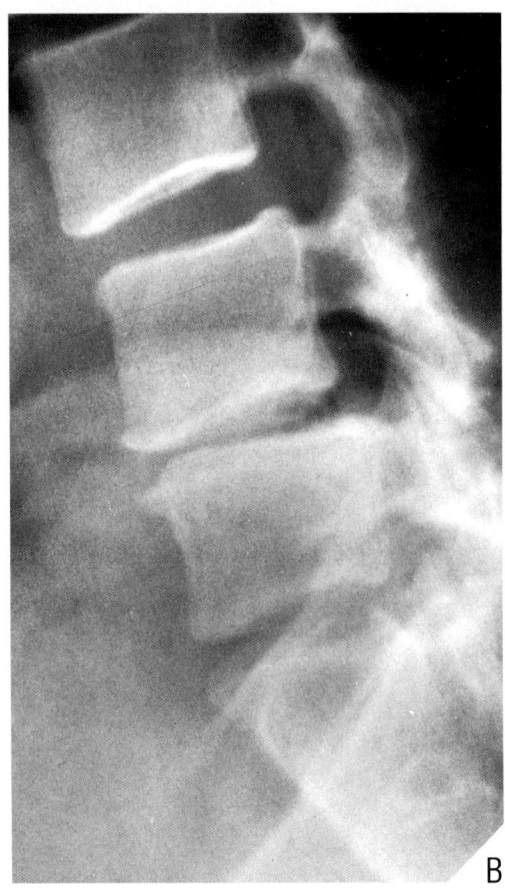

FIGURE 5.13 A 50-year-old man presented with chronic low back pain. **(A)** Standard lateral view of the lumbosacral spine in the neutral position shows narrowing of the L4–L5 disk space, indicating degenerative disk disease. There is no evidence of vertebral list. **(B)** Lateral view in flexion, however, demonstrates grade 1 spondylolisthesis at L4–L5.

Imaging of the Spine in Clinical Practice

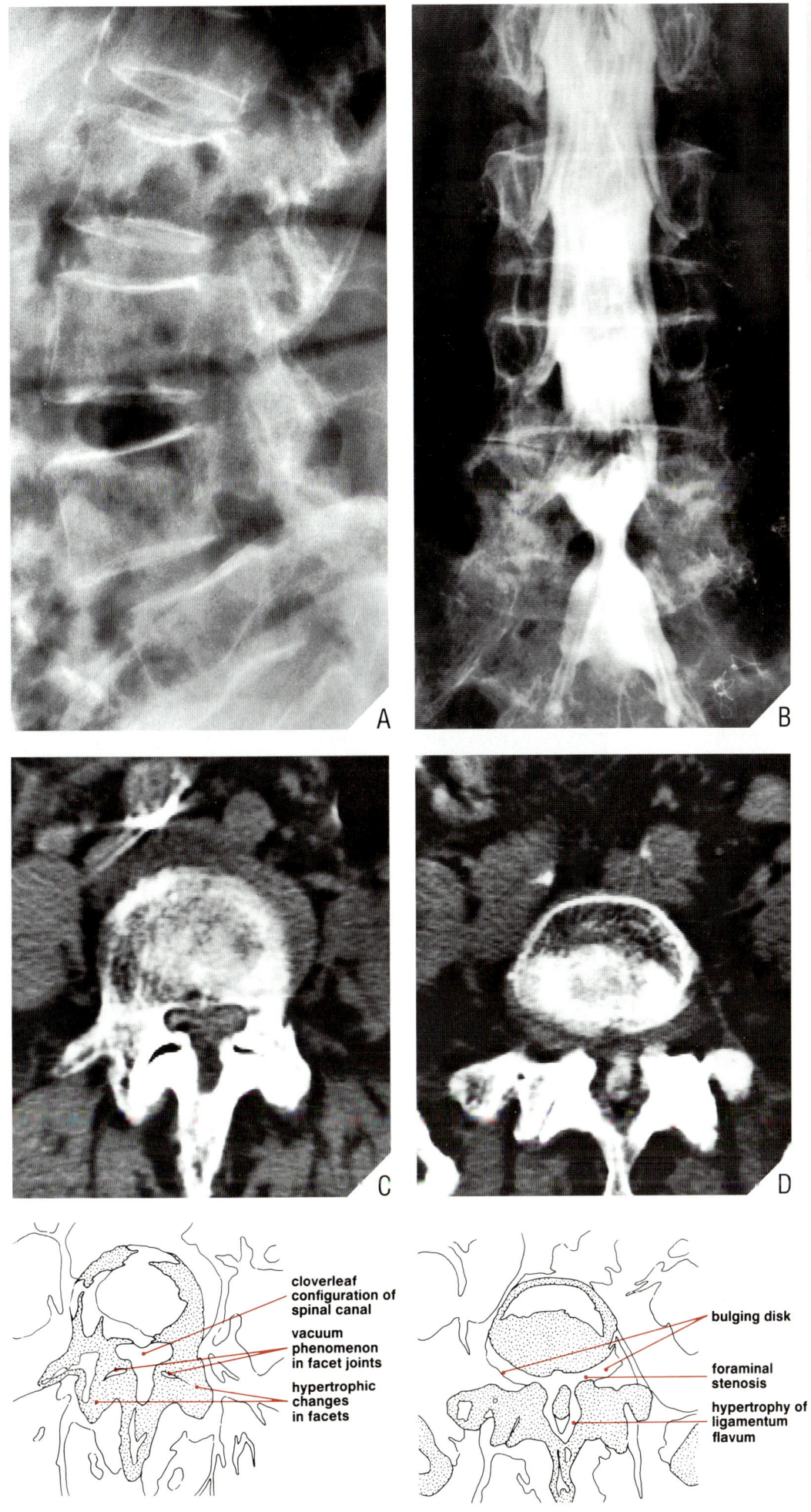

FIGURE 5.14 A 71-year-old woman was evaluated for severe low back pain. **(A)** Standard lateral view of the lumbar spine shows degenerative spondylolisthesis at the L4–L5 interspace. Note the short appearance of the pedicles. **(B)** A myelogram in the anteroposterior projection also discloses segmental narrowing of the thecal sac; the upper defect is related to spondylolisthesis, the lower to spinal stenosis. **(C,D)** CT sections demonstrate the details of the abnormalities—severe spinal and foraminal stenosis, hypertrophy of the ligamenta flava, and posterior bulging of the intervertebral disk. Note the cloverleaf configuration of the spinal canal secondary to marked hypertrophy of the facet joints. The vacuum phenomenon in the apophyseal joints is well demonstrated.

Degenerative Diseases of the Spine 5.9

attributed to developmental or acquired alterations in the neural arch that lead to instability and abnormal stress. The stress applied to the vertebra may result in decompensation of the ligaments, hypermobility, instability, and osteoarthritis of adjacent apophyseal joints.

Clinical symptoms associated with degenerative spondylolisthesis include low back pain, sciatic pain with signs of nerve root compression, and intermittent claudication. It should be noted, however, that many patients with degenerative spondylolisthesis are asymptomatic.

Radiographic findings of degenerative spondylolisthesis include osteoarthritic changes of the facet joints (joint narrowing, marginal eburnation, and osteophyte formation), anterior slippage of the superior vertebra on the inferior vertebra, and, in many instances, intervertebral vacuum phenomenon. The affected intervertebral disk space is invariably narrowed (see Figs. 5.8, 5.12).

Spinal Stenosis

Spinal stenosis is a much more severe complication of degenerative disease. The acquired form is caused by hypertrophy of the structures surrounding the spinal canal, such as the pedicles, laminae, articular processes, and the posterior aspect of the vertebral bodies, as well as the ligamentum flavum. This may or may not be complicated by posterior protrusion of the intervertebral disks. Iatrogenic spinal stenosis may develop after laminectomy secondary to subluxation in the facet joints, or after extensive posterior spinal fusion secondary to a build-up of bone on the anterior surface of the laminae. These alterations are usually apparent on plain film radiography; however, spinal stenosis can be better demonstrated by ancillary techniques, such as myelography, which can show the impingement of the thecal sac by hypertrophic changes of the posterior parts of the vertebral body and bulging disks (see Fig. 4.4). In general, the details of spinal stenosis are best delineated by CT (Fig. 5.14). In a normal subject, the sagittal diameter of the lumbar spinal canal exceeds 10 mm. If midsagittal measurement of the canal is less, spinal stenosis is confirmed. Magnetic resonance imaging is also an effective modality in evaluating spinal stenosis (Figs. 5.15, 5.16).

Spinal stenosis in the lumbar segment can be classified into three groups on the basis of the anatomic location: (1) stenosis of the spinal canal; (2) stenosis of the subarticular or lateral recesses; (3) stenosis of the neural foramina.

The causes of stenosis of the central canal are related to hypertrophic, osteoarthritic changes of the apophyseal joints, thickening of the ligamentum flavum, osteophytes arising from the vertebral bodies, and posterior disk protrusion. Bone hypertrophy at the site of the facet joints is a major cause of stenosis of the subarticular or lateral recesses, leading to encroachment on the neural elements in this region. Clinical manifestations of lateral recess syndrome include unilateral or bilateral leg pain,

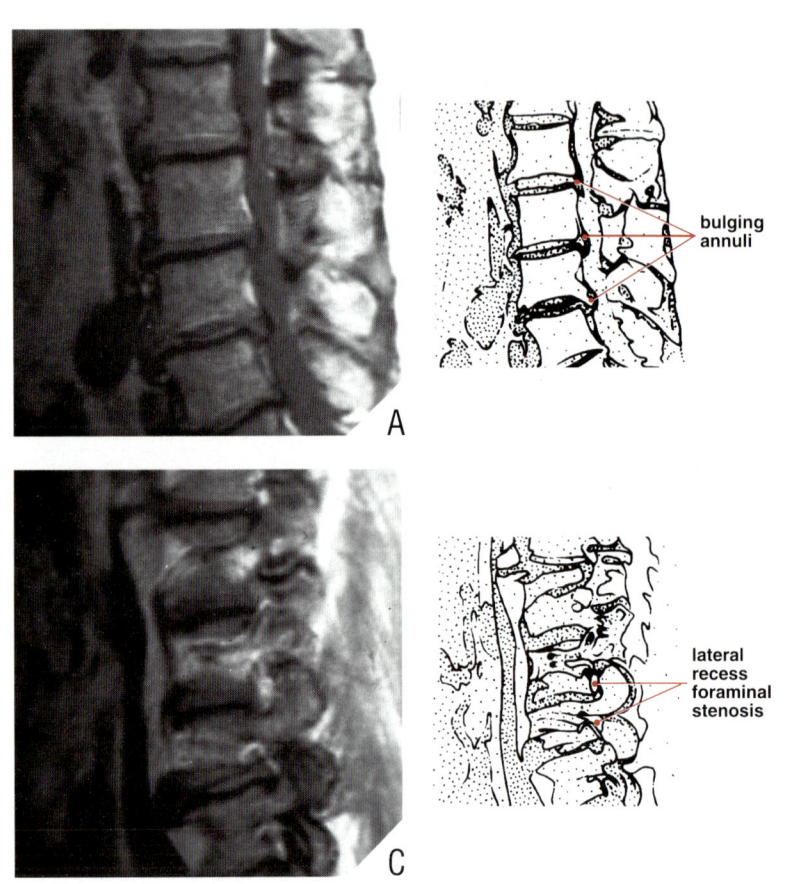

FIGURE 5.15 (A) Sagittal MRI (T1-weighted spin-echo image, TR800/TE20) shows narrowing of the intervertebral disk spaces associated with posterior bulging of annuli fibrosa. **(B)** GRASS image (flip angle 22.5°) demonstrates to better advantage bulging annuli compressing anterior aspect of the thecal sac. Note also dorsal compression of the sac due to ligamentous hypertrophy. The combined hypertrophic changes lead to spinal stenosis. **(C)** Parasagittal section (T1-weighted spin-echo image, TR800/TE20) demonstrates foreshortening of the neural foramina in cephalo-caudad dimension due to narrowing of the disk space and a narrowed sagittal dimension secondary to hypertrophy of the facet joints. **(D)** Axial MRI (T1-weighted spin-echo image, TR800/TE20) demonstrates hypertrophic changes of the facet joints. There is less epidural fat in the lateral recesses and neural foramina, secondary to degenerative hypertrophy of bony structures. The ligamentum flavum is slightly thickened. (Reproduced with permission from Beltran J: *MRI: Musculoskeletal System.* New York, Gower, 1990).

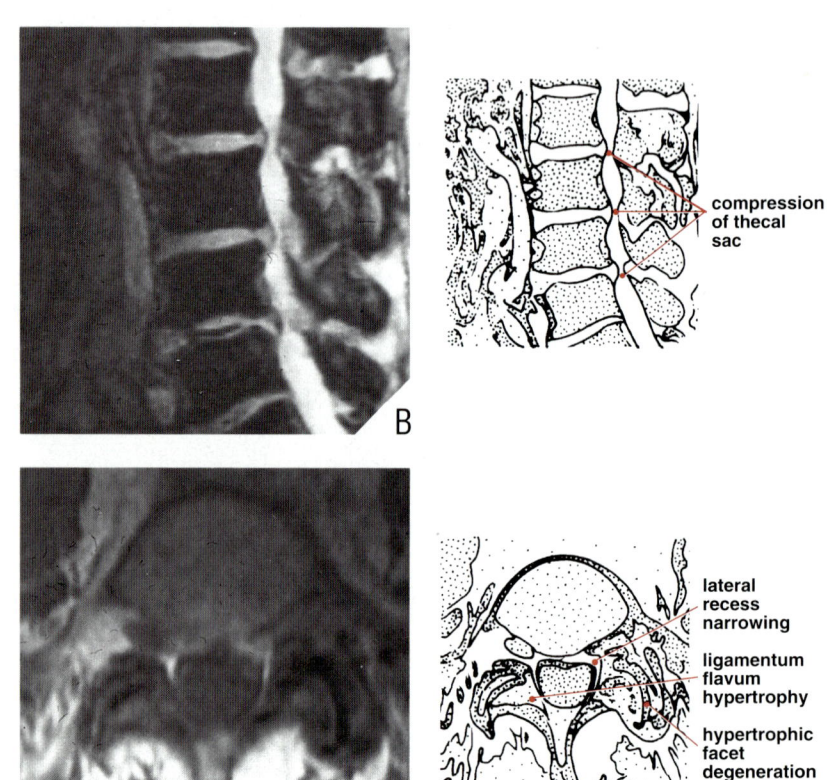

which is initiated or aggravated by long periods of standing or walking. These symptoms are usually relieved entirely by sitting or squatting.

Stenosis of the neural foramina is caused by hypertrophic changes and osteophytosis involving the vertebral body and articular process. Moreover, degenerative spondylolisthesis may be associated with distortion of the intervertebral foramen and may lead to compromise of the exiting nerve.

Cervical stenosis is typically secondary to either multiple-level spondylosis (ie, several osteophyte formations) or ossification of the posterior longitudinal ligament, or it is congenital (ie, secondary to congenitally short pedicles).

The patient with cervical stenosis will usually present with radiculopathy, myelopathy, or myeloradiculopathy. While radiculopathy is expressed by neck pain, arm pain, and possibly sensory and motor changes, myelopathy may be more subtle. Typically, the early stage of myelopathy is associated with gait disturbances or minor changes in the patient's bowel or bladder habits. These symptoms, if untreated, may progress to complete paralysis.

TREATMENT

Degenerative spine disease is often asymptomatic and, according to Mooney (1986), cannot be considered the major cause of chronic back pain. As Jackson and colleagues (1988) pointed out, neither is facet joint arthritis a major source of back pain.

More recently, McLain (personal communication) has demonstrated poor innervation of the facet joints, lumbar dorsal fascia, and paraspinal muscles, but rich innervation of the annulus, suggesting that the annulus is a more probable source of back pain because it possesses more pain receptors.

It appears, as Kahanovitz (1986) points out, that 90% of the patients with low back pain will recover from an episode of back pain in 6 to 12 weeks, regardless of the treatment administered. In other words, as the Quebec Task Force Study demonstrated, there are no scientific data to suggest that ice, heat, massage, ultrasound, or manipulation can benefit patients suffering from back or neck pain. Only patient education, aerobic training, and functional rehabilitation alter the natural history of back pain.

Therefore it seems that 10% of patients will go on to have chronic back pain. Of these, many will respond to an aggressive functional rehabilitation program. The remainder may or may not be candidates for surgical stabilization. Selection of surgical candidates is perhaps based more on art than on science. Relative contraindications to surgery include a history of tobacco abuse, an abnormal MMPI (Minnesota Multiphasic Personality Inventory) test, or inconsistent pain drawings. Diskography has recently gained wide acceptance despite the lack of firm scientific correlation for this technique. Many clinicians are attempting to correlate pain and diskographic injection as confirmation of spine stability.

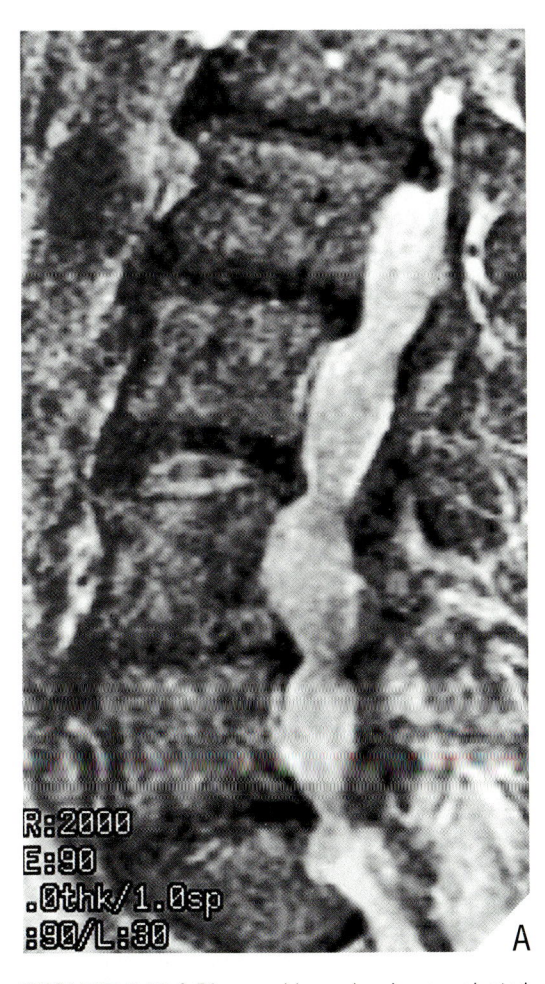

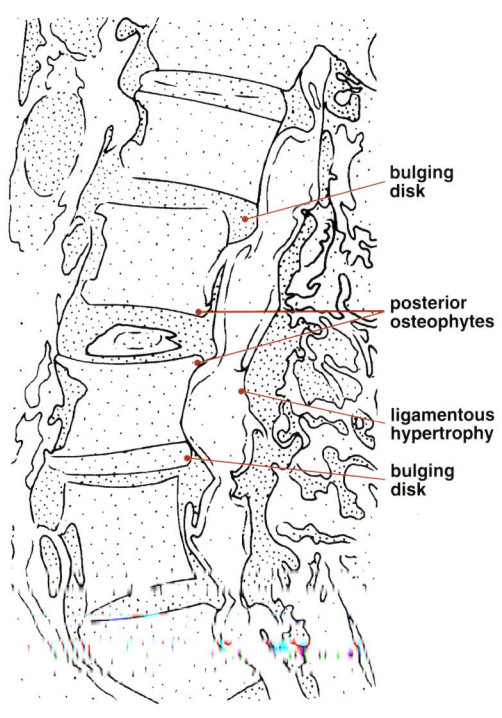

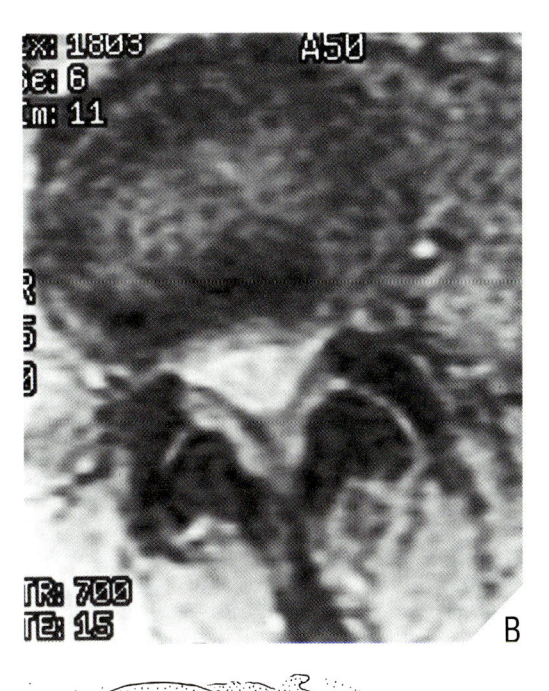

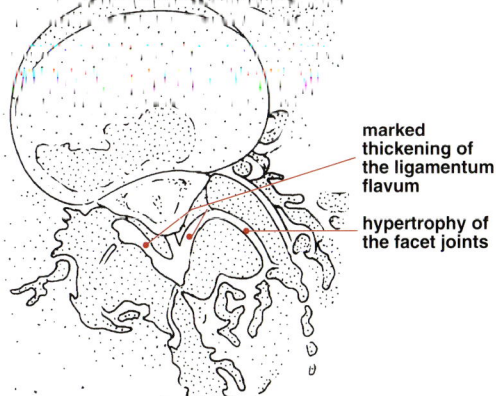

FIGURE 5.16 A 51-year-old man has been evaluated for possible spinal sternosis. (A) Sagittal T2-weighted MRI (SE, TR 2000/TE 90) shows significant narrowing of the ventrodorsal diameter of the spinal canal secondary to multiple bulging disks and posterior osteophytes. Also noted is compression of the thecal sac posteriorly, secondary to ligamentous hypertrophy. The lumbar portion of thecal sac assumed "washboard" configuration, typical for spinal stenosis. (B) Axial section demonstrates hypertrophy of the facet joints and marked thickening of the ligamentum flavum.

If surgical stabilization is elected, decisions regarding the choice of approach must be made. An anterior approach allows complete removal of the offending disk and also allows the surgeon to perform an anterior spine fusion. Alternatively, the surgeon of the future may be performing total disk replacements, as has been reported in eastern Europe.

Posterior fusion has been reported to have a greater success rate and allows for easier, more complete decompression of the neurologic structures (Jackson RT, et al., 1988).

Instrumentation may or may not be required. Instrumentation allows the maintenance of reduction when reduction of the spinal elements is essential. It also improves solidity of the fusion and time to achieve fusion.

Degenerative spondylolisthesis describes a radiographic diagnosis which may or may not be symptomatic. The patient may, however, present with symptoms secondary to disk instability (eg, back pain) or symptoms secondary to spinal stenosis (eg, leg pain, neurologic claudication).

Controversy exists regarding treatment of this condition. The authors of this text recommend disregarding the radiographic appearance of the spine and treating the symptoms. Patients presenting with isolated back pain are evaluated for lumbar fusion. If reduction is achieved on preoperative extension films, instrumentation will help to maintain reduction of maturing fusion masses. Instrumentation, however, should not be used to achieve a forceful reduction.

Patients presenting with leg pain or neurologic claudication with minimal or no back pain should undergo a neurologic decompression. The role of concomitant fusion is controversial. The authors of this text recommend fusion when significant back pain is present or in young patients with preservation of disk space who have had more than 50% of the posterior elements removed (all of one facet or 50% of each facet). If the patient is older, with an arthritic spine and significant disk space collapse, no fusion is performed but the patient is followed closely after surgery for the development of back pain and/or increased post-laminectomy spine deformity.

The treatment of spinal stenosis is dependent on its location and extent. If there is compromise of the canal posteriorly or if the canal compromise is secondary to multilevel anterior lesions, posterior decompression in the form of a laminectomy or laminoplasty is usually performed. In doing the decompression, we try to be as complete as possible and remove all structures necessary to insure complete neurologic decompression. If the stenosis is secondary to an anterior penetrating lesion, we perform an anterior decompression, ie, a complete anterior vertebrectomy.

When performing a laminectomy the question of posterolateral fusion versus no fusion often arises. In practice we generally recommend procedures according to the clinical presentation of the patient: if the patient presents with extremity pain, then a decompression procedure alone is performed; if the patient presents with both back pain and extremity pain, where back pain is a predominant complaint, then laminectomy and fusion are performed simultaneously.

Options for treatment of cervical stenosis include multiple-level diskectomy, multiple-level vertebrectomy, or posterior laminoplasty.

SUGGESTED READING

Beggs I: Radiological assessment of degenerative diseases of the cervical spine. *Semin Orthop* 2:63, 1987.

Bora FW Jr, Miller G: Joint physiology, cartilage metabolism, and the etiology of osteoarthritis. *Hand Clin* 3:325, 1987.

Brandt KD: Osteoarthritis. *Clin Geriatr Med* 4:279, 1988.

Davis MA: Epidemiology of osteoarthritis. *Clin Geriatr Med* 4:241, 1988.

Forestier J, Rotes Querol J: Senile ankylosing hyperostosis of the spine. *Ann Rheum Dis* 9:321, 1950.

Jackson RT, Jacobs RR, Monesano PX: 1988 Volvo Award in Clinical Sciences: Facet joint injections in low-back pain: A prospective statistical study. *Spine* 13:966, 1988.

Jacobs RR, Montesano PX, Jackson RP: Enhancement of lumbar spine fusion by use of translaminar facet joint screws. *Spine* 14:12, 1988.

Kahanovitz N: Lumbar spine. In *Orthopaedic Knowledge, Update 3*. American Academy of Orthopaedic Surgeons, 1990.

Kirkaldy-Willis WH, Farfan HG: Instability of the lumbar spine. *Clin Orthop* 165:110, 1982.

Knutsson F: The vacuum phenomenon in the intervertebral discs. *Acta Radiol* 23:173, 1942.

Kumpan W, Salomonowitz E, Seidl G, et al: The intervertebral vacuum phenomenon. *Skel Radiol* 15:444, 1986.

Lefkowitz DM, Quencer RM: Vacuum facet phenomenon: A computed tomographic sign of degenerative spondylolisthesis. *Radiology* 144:562, 1982.

Maldague BE, Noel HM, Malghem JJ: The intervertebral vacuum cleft: A sign of ischemic vertebral collapse. *Radiology* 129:23, 1978.

Mayer TG, Gatchel RJ, Kishino N, et al: 1985 Volvo Award in Clinical Sciences: Objective assessment of spine function following industrial injury: A prospective study with comparison group and one-year follow-up. *Spine* 10:482, 1985.

McAfee PC, Ullrich CG, Levinsohn EM, et al: Computed tomography in degenerative lumbar spinal stenosis. The value of multiplanar reconstruction. *RadioGraphics* 2:529, 1982.

Milgram JE: Recurrent articular spondylolisthesis: Common cause of vertebral instabilities, root pain, sciatica, and ultimately spinal stenosis. Early detection and blocking of specific dislocations. *Bull Hosp Jt Dis Orthop Inst* 46:47, 1986.

Mooney V: The presidential address to the International Society for the Study of the Lumbar Spine entitled "Where is the pain coming from?" *Spine* 7:754, 1986.

Norman A, Robbins H, Milgram JE: The acute neuropathic arthropathy—A rapid severely disorganizing form of arthritis. *Radiology* 90:1159, 1968

Pathria M, Sartoris DJ, Resnick D: Osteoarthritis of the facet joints: Accuracy of oblique radiographic assessment. *Radiology* 164:227, 1987.

Postachinni F, Pezzeri G, Montanaro A, et al: Computerized tomography in lumbar stenosis. *J Bone Joint Surg* 62B:78, 1980.

Pritzker KPH: Aging and degeneration in the lumbar intervertebral disc. *Orthop Clin North Am* 8:65, 1977.

Resnick D: Degenerative diseases of the vertebral column. *Radiology* 156:3, 1985.

Resnick D, Niwayama G: Entheses and enthesopathy. Anatomical, pathological and radiological correlation. *Radiology* 246:1, 1983.

Resnick D, Niwayama G, Goergen TG: Degenerative disease of the sacroiliac joint. *Invest Radiol* 10:608, 1975.

Resnick D, Shaul SR, Robins JM: Diffuse idiopathic skeletal hyperostosis (DISH): Forestier's disease with extraspinal manifestations. *Radiology* 115:513, 1975.

Schmorl G, Junghanns H: *The Human Spine in Health and Disease*, 2nd ed (translated by Besemann EF). New York, Grune & Stratton, 1971.

Schumacher HR: Articular cartilage in the degenerative arthropathy of hemochromatosis. *Arthritis Rheum* 25:1460, 1982.

Sokoloff L: Pathology and pathogenesis of osteoarthritis. In Hollander JL, McCarty DJ (eds): *Arthritis and Allied Conditions,* 8th ed. Philadelphia, Lea & Febiger, 1972.

Spitzer WO, LeBlanc FE, Dupuis M: Scientific approach to the assessment and management of activity-related spinal disorders. A monograph for clinicians. Report of the Quebec Task Force on Spinal Disorders. *Spine* 12:7S(suppl. 1), 1987.

Weisz GM: Value of computerized tomography in diagnosis of diseases of the lumbar spine. *Med J Aust* 1:216, 1982.

Weisz GM, Lee P: Spinal canal stenosis. *Clin Orthop* 179:134, 1983.

Weisz GM, Lee P: Spinal reserve capacity. A radiologic concept of lumbar canal stenosis. *Orthop Rev* 13:579, 1984.

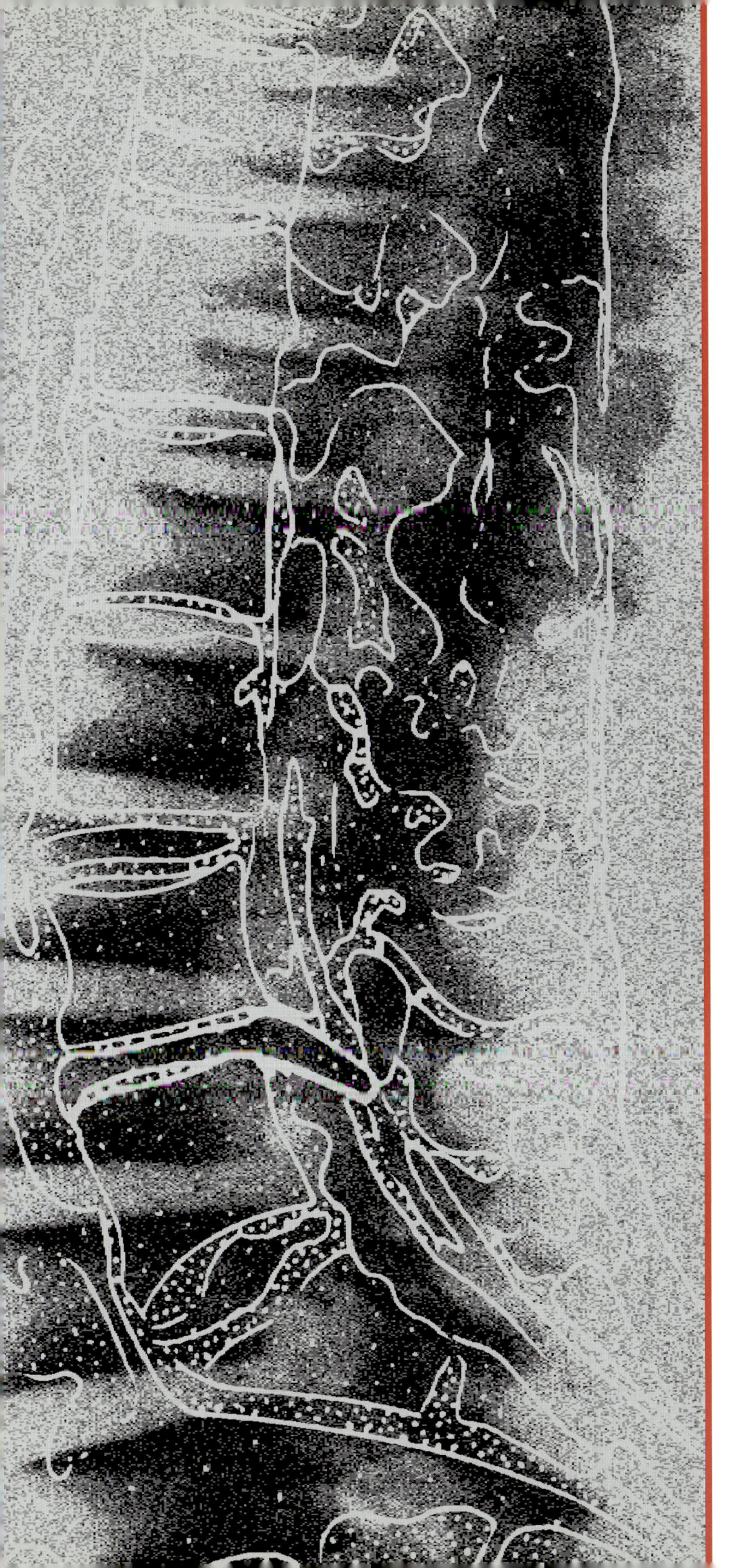

Inflammatory Arthritides of the Spine

6

The inflammatory arthritides comprise a group of differing and for the most part systemic disorders which have in common one important feature: inflammatory pannus eroding articular cartilage and bone (Fig. 6.1).

RHEUMATOID ARTHRITIS

Rheumatoid arthritis is a progressive, chronic, systemic inflammatory disease affecting primarily the synovial joints; women are affected three times more often than men. The course of the disease varies from patient to patient, and there is a striking tendency towards spontaneous remissions and exacerbations. The detection of rheumatoid factor(s), representing specific antibodies in the patient's serum, is an important diagnostic finding. Although the point is debatable, some investigators also include under this rubric a condition called *seronegative rheumatoid arthritis*, in which patients with absent rheumatoid factor nevertheless exhibit the typical clinical and radiographic picture of rheumatoid arthritis.

Rheumatoid factors, widely used for clinical diagnosis, are antigammaglobulin antibodies that are elaborated in part by rheumatoid synovium. Rheumatoid factors in synovial fluid are either of the IgG or IgM variety. They participate in pathogenesis of rheumatoid arthritis through the formation of local and circulating antigen–antibody complexes. These complexes activate the complement system, which releases mediators responsible for producing inflammation within the joint structures. The process initiating these events is as yet unknown. Since rheumatoid factors are sometimes found in the joint fluids of patients with nonrheumatoid disorders, their presence is not necessarily diagnostic of rheumatoid arthritis. However, finding high titers of these factors in a joint effusion strongly suggests the diagnosis of rheumatoid arthritis. After the onset of disease, it is often possible to identify rheumatoid factors in the synovial fluid before they can be detected in the serum, thus allowing early diagnosis.

Radiographic Features

Rheumatoid arthritis is characterized by a diffuse, usually multicompartmental, symmetric narrowing of the joint space associated with marginal or central erosions, periarticular osteoporosis, and periarticular soft tissue swelling; subchondral sclerosis is minimal or absent and there is no formation of osteophytes. The thoracic and lumbar segments of the spine are only rarely affected by rheumatoid arthritis. The cervical spine, however, is involved in approximately 50% of patients with this condition.

The most characteristic radiographic features of rheumatoid arthritis in the cervical spine can be observed in the odontoid process, the atlantoaxial joints, and the apophyseal joints. Erosive changes may be seen in the odontoid process (see Fig. 4.2) and apophyseal joints (Fig. 6.2). Subluxation in the atlantoaxial joint is a common finding, frequently accompanied by superior migration of the odontoid process. The other structures occasionally affected by the rheumatoid process include the intervertebral disks and adjacent vertebral bodies, which become involved as a result of synovitis extending from the joints of Luschka. Only a small percentage of patients

HIGHLIGHTS OF INFLAMMATORY ARTHRITIS

Large Joints

Morphology

1 diffuse joint-space narrowing
2 marginal or central erosions
3 absent or minimal subchondral sclerosis
4 lack of osteophytes
5 cystic lesions
6 osteoporosis
7 periarticular soft tissue swelling (symmetric, usually fusiform)

Small Joints

1 periarticular osteoporosis
2 joint-space narrowing
3 marginal erosions
4 boutonnière deformity
5 swan-neck deformity
6 subluxations and dislocations
7 soft tissue swelling (symmetric, fusiform)

Spine

1 erosion of anterior aspect of odontoid
2 atlantoaxial subluxation with cephalad migration of C-2
3 erosion and fusion of apophyseal joints
4 erosion and whittling of spinous processes
5 destruction of intervertebral disks
6 erosion of vertebral bodies

Distribution

Rheumatoid Arthritis

Psoriatic Arthritis and Reiter Syndrome*
Ankylosing Spondylitis**

*Reiter syndrome more often affects the hip and lower extremity

**Most frequently affected large joints are hips and glenohumeral articulations

Erosive Osteoarthritis
adult   juvenile

Rheumatoid Arthritis

Psoriatic Arthritis   Reiter Syndrome

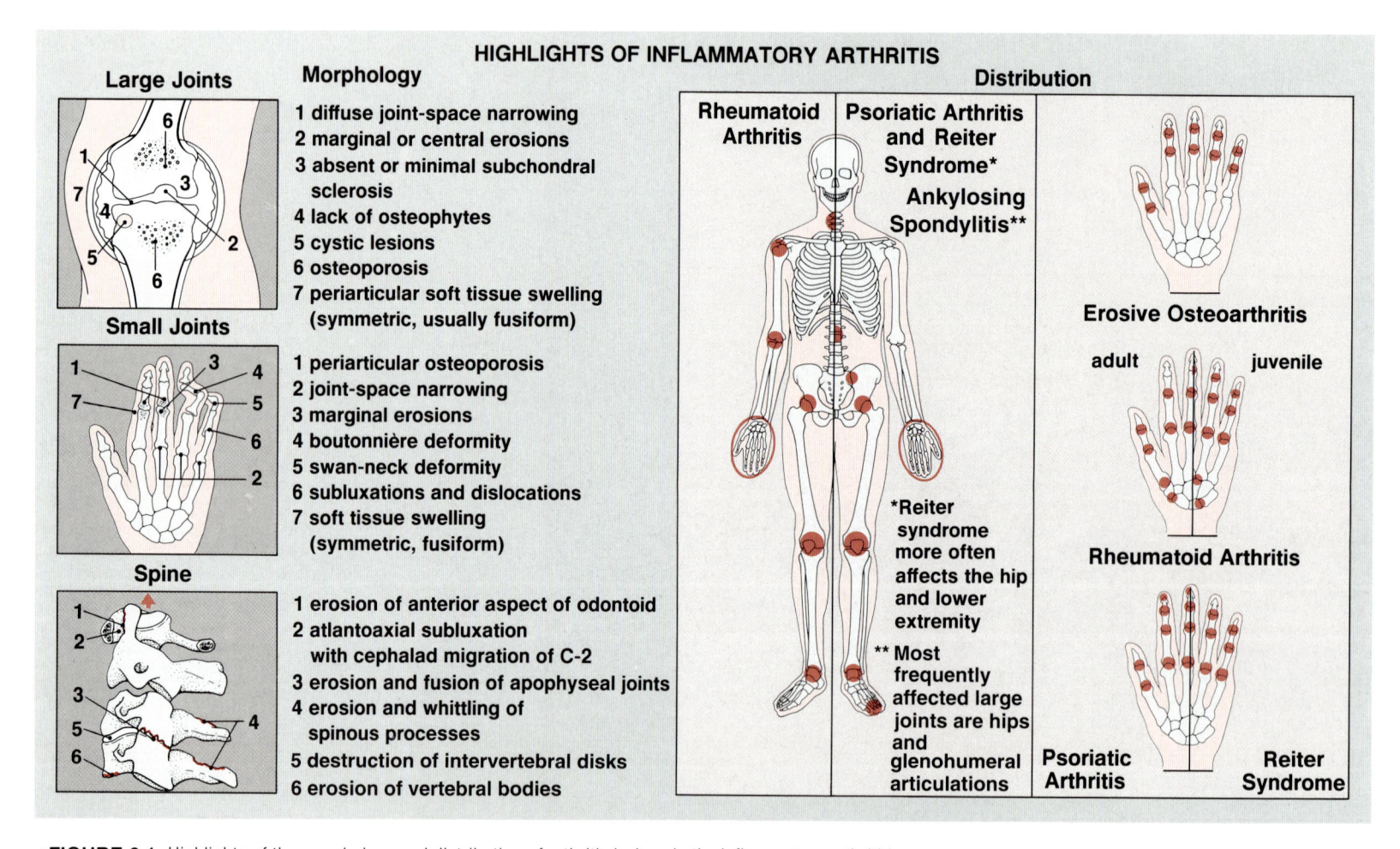

FIGURE 6.1 Highlights of the morphology and distribution of arthritic lesions in the inflammatory arthritides.

with cervical disease develop cervical myelopathy. Magnetic resonance imaging is an ideal modality for evaluating spinal cord involvement in these patients (see Fig. 4.5B).

Treatment of Cervical Instability

Cervical instability can be classified into three types: basilar invagination, C1–C2 instability, and subaxial subluxation or dislocation.

BASILAR INVAGINATION

In the past, lines such as those of Chamberlain, McRae, and McGregor (see Figs. 2.4–2.6) have been used to define basilar invagination. More recently, the Ranawat method (see Fig. 2.7) was found to be more useful because the landmarks are easier to locate radiographically. Indications for surgical stabilization include progressive invagination or declining neurologic status. These patients are often treated for 7 to 10 days with cervical traction, followed by occipito–cervical fusion. The neurologic status often improves with traction, as the odontoid process can be drawn out of the foramen magnum in this manner. However, if neurologic compromise persists, posterior decompression of the foramen magnum accompanied by a posterior C1 laminectomy may be required. In addition, an anterior transoral odontectomy is sometimes necessary.

C1–C2 INSTABILITY

C1–C2 instability is usually secondary to destruction of the transverse ligament by the inflammatory process. Atlantoaxial instability is treated by a posterior C1–C2 fusion, using either the Gallie or the Brook technique. The authors have not had good results using a Halifax clamp, and therefore, cannot recommend it. If the posterior elements are incompetent or absent, a posterior C1–C2 screw arthrodesis, as described by Magerl (1987), may be necessary. On the other hand, if the patient's bone is extremely osteopenic, an onlay fusion with halo immobilization must be performed.

SUBAXIAL SUBLUXATION OR DISLOCATION

These problems are treated by standard posterior wiring, such as the Bohlman triple-wire technique.

SERONEGATIVE SPONDYLOARTHROPATHIES

Ankylosing Spondylitis

Ankylosing spondylitis, known in the European literature as *Bekhterev disease* or *Marie–Strümpell disease*, is a chronic progressive inflammatory arthritis principally affecting the synovial joints of the spine and adjacent soft tissues, as well as the sacroiliac joints. The peripheral joints, such as hips, shoulders, and knees, may also be involved. This condition is seven times more common in men than in women, and usually occurs at a young age. Patients with ankylosing spondylitis frequently exhibit extraarticular features of disease, including iritis, pulmonary fibrosis, cardiac conduction defects, aortic incompetence, spinal cord compression, and amyloidosis. Low-grade fever, anorexia, fatigue, and weight loss may be present. Rheumatoid factor testing yields negative results in patients with

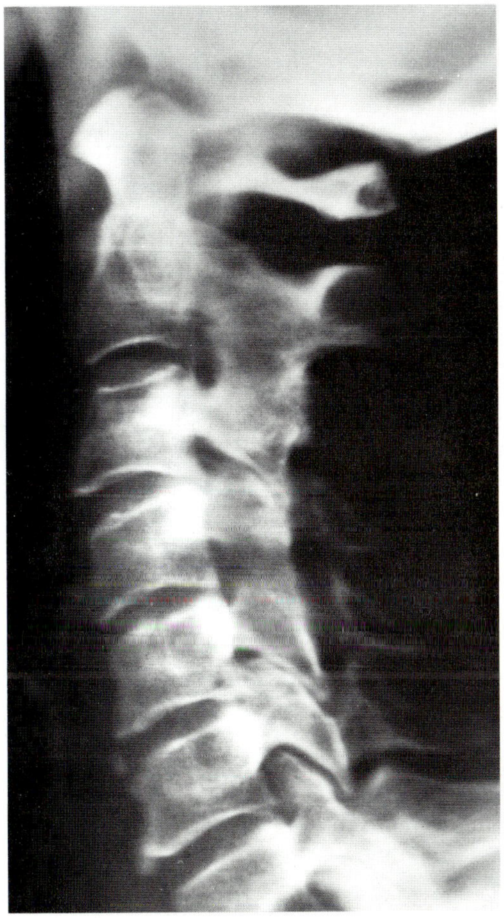

FIGURE 6.2 Lateral tomogram of the cervical spine in a 44-year-old woman demonstrates the erosions and narrowing of the apophyseal joints typical of rheumatoid arthritis.

ankylosing spondylitis, which is the prototype of the seronegative spondyloarthropathies. However, as many as 95% of these patients are positive for histocompatibility antigen HLA-B27. Histopathologically, ankylosing spondylitis is a diffuse proliferative synovitis of the diarthrodial joints, exhibiting features similar to those seen in rheumatoid arthritis.

Squaring of the anterior border of the lower thoracic and lumbar vertebrae is one of the earliest radiographic features of ankylosing spondylitis, best demonstrated on the lateral view of the spine (Fig. 6.3). As the condition progresses, syndesmophytes form, bridging the vertebral bodies (Fig. 6.4). The delicate appearance of these excrescences and their vertical, rather than horizontal, orientation distinguish them from the osteophytes of degenerative spine disease. Paravertebral ossifications are common in ankylosing spondylitis. When the apophyseal joints and vertebral bodies fuse late in the course of the disease, a radiographic hallmark of this condition, the "bamboo" spine, can be observed (Fig. 6.5). The sacroiliac joints are also invariably affected.

TREATMENT

In ankylosing spondylitis, not only does the spine fuse, but invariably it fuses in kyphosis. The kyphotic deformity can occur in the cervical, thoracic, or lumbar spine. Deformities of the cervical or lumbar spine are corrected by osteotomy. Cervical spine osteotomy is usually per-

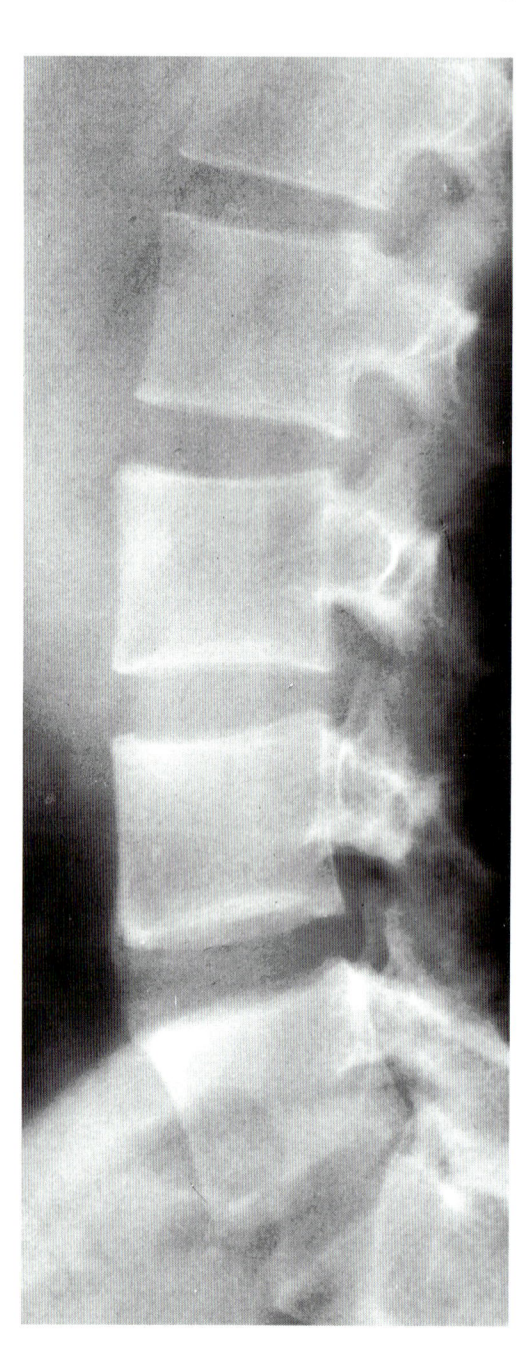

FIGURE 6.3 Lateral radiograph of the lumbar spine in a 28-year-old man demonstrates squaring of the vertebral bodies secondary to small osseous erosions at the corners. This finding is an early radiographic feature of ankylosing spondylitis. Note also the formation of syndesmophytes at the L4–L5 disk space.

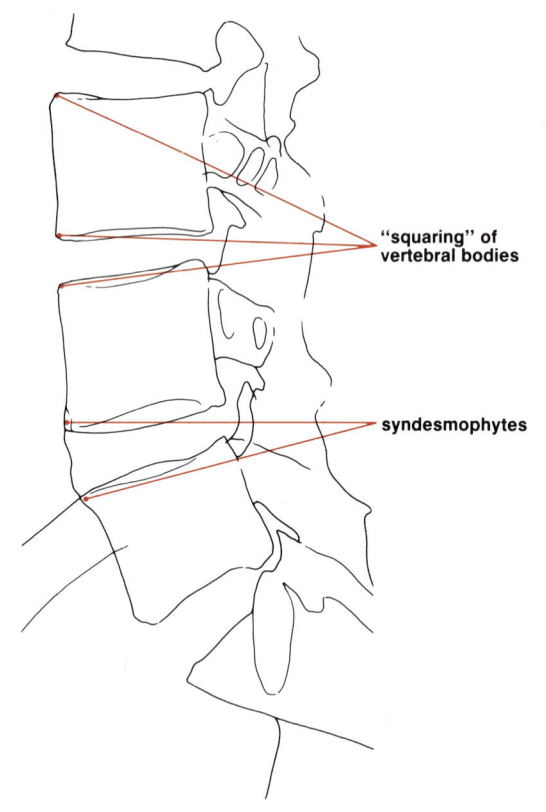

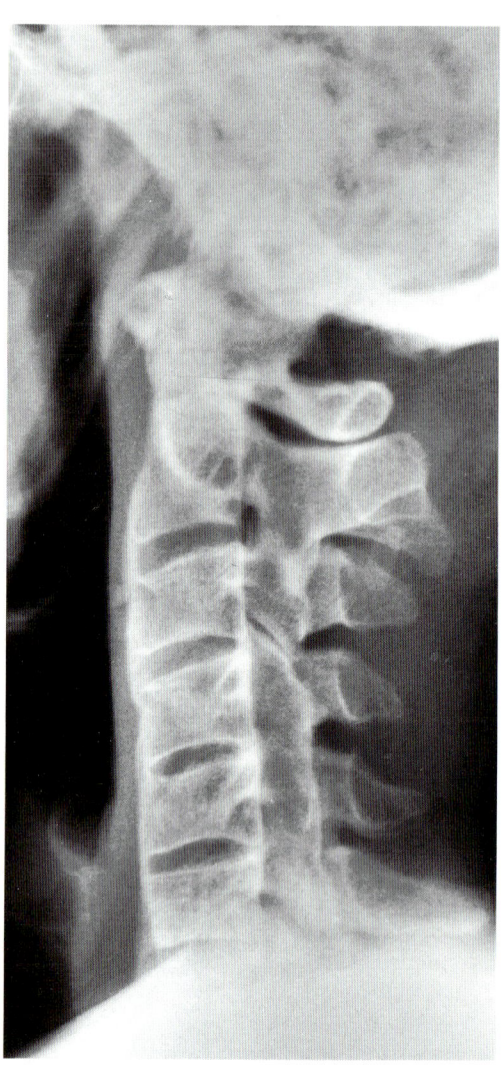

FIGURE 6.4 Lateral view of the cervical spine in a 31-year-old man demonstrates delicate syndesmophytes bridging the vertebral bodies, a common feature of ankylosing spondylitis. Note the fusion of several apophyseal joints.

Imaging of the Spine in Clinical Practice

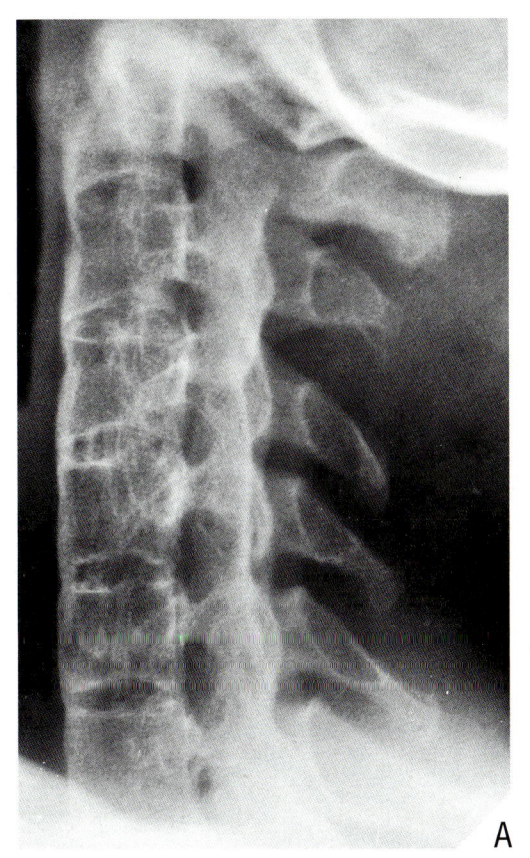

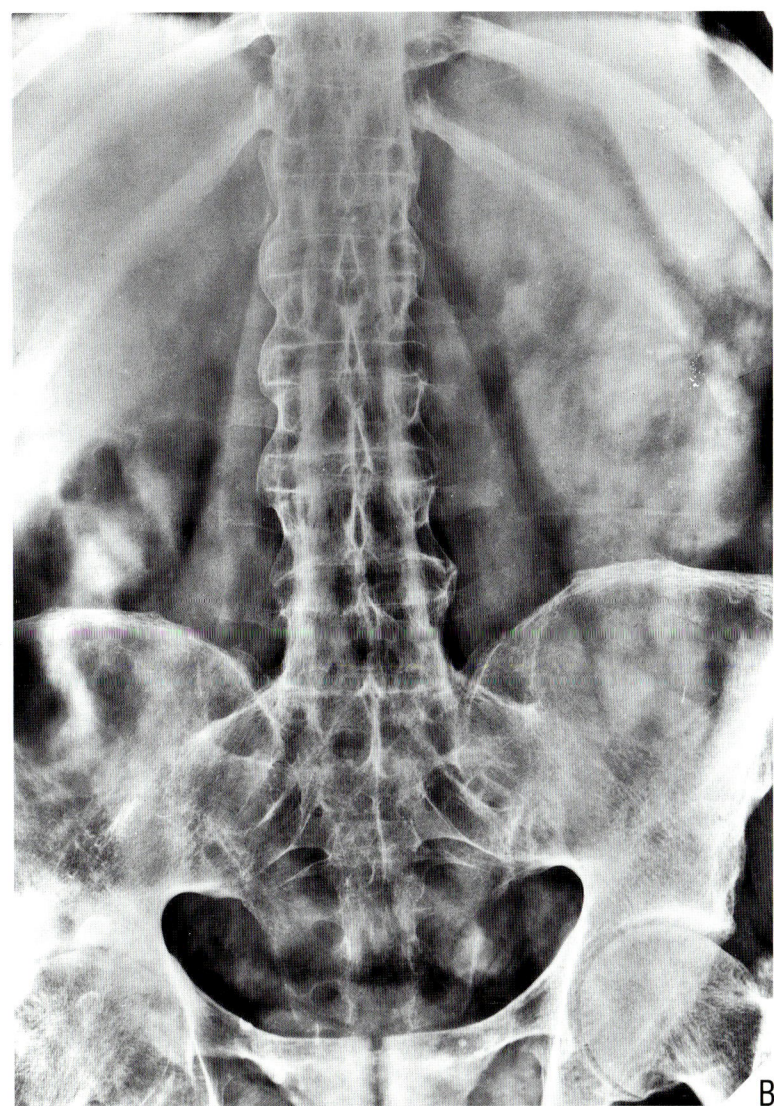

FIGURE 6.5 (A) Lateral film of the cervical spine in a 53-year-old man with advanced ankylosing spondylitis shows anterior syndesmophytes bridging the vertebral bodies and posterior fusion of the apophyseal joints, together with paravertebral ossifications, producing a "bamboo" spine appearance. The same phenomenon is seen on the anteroposterior **(B)** and lateral **(C)** projections of the lumbosacral spine. Note on the anteroposterior view the fusion of the sacroiliac joints and the involvement of both hip joints.

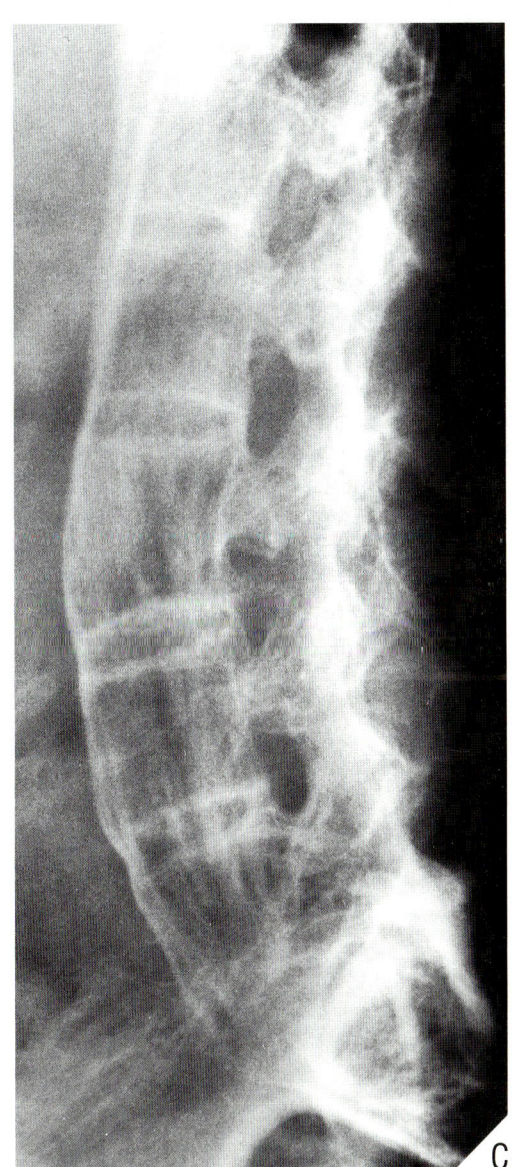

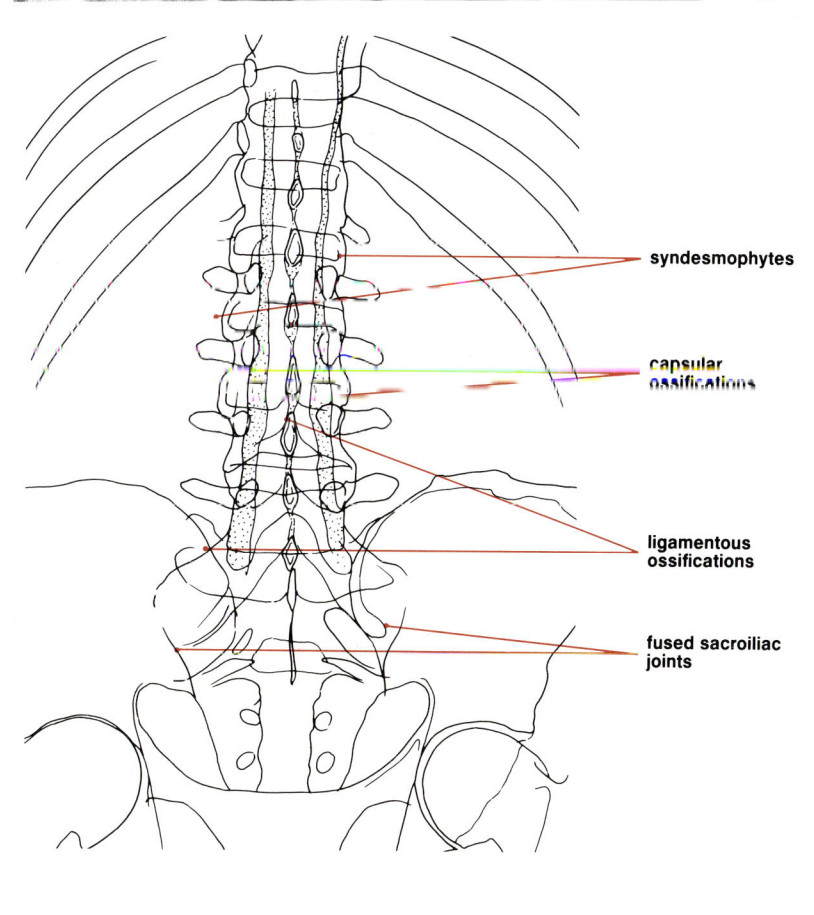

Inflammatory Arthritides of the Spine   6.5

formed at the C7–T1 junction (Fig. 6.6). Posterior laminectomy and bilateral facetectomy are also performed at the C7–T1 level, with the adjacent laminae (ie, the laminae of C6 and T2) undercut so that a closing wedge osteotomy can be achieved without impinging on the associated neural structures. The procedure is done either under local or general anesthesia with a "wake-up" test being performed at the time of osteotomy. Lumbar osteotomies are usually done at the L2–L3 junction; similar to the procedure in the cervical spine, the osteotomy is performed with the patient awake so that neurologic function can be closely monitored.

Thoracic kyphosis may or may not be accompanied by lumbar kyphosis. In concomitant thoracic and lumbar kyphosis, the corrective osteotomy is usually performed in the lumbar spine, as for treatment of an isolated lumbar kyphosis (Fig. 6.7).

In the immediate postoperative period, lateral films of the lumbar spine demonstrate three patterns of correction in the anterior spine after closure of the posterior wedge. Most commonly, there is a fracture of the ossified anterior longitudinal ligament associated with opening of the anterior disk space (Fig. 6.8A). Alternatively, the anterior longitudinal ligament may avulse a bone fragment from the lower of two adjacent vertebrae (Fig. 6.8B). The third pattern of correction is seen if the anterior longitudinal ligament remains intact, but there is a wedge compression fracture of the posterior portion of one of the vertebral bodies at the osteotomy site (Fig. 6.8C). Posterior fusion is usually solid at 9 months after surgery.

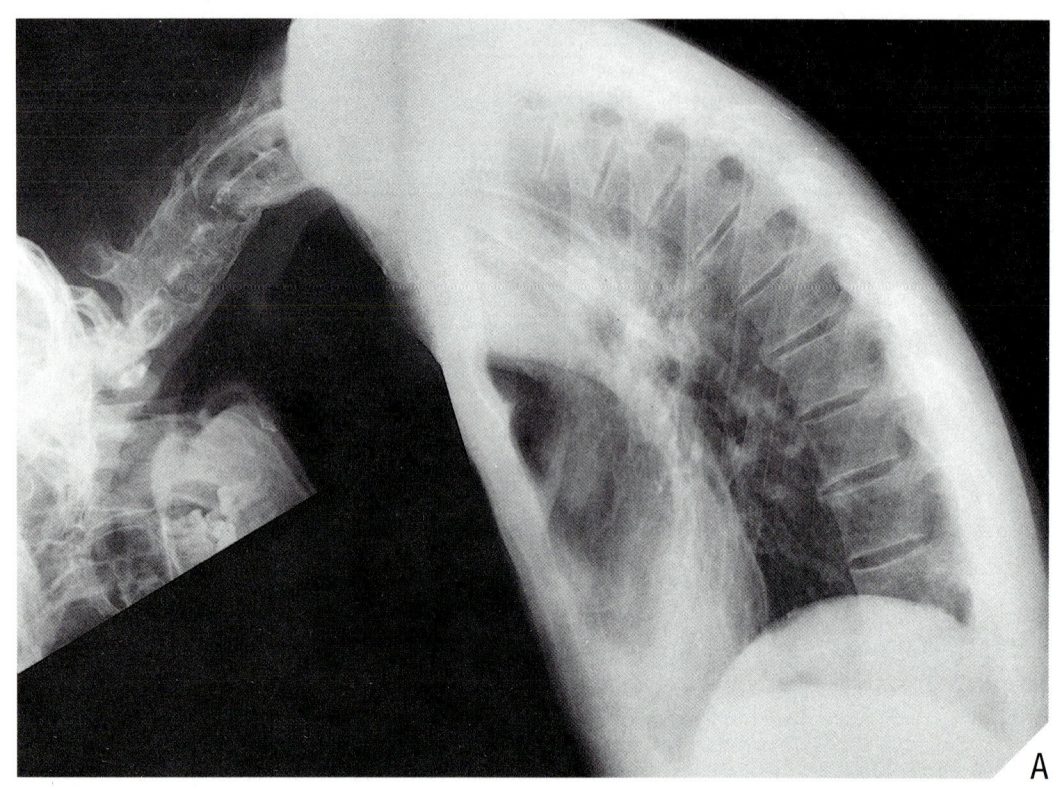

FIGURE 6.6 A 30-year-old man with advanced spinal deformity secondary to ankylosing spondylitis underwent a corrective osteotomy at the level of C6–C7. **(A)** Composed lateral view of the cervical and thoracic spine dramatically demonstrates the severity of the cervicothoracic kyphosis. **(B)** Lateral tomogram of the cervical spine using an equalizing wedge filter shows the site of osteotomy at the C6–C7 level. Note the degree of achieved correction. (Reproduced with permission from Gerscovich EO, Greenspan A, Montesano PX: Ankylosing spondylitis of the spine: A review of current methods of treatment and the radiologic appearance of the surgical correction. *Orthopedics;* in press)

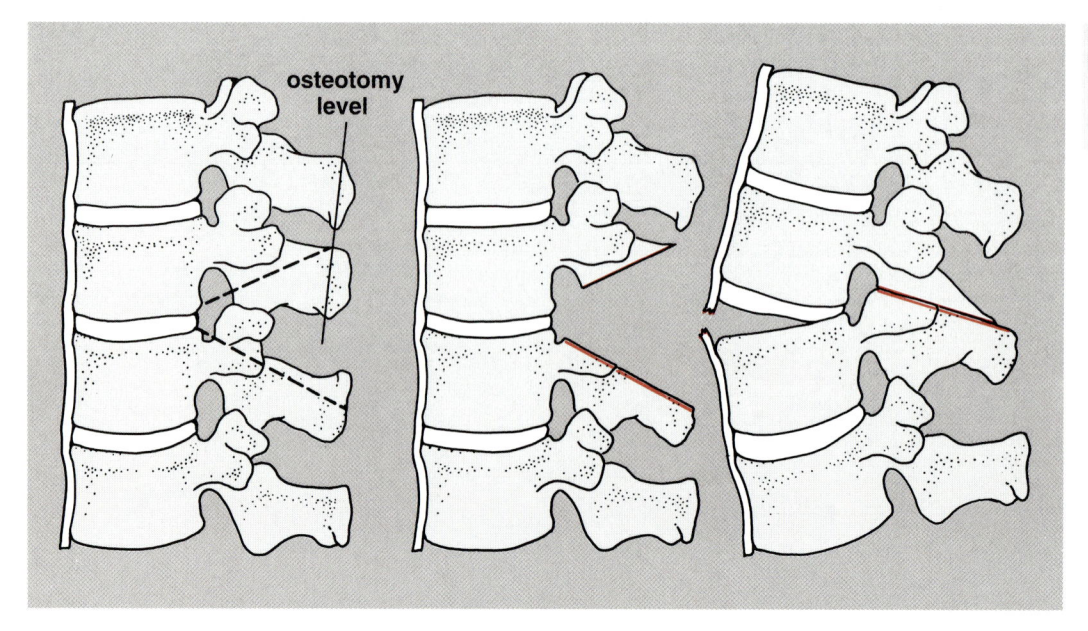

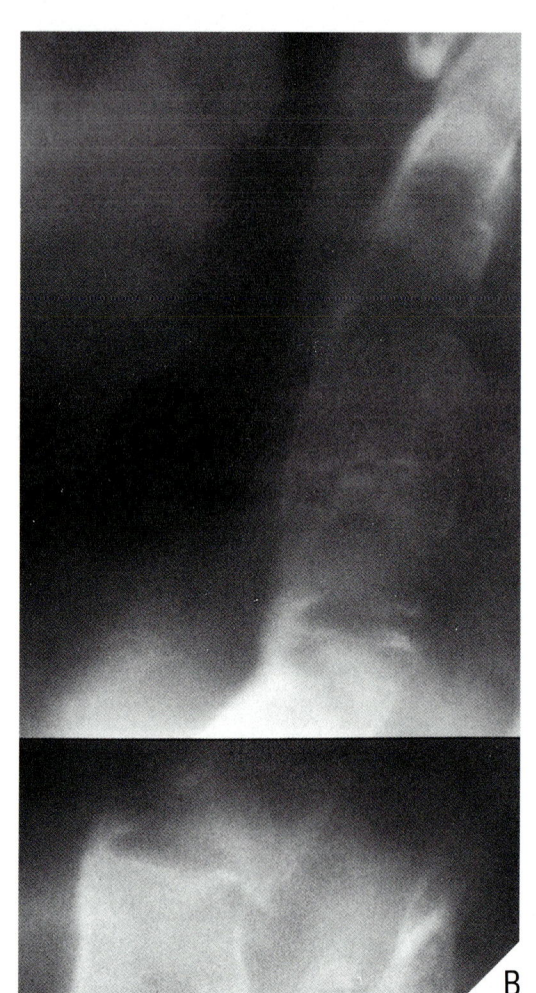

FIGURE 6.7 Correction of kyphosis in ankylosing spondylitis by extension osteotomy of the lumbar spine. (Modified from McMaster MJ: A technique for lumbar spinal osteotomy in ankylosing spondylitis. *J Bone Joint Surg* 67B:204, 1985)

Imaging of the Spine in Clinical Practice

Thoracic kyphosis with concomitant lumbar lordosis must be treated by multilevel thoracic osteotomies (Fig. 6.9). In general, no more than 10 degrees of correction is achieved at a single level, thus necessitating multiple osteotomies, usually six or more. This is regarded as the most dangerous of all the osteotomies as the ratio of cord to canal space is greatest at the level of the thoracic spine, leaving little or no extra space.

As an alternate method for correction of kyphosis in ankylosing spondylitis, Wilson and Levine (1969) introduced a pelvic osteotomy. The procedure consists of a one-stage bilateral iliac osteotomy similar to Salter's innominate osteotomy for the treatment of congenital dislocation of the hip. In this procedure the body is rotated backward over the caudal pelvic segment on a pivot in the osteotomy line. This shifts the body's center of gravity dorsally towards a more normal position. The procedure can be performed as a primary corrective procedure when lumbar osteotomy is

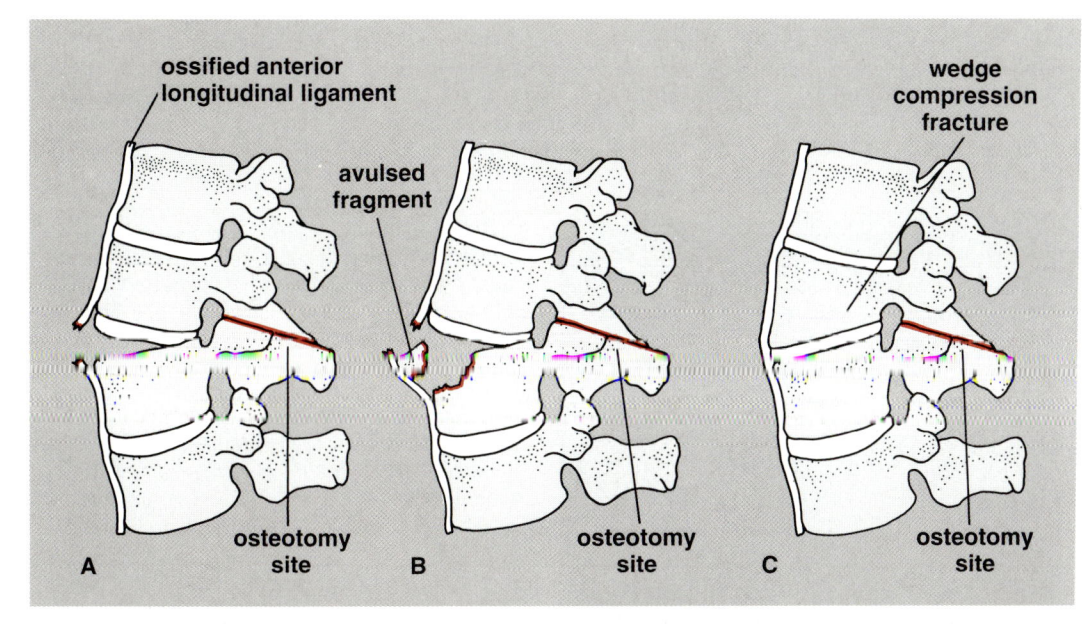

FIGURE 6.8 Three patterns of correction in the anterior spine following closure of posterior osteotomy. **(A)** Fracture of the ossified anterior longitudinal ligament with opening of the anterior portion of the disk space. **(B)** Fracture of the ossified anterior longitudinal ligament with an avulsed fragment of the lower vertebra. **(C)** Intact ligament with posterior fracture of one of the vertebrae at the osteotomy level. (Reproduced with permission from Gerscovich EO, Greenspan A, Montesano PX: Ankylosing spondylitis of the spine: A review of current methods of treatment and the radiologic appearance of the surgical correction. *Orthopedics*; in press)

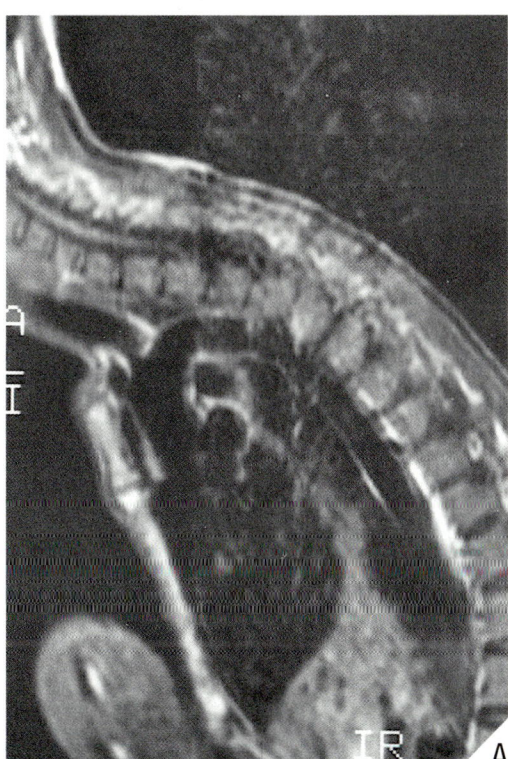

FIGURE 6.9 A 36-year-old man with a 15-year history of ankylosing spondylitis. **(A)** Sagittal MRI of cervicothoracic spine demonstrates advanced kyphosis. **(B,C)** After anterior diskectomy, corrective anterior wedge thoracic osteotomy at the multiple levels (T6–T12), and posterior osteotomy and spinal fusion at the T6–L1 level with Zielke system, significant correction of the spine has been achieved.

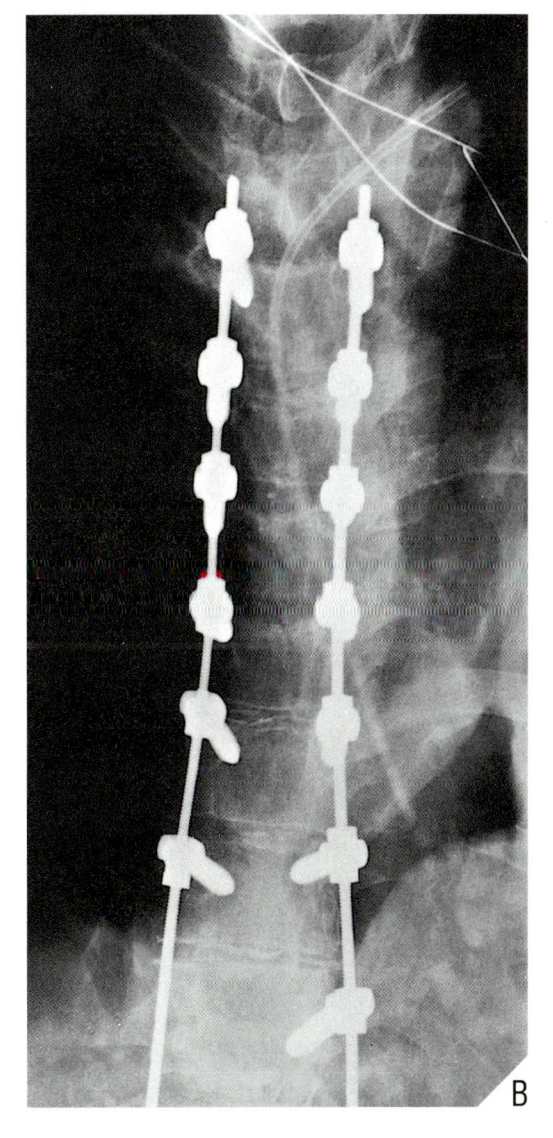

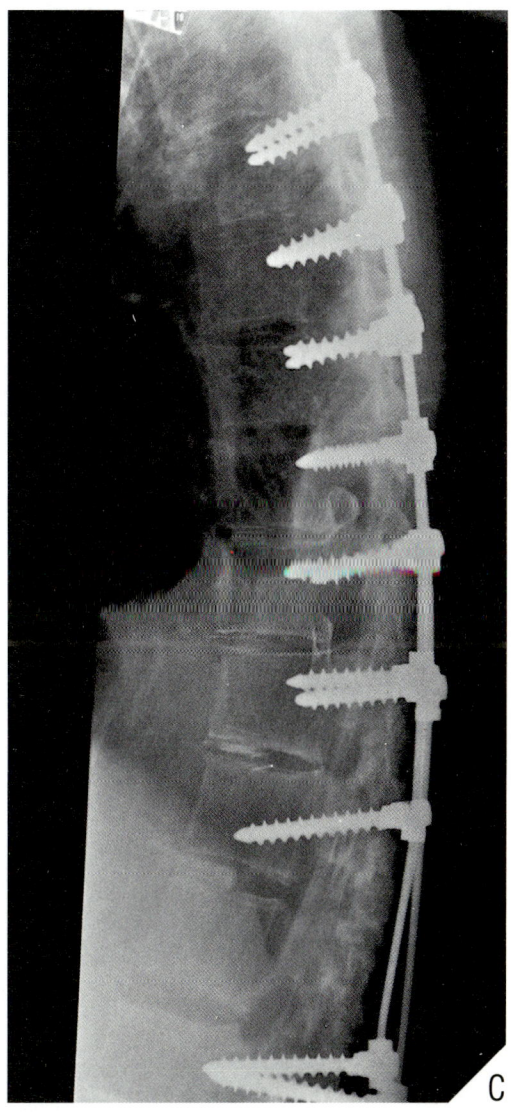

Inflammatory Arthritides of the Spine

contraindicated or when previous spinal corrective procedures have failed (Fig. 6.10). Pelvic osteotomy is a relatively safe procedure, yields good results, and is associated with little morbidity. Another of its advantages is that external immobilization with a plaster cast is not required.

Reiter Syndrome

Reiter syndrome is a clinical disease of infectious origin that affects males five times more often than females. It is characterized by arthritis, conjunctivitis, and urethritis. Also typical of Reiter syndrome is the presence of a mucocutaneous rash—keratoderma blennorrhagica. As in the case of ankylosing spondylitis, eye involvement is common and can include conjunctivitis, iritis, uveitis, and episcleritis. Approximately 60% to 80% of patients are positive for HLA-B27. This frequency varies according to the ethnic origin of the patient. Unlike ankylosing spondylitis, Reiter syndrome may be accompanied by unilateral sacroiliac disease.

Two types of Reiter syndrome have been identified: *sporadic* and *epidemic*. The sporadic (or endemic) type, which is common in the United States, is associated with nongonococcal urethritis, prostatitis, or hemorrhagic cystitis, and occurs almost exclusively in men. In Europe, a second type has been identified, an epidemic form associated with bacillary *(Shigella)* dysentery; it may also occur in women. There has been considerable research on the putative role of *Yersina enterocolitica* in epidemic Reiter syndrome, particularly in Scandinavia, where such infections are more prevalent than in North America.

Radiographically, Reiter syndrome is marked by peripheral, usually asymmetric, arthritis with a predilection for the joints of the lower limb. The foot is the most common site of involvement, particularly the metatar-

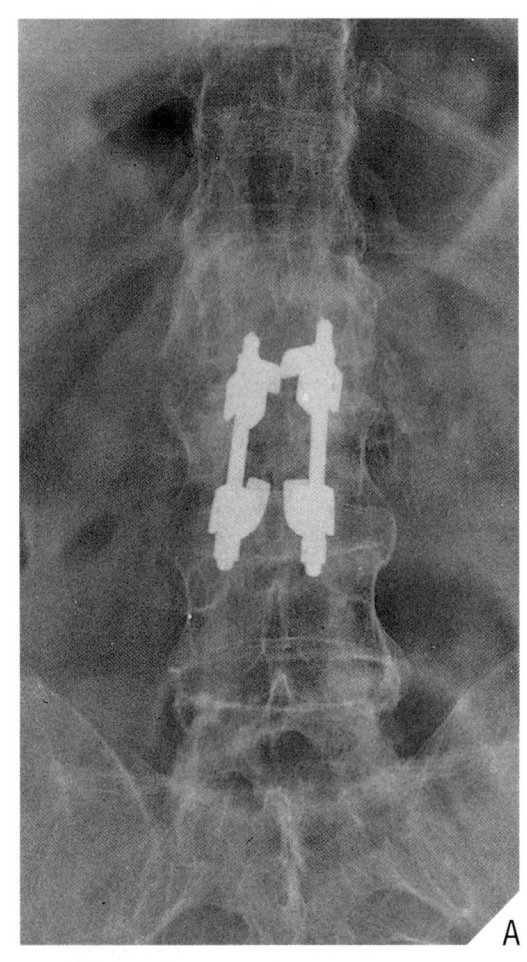

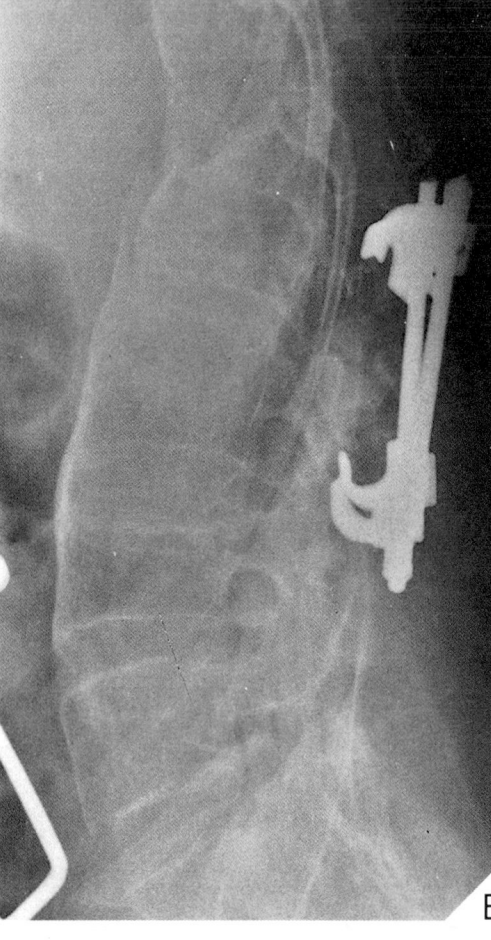

FIGURE 6.10 A 45-year-old man with ankylosing spondylitis diagnosed at age of 21 has been unsuccessfully treated by extension lumbar osteotomy at the level of L1–L3. Postoperative anteroposterior **(A)** and lateral **(B)** radiographs show persistence of thoracic kyphosis. Following pelvic osteotomy **(C,D)**, significant extension of lumbar spine has been achieved. (Reproduced with permission from Gerscovich EO, Greenspan A, Montesano PX: Ankylosing spondylitis of the spine: A review of current methods of treatment and the radiologic appearance of the surgical correction. *Orthopedics*; in press)

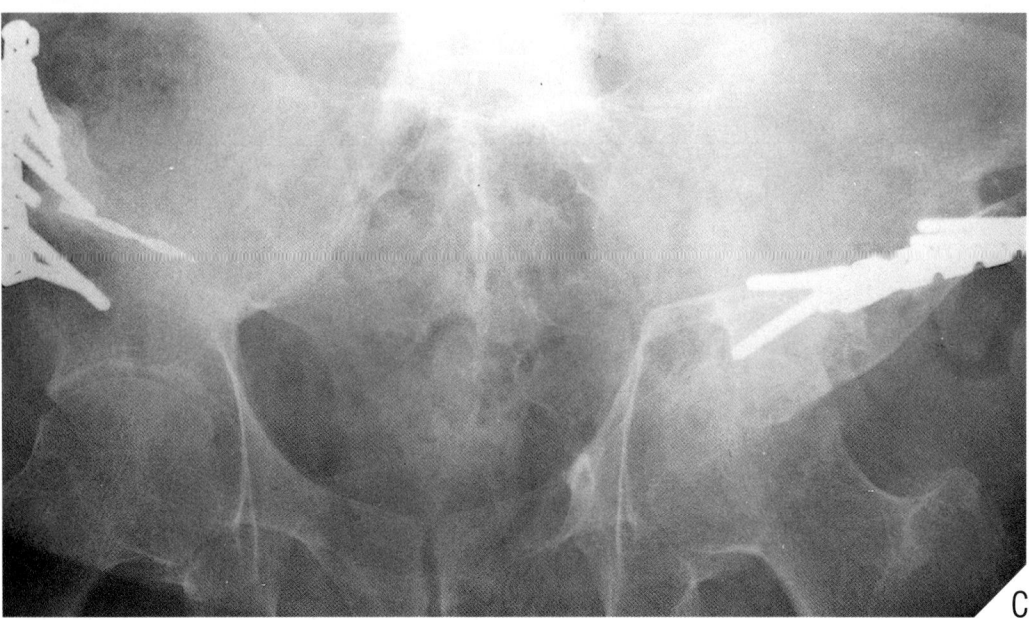

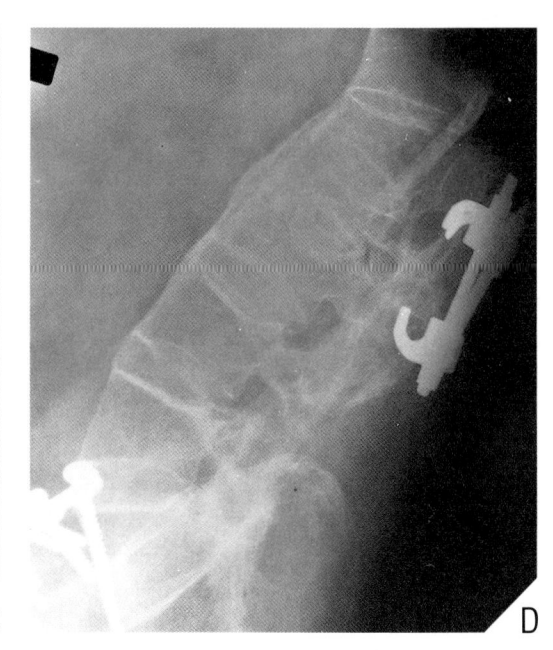

sophalangeal joints and the heels. Periosteal new bone formation is not uncommon. Involvement of the sacroiliac joints, which is frequently encountered, may be either asymmetric (unilateral or bilateral with one side more severely affected) or symmetric (bilateral) (Fig. 6.11). In the thoracic and lumbar spine, coarse syndesmophytes or paraspinal ossifications may be present, characteristically bridging adjacent vertebrae (Fig. 6.12).

Psoriatic Arthritis

Five specific subgroups of arthritic syndromes have been described in psoriatic arthritis. Subgroup 1, or *classic* psoriatic arthritis, is characterized by nail pathology with occasional involvement of the terminal tufts and by involvement of the distal and occasionally the proximal interphalangeal joints of the hand. Subgroup 2, well known for the "opera glass" deformity of the hand, is termed *arthritis mutilans* because of the extensive destruction of the phalanges and metacarpal joints including "pencil-in-cup" deformity; patients with arthritis mutilans often have sacroiliitis. Subgroup 3 is characterized by *symmetric polyarthritis* and may result in ankylosis of the proximal and distal interphalangeal joints. This form of psoriatic arthritis is often indistinguishable from rheumatoid arthritis. Subgroup 4 is characterized by *oligoarticular arthritis;* in contrast to subgroup 3, the joint involvement is asymmetric, usually involving the proximal and distal interphalangeal and metacarpophalangeal articulations. This is the most common subgroup of psoriatic arthritis; patients typically exhibit a "sausage-like" swelling of the digits. Subgroup 5 is a spondyloarthropathy that has features similar to those of ankylosing spondylitis.

The etiology of psoriatic arthritis is unknown, and its relationship to rheumatoid arthritis and spondyloarthropathies is still unsettled. It occurs in 5% to 7% of patients with psoriasis and predominantly involves the distal interphalangeal joints of the hands and feet, although other sites—the proximal interphalangeal joints, as well as the hips, knees, ankles, and spine—may be affected.

In general, there are few characteristic radiographic features of psoriatic arthritis that help in arriving at a correct diagnosis. In the phalanges of the hand or foot, a periosteal reaction in the form of a "fluffy" new bone has a periarticular location and, in association with erosions of the interphalangeal joints, it exhibits a "mouse ear" appearance. In arthritis mutilans, severe deformities such as the "pencil-in-cup" configuration and interphalangeal ankylosis, may be observed. In the heel, late-stage changes are characterized by the formation of broad-based osteophytes and the presence of erosions and a fluffy periostitis.

Psoriatic arthritis of the spine is associated with a particularly high incidence of sacroiliitis, which may be bilateral and symmetric, bilateral and asymmetric, or unilateral. As in Reiter syndrome, coarse asymmetric syndesmophytes and paraspinal ossification may be seen (Fig. 6.13).

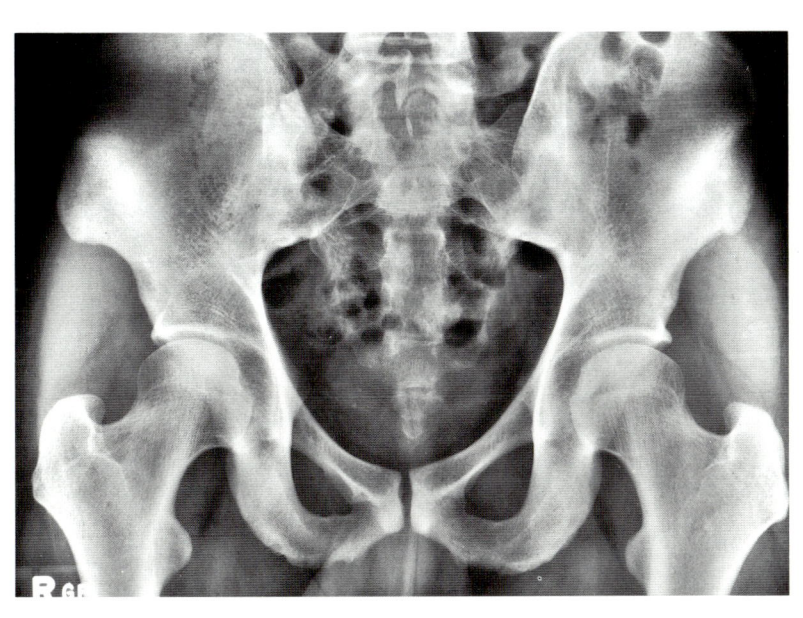

FIGURE 6.11 Anteroposterior view of a pelvis of a 28-year-old man with Reiter syndrome demonstrates symmetric bilateral involvement of the sacroiliac joints. More commonly, the involvement is asymmetric.

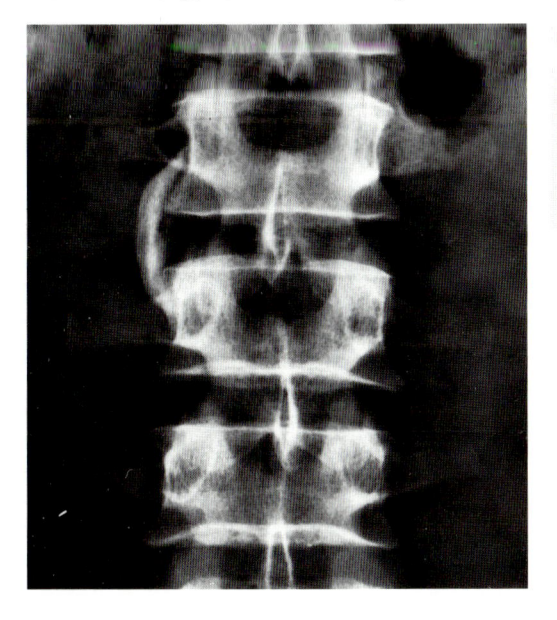

FIGURE 6.12 Anteroposterior radiograph of the lumbar spine of a 23-year-old man with Reiter syndrome shows a characteristic paraspinal ossification bridging the L2 and L3 vertebrae.

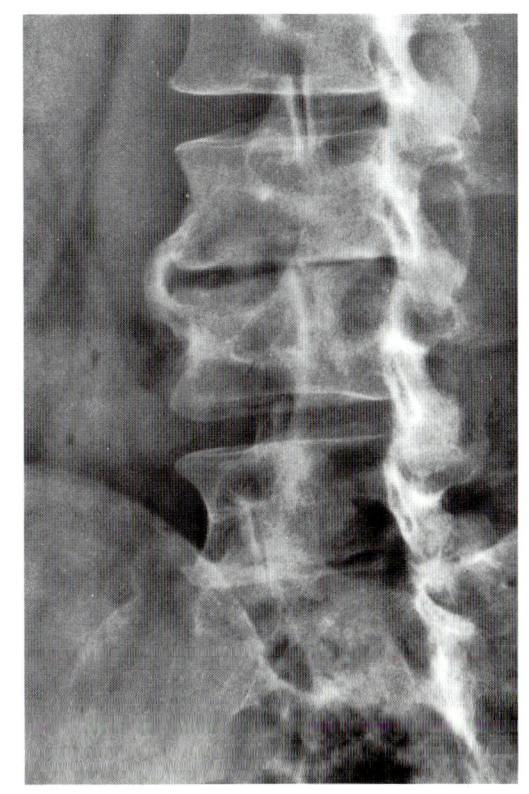

FIGURE 6.13 Oblique film of the lumbar spine in a 30-year-old man with psoriasis demonstrates a single, coarse syndesmophyte bridging the bodies of L3 and L4. The right sacroiliac joint is also affected.

Enteropathic Arthropathies

This group comprises arthritides associated with inflammatory intestinal diseases, such as ulcerative colitis, regional enteritis (Crohn disease), and intestinal lipodystrophy (Whipple disease), the last of which predominantly affects men in the fourth and fifth decades of life. The histocompatibility antigen HLA-B27 is present in most patients with enteropathic abnormalities. In all three conditions, the spine and the sacroiliac and peripheral joints may be affected. In the spine, squaring of the vertebral bodies and the formation of syndesmophytes are common features. Sacroiliitis, which is usually bilateral and symmetric, is radiographically indistinguishable from that seen in ankylosing spondylitis (Fig. 6.14). Patients may also exhibit a peripheral arthritis, the activity of which is generally correlated with the activity of the bowel disease.

Finally, it should be noted that arthritis may develop after intestinal bypass procedures. The synovitis is polyarticular and symmetric, but radiographically the lesions are nonerosive.

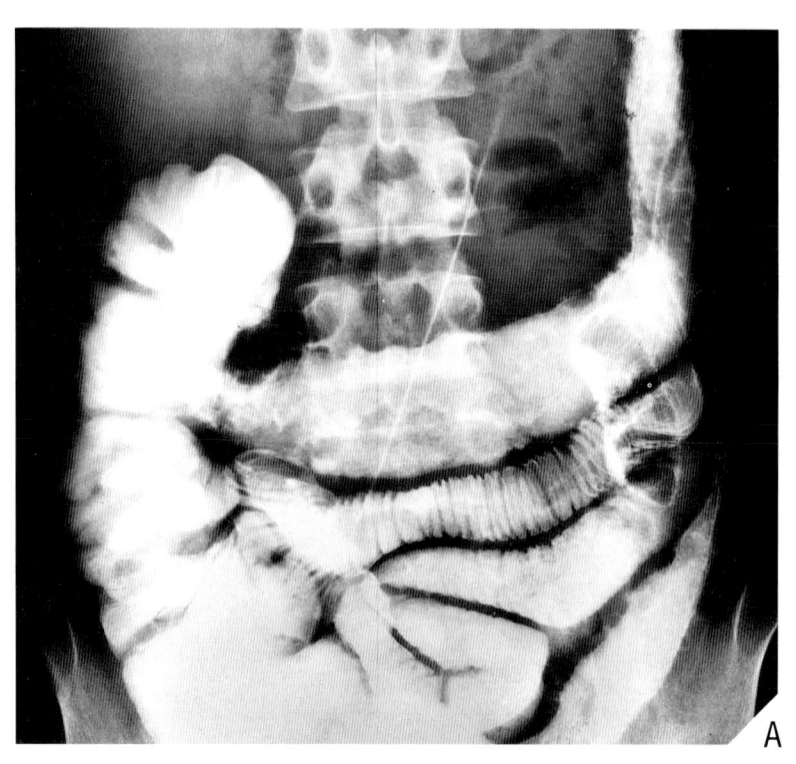

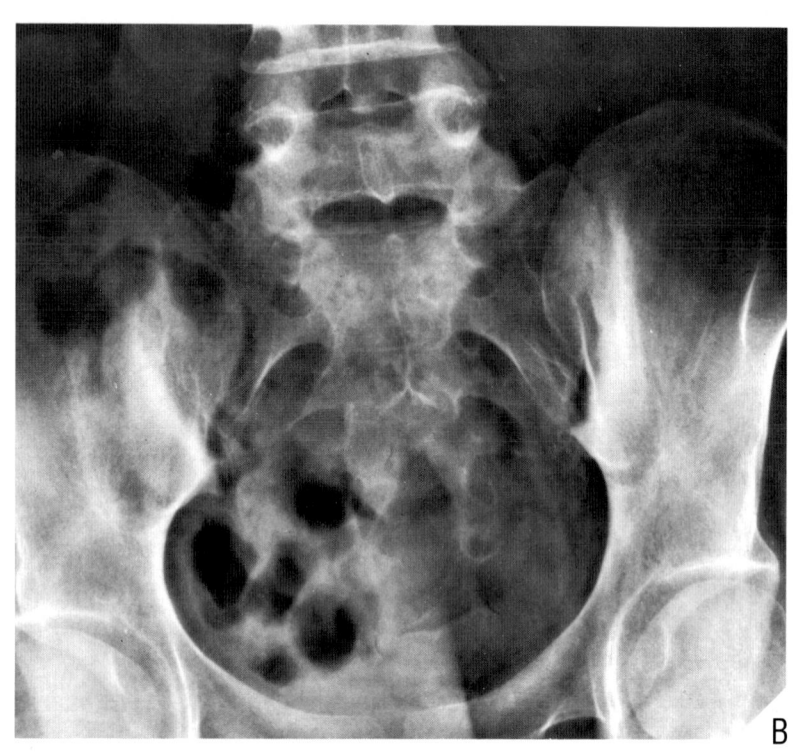

FIGURE 6.14 A 20-year-old woman with known ulcerative colitis developed severe low back pain localized to the sacroiliac joints. **(A)** Barium enema study shows extensive involvement of the transverse colon, consistent with ulcerative colitis. **(B)** Posteroanterior view of the pelvis shows symmetric, bilateral sacroiliitis similar to that seen in ankylosing spondylitis.

Suggested Reading

Ansell BM, Wigley RAD: Arthritic manifestations in regional enteritis. *Ann Rheum Dis* 23:64, 1964.

Arnett FC, Bias WB, Stevens MB: Juvenile-onset chronic arthritis. Clinical and radiographic features of a unique HLA-B27 subset. *Am J Med* 69:369, 1980.

Baker H, Godling DN, Thompson M: Psoriasis and arthritis. *Ann Intern Med* 58:909, 1963.

Berens DL: Roentgen features of ankylosing spondylitis. *Clin Orthop* 74:20, 1971.

Boyle AC: The rheumatoid neck. *Proc R Soc Med* 64:1161, 1971.

Breedveld FC, Algra PR, Vielvoye CJ, et al: Magnetic resonance imaging in the evaluation of patients with rheumatoid arthritis and subluxations of the cervical spine. *Arthritis Rheum* 30:624, 1987.

Clark RL, Muhletaler CA, Margulies SI: Colitic arthritis: Clinical and radiographic manifestations. *Radiology* 101:585, 1971.

Eastmond CJ, Woodrow JC: The HLA system and the arthropathies associated with psoriasis. *Ann Rheum Dis* 36:112, 1977.

Gerscovich EO, Greenspan A, Montesano PX: Ankylosing spondylitis of the spine: A review of current methods of treatment and the radiologic appearance of the surgical correction. *Orthopedics;* in press.

Jacobs RR, Montesano PX, Jackson RE: Enhancement of lumbar spine fusion by use of translaminar facet joint screws. *Spine* 14:12, 1989.

Kelly III JJ, Weisiger BB: The arthritis of Whipple's disease. *Arthritis Rheum* 6:615, 1963.

Killebrew K, Gold RH, Sholkoff SD: Psoriatic spondylitis. *Radiology* 108:9, 1973.

Magerl F, Seeman PS: Stable posterior fusion of the atlas and axis by transarticular screw fixation. In Kehr P, Weidner A (eds): *Cervical Spine.* Vienna, Springer-Verlag, 1987.

Martel W, Braunstein EM, Borlaza G, et al: Radiologic features of Reiter's disease. *Radiology* 132:1, 1979.

Martel W, Holt JF, Cassidy JT: The roentgenologic manifestations of juvenile rheumatoid arthritis. *Am J Roentgenol* 88:400, 1962.

Mathews JA: Atlanto–axial subluxation in rheumatoid arthritis. A 5-year follow-up study. *Ann Rheum Dis* 33:526, 1980.

McMaster MJ: A technique for lumbar spinal osteotomy in ankylosing spondylitis. *J Bone Joint Surg* 67B:204, 1985.

Park WM, O'Neil M, McCall IW: The radiology of rheumatoid involvement of the cervical spine. *Skel Radiol* 4:1, 1979.

Peterson CC Jr, Silbiger ML: Reiter's syndrome and psoriatic arthritis: Their roentgen spectra and some interesting similarities. *Am J Roentgenol* 101:860, 1967.

Pettersson H, Larson E-M, Holtas S: MR imaging of the cervical spine in rheumatoid arthritis. *AJNR* 9:573, 1988.

Ranawat CS, O'Leary P, Pellicci P, et al: Cervical spine fusion in rheumatoid arthritis. *J Bone Joint Surg* 61A(1003):103, 1979.

Resnick D: Common disorders of synovium-lined joints: Pathogenesis, imaging abnormalities, and complications. *AJR* 151:1079, 1988.

Resnick D, Niwayama G, Goergen TG: Comparison of radiographic abnormalities of the sacroiliac joint in degenerative disease and ankylosing spondylitis. *Am J Roentgenol* 128:189, 1977.

Resnik CS, Resnick D: Radiology of disorders of the sacroiliac joints. *JAMA* 253:2863, 1985.

Styblo K, Bossers GT, Slot GH: Osteotomy for kyphosis in ankylosing spondylitis. *Acta Orthop Scand* 56:294, 1985.

Weissman BN, Aliabado P, Weinfeld MS, et al: Prognostic features of atlantoaxial subluxation in rheumatoid arthritis patients. *Radiology* 144:745, 1982.

Wilson PD, Levine DB: Compensatory pelvic osteotomy for ankylosing spondylitis. *J Bone Joint Surg* 51A:142, 1969.

Wolfe BK, O'Keefe D, Mitchell DM, et al: Rheumatoid arthritis of the cervical spine: Early and progressive radiographic features. *Radiology* 165:145, 1987.

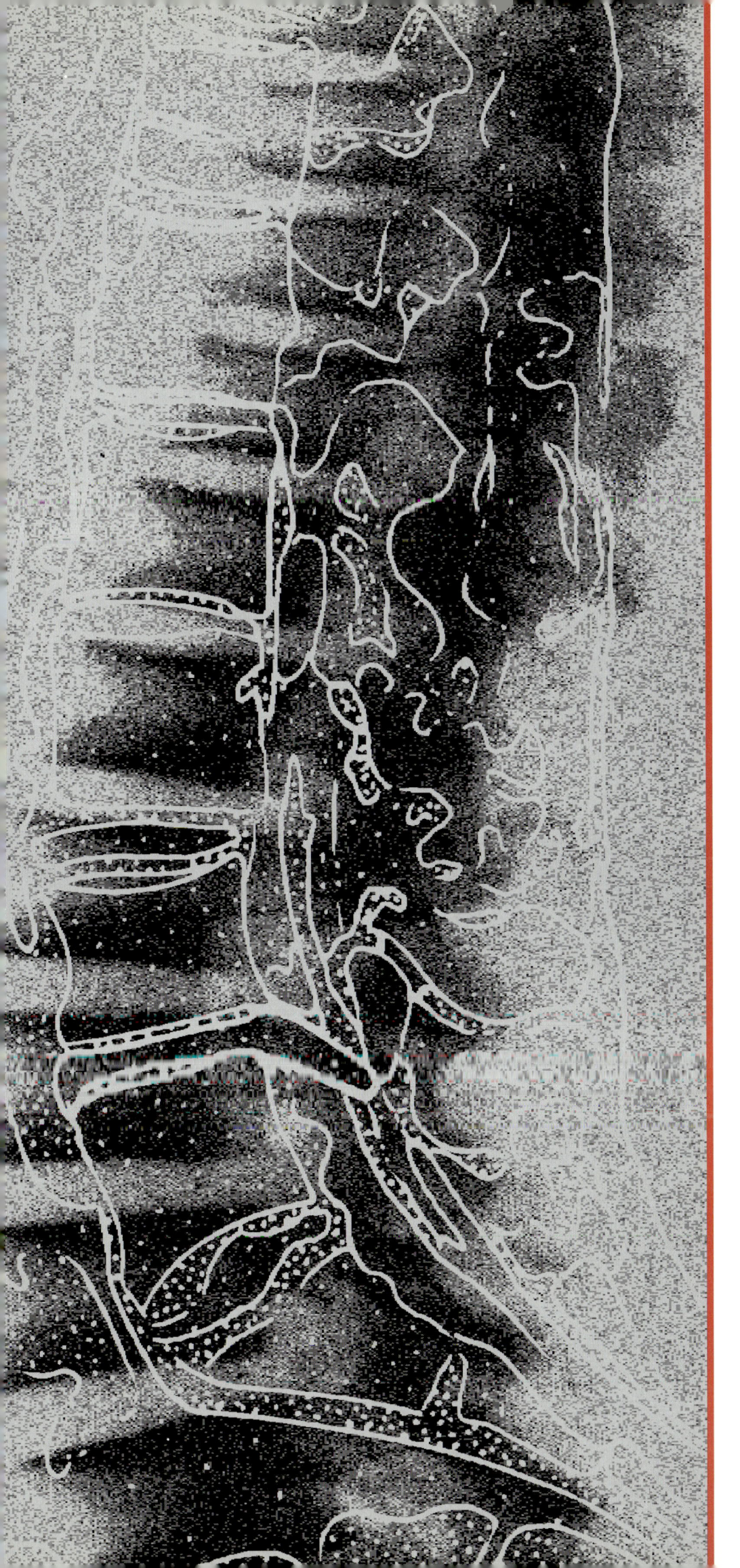

Miscellaneous Arthropathies Affecting the Spine

7

ALKAPTONURIA (OCHRONOSIS)

Alkaptonuria is a rare inherited disease which is transmitted as an autosomal recessive trait and is characterized by metabolic abnormality resulting from the absence of the enzyme homogentisic acid oxidase. This enzyme takes part in the normal degradation pathway for the aromatic amino acids tyrosine and phenylalanine. As a consequence of its absence, significant amounts of homogentisic acid accumulate in various organs, with a predilection for connective tissues. The articular cartilage is affected because the abnormal pigment, a polymer of homogentisic acid, is deposited in the joints, resulting in arthropathy. As a rule, ochronotic arthropathy is a manifestation of long-standing alkaptonuria. The condition affects males and females equally. The clinical signs include mild pain and a decreased range of motion in various joints. Radiography demonstrates dystrophic calcifications that most commonly involve the intervertebral disks, cartilage, tendons, and ligaments (Fig. 7.1). Osteoporosis is usually present. Disk spaces are narrowed, with occasional vacuum phenomena. The extraspinal abnormalities are limited to involvement of sacroiliac joints, symphysis pubis, and large peripheral joints. The joint spaces are narrowed, and there is evidence of periarticular sclerosis with occasional appearance of small osteophytes. Tendinous calcifications and ossifications may occur, leading occasionally to tendon rupture. The radiographic findings may mimic those of degenerative joint disease or CPPD.

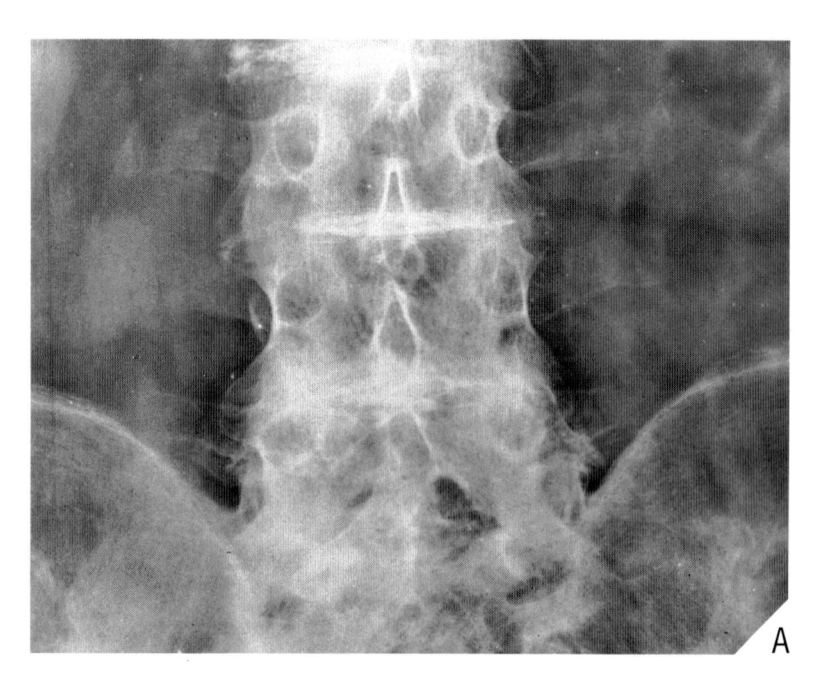

HYPERPARATHYROIDISM ARTHROPATHY

Hyperparathyroidism is caused by overactivity of the parathyroid glands, which produce parathormone (PTH). Increased production of this hormone is secondary to either hyperplasia of glands or adenoma; only in very rare instances is hyperparathyroidism associated with parathyroid carcinoma. Excessive secretion of PTH, which acts on the kidneys and bone, leads to disturbances in calcium and phosphorus metabolism, resulting in hypercalcemia, hyperphosphaturia, and hypophosphatemia. Renal excretion of calcium and phosphate is increased, and serum levels of calcium are elevated, whereas those of phosphorus are reduced; serum levels of alkaline phosphatase are also elevated. The most characteristic features, subperiosteal and subchondral resorption of bone, may appear at the margins of certain joints, thus accounting for the articular manifestations or "arthropathy" of hyperparathyroidism. The arthropathy is often noted at the acromioclavicular joint, the sternoclavicular and sacroiliac articulations, and at the symphysis pubis; only rarely does it affect the metacarpophalangeal and interphalangeal joints. The other noteworthy feature of hyperparathyroidism arthropathy is chondrocalcinosis, which is a deposition of calcium in the articular and fibrocartilage. Chondrocalcinosis may mimic degenerative joint disease and calcium pyrophosphate dihydrate crystal deposition arthropathy. It can be distinguished from the calcification of degenerative joint disease by the absence of arthritic changes in the joint, and from calcium pyrophos-

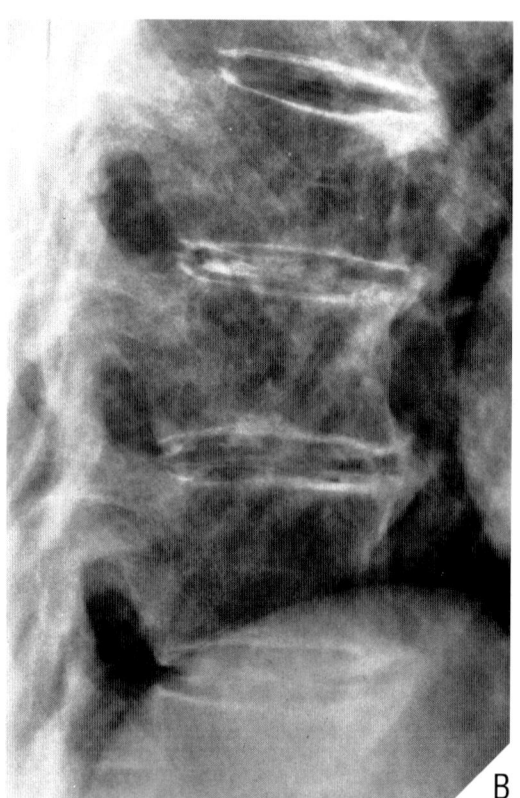

FIGURE 7.1
Anteroposterior (**A**) radiograph of the lumbar and lateral (**B**) radiograph of the thoracic spine of a 64-year-old woman with a clinical diagnosis of alkaptonuria demonstrate narrowing of several intervertebral disk spaces associated with marginal anterior osteophytes and moderate osteoporosis. Characteristic calcifications of multiple intervertebral disks is a hallmark of ochronosis. (Courtesy of Dr. J. Tehranzadeh, Orange, CA)

phate dihydrate crystal deposition by the presence of osteopenia and other typical features of hyperparathyroidism.

In primary hyperparathyroidism the spine is affected by osteopenia. Only in rare instances does a localized area of massive bone resorption associated with brown tumor give rise to local symptoms. Back pain secondary to vertebral compression fractures is occasionally a presenting symptom.

In secondary hyperparathyroidism, chronic renal failure is usually accompanied by bone abnormalities. The lesions include increased bone resorption and increased bone deposition. The latter manifest as sclerotic changes in the spine giving rise to a typical banded appearance referred to as a "rugger jersey" spine (Fig. 7.2).

GOUT

Gout is a metabolic disorder characterized by recurrent episodes of arthritis associated with the presence of monosodium urate monohydrate crystals in the synovial fluid leukocytes and, in many cases, gross deposits of sodium urate (tophi) in periarticular soft tissues. Serum uric acid concentrations are elevated. The majority of patients are male, but gouty arthritis is seen in postmenopausal women as well.

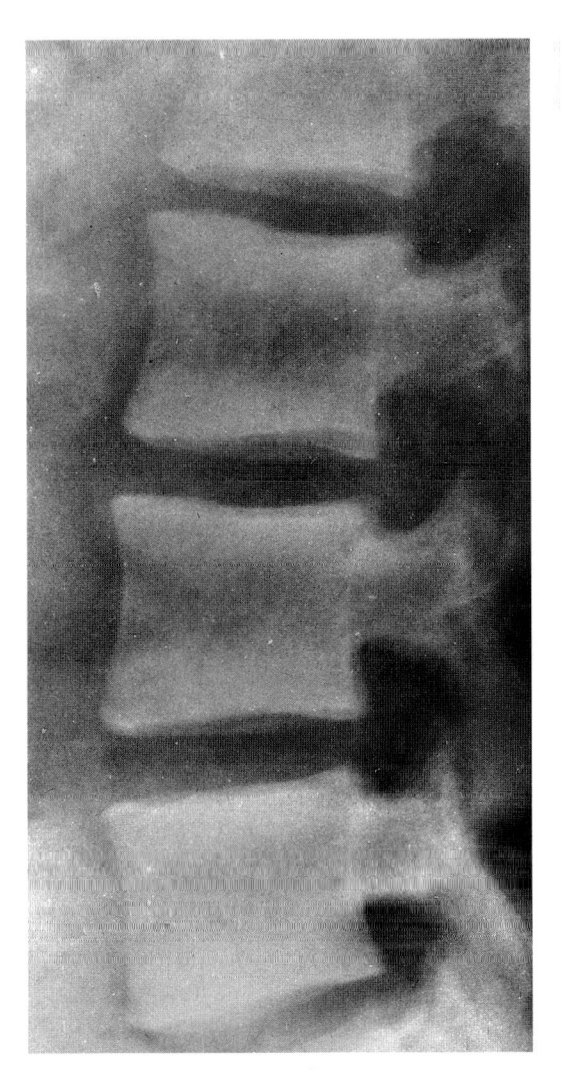

The great toe is the most common site of involvement in gouty arthritis; the condition known as *podagra*, which involves the first metatarsophalangeal joint, occurs in about 75% of patients. Other frequently affected sites include the ankle, knee, elbow, and wrist. The spine is affected in gout only in extremely rare instances.

Hyperuricemia

An increased miscible pool of uric acid with resulting hyperuricemia can occur in two principal ways. First, urate is produced in such large quantities that even though excretion routes are of normal capacity, they are inadequate to handle the excessive load. Second, the capacity for uric acid cannot be eliminated.

In 25% to 30% of gouty patients, a primary defect in the rate of purine synthesis causes excessive uric acid formation, as reflected in excessive urinary uric acid excretion (over 600 mg/day) measured while

FIGURE 7.2 A 17-year-old boy with chronic renal failure developed secondary hyperparathyroidism. Lateral radiograph of the lumbar spine demonstrates sclerotic bands adjacent to the vertebral endplates—the so-called rugger-jersey spine.

the patient is maintained on a standard purine-free diet. Increased production can also be seen in gout secondary to myeloproliferative disorders associated with increased destruction of cells and result in increased breakdown of nucleic acids. Decreased excretion occurs in primary gout in patients with a dysfunction in the renal tubular capacity to secrete urate and in patients with chronic renal disease. In most patients, however, there is evidence of both uric acid overproduction and diminished renal excretion of uric acid.

The chance of development of gouty arthritis in hyperuricemic individuals should increase in proportion to the duration and, even more, to the degree of hyperuricemia. Monosodium urate, however, has a marked tendency to form relatively stable supersaturated solutions; therefore, the proportion of hyperuricemic patients who actually develop gouty arthritis is relatively low. The clinical development of gouty arthritis in the hyperuricemic subject is also substantially influenced by other factors, such as binding of urate to plasma proteins or the presence of promoters or inhibitors of crystallization.

Radiographic Features

Gouty arthritis has several characteristic radiographic features. Erosions, which are usually sharply marginated, are initially periarticular in location and are later seen to extend into the joint; an "overhanging edge" of erosion is a frequent identifying feature. Usually, there is a striking lack of osteoporosis, which helps differentiate this condition from rheumatoid arthritis. The reason for the absence of osteoporosis is that the duration of an acute gouty attack is too short to allow the development of the disuse osteoporosis so often seen in patients with rheumatoid arthritis. If erosion involves the articular end of the bone and extends into the joint, part of the joint is usually preserved. In chronic tophaceous gout, sodium urate deposits in and around the joint are seen, creating a dense mass in the soft tissues called a tophus, which frequently exhibits calcifications. Characteristically, tophi are randomly distributed and are usually asymmetric. Periarticular and articular erosions, unlike those in rheumatoid arthritis, are also asymmetric in distribution. Tkach (1970) observed thoracic osteophytosis in patients with documented gouty arthritis. Urate deposition in the spine is, however, rare. Erosions of the odontoid process and end-plates of the vertebral bodies, disk space narrowing, and vertebral subluxation have been reported. Burnham and colleagues (1977) and Forrester and co-workers (1978) described erosions of the posterior elements of the lumbar spine in patients with gout.

CPPD Crystal Deposition Disease

Clinical Features

Resulting from the intra-articular presence of calcium pyrophosphate dihydrate (CPPD) crystals, CPPD crystal deposition disease affects men and women equally; most commonly, patients are middle-aged and older. The condition may be asymptomatic, in which case it is commonly referred to as *chondrocalcinosis;* when symptomatic, it is called *pseudogout.* There is, however, a great deal of confusion about these terms, and they are often misused.

In an effort to explain the relationship between chondrocalcinosis, calcium pyrophosphate arthropathy, and the pseudogout syndrome, Resnick has proposed an integration of these terms under the rubric CPPD crystal deposition disease. *Chondrocalcinosis,* a condition in which calcification of the hyaline (articular) cartilage or fibrocartilage (menisci) occurs, may be seen in other conditions as well, such as gout, hyperparathyroidism, hemochromatosis, hepatolenticular degeneration (Wilson disease), and degenerative joint disease. Calcium pyrophosphate arthropathy refers to CPPD crystal deposition disease affecting the joints and producing structural damage to the articular cartilage. It displays distinctive radiographic abnormalities such as narrowing of the joint space, subchondral sclerosis, and osteophytosis. The pseudogout syndrome represents a condition in which symptoms such as acute pain are similar to those seen in gouty arthritis; however, it does not respond to the usual treatment (colchicine) for the latter disease.

Calcium pyrophosphate crystals, the pathogens in pseudogout, range up to 10μ in length. As in gout, many intracellular crystals are seen during an acute episode. Pyrophosphate crystals are positively birefringent in that they are blue when the longitudinal axis of the crystal is parallel to the slow vibrations axis of the red compensator and yellow when it is perpendicular.

Radiographic Features

Radiographically, the arthritic changes encountered in this condition are similar to those seen in osteoarthritis, but the wrist, elbow, shoulder, ankle, and the femoropatellar joint compartment are also characteristically involved. In the spine, fibrocartilaginous calcifications are rarely seen. Occasionally they may be observed within intervertebral disks, particularly in anulus fibrosus. In case of spinal involvement, disk space narrowing is a common radiographic finding, and it may be associated with vertebral sclerosis. Calcification of articular cartilage in the sacroiliac joints is infrequently seen.

As mentioned above, CPPD crystal deposition disease is characterized by calcification of the articular cartilage and menisci; the tendons, ligaments, and joint capsule may exhibit calcifications as well. The mineral deposits are associated with a tissue reaction characterized by the presence of histiocytes and multinucleated giant cells, and sometimes with bone and cartilage formation. The differential diagnosis should include tumoral calcinosis, a disorder characterized by the presence of single or multiple lobulated cystic masses in the soft tissues, usually near the major joints, containing chalky material consisting of calcium phosphate, calcium carbonate, or hydroxyapatite. The calcified deposits fail to show a crystalline appearance when examined by polarization microscopy. In this condition, the masses are painless and usually occur in children and adolescents, the majority of whom are black.

Hemochromatosis

Hemochromatosis is a rare disorder characterized by iron deposition in various organs, particularly the liver, skin, and pancreas. It may be primary (endogenous or idiopathic), due to an error in metabolizing iron, or secondary, due to iron overload. Idiopathic hemochromatosis may be familial and has been linked with histocompatibility antigens HLA-A3, HLA-B7, and HLA-B14. The secondary form of hemochromatosis is related to iron overload (such as transfusions or dietary intake) and may be associated with alcohol abuse. Hemochromatosis affects males ten times more frequently than females. It is generally diagnosed between the ages of 40 and 60 on the basis of markedly elevated serum iron levels. For confirmation, biopsy of the liver or synovium may be performed. Fifty percent of patients with hemochromatosis will develop a slowly progressing arthritis, starting in the small joints of the hands, but eventually the large joints as well as intervertebral disks in the cervical and lumbar region may become affected. However, the most common manifestation of hemochromatosis in the spine is osteoporosis. The incidence of this finding varies from 25% to 58%. Patients with this type of osteoporosis are usually asymptomatic, although occasionally pathologic vertebral fractures may result.

In the hand, the second and third metacarpophalangeal joints are characteristically affected although other small joints such as the interphalangeal and carpal articulations may also be involved. Degenerative changes may also be seen in the shoulders, knees, hips, and ankles. Loss of the articular space, eburnation, subchondral cyst formation, and osteophytosis are the most prominent radiographic features of hemochromatosis. The changes may occasionally mimic those seen in CPPD crystal deposition disease and rheumatoid arthritis.

Arthritis Associated with AIDS

An increased prevalence of rheumatologic disorders has recently been described in patients with HIV infection. Berman and colleagues (1988) stated that 71% of patients infected with HIV virus had rheumatic complaints, including arthralgias, Reiter syndrome, psoriatic arthritis, myositis, vasculitis, and undifferentiated articular syndromes. Solomon and colleagues (1988) found that patients with HIV infection demonstrated a 144-fold increase in the prevalence of Reiter syndrome and a 10- to 40-fold increase in the prevalence of psoriasis, compared with the general population. It is interesting to note that arthritis was seen during various stages of HIV infection and often preceded clinical manifestations of AIDS. The arthritis was more severe and was unresponsive to conventional treatment with nonsteroidal anti-inflammatory medications. Several hypotheses have been suggested to explain the coexistence of inflammatory arthritis and HIV infection. One of these suggests that Reiter syndrome entails an interaction between a genetic predisposition (eg, HLA B27 locus) and environmental factors, most often venereal infections. The immune system also plays a role in the pathogenesis of Reiter syndrome. Likewise, the pathogenesis of psoriatic arthritis may entail genetic predisposition (eg, HLA-B27 or HLA-B38 locus). Because infection with HIV virus is commonly followed by the development of immunodeficiency syndrome, it is possible that the altered immune mechanism noted in patients with AIDS triggered the onset of Reiter syndrome or psoriatic arthritis in genetically predisposed patients. A second hypothesis suggests that HIV-related immunodeficiency causes susceptibility to infection by a variety of bacterial and viral organisms which, in turn, trigger the onset of arthritis in a genetically predisposed patient. A third hypothesis implies that there might be yet undiscovered common epidemiologic factors that may predispose an individual to the onset of both HIV infection and arthritis. Finally, the arthritis may reflect a direct action of HIV infection on synovial tissues. As Rosenberg and colleagues (1989) have pointed out, radiographic documentation of seronegative arthritis should raise the possibility of HIV-associated arthritis as part of the differential diagnosis, particularly in patients with known risk factors for HIV infection.

Infectious Arthritis

Infectious arthritides demonstrate invariably a positive radionuclide bone scan, particularly when indium-labeled white cells are used as a tracer (see Chapter 1), and a very similar radiographic picture, including joint effusion and destruction of cartilage and subchondral bone with consequent joint-space narrowing. However, certain clinical and radiographic features are characteristic of individual infectious processes as demonstrated at various target sites. In general, however, infectious arthritis is characterized by the complete destruction of both articular ends of the bones forming the joint. In the spine, the most common form of infection is an infected disk ("diskitis"). A detailed description of pyogenic arthritis, fungal arthritis, and other infectious arthritides caused by viruses and spirochetes is provided in the section on infections (Chapter 13).

Suggested Reading

Anderson HC: Mechanisms of pathologic calcification. *Rheum Dis Clin North Am* 14:303, 1988.

Baker ND: Hemochromatosis. In Taveras JM, Ferrucci JT (eds): *Radiology—Diagnosis, Imaging, Intervention.* Philadelphia, J B Lippincott, 1986.

Barthelemy CR, Nakayama DA, Carrera GF, et al: Gouty arthritis: A prospective radiographic evaluation of sixty patients. *Skeletal Radiol* 11:1, 1984.

Berman A, Espinoza LR, Diaz JD, et al: Rheumatic manifestations of human immunodeficiency virus infection. *Am J Med* 85:59, 1988.

Burnham J, Fraker K, Steinbach H: Pathologic fracture in an unusual case of gout. *Am J Roentgenology* 129:1116, 1977.

Dalinka MK, Reginato AJ, Golden DA: Calcium deposition diseases. *Semin Roentgenol* 17:39, 1982.

Forrester DM, Brown JC, Nesson JW: *The Radiology of Joint Disease,* 2nd ed. Philadelphia, W B Saunders, 1978.

Hall MC, Selin G: Spinal involvement in gout. *J Bone Joint Surg* 42A:341, 1976.

Jensen PS: Chondrocalcinosis and other calcifications. *Radiol Clin North Am* 26:1315, 1988.

Genant HK: Roentgenographic aspects of calcium pyrophosphate dihydrate crystal deposition disease (pseudogout). *Arthritis Rheum* 19:307, 1976.

Hrisch JH, Killien FC, Troupin RH: The arthropathy of hemochromatosis. *Radiology* 118:591, 1976.

Justesen P, Andersen PE Jr: Radiologic manifestations in alkaptonuria. *Skel Radiol* 11:204, 1984.

Resnick CS, Resnick D: Crystal deposition disease. *Semin Arthritis Rheum* 12:390, 1983.

Rosenberg ZA, Norman A, Solomon G: Arthritis associated with HIV infection: Radiographic manifestations. *Radiology* 173:171, 1989.

Rubenstein J, Pritzker KPH: Crystal-associated arthropathies. *AJR* 152:685, 1989.

Schumacher HR Jr: Crystals, inflammation, and osteoarthritis. *Am J Med* 83:11, 1987.

Schumacher HR Jr: Hemochromatosis and arthritis. *Arthritis Rheum* 7:41, 1964.

Solomon G, Brancato LJ, Itescu S, et al: Arthritis, psoriasis, and related syndromes associated with HIV infection (abstr). *Arthritis Rheum* 31(suppl 4): S-12, 1988.

Tkach S: Gouty arthritis of the spine. *Clin Orthop* 71:81, 1970.

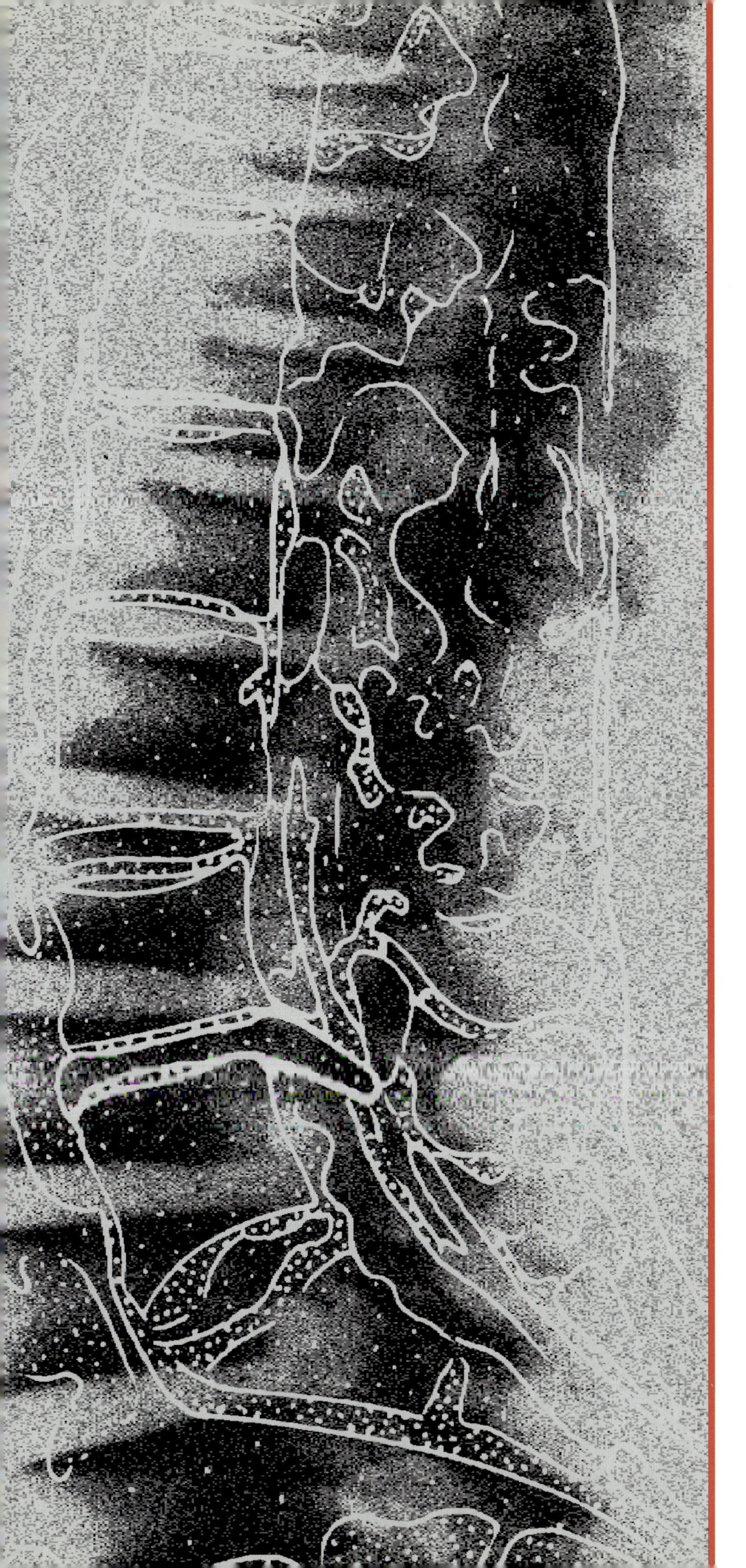

Radiologic Evaluation of Tumors and Tumor-like Lesions

8

CLASSIFICATION

Tumors, including tumor-like lesions, can be divided into two general groups: benign and malignant. The latter group can be further subclassified into primary malignant tumors, secondary malignant tumors (from the transformation of benign conditions), and metastatic tumors (Fig. 8.1). All of these lesions can be still further classified according to their tissue of origin (Fig. 8.2).

For proper understanding of the terminology, it is important to redefine certain terms applied to tumors and tumor-like lesions.

The term *tumor* usually means *mass;* in common radiologic and orthopedic parlance, however, it is the equivalent of the term *neoplasm*. By definition, a neoplasm should demonstrate autonomous growth; if it can also give rise to local or remote metastases, it is defined as a *malignant neoplasm* or *malignant tumor*. In addition to these definitions (and not dealt with in this chapter) are specific histopathologic criteria for defining a tumor as benign or malignant. It is nevertheless worth mentioning that certain giant-cell tumors, despite a "benign" histopathological appearance, may produce distant metastases, and that certain cartilage tumors, despite a "benign" histopathologic pattern, can behave locally like malignant neoplasms, even though this is detectable only by radiography. Moreover, certain lesions discussed here and termed *tumor-like lesions* are not true neoplasms but rather have a developmental or inflammatory origin. They are included in this chapter because they display a radiographic pattern that is almost indistinguishable from that of true neoplasms. Their etiology is, in some cases, still a matter of debate.

RADIOLOGIC IMAGING MODALITIES

The radiologic modalities most often used in analyzing tumors and tumor-like lesions of the spine include:

- conventional radiography
- magnification radiography
- tomography
- angiography (usually arteriography)
- computed tomography (CT)
- magnetic resonance imaging (MRI)
- scintigraphy (radionuclide bone scan)
- fluoroscopy- or CT-guided percutaneous soft tissue and bone biopsy.

In most instances, standard radiographic views specific for the anatomic site of the vertebral column under investigation, in conjunction with conventional tomography, are sufficient for correct diagnosis (Fig. 8.3), which can be subsequently confirmed by biopsy and histologic examination. Chest radiography may also be required in cases of suspected metastasis, the most frequent complication of malignant lesions. This should be done before any treatment of a malignant primary bone tumor is undertaken, since most malignancies of bone metastasize to the lung. Magnification radiography may reveal small details not sufficiently outlined on routine films. Although CT by itself is rarely helpful in making a specific diagnosis, it can provide a precise delineation of the extent of a vertebral lesion (Fig. 8.4) and may also demonstrate breakthrough of the cortex and the involvement of surrounding soft tissues. Contrast enhancement of CT images aids in the identification of major neurovascular structures as well as vascularized lesions, and facilitates evaluation of the relationship between the tumor and the surrounding soft tissues and neurovascular structures.

Arteriography is used mainly to map out bone lesions and to assess the extent of disease. It can also demonstrate the vascular supply of a tumor, locate vessels suitable for preoperative intra-arterial chemotherapy, and delineate the area suitable for open biopsy, since the most vascular area of a tumor contains the most aggressive component of the lesion. Occasionally, arteriography can be used to demonstrate abnormal tumor vessels, corroborating findings of plain-film radiography and tomography. It can be combined with an interventional procedure, such as embolization of hypervascular tumors, before further treatment (Fig. 8.5).

Myelography may be helpful in identifying tumors that invade the vertebral column and the thecal sac (Fig. 8.6).

MRI is indispensable in evaluation of bone and soft tissue tumors. Particularly in the latter, MRI offers distinct advantages over CT. There is improved visualization of tissue planes surrounding the lesion, and neurovascular involvement can be evaluated without the use of intravenous contrast. For the evaluation of intra- and extraosseous extension of a tumor, MR imaging is crucial because it can determine with high accuracy the presence or absence of soft tissue invasion by a tumor (Fig. 8.7). T1-weighted spin-echo images enhance tumor contrast with bone, bone marrow and fatty tissue, whereas T2-weighted SE images enhance tumor contrast with muscle and accentuate peritumoral edema. On the other hand, in comparison with CT, MR images do not clearly depict or allow characterization of calcification in the tumor matrix; in fact, large amounts of calcification or ossification may be almost undetectable. Moreover, MRI is less satisfactory than CT, or even plain films and tomography, for demonstrating

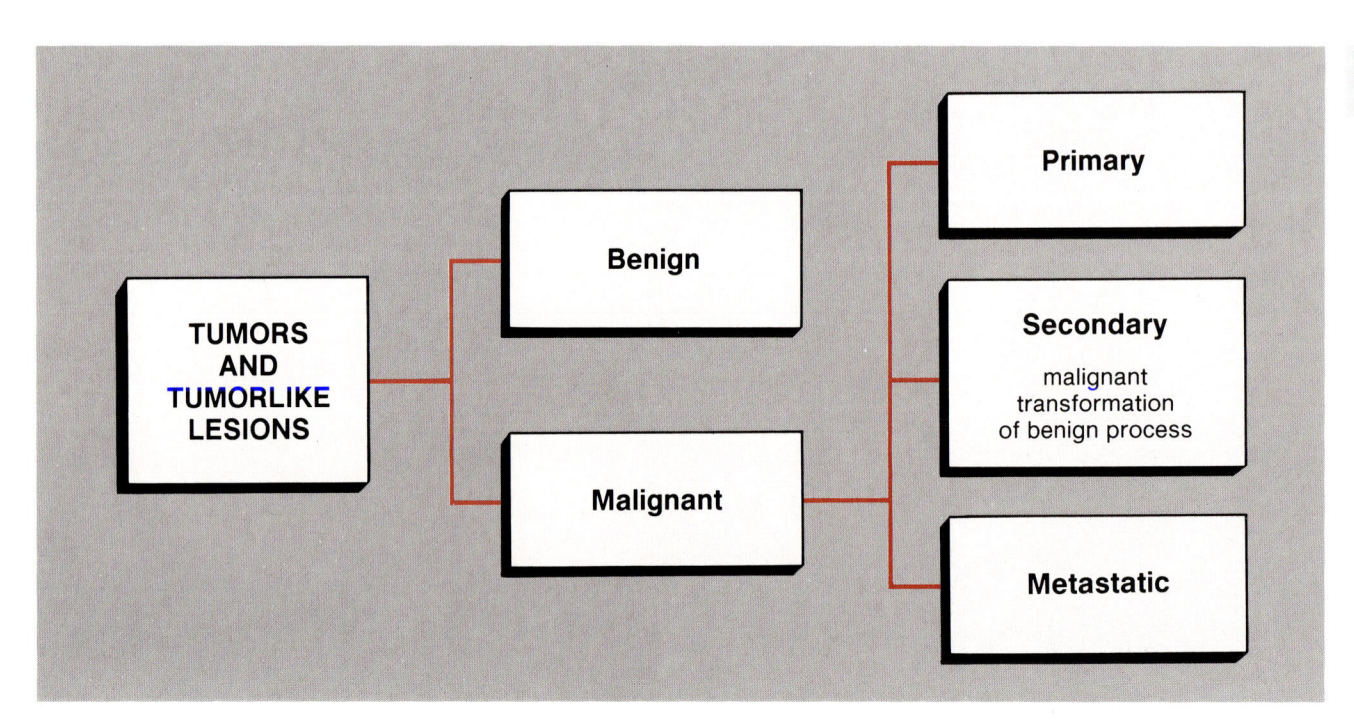

FIGURE 8.1
Classification of tumors and tumor-like lesions.

FIGURE 8.2 CLASSIFICATION OF TUMORS AND TUMOR-LIKE LESIONS BY TISSUE OF ORIGIN

TISSUE OF ORIGIN	BENIGN LESION	MALIGNANT LESION
Bone-forming (osteogenic)	Osteoma Osteoid osteoma Osteoblastoma	Osteosarcoma (and variants) Juxtacortical osteosarcoma (and variants)

Cartilage-forming (chondrogenic)	Enchondroma (chondroma)
	Periosteal (juxtacortical) chondroma
	Enchondromatosis (Ollier disease)
	Osteochondroma (osteocartilaginous exostosis, single or multiple)
	Chondroblastoma
	Chondromyxoid fibroma
		Chondrosarcoma (central)
		  Conventional
		  Mesenchymal
		  Clear cell
		  Dedifferentiated
		Chondrosarcoma (peripheral)
		  Periosteal (juxtacortical)

Fibrous, osteofibrous, and fibrohistiocytic (fibrogenic)	Fibrous cortical defect (metaphyseal fibrous defect) Nonossifying fibroma Benign fibrous histiocytoma Fibrous dysplasia (mono- and polyostotic) Periosteal desmoid Desmoplastic fibroma Osteofibrous dysplasia (Kempson-Campanacci lesion) Ossifying fibroma (Sissons lesion)	Fibrosarcoma Malignant fibrous histiocytoma
Vascular	Hemangioma Glomus tumor Cystic angiomatosis	Angiosarcoma Hemangioendothelioma Hemangiopericytoma
Hematopoietic, reticuloendothelial, and lymphatic	Giant-cell tumor (osteoclastoma) Eosinophilic granuloma Lymphangioma	Malignant giant-cell tumor Histiocytic lymphoma Hodgkin lymphoma Leukemia Myeloma (plasmacytoma) Ewing sarcoma
Neural (neurogenic)	Neurofibroma Neurilemoma	Malignant schwannoma Neuroblastoma Primitive neuroectodermal tumor (PNET)
Notochordal		Chordoma
Fat (lipogenic)	Lipoma	Liposarcoma
Unknown	Simple bone cyst Aneurysm bone cyst Intraosseous ganglion	Adamantinoma

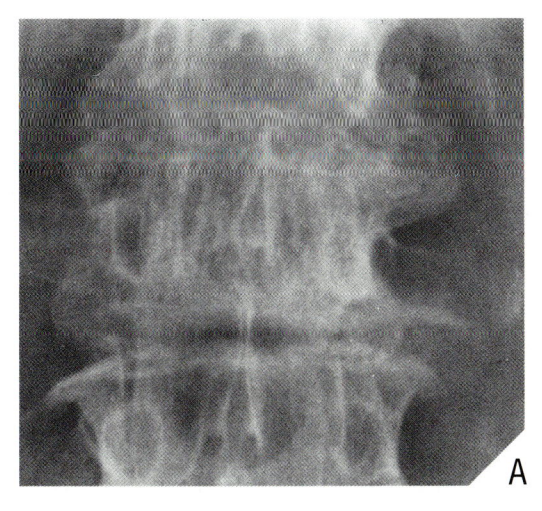

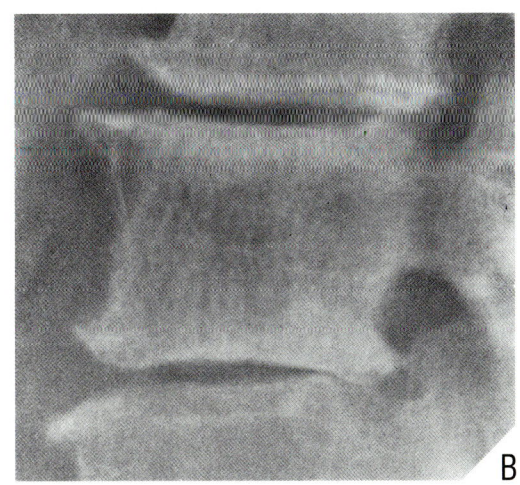

FIGURE 8.3 Anteroposterior **(A)** and lateral **(B)** views of the lumbar spine show characteristic radiographic appearance of vertebral hemangioma. The presence of coarse, vertical striations (so-called corduroy pattern) is almost pathognomonic for this lesion.

Radiologic Evaluation of Tumors and Tumor-like Lesions

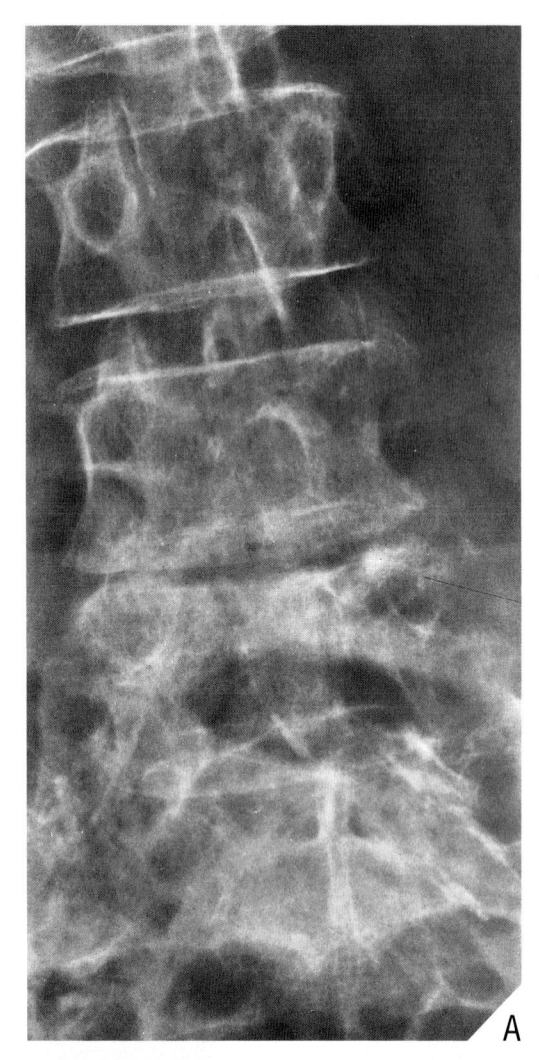

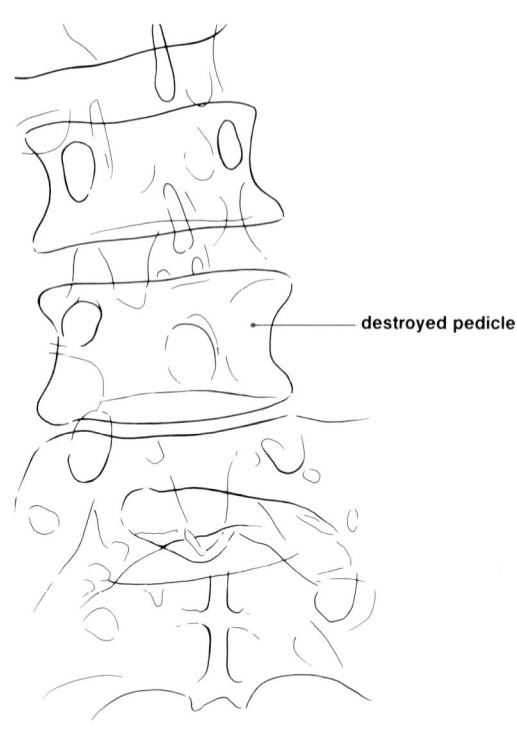

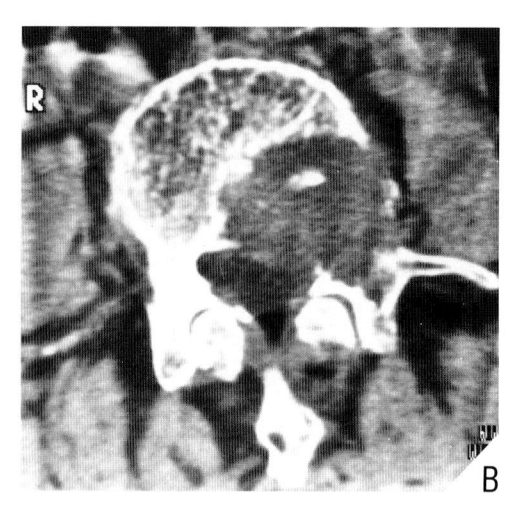

FIGURE 8.4 (A) Anteroposterior plain film of the lumbar spine in a 67-year-old woman who presented with lower back pain of four months' duration demonstrates destruction of the left pedicle of the L4 vertebra. **(B)** CT section shows extension of the tumor into the vertebral body.

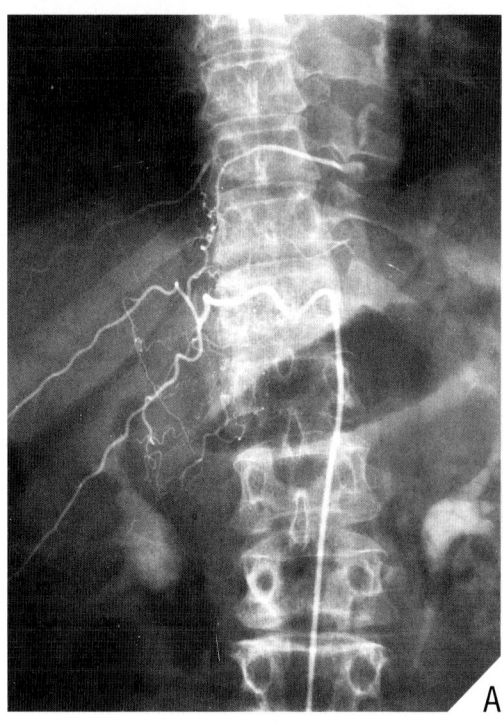

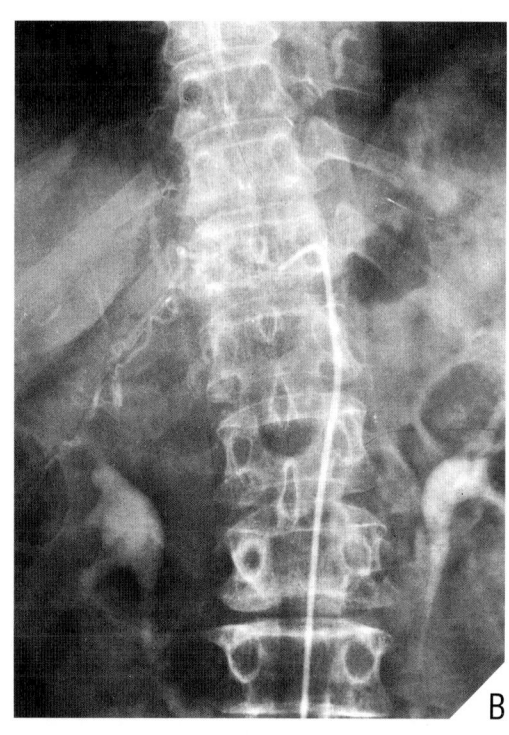

FIGURE 8.5 A 73-year-old woman presented with a collapsed T11 vertebra, which showed in addition a corduroy-like pattern suggestive of hemangioma. Vertebral angiography was performed. **(A)** Arteriogram of the eleventh right intercostal artery outlines a vascular paraspinal mass associated with hemangioma and indicates extension of the lesion into the soft tissues. **(B)** After embolization, the lesion shows a marked decrease in vascularity. Subsequently, the patient underwent decompression laminectomy and anterior fusion at T10–T11 using a fibular strut graft.

Imaging of the Spine in Clinical Practice

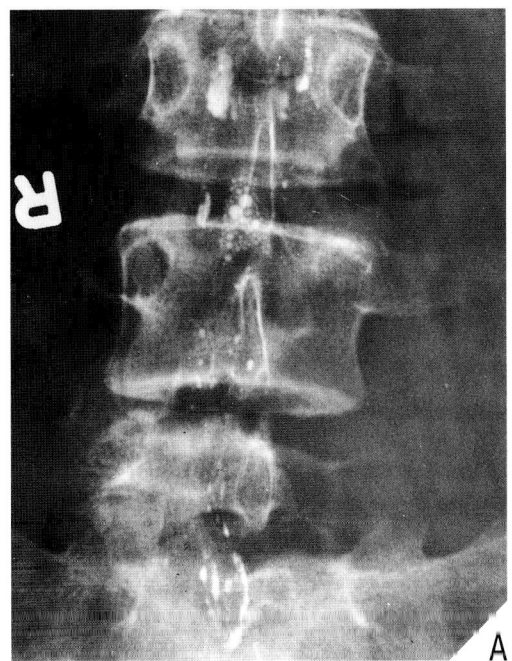

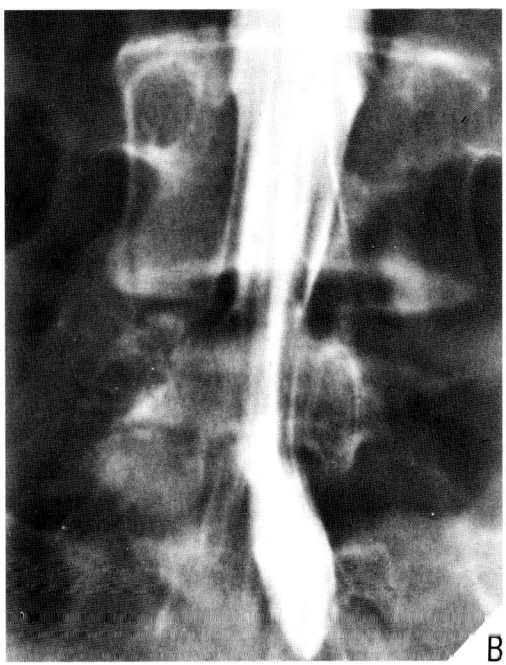

FIGURE 8.6 Initial radiographic examination of the lumbar spine of this 14-year-old girl with an 18-month history of lower back pain and sciatica of the left leg did not disclose any abnormalities; myelography was performed because of suspected herniation of a lumbar disk, but it was inconclusive. A repeat study was requested when the symptoms became more severe after 3 months. **(A)** Plain film of the lumbosacral spine shows destruction of the left pedicle and the left part of the L5 body (note the residual contrast agent in the subarachnoid space). A repeat myelogram using a water-soluble contrast (metrizamide) shows, on the anteroposterior view **(B)**, extradural compression of the thecal sac on the left side, with displacement of the nerve roots. Biopsy confirmed the radiographic diagnosis of an aneurysmal bone cyst.

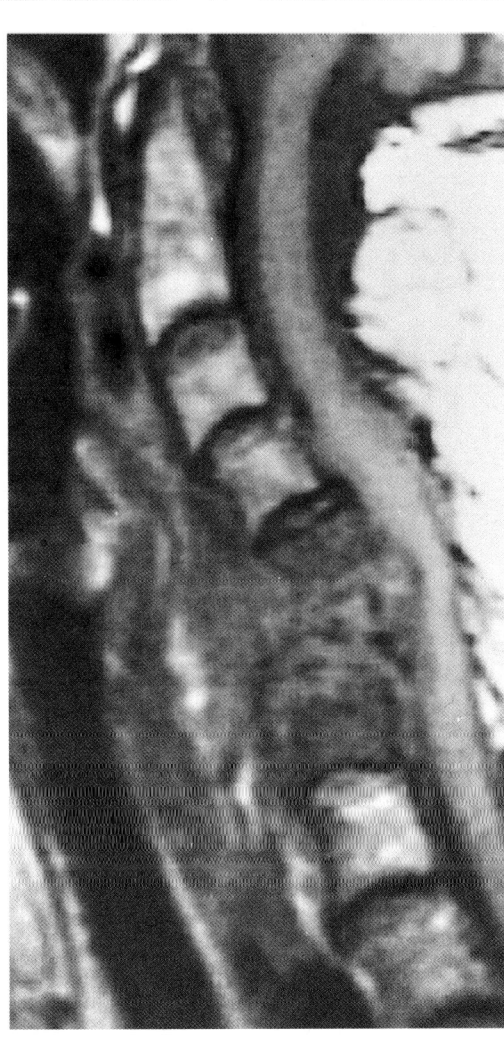

FIGURE 8.7 Sagittal spin-echo T1-weighted MRI depicts, with high accuracy, the soft tissue extension of metastatic adenocarcinoma to the vertebrae C5, C6, and C7. The compression of the spinal cord by the tumor is well demonstrated.

cortical destruction. It is important to realize that both MRI and CT have their own advantages and disadvantages, and circumstances exist in which either can be the preferential or complementary study. It is even more important to remember that the value of both MRI and CT is greatly enhanced when the surgeon communicates the type of information needed to the radiologist who will perform and interpret the study.

Several investigators have recently stressed the advantage of MRI contrast enhancement with intravenous injection of gadopentate dimeglumine (gadolinium diethylenetriamine-pentaacetic acid or Gd-DTPA). Enhancement was found to give better delineation of the tumor's richly vascularized parts and of compressed tissue immediately surrounding the tumor. The contrast studies also improved the differentiation of necrotic tissue from viable areas in various malignant tumors.

According to recent investigations, MRI may have an additional application in the evaluation of tumor response to radiation and chemotherapy and in evaluating local recurrence. On gadolinium-enhanced T1-weighted images, signal intensity remains low in avascular, necrotic areas of tumor, whereas it increases in viable tissue. Although static MR imaging was of little value for assessment of response to the treatment, dynamic MR imaging using Gd-DTPA as a contrast enhancement had the highest degree of accuracy (85.7%) and was superior to scintigraphy, particularly in patients who were receiving intra-arterial chemotherapy. In general, drug-sensitive tumors display slower uptake of Gd-DTPA after preoperative chemotherapy than do nonresponsive lesions. The rapid uptake of Gd-DTPA by malignant tissues may be due to increased vascularity and more rapid perfusion of the contrast material through an expanded interstitial space. The latest observation suggests that MR spectroscopy may also be useful in the evaluation of patients undergoing chemotherapy.

It must be stressed that most of the time MRI is not suitable for establishing the precise nature of a bone tumor. In particular, too much faith has been placed in MRI as a method for distinguishing benign from malignant lesions. Trials using combined ^{1}H MR imaging and ^{31}P MR spectroscopy failed to distinguish most benign lesions from malignant tumors. Despite the utilization of various criteria, the application of MRI

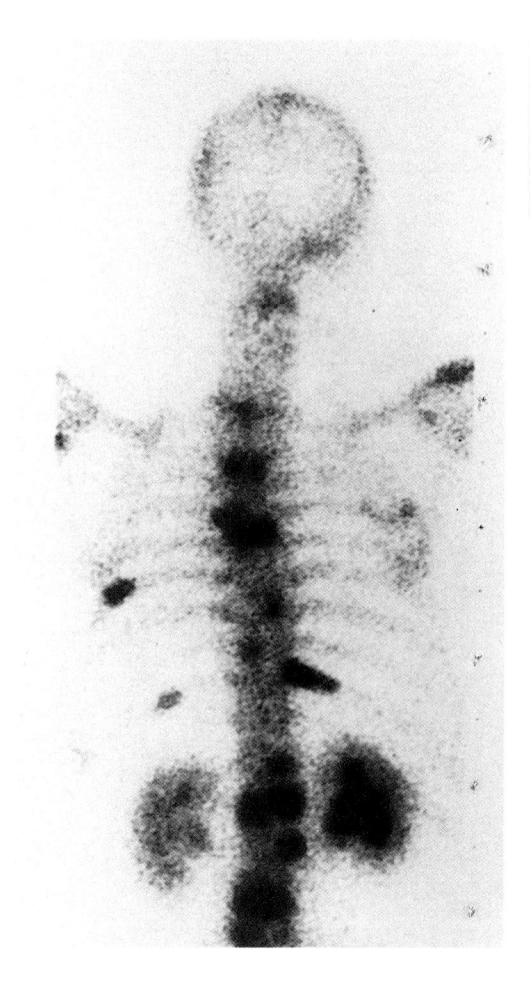

FIGURE 8.8 A radionuclide bone scan obtained after administration of 15 mCi (555 MBq) of technetium-99m-labeled methylene diphosphonate in a patient with carcinoma of the prostate shows increased uptake of a tracer in several vertebrae affected by metastatic process. (Courtesy of Robert C. Stadalnik, M.D., Sacramento, CA.)

to tissue diagnosis has rarely achieved satisfactory results because, in general, the small number of protons in calcified structures renders MRI less useful in evaluation of bone lesions. Valuable evidence concerning the production of the tumor matrix can be missed by this modality because of its unsatisfactory demonstration of small calcified structures. Moreover, as several investigations have shown, MRI is an imaging modality of low specificity. T1 and T2 measurements are usually of limited value for histologic characterization of musculoskeletal tumors. Quantitative determination of relaxation times has not proven clinically valuable in identifying various tumor types, although it is an important technique in the staging of osteosarcoma or chondrosarcoma. In particular, T2-weighted images are crucial in delineating extraosseous extension of tumor and peritumoral edema, as well as in assessing the involvement of major neurovascular bundles. Necrotic areas change from low-intensity signal in the T1-weighted image to a very bright intense signal in the T2-weighted images and can be differentiated from viable, solid tumor tissue. Although MR imaging cannot predict the histology of bone tumors, it may occasionally be useful for distinguishing benign from pathologic fracture.

The radionuclide bone scan is an indicator of mineral turnover. Because there is usually enhanced deposition of bone-seeking radiopharmaceuticals in areas of bone undergoing change and repair, scintigraphy is useful in localizing tumors and tumor-like lesions of the vertebral column, particularly in such conditions as eosinophilic granuloma or metastatic cancer, in which more than one lesion is present (Fig. 8.8). It also plays an important role in localizing small lesions, such as osteoid osteomas, which may not always be visible on plain-film studies. In most instances radionuclide bone scanning cannot distinguish benign lesions from malignant tumors, since increased blood flow with consequently increased isotope deposition and increased osteoblastic activity is present in both benign and malignant conditions. However, scintigraphy can sometimes achieve such differentiation in benign lesions that do not absorb the radioactive isotope. In addition, the radionuclide bone scan is occasionally useful for differentiating multiple myeloma, which usually shows no significant uptake of the tracer, from metastatic cancer, which usually does.

In addition to ^{99m}Tc-labeled phosphate compounds for routine radionuclide scans, occasionally ^{67}Ga is useful for detection and staging of bone and soft tissue neoplasms. Gallium in the body is handled much like iron, in that the protein transferrin carries it in the plasma and it competes for extravascular iron-binding proteins such as lactoferrin. The dosage for adults ranges from 3 mCi (111 MBq) to 10 mCi (370 MBq) per study. The exact mechanism of tumor uptake of gallium remains unsettled, and its uptake varies with tumor type. In particular, Hodgkin lymphomas and histiocytic lymphomas are prone to significant gallium uptake.

Percutaneous bone and soft tissue biopsy done in the radiology department has in recent years gained a place in the diagnostic workup for various neoplastic diseases, including bone tumors. In patients with primary bone neoplasms it allows rapid histologic diagnosis. It also aids in assessment of the effects of chemotherapy and radiation therapy, and helps to locate the site of the primary tumor in cases of metastatic disease. In addition, percutaneous bone and soft tissue biopsy performed in the radiology suite is simple and inexpensive compared with biopsy done in the operating room.

Finally, it is important to compare recent radiologic studies with earlier films; this point cannot be sufficiently emphasized. Such comparison can reveal not only the nature of a bone lesion, but also its aggressiveness—a critical factor in a diagnostic workup.

TUMORS AND TUMOR-LIKE LESIONS OF THE SPINE

Diagnosis

CLINICAL INFORMATION

The age of the patient is the single most important item of clinical data in the radiographic establishment of tumor diagnosis. Certain tumors have a predilection for specific age groups (Fig. 8.9). Aneurysmal bone cysts, for example, rarely occur beyond the age of 20 years, and giant-cell tumors, as a rule, occur only after the skeletal maturity. Other lesions may have different radiographic presentations or may arise in different locations in patients of different ages.

Also important in the clinical differentiation of lesions with similar radiographic presentations, such as eosinophilic granuloma, osteomyelitis, and Ewing sarcoma, is the duration of the patient's symptoms. In eosinophilic granuloma, the amount of bone destruction visible on radiograph after 1 week of symptoms is usually the same as that seen after 4 to 6 weeks of symptoms in osteomyelitis and 3 to 4 months in Ewing sarcoma.

The growth rate of the tumor may be an additional helpful factor in differentiating malignant (usually rapidly growing) from benign (usually slowly growing) tumor.

IMAGING MODALITIES

With so many imaging modalities available to diagnose and further characterize the bone tumors, radiologists and clinicians are frequently uncertain how to proceed in a given case, concerning the modality of choice for a particular problem, the order of preference in which a modality should be used, and when to stop. It is important to keep in mind that the choice of techniques for imaging a musculoskeletal tumor should be dictated not only by the clinical presentation but also by equipment availability, expertise, cost, and restrictions applicable to individual patients (for example, an allergy to ionic or nonionic iodinated contrast agents may preclude the use of myelography; the presence of a pacemaker may preclude the use of MRI; a physiologic state such as pregnancy, which precludes the use of ionized radiation, favors, for instance, sonography). Some of these problems are discussed in general in Chapter 1. Here, an attempt is made to provide general guidelines for bone and soft tissue tumors. In the evaluation of bone tumors, plain radiography and tomography are still the gold standard for diagnostic purposes. The most important principle is that results obtained by one or more ancillary techniques must always be compared with plain-film studies. The choice of imaging technique is usually dictated by the type of tumor suspected. For instance, when osteoid osteoma is suspected on the basis of clinical history, plain film radiography followed by scintigraphy constitutes the primary method of choice. Once the lesion has been localized to a particular vertebra, CT should be employed for specific localization and to obtain quantitative information (ie, measurements). On the other hand, when a paravertebral soft tissue tumor is suspected, the primary modality should be an MRI study, since this is the only technique that can accurately localize and characterize

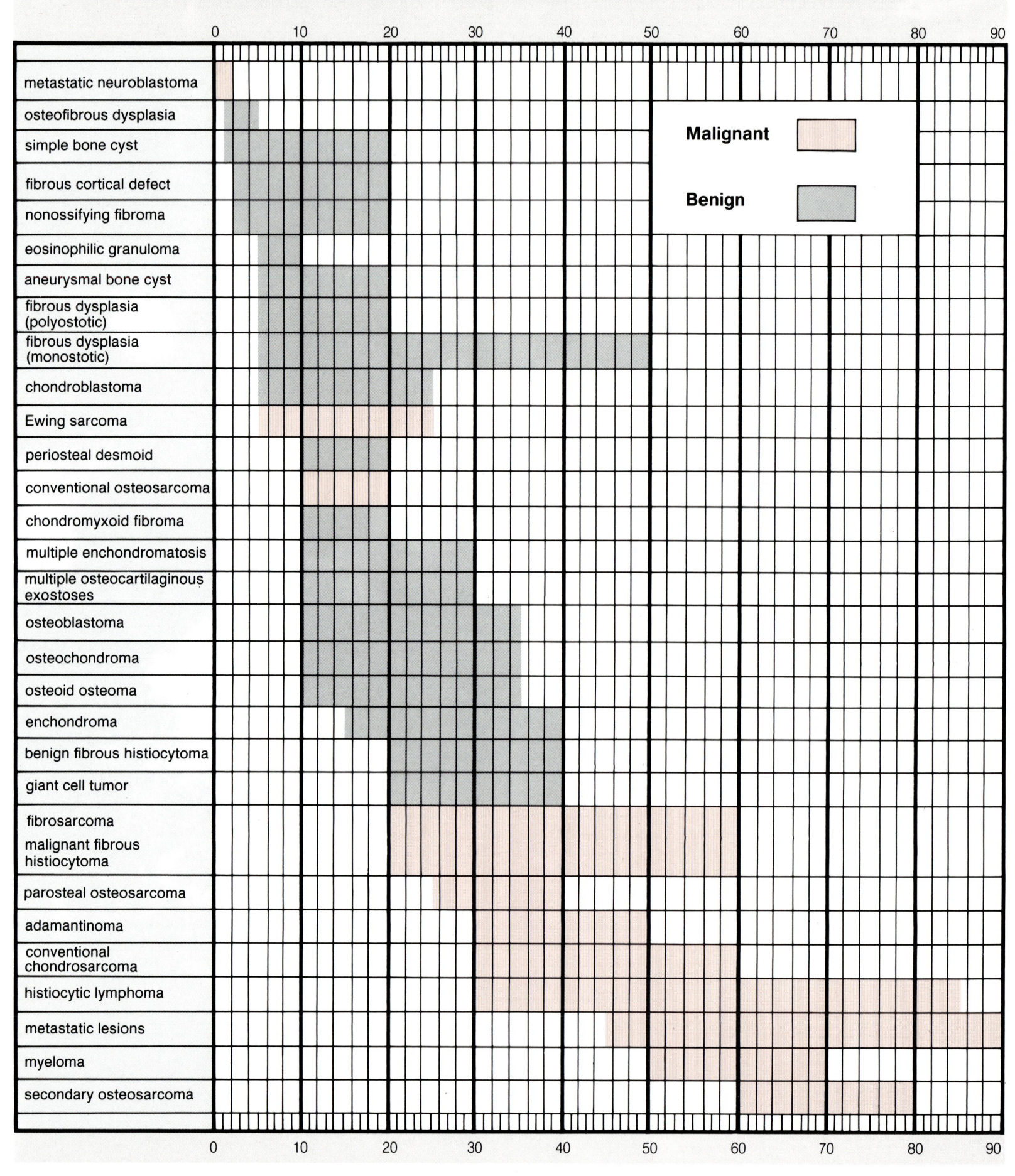

FIGURE 8.9 Peak age incidence of benign and malignant tumors and tumor-like lesions. (Sources: Dahlin DC, Unni KK: *Bone Tumors: General Aspects and Data on 8542 Cases,* 3rd ed. Springfield, IL, Charles C Thomas, 1986; Huvos AG: *Bone Tumors. Diagnosis, Treatment and Prognosis.* Philadelphia, W B Saunders, 1979; Jaffee HL: *Tumors and Tumorous Conditions of the Bones and Joints.* Philadelphia, Lea & Febiger, 1968; Mirra JM, Picci P, Gold RH: *Bone Tumors: Clinical, Radiologic and Pathologic Correlations.* Phildelphia, Lea & Febiger, 1989; Schajowicz F: *Tumors and Tumorlike Lesions of Bone and Joints.* New York, Springer-Verlag, 1981; Wilner D: *Radiology of Bone Tumors and Allied Disorders.* Philadelphia, Lea & Febiger, 1982).

Imaging of the Spine in Clinical Practice

soft tissue lesions. Likewise, if plain films are suggestive of a malignant tumor arising in the vertebral column, MRI or CT should then be employed to evaluate the extent of intraosseous tumor and extraosseous involvement.

In some instances, the use of CT over MRI is dependent on the features visible on plain radiographs: if there is no definite evidence of soft tissue extension, CT may be superior to MRI for detecting subtle cortical erosions and periosteal reaction, providing at the same time an excellent means of determining the intraosseous extension of the tumor. On the other hand, if plain radiographs suggest cortical destruction and soft tissue mass, MRI would be the preferred modality, since it provides exquisite soft tissue contrast and can determine the extraosseous extension of the tumor and involvement of the neural structures much better than CT.

In evaluating the results of radiotherapy and chemotherapy in treatment of malignant tumors, dynamic MR imaging using Gd-DTPA for contrast enhancement is far superior to scintigraphy, CT, or even plain MR imaging.

Figure 8.10 depicts one of the many algorithms helpful for evaluating the vertebral lesions discovered on standard plain radiographs. Note that the proper order of the use of various imaging modalities depends upon two main factors: (1) whether the plain film findings are or are not diag-

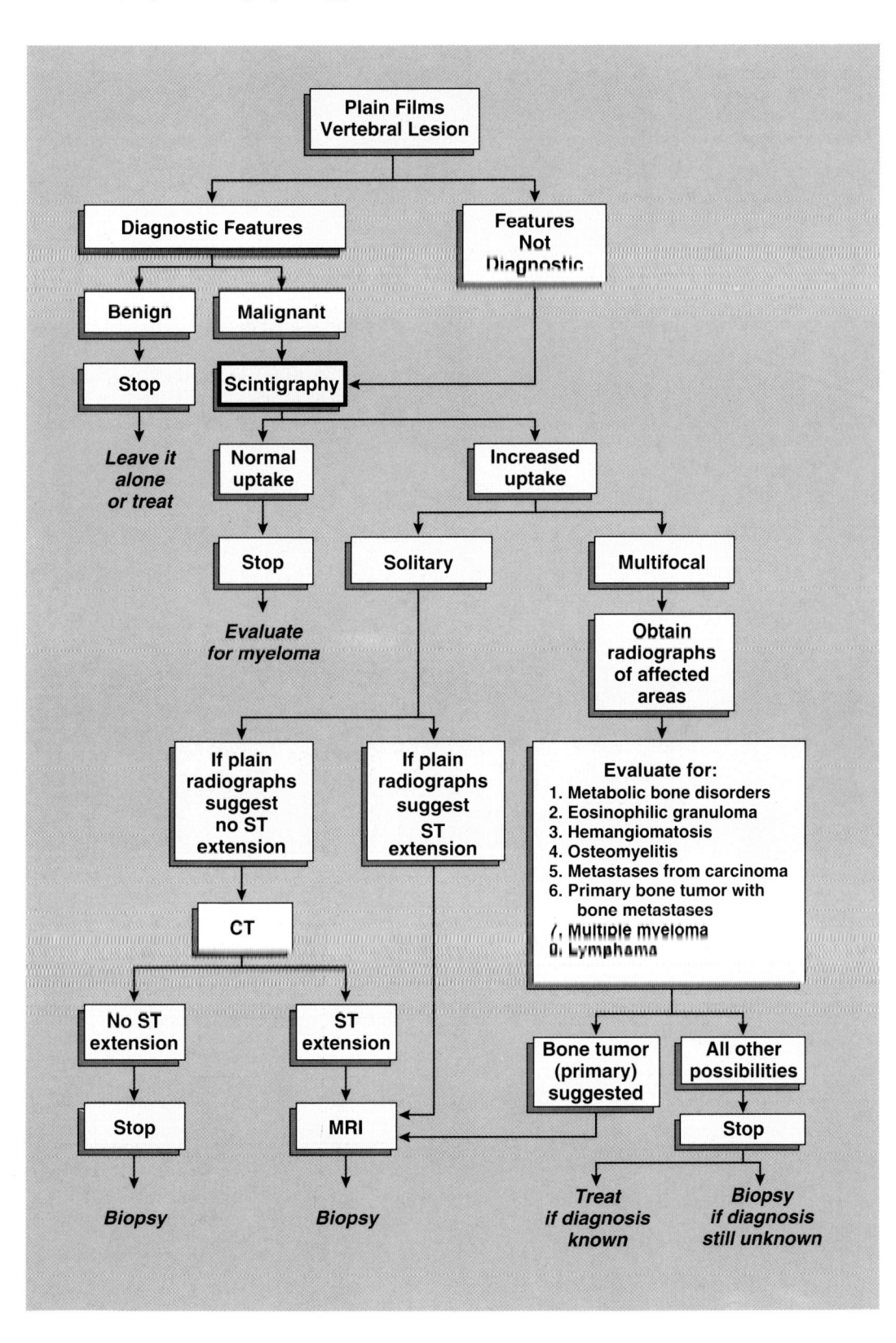

FIGURE 8.10 Evaluation of vertebral lesion discovered on standard radiographs.

nostic for any particular tumor; and (2) upon the lesion's uptake of a tracer on radionuclide bone scanning. Here scintigraphy plays a crucial role, dictating further steps in utilizing different techniques.

SITE OF THE LESION

The site of a vertebral bone lesion is an important factor, since some tumors have a predilection for specific sites. For instance, the benign lesions such as osteoid osteoma, osteoblastoma, osteochondroma, and aneurysmal bone cyst usually affect the posterior elements of a vertebra. On the other hand, most of the malignant lesions, such as osteosarcoma, chondrosarcoma, myeloma, and metastatic carcinoma, affect the vertebral body (Fig. 8.11).

BORDERS OF THE LESION

Evaluation of the borders or margins of a lesion is crucial to determining whether it is slow growing or fast growing (aggressive). Slow-growing lesions, which are usually benign, have sharply outlined sclerotic borders or a narrow zone of transition (Fig. 8.12), whereas malignant or aggressive lesions typically have indistinct borders or a wide zone of transition, with either minimal or no reactive sclerosis (see Fig. 8.17). It must be

FIGURE 8.11 Distribution of various tumors and tumor-like lesions in a vertebra. Malignant lesions are seen predominantly in its anterior part (body), while benign lesions predominate in its posterior elements (neural arch).

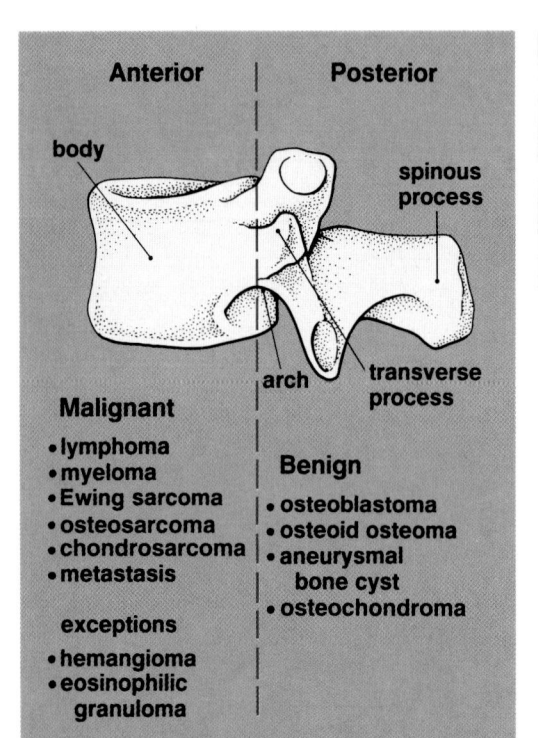

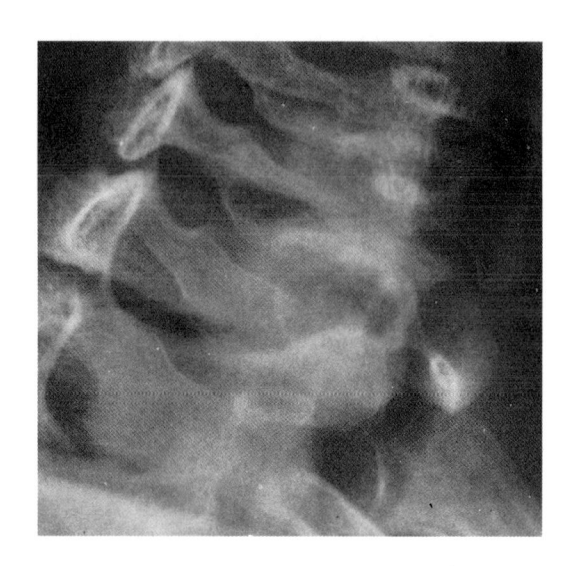

FIGURE 8.12 A sharply outlined sclerotic border marks benign lesions, as illustrated in this example of osteoblastoma affecting pedicle of C6 vertebra.

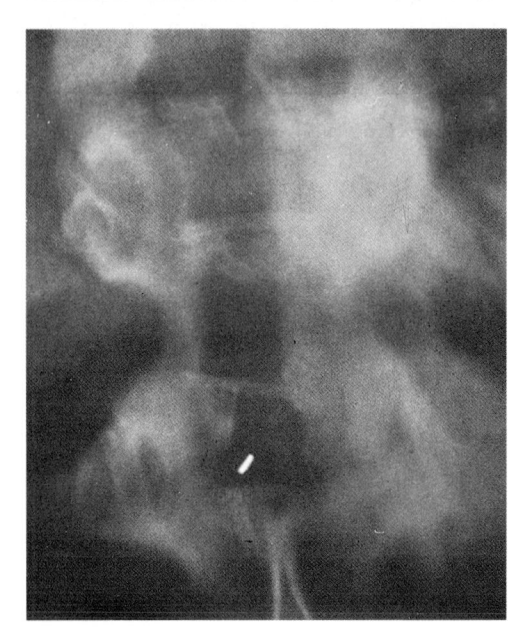

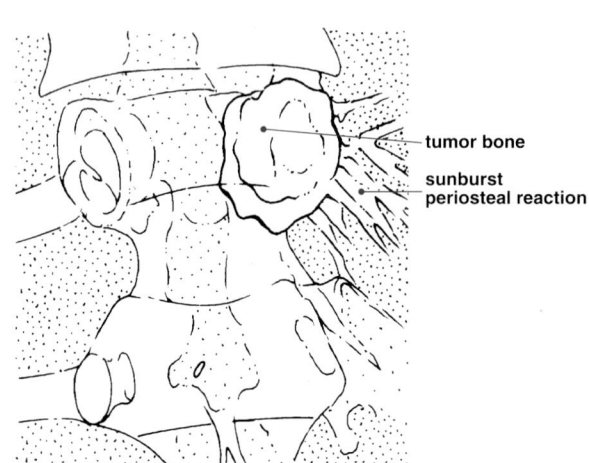

FIGURE 8.13 Osteosarcoma is typified by the presence of tumor bone. Extension to the soft tissues and "sunburst" periosteal reaction are the corroborative features of this malignant osteoblastic tumor. (Reprinted with permission from Bullough PG, Boachie-Adjei O: *Atlas of Spinal Diseases*. New York, Gower, 1988.)

Imaging of the Spine in Clinical Practice

emphasized that treatment can alter the appearance of malignant bone tumors; after radiation or chemotherapy they may exhibit significant sclerosis, as well as a narrow zone of transition.

Type of Matrix

All bone tumors are composed of characteristic tissue components: the tumor matrix. Usually only two of these—osteoblastic and cartilaginous tissue—can be clearly demonstrated radiographically. If bone or cartilage is identified within a tumor, one can assume that it is either osteoblastic or cartilaginous in origin. The identification of tumor-bone within or adjacent to the area of destruction should alert the radiologist to the possibility of osteosarcoma. However, the deposition of new bone may also be caused by a reparative process secondary to bone destruction—so called reactive sclerosis—rather than by production of osteoid or bone by malignant cells. Tumor-bone is often radiographically indistinguishable from reactive bone; however, fluffy, cotton- or cloud-like densities within the affected bone structure and in the adjacent soft tissue should suggest the presence of tumor-bone, and therefore, a diagnosis of osteosarcoma (Fig 8.13).

Cartilage is identified by the presence of typically popcorn-like, punctate, annular, or comma-shaped calcifications. Since cartilage usually grows in lobules, a tumor of cartilaginous origin is often suggested by lobulated growth (Fig. 8.14).

Type of Bone Destruction

The type of bone destruction caused by a tumor is primarily related to the rate of tumor growth. Although not pathognomonic for any specific neoplasm, the types of destruction which could be described as geographic (Fig. 8.15), moth-eaten (Fig. 8.16), or permeative (Fig. 8.17), might suggest not only a benign or malignant neoplastic process but sometimes even the histologic type of the tumor, as in the permeative type of bone destruction characteristically produced by the so-called round cell tumors.

Periosteal Response

The periosteal reaction to a neoplastic process in bone is usually categorized as uninterrupted or interrupted. The first type of reaction is marked by solid layers of periosteal density, indicating a longstanding benign process such as that seen in osteoid osteoma and osteoblastoma (Fig. 8.18).

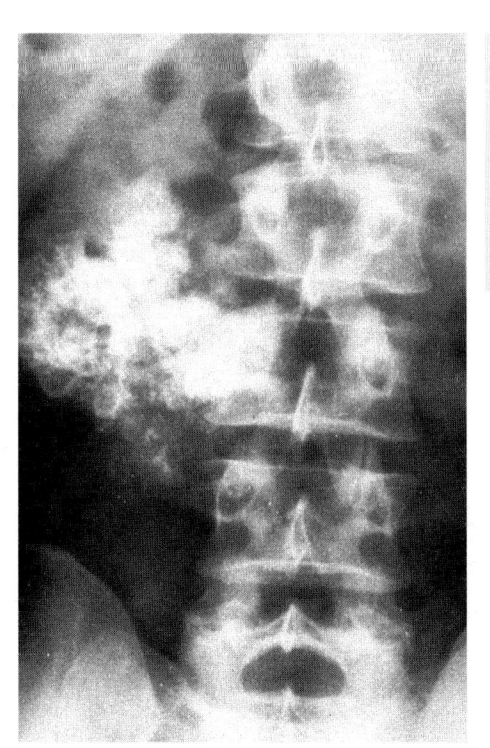

FIGURE 8.14 Anteroposterior radiograph of lumbar spine shows a large calcified mass with lobulated borders. On biopsy this lesion proved to be a chondrosarcoma. (Reprinted with permission from Bullough PG, Boachie-Adjei O: *Atlas of Spinal Diseases*. New York, Gower, 1988.)

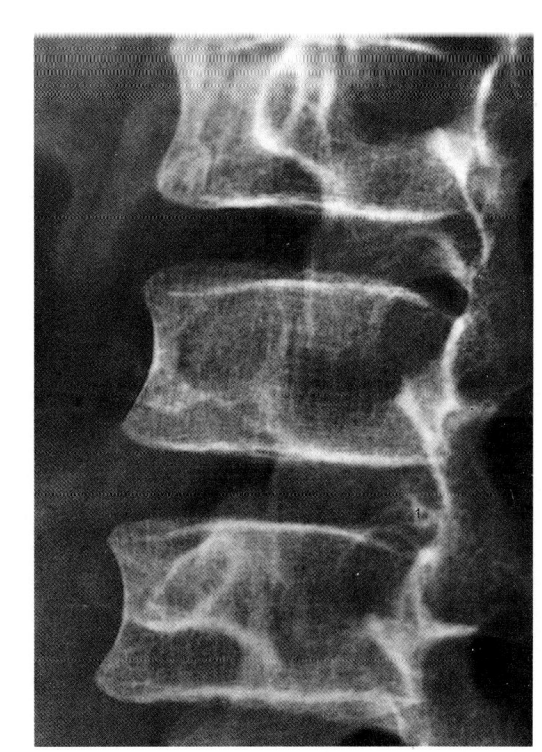

FIGURE 8.15 Geographic type of bone destruction is present in the pedicle of L3 affected by aneurysmal bone cyst.

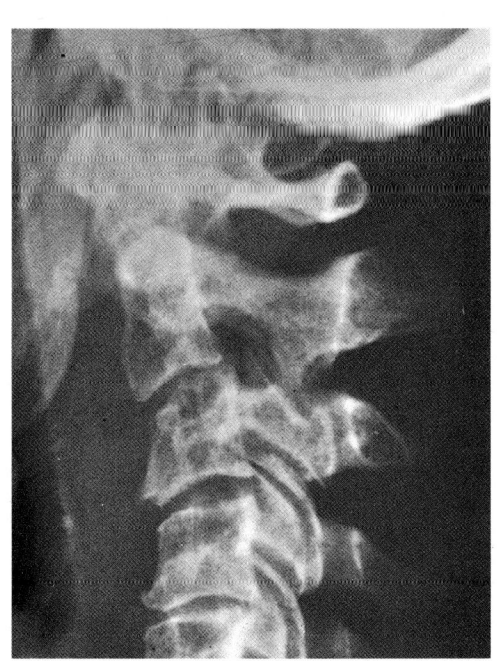

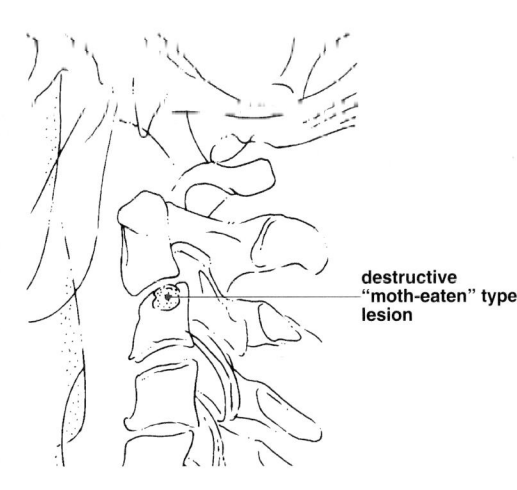

FIGURE 8.16 Moth-eaten type of bone destruction is usually characteristic for malignant tumors. In this example of a large-cell lymphoma affecting the vertebral body of C3.

Radiologic Evaluation of Tumors and Tumor-like Lesions

Uninterrupted reaction is also seen in non-neoplastic processes such as eosinophilic granuloma and osteomyelitis. The interrupted type of periosteal reaction suggests malignancy and a highly aggressive nonmalignant process. It may appear as a sunburst pattern (see Fig. 8.13) or a lamellated (onion-skin) pattern, and is commonly seen in malignant primary tumors such as osteosarcoma or Ewing sarcoma. However, in vertebral lesions it is unusual to see any significant degree of periosteal reaction.

Soft Tissue Extension

With few exceptions—such as giant-cell tumors, aneurysmal bone cysts, and osteoblastoma—benign tumors and tumor-like lesions of bone usually do not exhibit soft tissue extension. Almost invariably, therefore, a soft tissue mass indicates an aggressive lesion and one that is in many instances malignant (Fig. 8.19). It should be kept in mind, however, that non-neoplastic conditions such as osteomyelitis also exhibit a soft tissue

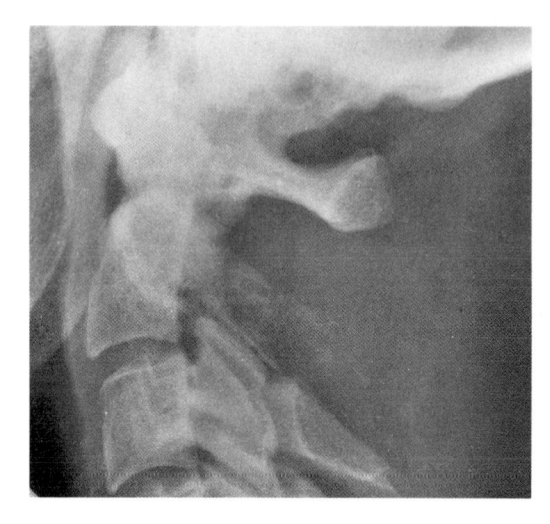

FIGURE 8.17 Permeative type of bone destruction is a radiographic hallmark of malignant tumors, in this example of a chordoma, affecting the body and spinous process of C2. Note also the ill-defined margin (wide zone of transition) of the lesion and lack of reactive sclerosis.

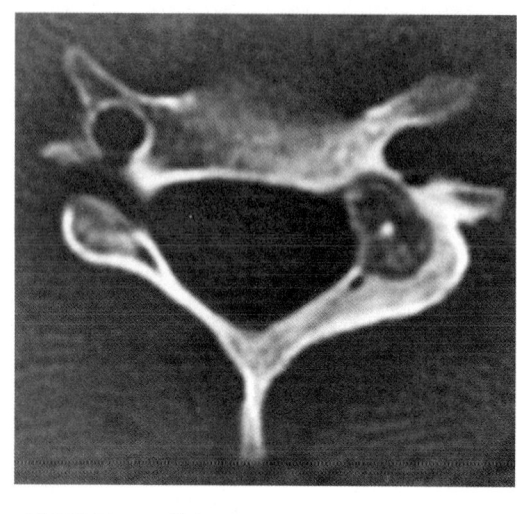

FIGURE 8.18 Uninterrupted, solid periosteal reaction is usually the characteristic feature of a benign tumor, in this example an osteoid osteoma localized to the lamina and pedicle of C6.

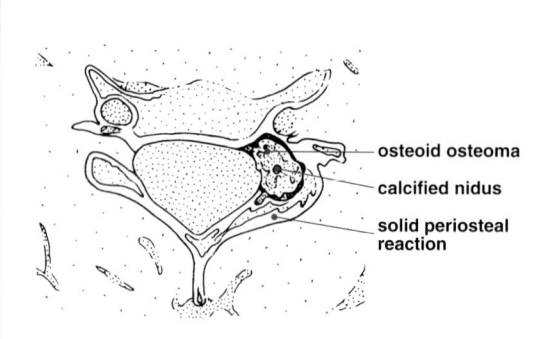

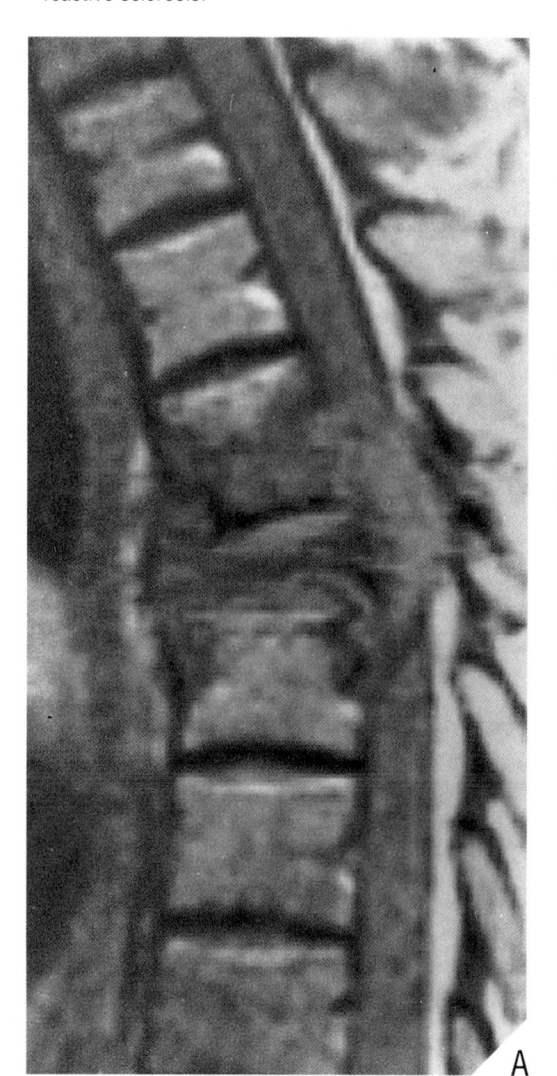

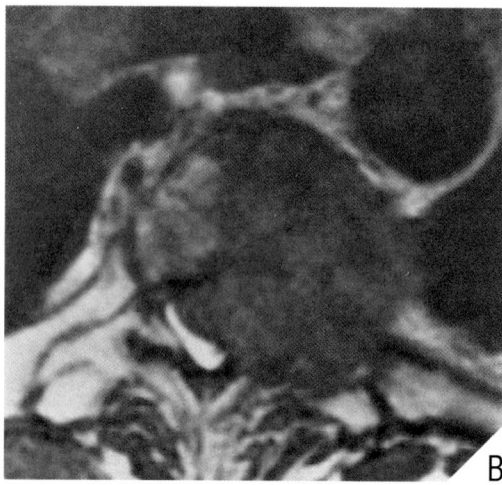

FIGURE 8.19 Sagittal **(A)** and axial **(B)** MRI demonstrate destruction of the vertebral bodies of T9 and T10 associated with a large paraspinal soft tissue mass extending anteriorly and posteriorly. The biopsy of the mass revealed metastatic adenocarcinoma.

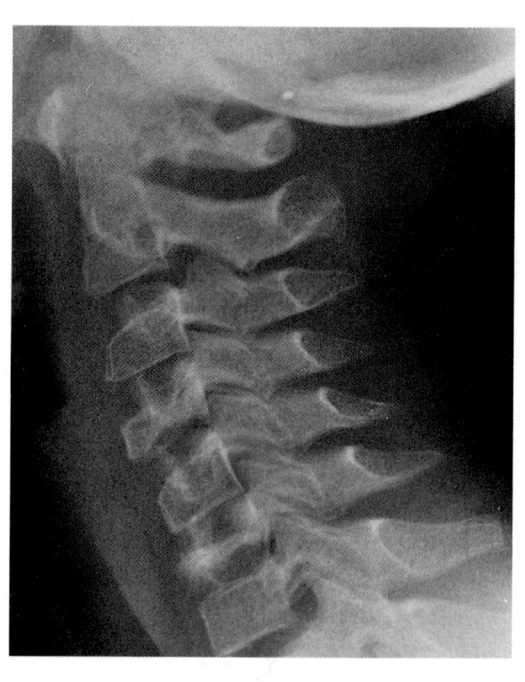

FIGURE 8.20 Pathologic fractures of the vertebrae C4 and C6 are seen in a 4-year-old boy with multifocal eosinophilic granuloma.

Imaging of the Spine in Clinical Practice

component, but the involvement of the soft tissues is usually poorly defined, with obliteration of fatty tissue layers. In malignant processes, on the other hand, the tumor mass is sharply defined, extending through the destroyed cortex with preservation of the tissue planes.

Multiplicity of Lesions

A multiplicity of malignant lesions usually indicates metastatic disease, multiple myeloma, or lymphoma. Very rarely do primary malignant lesions, such as an osteosarcoma and Ewing sarcoma, present as multifocal disease. Benign lesions, on the other hand, tend to involve multiple sites, as in eosinophilic granulomas and *hemangiomas*.

Benign Versus Malignant Nature

Although it is sometimes very difficult to distinguish benign from malignant bone lesions on the basis of radiography alone, certain characteristic features favor one classification or the other. Benign tumors are usually characterized by well-defined sclerotic borders, a geographic type of bone destruction, solid, uninterrupted periosteal reaction, and no soft tissue mass. Malignant lesions, on the other hand, tend to exhibit poorly defined borders with a wide zone of transition, a moth-eaten or permeative pattern of bone destruction, an interrupted periosteal reaction of the sun burst or onion-skin type, and an adjacent soft tissue mass. It should be kept in mind, however, that some benign lesions, such as an aneurysmal bone cyst or giant-cell tumor, may also exhibit aggressive features.

Management

When all clinical and radiographic data for the patient with a bone lesion have been analyzed, the most important diagnostic decision to be made is whether the lesion is definitely benign and not to be biopsied, but rather completely ignored—a so-called "don't touch" lesion—or whether it has an aggressive or ambiguous appearance and should therefore be further investigated via percutaneous or open biopsy. The results of the histopathologic examination of a specimen will determine whether the further management of a given case should be surgical, chemotherapeutic, radiotherapeutic, or a combination of these.

Monitoring the Results of Treatment

Five modalities—plain film radiography; CT; MRI; scintigraphy; and arteriography—are commonly used to monitor the results of treatment for bone tumors. Of these, plain film radiography is used mainly to document the results of surgical resection of benign lesions, such as osteochondroma or osteoid osteoma, or for followup after curettage of benign tumors or tumor-like lesions and application of bone grafts. The effectiveness of chemotherapy is best monitored by a combination of plain film radiography, arteriography, and MRI. Recurrence or metastatic spread of a tumor can be effectively shown at an early stage by scintigraphy, CT, or MRI.

Complications of Tumors and Tumor-like Lesions

Although the most frequent direct complication of malignant bone tumors is metastasis, particularly to the lung, the most serious complication of some benign lesions is their potential for malignant transformation. Moreover, some benign lesions, such as those seen in multiple cartilaginous exostoses and enchondromatosis, may cause severe growth disturbance. In general, however, the most common complication of tumors and tumor-like lesions is pathologic fracture. Although not a diagnostic factor, this may complicate both benign and malignant lesions. Among the lesions with a high potential for pathologic fracture are eosinophilic granuloma (Fig. 8.20), hemangioma, and multiple myeloma. Occasionally, pathologic fracture is the first sign of a neoplastic process.

Suggested Reading

Ayala AG, Zornosa J: Primary bone tumors: Percutaneous needle biopsy. *Radiology* 149:675, 1983.

Bloem JL, Bluemm RG, Taminiau AHM, et al: Magnetic resonance imaging of primary malignant bone tumors. *RadioGraphics* 7:425, 1987.

Dahlin DC, Unni KK: *Bone Tumors: General Aspects and Data on 8542 Cases*, 3rd ed. Springfield, IL, Charles C Thomas, 1986.

Edeiken J: *Roentgen Diagnosis of Diseases of Bone*, 3rd ed. Baltimore, Williams & Wilkins, 1981.

Edeiken J, Hodes PJ, Caplan LH: New bone production and periosteal reaction. *AJR* 97:708, 1966.

Ehman RL, Berquist TH, McLeod RA: MR Imaging of the musculoskeletal system: A 5-year appraisal. *Radiology* 166:313, 1988.

Greenspan A, Klein MJ: Radiology and pathology of bone tumors. In Lewis MM (ed): *Musculoskeletal Oncology—A Multidisciplinary Approach*. Philadelphia, W B Saunders, 1992.

Huvos AG: *Bone Tumors. Diagnosis, Treatment and Prognosis*. Philadelphia, W B Saunders, 1979.

Jaffee HL: *Tumors and Tumorous Conditions of the Bones and Joints*. Philadelphia, Lea & Febiger, 1968.

Kricun ME: Radiographic evaluation of solitary bone lesions. *Orthop Clin North Am* 14:39, 1983.

Lichtenstein L: *Bone Tumors*, 5th ed. St. Louis, Mosby, 1977.

Lodwick GS: A systematic approach to the roentgen diagnosis of bone tumors. In *Tumors of Bone and Soft Tissue*. Chicago, Year Book Medical Publishers, 1965.

Lodwick GS: The bones and joints. In Hodes PJ (ed): *Atlas of Tumor Radiology*. Chicago, Year Book Medical Publishers, 1971.

Lodwick GS, Wilson AJ, Farell C, et al: Determining growth rates of focal lesions of bone from radiographs. *Radiology* 134:577, 1980.

Mink J: Percutaneous bone biopsy in the patient with known or suspected osseous metastases. *Radiology* 161:191, 1986.

Mirra JM, Picci P, Gold RH: *Bone Tumors: Clinical, Radiologic and Pathologic Correlations*. Philadelphia, Lea & Febiger, 1989.

Moser RP, Madewell JE: An approach to primary bone tumors. *Radiol Clin North Am* 25:1049, 1987.

Murray RO, Jacobson HG: *The Radiology of Bone Diseases*, 2nd ed. New York, Churchill Livingstone, 1977.

Norman A: The radiologic approach to bone tumors. In *Bone and Joints*. Baltimore, Williams & Wilkins, 1976, p. 196.

Schajowicz F: *Tumors and Tumorlike Lesions of Bone and Joints*. New York, Springer-Verlag, 1981.

Spjut HJ, Dorfman HD, Fechner RE, et al: Tumors of bone and cartilage. In *Atlas of Tumor Pathology*, Fas 5. Washington, DC, Armed Forces Institute of Pathology, 1971.

Wilner D: *Radiology of Bone Tumors and Allied Disorders*. Philadelphia, Lea & Febiger, 1982.

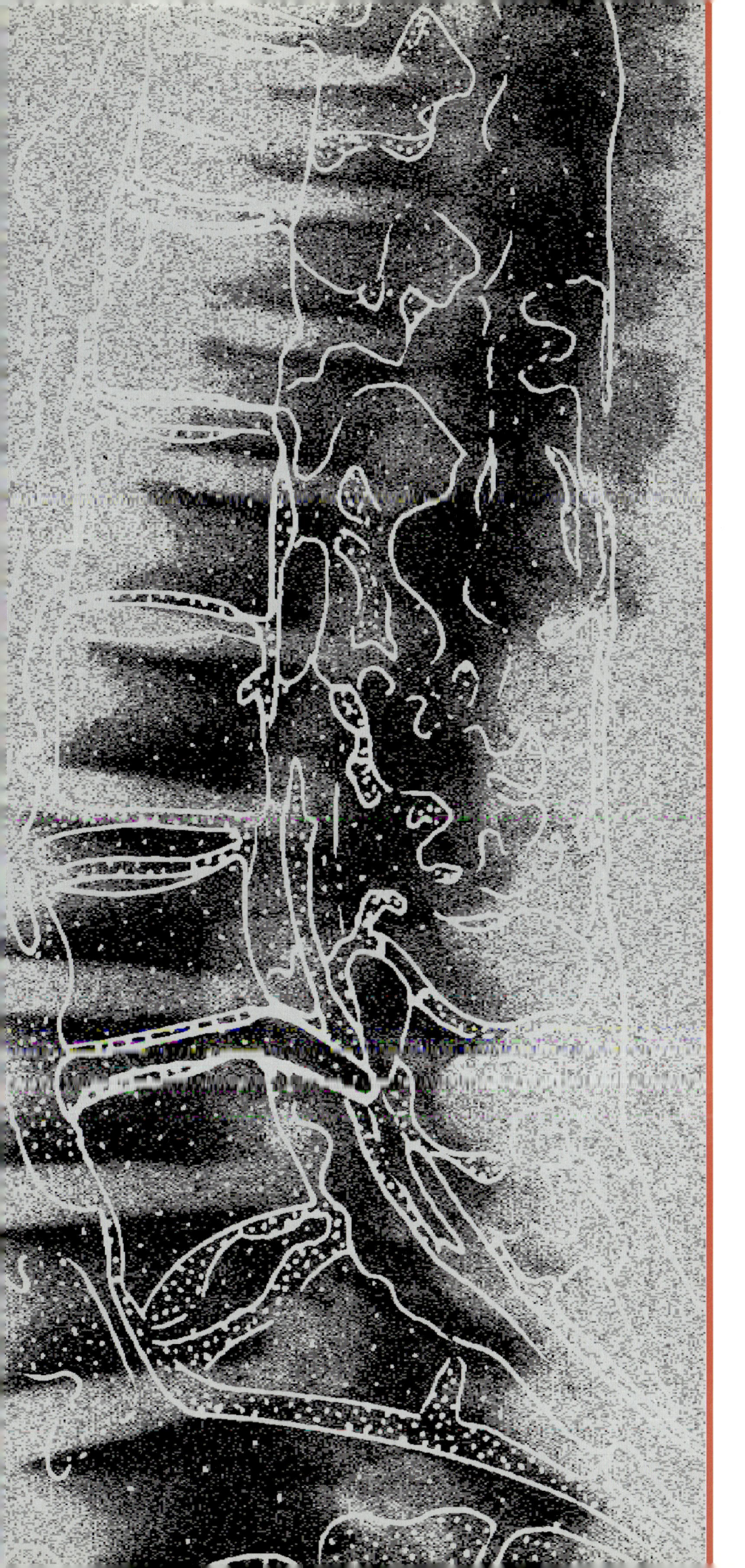

Benign Lesions of the Vertebral Column

9

OSTEOID OSTEOMA

The most important clinical symptom of osteoid osteoma is pain that is more severe at night and is dramatically relieved by salicylates (aspirin) within about 20 to 25 minutes. This typical history can be elicited in more than 75% of cases and serves as an important clue to the diagnosis. Osteoid osteoma occurs in the young, usually in the second to third decades (most commonly between the ages of 10 and 35 years). Its sites of predilection are the long bones, particularly the femur and tibia, but the spine is not infrequently affected.

Osteoid osteoma is a benign osteoblastic lesion characterized by a nidus, which may be purely radiolucent or may have a sclerotic center. The nidus usually measures less than 1 cm in diameter and is often surrounded by a zone of reactive bone formation. Very rarely, an osteoid osteoma may have more than one nidus, in which case it is called a *multicentric* or *multifocal* osteoid osteoma.

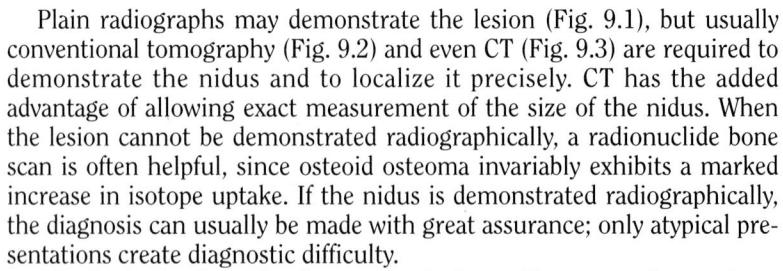

Plain radiographs may demonstrate the lesion (Fig. 9.1), but usually conventional tomography (Fig. 9.2) and even CT (Fig. 9.3) are required to demonstrate the nidus and to localize it precisely. CT has the added advantage of allowing exact measurement of the size of the nidus. When the lesion cannot be demonstrated radiographically, a radionuclide bone scan is often helpful, since osteoid osteoma invariably exhibits a marked increase in isotope uptake. If the nidus is demonstrated radiographically, the diagnosis can usually be made with great assurance; only atypical presentations create diagnostic difficulty.

Histologically, the nidus is composed of osteoid, or sometimes mineralized immature bone. It is a small, well-circumscribed, and self-limited lesion. Its microtrabeculae and irregular islets of osteoid matrix and bone are surrounded by a richly vascular fibrous stroma in which osteoblastic and osteoclastic activity is often prominent. The perilesional sclerosis is composed of dense bone displaying a variable maturation pattern.

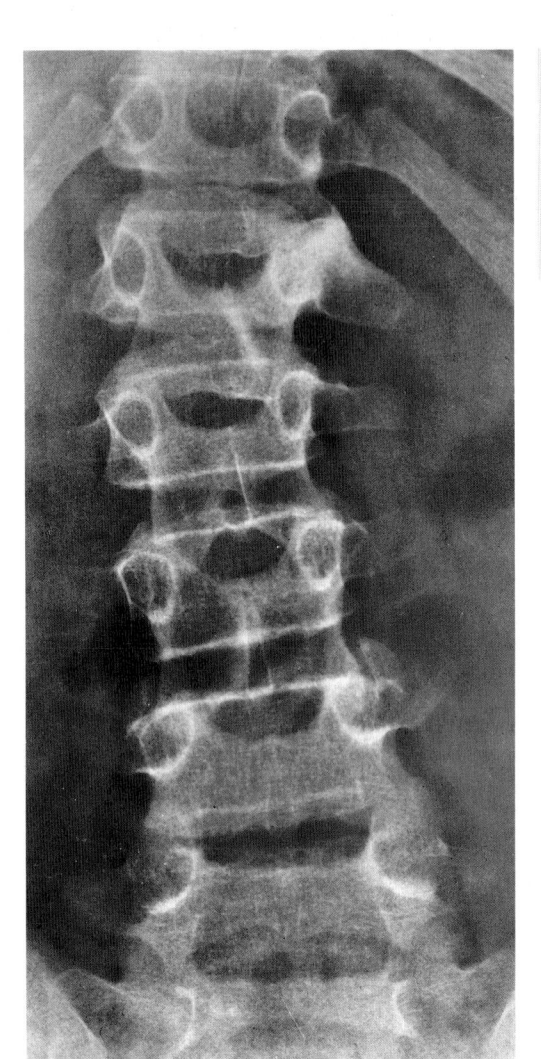

FIGURE 9.1 Anteroposterior plain film of the spine shows an osteoid osteoma in the left pedicle of L1 in a 12-year-old boy. Note the shallow-curve scoliosis with concavity directed toward the lesion.

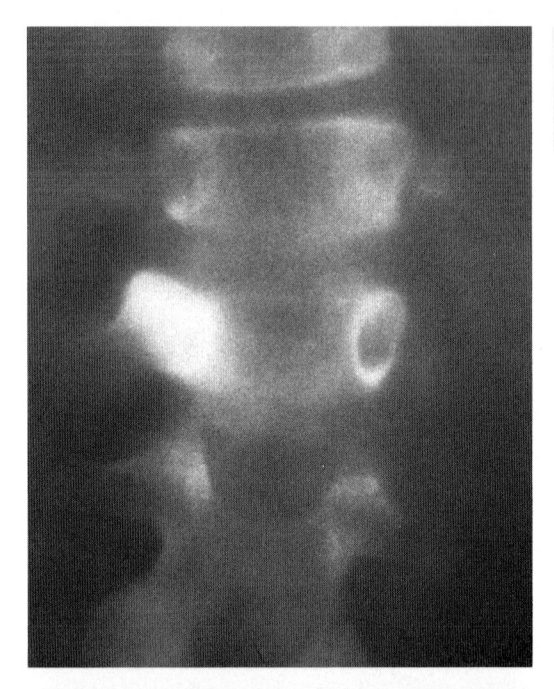

FIGURE 9.2 Tomographic examination delineates osteoid osteoma in the left pedicle of L1 vertebra.

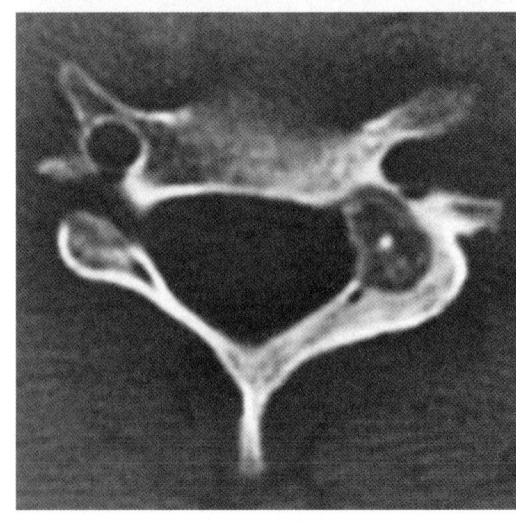

FIGURE 9.3 A 10-year-old girl presented with pain in the left side of the neck, which was more severe at night. Plain radiographs of the cervical spine were ambiguous. Radionuclide bone scan showed increased uptake of the tracer at the level of C6. Computed tomography section demonstrates the lesion of osteoid osteoma, located in the left pedicle of C6, extending into the lamina.

Imaging of the Spine in Clinical Practice

Differential Diagnosis

It must be emphasized that even when an apparent osteoid osteoma exhibits a classic radiographic appearance, the differential diagnosis should include a bone abscess (Brodie abscess) and a bone island. A bone abscess may have a similar radiographic appearance, but a linear, serpentine tract extending from the abscess cavity towards the vertebral endplate can usually be detected. A bone island usually shows no increase in isotope uptake on radionuclide bone scanning.

Complications

Osteoid osteoma may be occasionally accompanied by complications. A vertebral lesion, particularly in the neural arch, may lead to painful scoliosis, with the concavity of the curvature directed towards the side of the lesion (see Fig. 9.1).

Treatment

The treatment of osteoid osteoma consists of complete en bloc resection of the nidus. The resected specimen and the involved bone should be radiographed promptly to exclude the possibility of incomplete resection, which may lead to recurrence.

OSTEOBLASTOMA

Osteoblastoma, which accounts for approximately 1% of all primary bone tumors and 3% of all benign bone tumors, is a lesion histologically very similar to osteoid osteoma, but it is grossly characterized by a larger size (>1.5 cm in diameter and usually >2 cm). The patient's age at which it arises is also similar to that of osteoid osteoma: 75% of osteoblastomas occur in the first, second, and third decades. Although the long bones are frequently involved, the lesion has a predilection for the vertebral column. Its clinical presentation, however, is different from that of osteoid osteoma: some patients are asymptomatic, and when pain is present, it is not readily relieved by salicylates.

Plain film radiography and conventional tomography are usually sufficient to demonstrate the lesion and to suggest the diagnosis (Fig. 9.4). On the rare occasions when the tumor penetrates the cortex and extends into the soft tissues, CT or MRI may demonstrate these features (Fig. 9.5).

Osteoblastoma has three distinctive radiographic presentations:

1. A giant osteoid osteoma: the lesion is usually greater than 2 cm in diameter, exhibits less reactive sclerosis and, can have a more prominent periosteal response than osteoid osteoma.

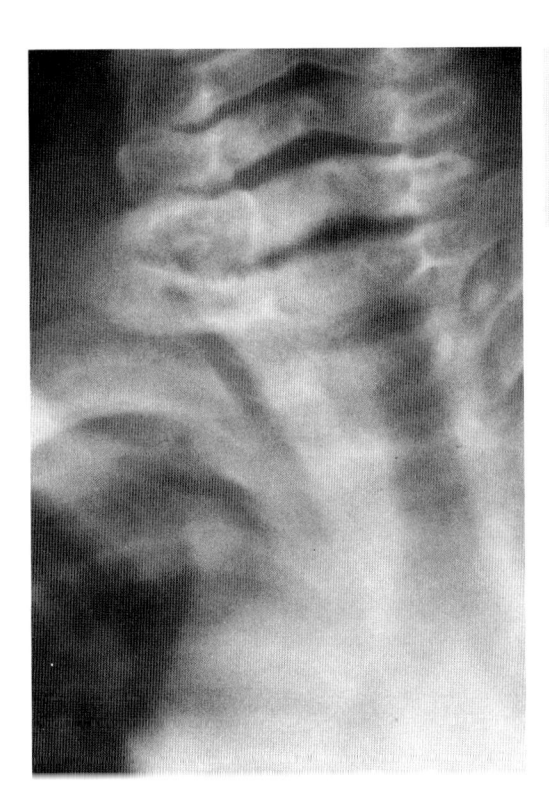

FIGURE 9.4 Tomographic section of the cervical spine shows an expanding "blow-out" lesion with several small central opacities in the right lamina of C6.

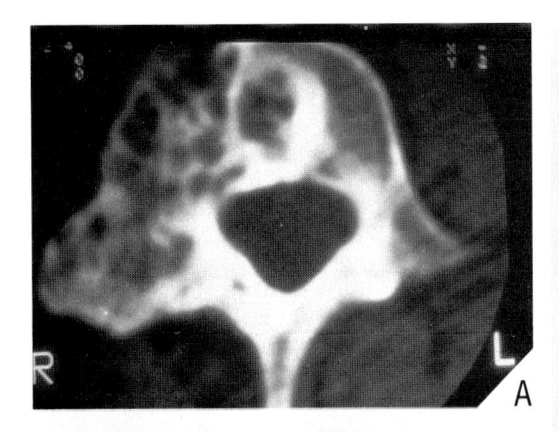

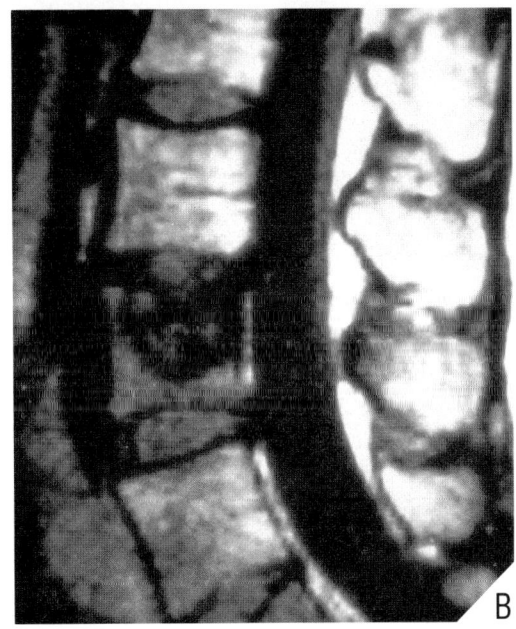

FIGURE 9.5 A 16-year-old girl has been diagnosed as having osteoblastoma affecting body and right pedicle of L4 **(A)** CT section demonstrates a large, lobulated lesion breaking through the anterolateral cortex on the right side. **(B)** T1-weighted sagittal MRI shows the lesion violating the superior endplate of L4, extending posteriorly into the disk space. (Courtesy of Lynn S. Steinbach, M.D., San Francisco, CA)

2. A blow-out expansion similar to an aneurysmal bone cyst, with small radiopacities in the center: this pattern is particularly common in lesions involving the spine (see Fig. 9.4).
3. An aggressive lesion simulating a malignant tumor (Fig. 9.6).

Differential Diagnosis

Histologic differentiation between osteoid osteoma and osteoblastoma can be very difficult; in a considerable number of patients this is impossible. Both are osteoid-producing lesions; in the typical osteoblastoma, however, the bone trabeculae are broader and longer and seem less densely packed and less coherent than those in osteoid osteoma.

The differential diagnosis of osteoblastoma should include a possible bone abscess. The latter lesion is usually marked by a serpentine tract. Aggressive osteoblastoma (see Fig. 9.6) should be differentiated from osteosarcoma, in which case tomography and CT may be helpful. CT may also be helpful in the differential diagnosis of lesions located in complex anatomic regions such as the vertebrae.

Treatment

The treatment for osteoblastoma is similar to that for osteoid osteoma: wide resection should be performed. Larger lesions may also require bone grafting and internal fixation.

OSTEOCHONDROMA

Also known as *osteocartilaginous exostosis*, osteochondroma is characterized by a cartilage-capped bony projection on the external surface of a bone. It is the most common benign lesion of bone, usually diagnosed before the third decade of life. Osteochondroma, which has its own growth plate, usually stops growing at skeletal maturity. The most common sites of involvement are the metaphyses of long bones, particularly the region around the knee and the proximal humerus. The spine is only occasionally affected (Fig. 9.7). Of the 880 solitary osteochondromas in the radiologic archives of the Armed Forces Institute of Pathology, 0.8% involved cervical spine, 0.9% the thoracic spine, and 1.1% the lumbar

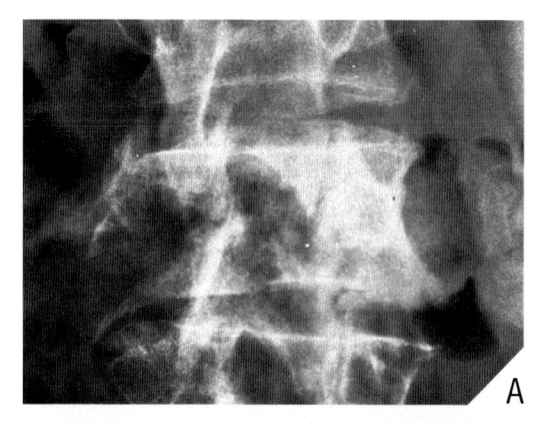

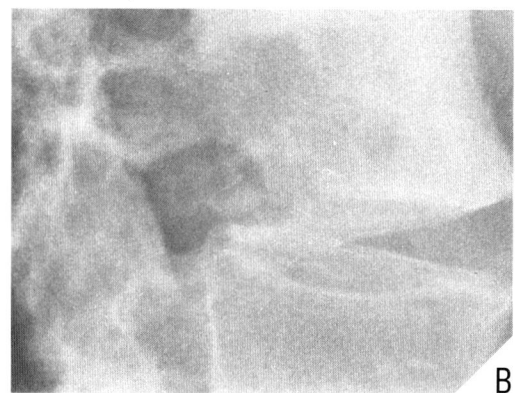

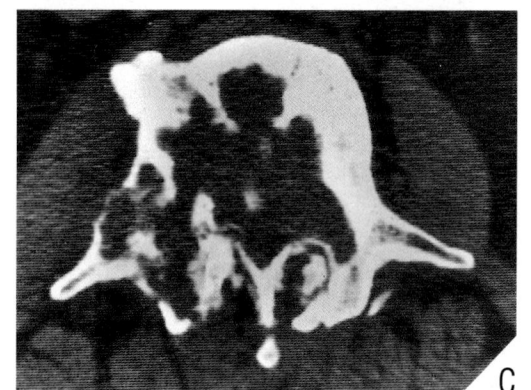

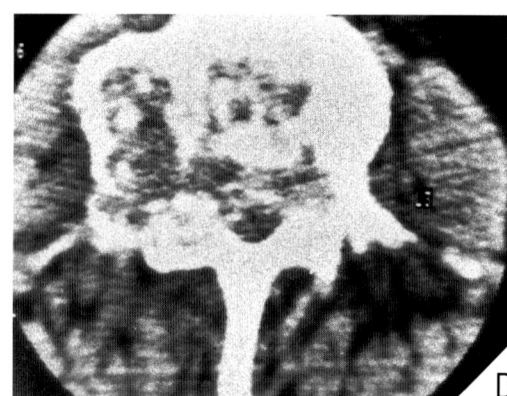

FIGURE 9.6 A 65-year-old man presented with insidious onset of pain in the lower back radiating to the right lower extremity. **(A)** Anteroposterior view of the lumbar spine shows an aggressive, destructive lesion affecting the right half of the vertebral body of L3 with suggestion of new bone formation at the periphery of the lesion. **(B)** Lateral radiograph shows extension of the tumor to the pedicle, the lamina, and intervertebral foramen. CT section through L3, filmed using bone window **(C)** and soft tissue window **(D)**, demonstrate focal areas of bone formation within the lytic tumor. The aggressive appearance of the lesion prompted differential diagnosis of plasmacytoma, chordoma, lymphoma, and, metastasis. Subsequent biopsy revealed an aggressive osteoblastoma, a very unusual occurrence in this age group.(Courtesy of Ibrahim F. Abdelwahab, M.D., New York, NY)

spine. In the spine the lesion is located close to the secondary ossification centers, near the tip of the spinous process, the vertebral arch, the pedicle, and close to the costovertebral joint.

The radiographic presentation of osteochondroma is characteristic: the lesion may be pedunculated, with a slender pedicle usually directed away from the neighboring growth plate, or it may be sessile, with a broad base attached to the cortex. The most important characteristic feature of either type of lesion is uninterrupted merging of the cortex of the host bone with the cortex of the osteochondroma. In addition, there is communication between the medullary portion of the lesion and the medullary cavity of the adjacent bone. These are important features that distinguish this lesion from the occasionally similar-appearing bone masses of osteoma, periosteal chondroma, juxtacortical osteosarcoma, soft tissue osteosarcoma, and juxtacortical myositis ossificans. The other characteristic feature of osteochondroma is the presence of calcifications in the chondro–osseous portion of the stalk of the lesion. Histologically, the cap of osteochondroma is composed of hyaline cartilage arranged similarly to that of a growth plate. A zone of calcifications in the chondro–osseous portion of the stalk corresponds to the zone of provisional calcification in the physis. Beneath this zone vascular invasion takes place and replacement of the calcified cartilage by new bone formation, which undergoes maturation and merges with the cancellous bone of the host bone medullary cavity.

Complications

Osteochondroma may be complicated by a number of secondary abnormalities—pressure on nerves or blood vessels, fracture through the lesion, and inflammatory changes of the bursa exostotica covering the cartilaginous cap.

The least common complication of osteochondroma, occurring in solitary lesions in less than 1% of cases, is malignant transformation to chondrosarcoma. Nevertheless, it is important to recognize this complication at an early stage. The chief clinical features that suggest malignant transformation of an osteochondroma are pain (in the absence of a fracture, bursitis, or pressure on nearby nerves) and a growth spurt or continued growth of the lesion beyond the age of skeletal maturity. Certain radiographic features have also been identified that may help in the determination of malignancy (Fig. 9.8).

The most reliable imaging modalities for evaluating the possible malignant transformation of an osteochondroma are plain radiography, conventional tomography, and MRI; the results of radionuclide bone scanning, which may show increased uptake of radiopharmaceutical at the site of the lesion, may not be reliable. The plain film usually demonstrates whether or not the calcifications in an osteochondroma are contained within the stalk of the lesion—a clear indication of benignity—but conventional tomography can occasionally also be helpful in this respect. Similarly, CT can show dispersed calcifications in the cartilaginous cap and increased thick-

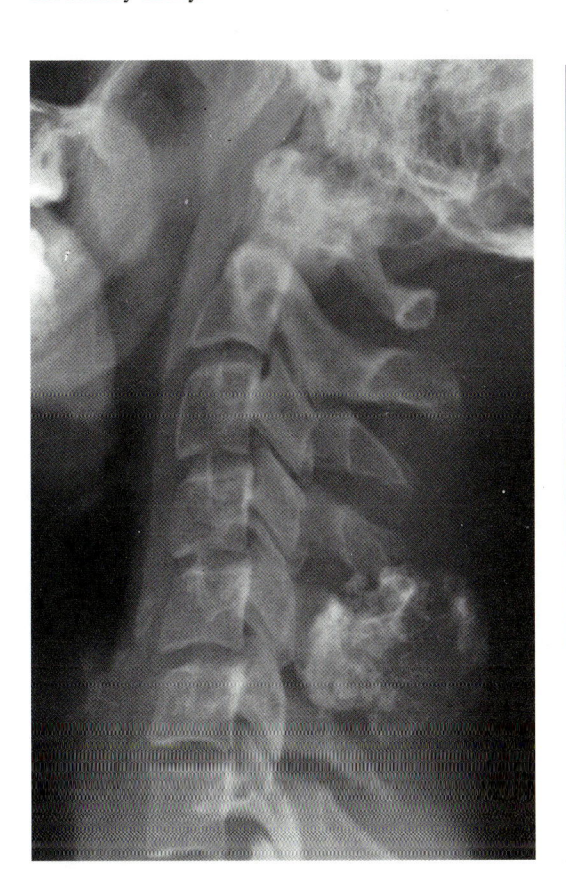

FIGURE 9.7 A 24-year-old man presented with a mass in the posterior neck. Lateral radiograph of the cervical spine shows an osteochondroma arising from the lamina of C5.

FIGURE 9.8 CLINICAL AND RADIOLOGIC FEATURES SUGGESTING MALIGNANT TRANSFORMATION OF OSTEOCHONDROMA

CLINICAL FEATURES	RADIOLOGIC FINDINGS	IMAGING MODALITY
Pain (in the absence of fracture, bursitis, or pressure on nearby nerves)	Enlargement of the lesion	Plain films (comparison with earlier radiographs)
Growth spurt (after skeletal maturity)	Development of a bulky carilaginous cap, usually 2 to 3 cm thick	CT, MRI, sonography
	Dispersed calcifications in the cartilaginous cap	Conventional tomography
	Development of a soft tissue mass with or without calcifications	Plain films, CT, MRI
	Increased uptake of isotope after closure of growth plate (not always reliable)	Scintigraphy

ness of the cap, cardinal signs of malignant transformation of the lesion, as Norman and Sissons (1984) have pointed out. Malghem and colleagues (1992) pointed out the usefulness of application of ultrasonography in measuring the thickness of cartilaginous cap.

The unreliability of radionuclide imaging is related to the fact that even benign exostoses exhibit increased uptake of radiopharmaceutical owing to endochondral ossification. Exostotic chondrosarcoma is also marked by uptake of isotope, related to active ossification, osteoblastic activity, and hyperemia within the cartilage and bony stalk of the tumor. Therefore, although the uptake is more intense in exostotic chondrosarcomas than in benign exostoses, various investigations have demonstrated that this is not always a reliable feature for distinguishing these lesions.

Treatment

Solitary lesions of osteochondroma usually can be monitored if they do not cause clinical problems. Surgical resection is indicated if (1) the lesion becomes painful, (2) there is suspected encroachment on adjacent nerves or blood vessels, (3) pathologic fracture occurs, or (4) there is uncertainty about the diagnosis.

MULTIPLE OSTEOCARTILAGINOUS EXOSTOSES

This condition is classified by some authorities in the category of bone dysplasias; it is a hereditary, autosomal-dominant disorder. The knees, ankles, and shoulders are the sites most frequently affected by the development of multiple osteochondromas, but occasionally the lesion may be seen in the spine. The radiographic features are similar to those of single osteochondromas, but the lesions are more frequently of the sessile type.

The pathologic features of multiple osteochondromas are the same as those of solitary lesions.

Complications

There is a greater incidence of growth disturbance in multiple osteocartilaginous exostoses than in single osteochondromas. Malignant transformation to chondrosarcoma is also more common, occurring in 5% to 15% of cases; lesions at the shoulder girdle and around the pelvis are at greater risk for transformation. The clinical and radiographic signs of this complication are identical to those in malignant transformation of a solitary osteochondroma.

Treatment

Multiple osteochondromas are treated individually. Like solitary lesions, they are likely to recur in younger children, and surgery may be deferred to a later date.

ENCHONDROMA (CHONDROMA)

This benign lesion is characterized by the formation of mature hyaline cartilage. When located centrally in the bone it is termed an *enchondroma;* when the location is extracortical (periosteal) it is called a *chondroma* (periosteal or juxtacortical). Although they can arise at any age, enchondromas are usually seen in patients in their second through fourth decades. There is no sex predilection. The short tubular bones of the hand (phalanges and metacarpals) are the most frequent sites of occurrence, although the lesions may also arise in the long tubular bones. The spine is a rare site of occurrence: of 725 solitary enchondromas in the files of the AFIP, only 0.3% were found in the cervical spine and 0.1% in the lumbar spine. Enchondromas are often asymptomatic; a pathologic fracture through the tumor often calls attention to the lesion.

In most instances, plain film radiography and conventional tomography can demonstrate the lesion. In the short bones and in the vertebra the lesion is often entirely radiolucent, whereas in the long bones it may display visible calcifications. If the calcifications are extensive, enchondromas are called *calcifying*. The lesions can also be recognized by scalloping of the inner cortical margins, since the cartilage in general grows in a lobular pattern.

CT and MRI may further delineate the tumor and localize it more precisely in the bone. On spin-echo T1-weighted MR images enchondromas demonstrate low signal intensity, whereas on T2-weighted images they demonstrate high signal intensity. The calcifications within the tumor will image as low signal intensity structures on all sequences. It must be stressed, however, that usually neither CT nor MRI is suitable for establishing the precise nature of a cartilaginous lesion, nor can CT and MRI distinguish benign from malignant lesions. Despite the use of various criteria, the application of MRI to the tissue diagnosis of cartilaginous lesions has not yielded satisfactory results.

Periosteal chondroma is a slow-growing, benign cartilaginous lesion that arises on the surface of a bone. It occurs in children as well as adults, with no sex predilection. There is usually a history of pain and tenderness, often accompanied by swelling at the site of the lesion, which is most commonly located in the proximal humerus. As the tumor enlarges, radiography shows it to be eroding the cortex in a "saucer-like" fashion, producing a solid buttress of periosteal new bone. The lesion has a sharp sclerotic inner margin demarcating it from the buttress of periosteal new bone. Scattered calcifications are often present within the lesion. This variant of benign cartilaginous lesion, to our knowledge, has not been reported in the spine.

Histologically, enchondroma consists of lobules of hyaline cartilage of variable cellularity. It can be recognized by the features of its intercellular matrix, which is uniformly translucent and contains relatively little collagen. The tissue is sparsely cellular and the cells contain small, dark-staining nuclei. The tumor cells are located in round spaces known as *lacunae*.

Complications

Aside from pathologic fracture, the single most important complication of enchondroma is malignant transformation to chondrosarcoma. With solitary enchondromas, this occurs almost exclusively in a long or flat bone and almost never in a short tubular bone. The radiographic signs of transformation include thickening of the cortex, destruction of the cortex, and a soft tissue mass. The development of pain at the site of the lesion in the absence of fracture is an important clinical sign.

Treatment

Curettage of the lesion with the application of a bone graft is the most common method of treatment.

ENCHONDROMATOSIS (OLLIER DISEASE)

Enchondromatosis is a condition characterized by multiple enchondromas, usually in the region of the metaphysis and diaphysis. When the skeleton is extensively affected, frequently with predominantly unilateral distribution, the term *Ollier disease* is applied. Involvement of the spine is occasionally seen (Fig. 9.9). The clinical manifestations of multiple enchondromas, such as knobby swellings of the digits or gross disparity in the length of the forearms or legs, are frequently recognized in childhood and adolescence; the disease has a strong preference for one side of the body. The disorder has no hereditary or familial tendency. Some investigators claim that it is not a neoplastic lesion but rather represents a developmental bone dysplasia.

The pathogenesis of Ollier disease is unknown. Two hypotheses have been suggested for the mechanism of enchondroma formation: one implicates ectopic rests of chondroblasts, the other the failure of chondrocytes and the failure of the growth plate to mature.

Plain film radiography is usually sufficient to demonstrate the typical features of enchondromatosis. Characteristically, interference of the lesion with the growth plate causes foreshortening of the limbs. Deformity of the bones is marked by radiolucent masses of cartilage, often in the hand and foot, containing foci of calcification.

Histologically, the lesions of enchondromatosis are essentially indistinguishable from those of solitary enchondromas, although on occasion they tend to be more cellular.

Complications

The most frequent and severe complication of Ollier disease is malignant transformation to chondrosarcoma. In contrast to solitary enchondromas, even lesions in the short tubular bones may undergo sarcomatous change. This is particularly true in patients with Maffucci syndrome, a congenital, nonhereditary disorder characterized by enchondromatosis and soft tissue hemangiomatosis. The skeletal lesions in this syndrome have the same distribution as those in Ollier disease, with a similarly strong predilection for one side of the body. Maffucci syndrome is recognized radiographically by multiple calcified phleboliths.

CHONDROBLASTOMA

Also known as *Codman tumor*, chondroblastoma is a benign lesion that occurs before skeletal maturity, characteristically presenting in the epiphyses of long bones such as the humerus, tibia, and femur. It represents less than 1% of all primary bone tumors. This tumor rarely occurs in the spine. It is usually eccentric, possessing a sclerotic border, and often exhibiting scattered calcifications of the matrix (25% of cases). In most cases, plain films and conventional tomography will demonstrate the lesion, but CT scan can aid in delineation of the calcifications when they are not visible by standard radiography.

Histologically, chondroblastoma is composed of uniform large round cells with ovoid nuclei and clear cytoplasm. Multinucleated osteoclast-like giant cells are a frequent finding. The matrix shows characteristic fine calcifications surrounding opposing chondroblasts, with a spatial arrangement resembling the hexagonal configuration of chicken wire.

Chondroblastoma treatment consists of wide resection and bone grafting.

CHONDROMYXOID FIBROMA

Chondromyxoid fibroma is a rare tumor of cartilaginous derivation, characterized by the production of chondroid, fibrous, and myxoid tissues in variable proportions; it accounts for 0.5% of all primary bone tumors and 2% of all benign bone tumors. The lesion occurs predominantly between ages 10 and 30, and affects males more than females. It has a predilection for the bones of the lower extremities, with preferred sites in the proximal tibia (32%) and distal femur (17%). The spine is an extremely rare site of occurrence since out of 340 cases of chondromyxoid fibromas reported in the literature, only 3 involved the spine (Huvous, 1991).

Its clinical symptoms include local swelling and pain, which is occasionally due to pressure on adjacent neurovascular structures by a peripherally located mass.

Its characteristic radiographic picture is that of an eccentrically located radiolucent lesion in the bone, with a sclerotic scalloped margin often eroding or ballooning out the cortex. The lesion may range from 1 to 10 cm in size, with an average of 3 to 4 cm. Calcifications are not apparent radiographically, but focal microscopic calcifications have been reported in as many as 27% of cases.

Pathologically, the most important feature of the lesion is its lobular or pseudolobular arrangement into zones of varying cellularity. The center of the lobule is hypocellular. Within the matrix, loosely arranged spindle-shaped and stellate cells with elongated processes are present. The periphery of the lobule is densely cellular, containing a mixture of mononuclear spindle-shaped and polyhedral stromal cells with a variable number of multinucleated giant cells.

Treatment usually consists of curettage and a bone graft. Recurrences are not infrequent, with the reported rate between 20% and 80%.

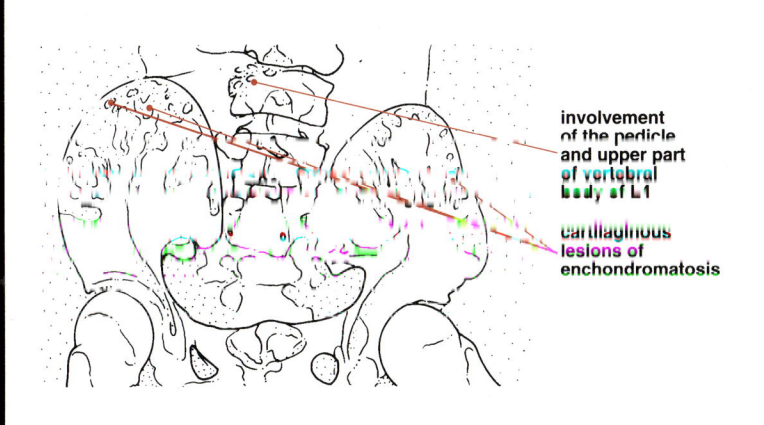

FIGURE 9.9 Anteroposterior radiograph of the upper pelvis shows crescent-shaped and ring-like calcifications in tongues of cartilage extending from the iliac crests in this 17-year-old boy with Ollier disease, extensively affecting almost the entire skeleton. Note involvement of the right pedicle and the upper part of the vertebral body of L4.

Aneurysmal Bone Cyst

Aneurysmal bone cysts arise predominantly in children; 90% of these lesions occur in patients under 20 years of age. The metaphyses of long bones are a frequent site of predilection, although aneurysmal bone cysts are sometimes seen in the diaphysis of a long bone, in flat bones such as the scapula or pelvis, and in the vertebrae. Approximately 15% of all aneurysmal bone cysts occur in the spine. When this lesion occurs in the spine it has a predilection for the posterior vertebral arch and spinous process (Fig. 9.10). Rarely the lesion may extend into the vertebral body (Fig. 9.11). Occasionally multiple vertebrae may be affected. Extradural cord compression is fairly common (Fig. 9.12), and may cause neurologic complications. Aneurysmal bone cysts can develop *de novo* or as a result of cystic changes in a preexisting lesion such as a chondroblastoma, osteoblastoma, giant-cell tumor, or fibrous dysplasia. The radiographic hallmark of an aneurysmal bone cyst is a multicystic, eccentric expansion ("blowout") of the bone, with a buttress or thin shell of periosteal response. Although plain radiographs usually suffice for evaluating the lesion (see Fig. 9.10), conventional tomography, CT, MRI, and scintigraphy can be of further assistance; CT is particularly helpful in determining the integrity of the cortex. Occasionally, myelography can demonstrate the pressure effect on the thecal sac (see Fig. 9.12).

Histologically, the lesion consists of multiple blood-filled sinusoid spaces alternating with more solid areas. The solid tissue is composed of

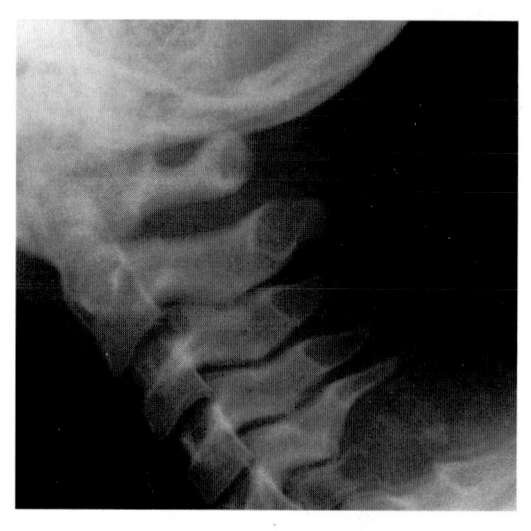

FIGURE 9.10 Lateral radiograph of the cervical spine of a 19-year-old man who presented with neck pain shows a large, lytic, expansile lesion in the spinous process of C6. The lesion, which on biopsy proved to be an aneurysmal bone cyst, is contained by a thin shell of cortical bone. (Reproduced with permission from Bullough PG, Boachie-Adjei O: *Atlas of Spinal Diseases.* New York, Gower, 1988)

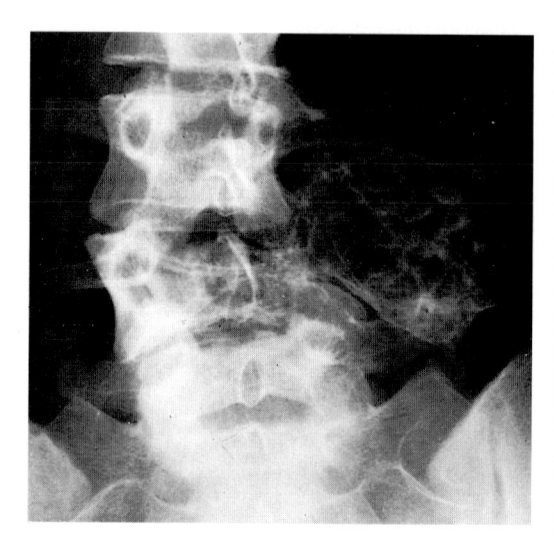

FIGURE 9.11 Anteroposterior view of the lower lumbar spine demonstrate "blow-out" expansion of the left transverse process of L4 by an aneurysmal bone cyst. The lesion extended into the left pedicle and vertebral body, resulting in compression fracture. The mild scoliotic deformity has developed as a result of the lesion. (Reproduced with permission from Bullough PG, Boachie-Adjei O: *Atlas of Spinal Diseases.* New York, Gower, 1988)

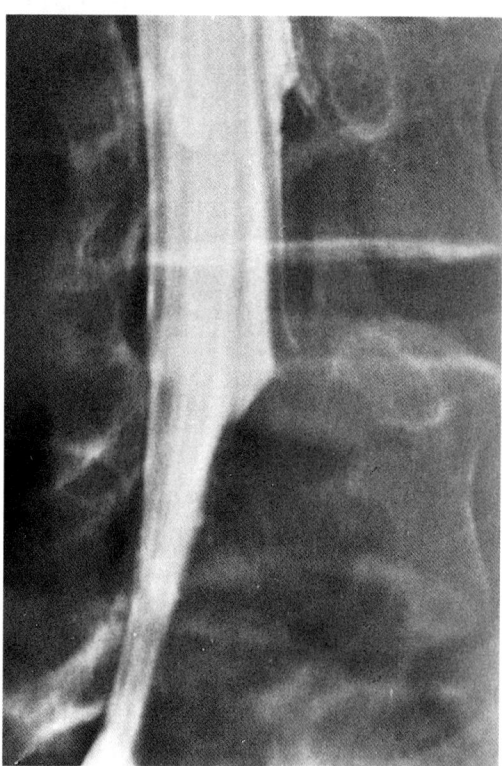

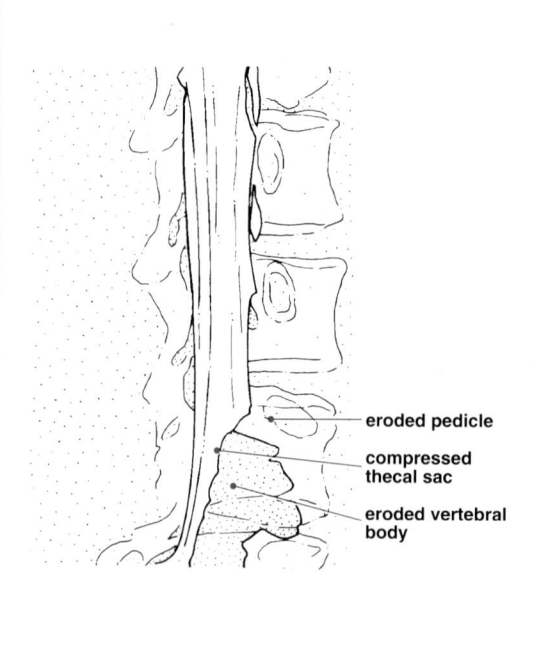

FIGURE 9.12 A 20-year-old woman had a myelogram performed as one of the tests to evaluate her complaints of lower back pain. A large lytic lesion is seen eroding the left pedicle of L5 and extending into the vertebral body, causing compression of the contrast-filled thecal sac. The biopsy revealed an aneurysmal bone cyst.

Imaging of the Spine in Clinical Practice

fibrous elements containing many multinucleated giant cells, and is richly vascular. The sinusoids have fibrous walls, often containing osteoid tissue or even mature bone.

Treatment

The treatment for aneurysmal bone cyst consists of surgical removal of the entire lesion. Bone grafting to repair the resulting defect is sometimes necessary. Recurrence of the lesion is frequent, however.

GIANT-CELL TUMOR

Also known as *osteoclastoma,* giant-cell tumor is an aggressive lesion characterized by richly vascularized tissue containing many uniformly distributed giant cells of osteoclast type. Sixty percent of these lesions occur in long bones, and almost all are localized to the articular end of the bone. Preferred sites include the proximal tibia, distal femur, distal radius, and proximal humerus. The incidence of giant-cell tumor in the spine has been reported to be 5% of all such tumors. Although giant-cell tumors may occur anywhere in the vertebral column, they are most common in the lumbar segment and the sacrum. The lesion has a predilection for the vertebral bodies. Clinically, in these locations, these tumors are likely to present with neurologic symptoms, the extent of which depends on the aggressiveness of the lesion and its location in the vertebra. Giant-cell tumors arise almost exclusively after skeletal maturity, when the growth plate is obliterated. Most patients are between 20 and 40 years of age; there is a female predominance of 2:1.

The radiographic features of giant-cell tumor in a long tubular bone are characteristic. It is a purely osteolytic, radiolucent lesion lacking sclerotic margins and usually lacking periosteal reactions. Scintigraphy may show more intense uptake of the tracer around the periphery of the lesion than within the lesion itself, which has been called the "donut configuration," presumably due to the hyperemic changes in the area surrounding the tumor. A soft tissue mass may also be present, and CT scan or MRI is usually required for adequate evaluation. Unlike lesions in the long bones, giant-cell tumors located in the spine and sacrum have no recognizable radiographically diagnostic characteristics. They tend to erode and replace the bone partly or completely, and they may extend into the pedicles and neural arches (Fig. 9.13). Frequently they destroy the cortex and extend

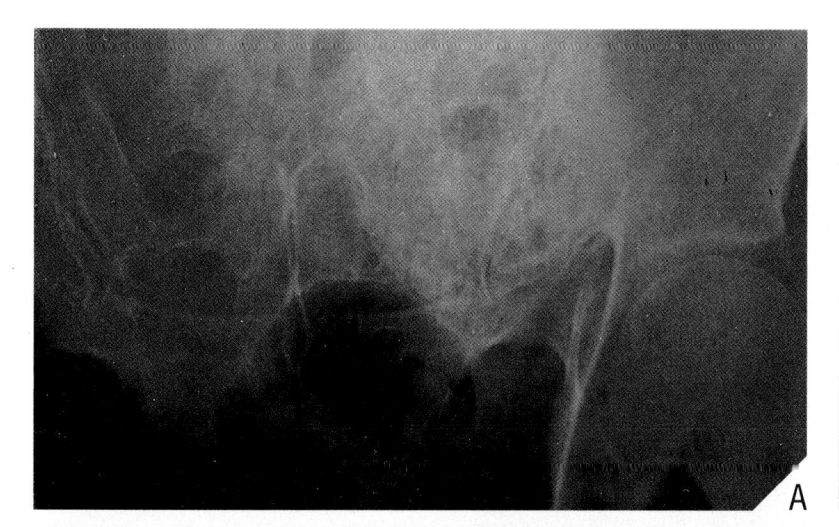

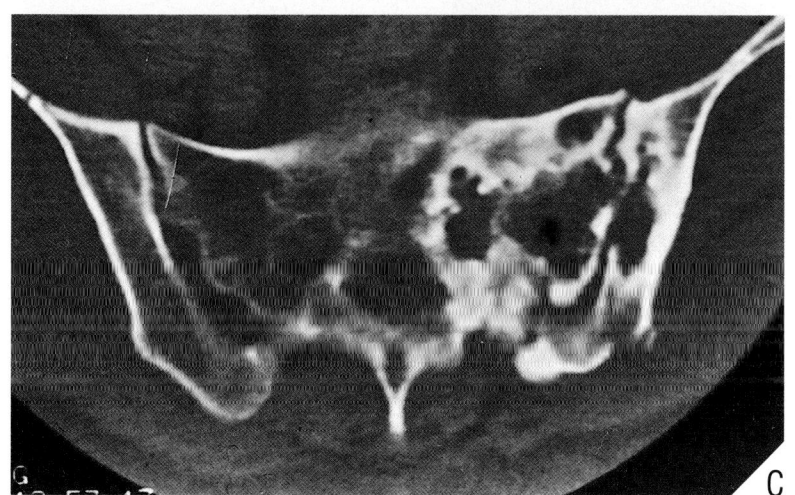

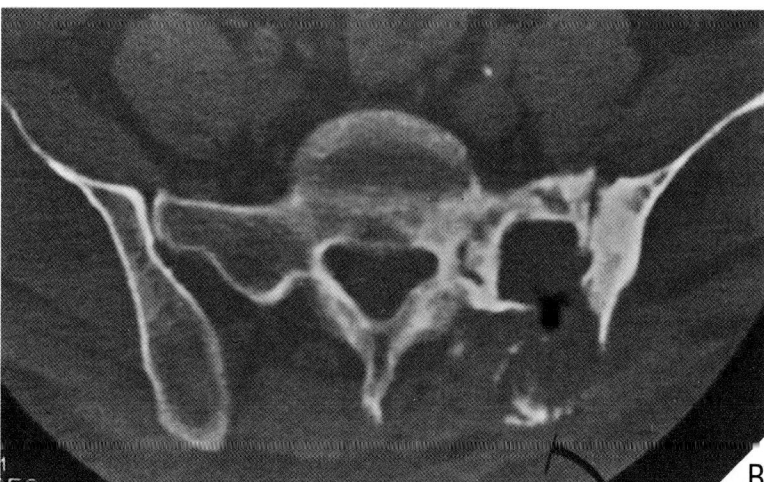

FIGURE 9.13 Anteroposterior radiograph of the pelvis (**A**) of a patient with giant-cell tumor shows a large sclerotic lesion involving the body of S1 and S2, and extending into the pedicles and across the sacroiliac joint, into the adjacent wing of the ilium. A CT section through S1 (**B**) shows extensive involvement of the transverse process and of the posterior wing of the ilium, the cortex of which has been breached. The intense sclerosis about this lesion results from reactive new bone formation secondary to pathologic fracture. (**C**) A CT section through S2 again shows the extent of lesion and the involvement of both the sacrum and the ilium. (Reproduced with permission from Bullough PG, Boachie-Adjei O: *Atlas of Spinal Diseases.* New York, Gower, 1988.)

into the adjacent soft tissue. From 5% to 10% of giant-cell tumors are malignant. However, because they have no characteristic radiographic features, malignant lesions cannot be diagnosed radiologically.

Histologically, giant-cell tumor is composed of a related dual population of mononuclear stromal cells and multinucleated giant cells. The background of the tumor contains a variable amount of collagen.

Differential Diagnosis

In elderly individuals, giant-cell tumors can easily be confused with metastatic disease, plasmacytoma, malignant fibrous histiocytoma, fibrosarcoma, or chondrosarcoma. In younger patients, they can mimic aneurysmal bone cysts.

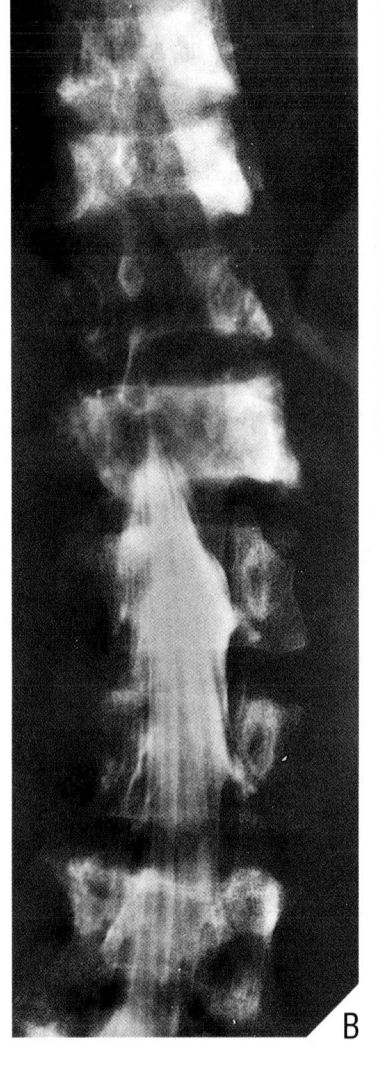

Complications and Treatment

Very rarely, giant-cell tumor may complicate cases of Paget disease, and multiple giant-cell tumors in Paget disease have also been reported (Fig. 9.14). The treatment of benign giant-cell tumors of the vertebra consists of wide resection with secondary implantation of an allograft. Some authorities recommend cryosurgery with liquid nitrogen (Marcove); others recommend heat and the use of methylmethacrylate to pack the tumor bed after intralesional excision. Recurrences are common and can be recognized on radiographs by resorption of the bone graft and the appearance of radiolucent areas similar to those in the original tumor. Good healing and lack of recurrence are demonstrated by incorporation of the bone graft into the normal bone. Especially after radiation therapy, recurrent lesions may undergo malignant transformation to fibrosar-

FIGURE 9.14 (A) Anteroposterior radiograph of the lower lumbar spine and pelvis and radionuclide bone scan (*inset*) demonstrate extensive involvement of the skeleton by Paget disease in this 59-year-old woman. **(B)** The patient subsequently developed severe back pain, and an extradural block was diagnosed on myelography, which required decompression laminectomy at the level of T10–T12. **(C)** Six months later, because of radiculopathy, a further decompression was indicated at L5–S1. Histologic examination of tissues obtained during two decompression procedures revealed conventional giant-cell tumor. (Reproduced with permission from Bullough PG, Boachie-Adjei O: *Atlas of Spinal Diseases.* New York, Gower, 1988)

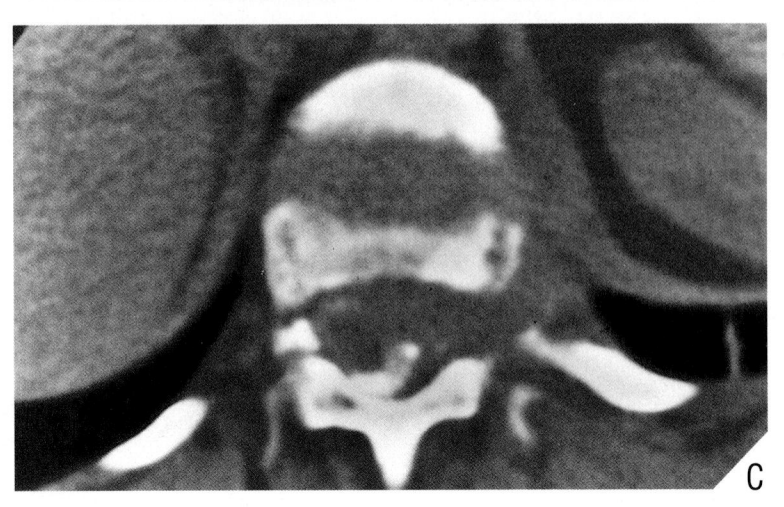

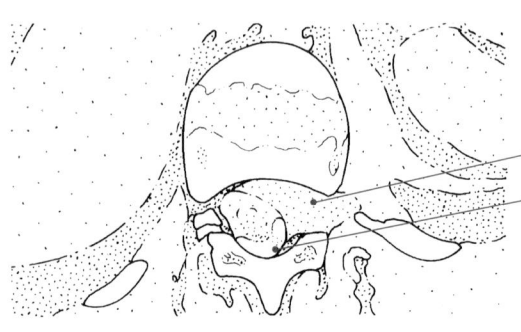

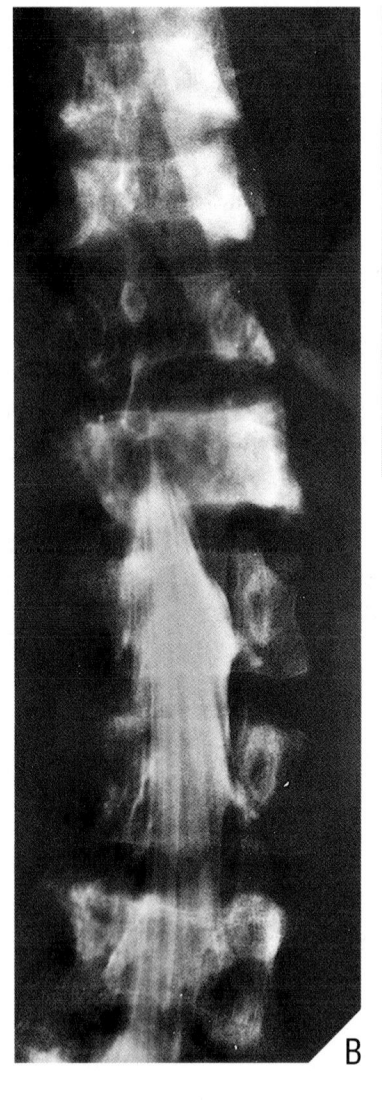

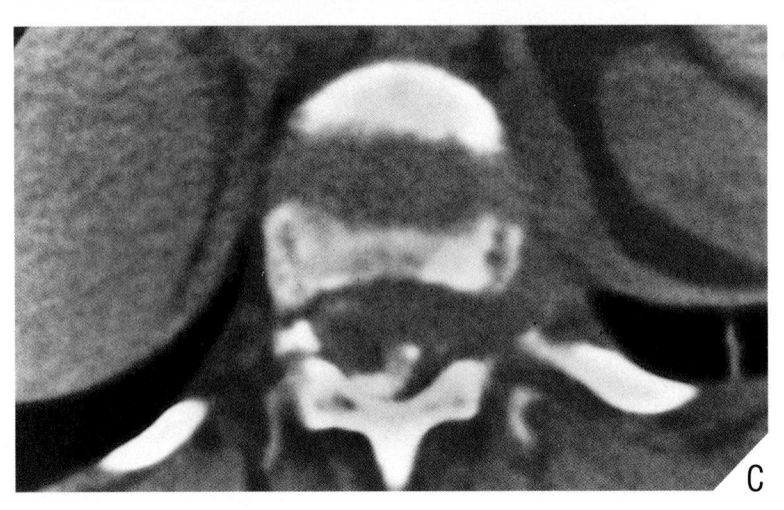

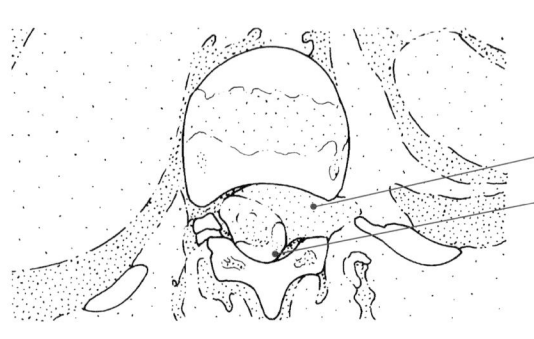

Imaging of the Spine in Clinical Practice

coma, malignant fibrous histiocytoma, or osteosarcoma. Even histologically, benign lesions occasionally produce distant metastases.

Hemangioma

A hemangioma is a benign lesion of bone arising from newly formed blood vessels. Some investigators consider these lesions benign neoplasms, whereas others classify them as congenital vascular malformations. They are classified, according to the type of vessels in the lesion, as *capillary, cavernous, venous,* or *mixed*.

The incidence of hemangiomas seems to increase with age, being highest after middle age. Women are affected twice as often as men. The most common sites are the spine, particularly the thoracic segment, and the skull. In the spine, the lesion typically involves a vertebral body, although it may extend into the pedicle or lamina (Fig. 9.15) and, rarely, to the spinous process. Occasionally, multiple vertebrae are affected. Most hemangiomas of the vertebral column are asymptomatic and are discovered incidentally. Symptoms occur when the lesion in an affected vertebra compresses the nerve roots or spinal cord secondary to epidural extension (Fig. 9.16). This neurologic complication is more commonly associated with lesions in the midthoracic spine. Another mechanism considered

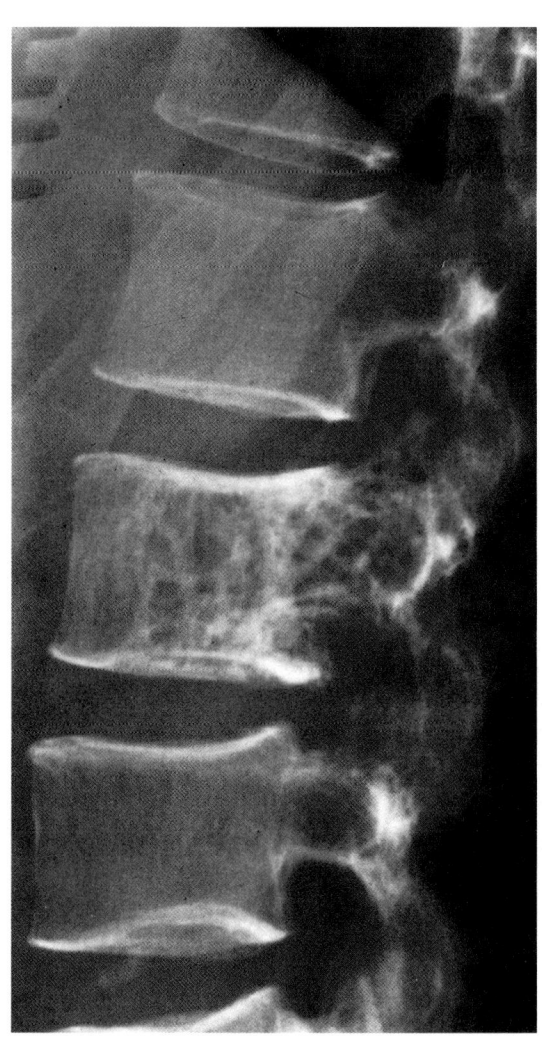

FIGURE 9.15 Hemangioma in the L1 vertebral body extends into the pedicle and lamina. Note the characteristic coarse, vertical striations ("corduroy-cloth" pattern).

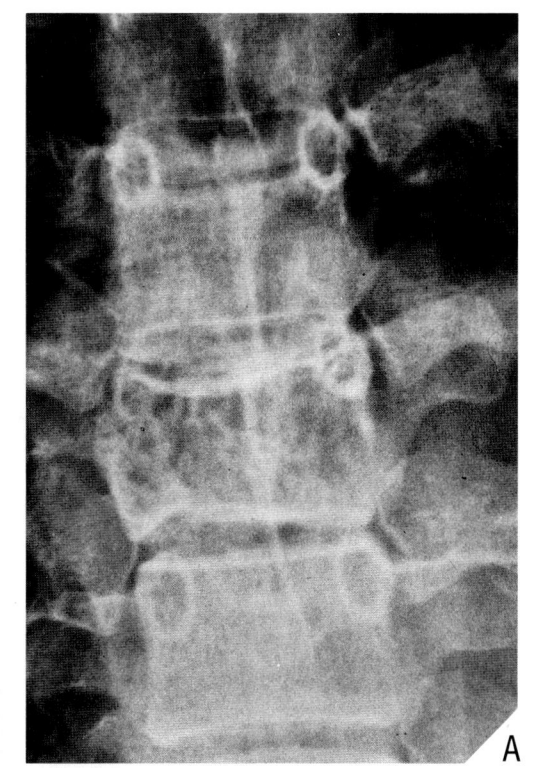

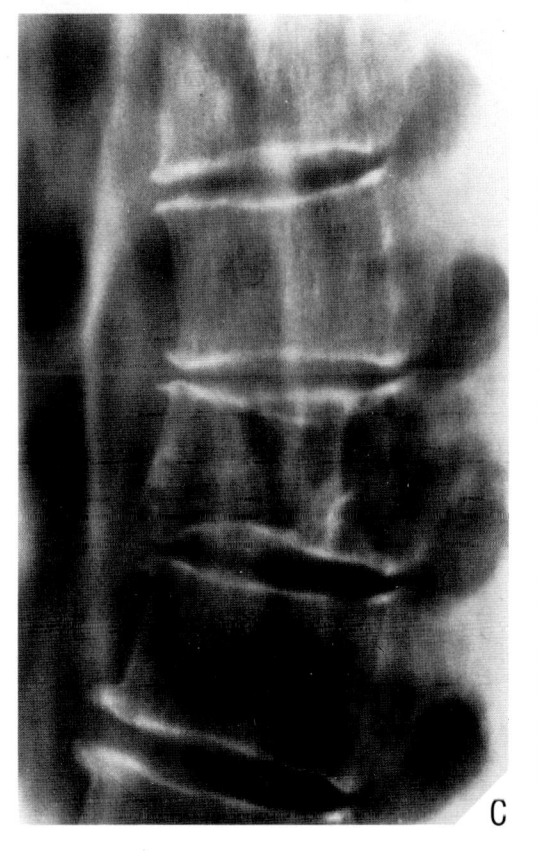

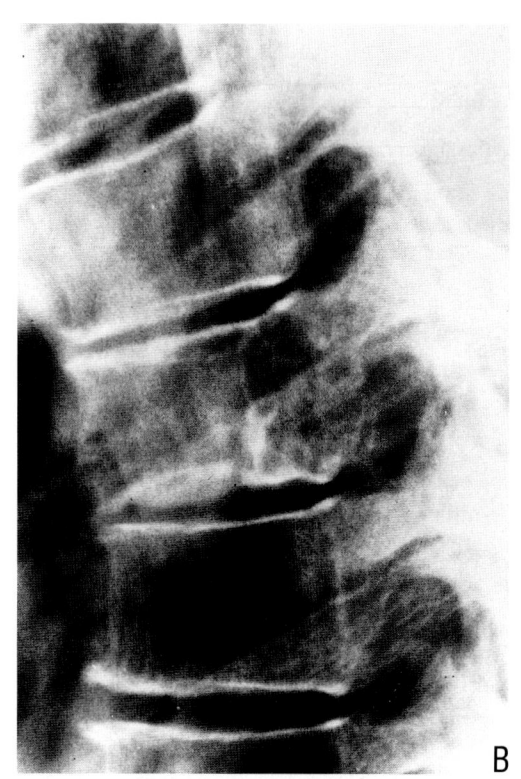

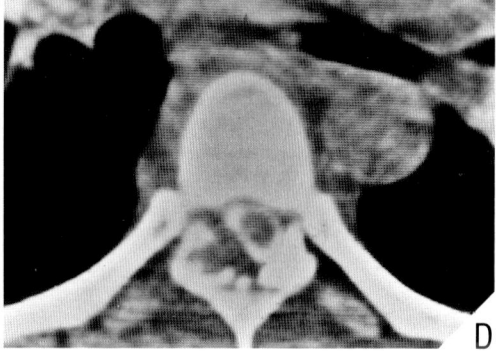

FIGURE 9.16 A 39-year-old presented with complaints of back pain and decreased sensation and strength in the right upper extremity. Anteroposterior **(A)** and lateral **(B)** radiographs of the thoracic spine show a radiolucent lesion involving the body of T6 and extending into the pedicle. **(C)** Lateral tomographic cut demonstrates ballooning of the posterior cortex of the vertebra and extension of the lesion into the posterior elements. **(D)** On CT scan, a soft tissue mass encroaching on the spinal canal and displacing the spinal cord is evident. Biopsy revealed a hemangioma. (Reproduced with permission from Greenspan A, et al: Hemangioma of the T6 vertebra with a compression fracture, extradural block and spinal cord compression. Case report #242. *Skel Radiol* 10:183, 1983)

responsible for compression of the cord, although seen less frequently, is fracture of the involved vertebral body with formation of an associated soft tissue mass or hematoma.

Hemangioma is typified radiographically by the presence of coarse vertical striations. In a vertebral body, this pattern is referred to as "honeycombing" or "corduroy cloth" (see Fig. 9.15), and in the skull as a "spoke-wheel" configuration. In the spine, this pattern is considered virtually pathognomonic for hemangioma; CT examination characteristically shows the pattern as multiple dots, which represent a cross section of reinforced trabeculae (Fig. 9.17). In the long and short tubular bones, hemangiomas exhibit a typical lace-like pattern and honeycombing.

Histologically, most hemangiomas consist of simple endothelium-lined channels, morphologically identical to capillary endothelium. Some or all of the vascular channels may be enlarged and may have a sinusoid-like appearance, in which case the lesion is referred to as the cavernous type.

Differential Diagnosis

The differential diagnosis of hemangioma in the spine should include Paget disease, eosinophilic granuloma, myeloma, and metastatic lesions. The characteristic "picture frame" appearance of a vertebra affected by Paget disease, as well as its larger than normal size, allows distinction from involvement of a vertebra by hemangioma. The lesion of myeloma in a vertebra, unlike that of hemangioma, is purely radiolucent—as are metastatic lesions—and displays no vertical striations.

Treatment

Asymptomatic hemangiomas do not require treatment. Symptomatic lesions are usually treated with radiation therapy to ablate the venous channels that form the lesions. Embolization, vertebrectomy, spinal fusion, or a combination of these are also used in treatment.

LYMPHANGIOMA

Lymphangioma is rare benign tumor of bone, composed of newly formed lymph vessels, usually in the form of dilated cystic spaces, that occasionally may affect the spinal column. It occurs twice as frequently in males than in females, usually in the first to third decade of life. Its most frequent presentation is as a painful swelling after a pathologic fracture of a vertebra. Its association with other soft tissue and visceral abnormalities, lymphedema, and chylous pleural effusion have been reported.

Radiographically, lymphangioma may mimic hemangioma or it may present as solitary or multiple areas of bone rarefaction surrounded by a zone of reactive sclerosis.

The pathologic appearance is that of dilated lymph vessels or cystic endothelium channels.

LIPOMA

Lipoma is a rare primary lesion of the vertebral column. Intraspinal lipomatous tumors constitute 1% of the total number of spinal axis neoplasms. The sacrum is the predilected site of involvement. More commonly, however, the involvement of the epidural space and intradural elements may lead to neurologic symptoms. Radiographically, the lipomatous tumors appear as radiolucent lesions with sclerotic borders, at times with vertical trabeculation in the vertebral body. Occasionally the vertebral body sclerosis may be present.

Treatment consists of surgical resection of the fatty masses, with particular care to preserve the neural elements.

NON-NEOPLASTIC LESIONS SIMULATING TUMORS

Some non-neoplastic conditions that may mimic bone tumors include intraosseous ganglion, "brown tumor" of hyperparathyroidism, and eosinophilic granuloma.

"Brown Tumor" of Hyperparathyroidism

Hyperparathyroidism is caused by excess secretion of parathormone by overactive parathyroid glands. Not infrequently, patients with this disorder present with solitary or multiple lytic lesions, most commonly in the

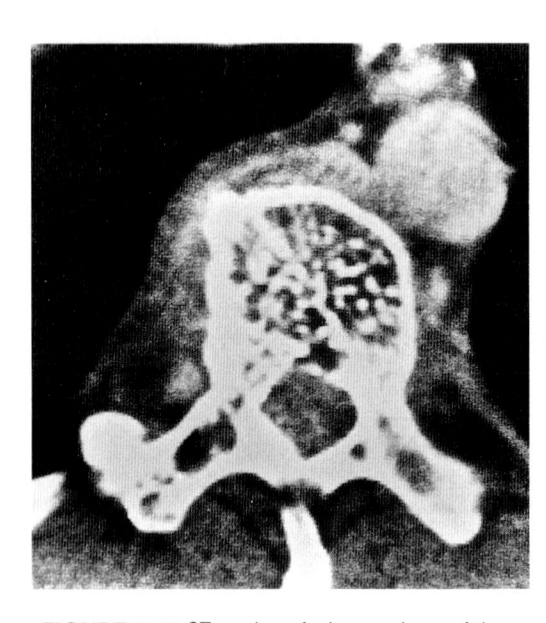

FIGURE 9.17 CT section of a hemangioma of the T10 vertebra demonstrates coarse dots that represent reinforced vertical trabeculae of the cancellous bone, typical of this lesion.

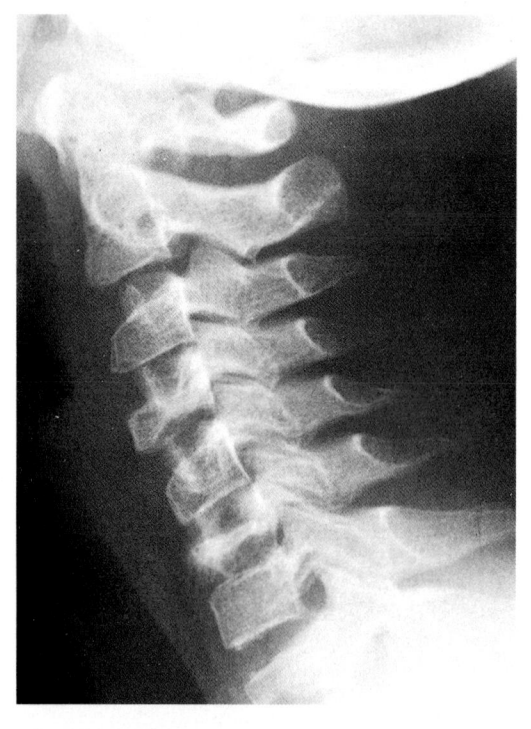

FIGURE 9.18 In this 6-year-old boy, eosinophilic granuloma affected multiple sites. Note the collapsed vertebral bodies of C4 and C6.

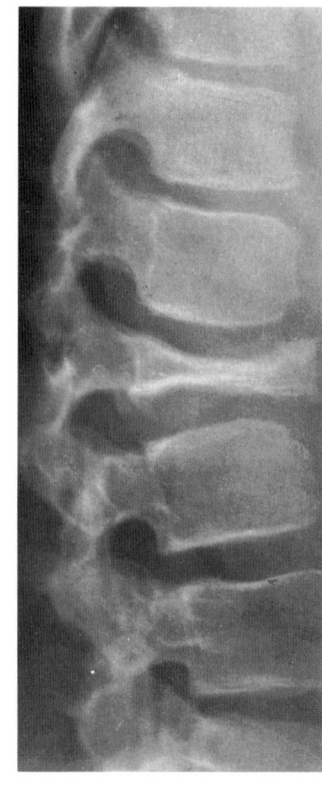

FIGURE 9.19 Vertebra plana in eosinophilic granuloma represents collapse of a vertebral body secondary to the destruction of bone by a granulomatous lesion. Note the preservation of the intervertebral disk spaces.

Imaging of the Spine in Clinical Practice

long and short tubular bones; only occasionally does brown tumor affect the vertebral body. On radiographic examination the lesions may resemble a tumor. This lesion is called a "brown tumor" because, in addition to fibrous tissue, it contains decomposing blood, which gives specimens obtained for pathologic examination a brown coloration. The correct diagnosis can be made on plain films by observing associated abnormalities, including a decrease in bone density (osteopenia); subperiosteal bone resorption, which is best seen on the radial aspect of the proximal and middle phalanges of the second and third fingers; a granular "salt-and-pepper" appearance of the cranial vault; resorption of the acromial ends of the clavicles; and soft tissue calcifications. Because hypersecretion of PTH causes a disturbance of calcium and phosphorus metabolism, the serum calcium concentration is usually high (hypercalcemia) and the serum phosphorus concentration is low (hypophosphatemia). These laboratory findings usually confirm the diagnosis.

Eosinophilic Granuloma

A non-neoplastic condition, eosinophilic granuloma belongs to the group of disorders known as *reticuloendothelioses* or *histiocytoses X* according to Lichtenstein's proposed nomenclature. These disorders include two other conditions, Hand–Schüller–Christian disease (xanthomatosis) and Letterer–Siwe disease (nonlipid reticulosis). The concept that all three entities represent different clinical manifestations of a single pathologic disorder, which is characterized by granulomatous proliferation of the reticulum cell, has gained wide acceptance.

Eosinophilic granuloma may manifest with either solitary or multiple lesions (Fig. 9.18). It is most often seen in children between 1 and 15 years of age, with a peak incidence between ages 5 and 10. The most frequently affected sites are the skull, ribs, pelvis, spine, and long bones. In the spine, collapse of a vertebral body, the so-called vertebra plana, is a characteristic manifestation of the disease (Fig. 9.19). This finding was long mistakenly interpreted as representing osteochondrosis of the vertebra and was given the eponymous name of *Calvé disease*.

Eosinophilic granuloma may mimic a malignant round-cell tumor, such as lymphoma or Ewing sarcoma. In its later stages the lesion becomes more sclerotic, with dispersed radiolucencies. The distribution of the lesion and the detection of silent sites in the skeleton are best identified by a radionuclide bone scan, which can also be very helpful in differentiating eosinophilic granuloma from Ewing sarcoma (which rarely presents with multiple foci).

Histologically, eosinophilic granuloma is composed of a variable admixture of two cell types: (1) eosinophilic leukocytes possessing bilobar nuclei and coarse, eosinophilic cytoplasmic granules; and (2) histiocytes, eosinophilic granuloma cells now proven to be identical to the Langerhans histiocytes present in skin.

SUGGESTED READING

Abdelwahab IF, Frankel VH, Klein MJ: Aggressive osteoblastoma of the third lumbar vertebra. Case report. *Skel Radiol* 15:164, 1986.

Baker ND, Greenspan A, Klein MJ, et al: Symptomatic vertebral hemangiomas: A report of four cases. *Skel Radiol* 15:458, 1986.

Bloem JL, Mulder JD: Chondroblastoma: A clinical and radiological study of 104 cases. *Skel Radiol* 14:1, 1985.

Bullough PG, Boachie-Adjei O: Atlas of Spinal Diseases. New York, Gower, 1988.

Camins MB, Rosenblum B, Harrison MJ: Osseous lesions of the vertebral axis and tumors of the cervical spine. In Lewis MM (ed): *Musculoskeletal Oncology—A Multidisciplinary Approach*. Philadelphia, W B Saunders, 1992.

Carrasco CH, Murray JA: Giant cell tumors. *Orthop Clin North Am* 20:385, 1989.

Dahlin DC: *Bone Tumors: General Aspects and Data on 6221 Cases*, 3rd ed. Springfield, IL, Charles C Thomas, 1981.

Freiberger RH, Loitman BS, Halpern M, et al: Osteoid osteoma: Report of 80 cases. *Am J Roentgenol* 82:194, 1959.

Greenspan A, Klein MJ, Bennett AJ, et al: Hemangioma of the T6 vertebra with a compression fracture, extradural block and spinal cord compression. Case report #242. *Skel Radiol* 10:183, 1983.

Helms CA: Osteoid osteoma. The double density sign. *Clin Orthop* 222:167, 1987.

Hudson TM, Chew FS, Manaster BJ: Scintigraphy of benign exostoses and exostotic chondrosarcomas. *Am J Roentgenol* 140:581, 1983.

Hudson TM, Hawkins IF Jr: Radiological evaluation of chondroblastoma. *Radiology* 139:1, 1981.

Hudson TM, Schiebler M, Springfield DS, et al: Radiology of giant cell tumors of bone: Computed tomography, arthrotomography, and scintigraphy. *Skel Radiol* 11:85, 1984.

Hudson TM, Springfield DS, Spanier SS, et al: Benign exostoses and exostotic chondrosarcomas: Evaluation of cartilage thickness by CT. *Radiology* 152:595, 1984.

Huvous AG: *Bone Tumors. Diagnosis, Treatment and Prognosis*, 2nd ed. Philadelphia, W B Saunders, 1991.

Jackson RP: Recurrent osteoblastoma: A review. *Clin Orthop* 131:229, 1987.

Jaffe HL: Osteoid osteoma. *Arch Surg* 31:709, 1935.

Jaffe HL: Aneurysmal bone cyst. *Bull Hosp Jt Dis Orthop Inst* 11:3, 1950.

Jaffe HL: Benign osteoblastoma. *Bull Hosp Jt Dis Orthop Inst* 17:141, 1956.

Kenney PJ, Gilula LA, Murphy WA: The use of computed tomography to distinguish osteochondroma and chondrosarcoma. *Radiology* 139:129, 1981.

Klein MH, Shankman S: Osteoid osteoma: Radiologic and pathologic correlation. *Skel Radiol* 21:23, 1992.

Kroon HM, Schurmans J: Osteoblastoma: Clinical and radiologic findings in 98 new cases. *Radiology* 175:783, 1990.

Laredo JD, Reizine D, Bard M, et al: Vertebral hemangioma: Radiographic evaluation. *Radiology* 161:183, 1986.

Lewis MM, Sissons H, Norman A, et al: Benign and malignant cartilage tumors. In Griffin PP (ed): *Instructional Course Lectures AAOS*, Vol 36. Chicago, American Academy of Orthopaedic Surgeons, 1987.

Malghem J, Vande Berg B, Noël H, et al: Benign osteochondromas and exostotic chondrosarcomas: Evaluation of cartilage cap thickness by ultrasound. *Skel Radiol* 21:33, 1992.

Marsh BW, Bonfiglio M, Brady LP, et al: Benign osteoblastoma: Range of manifestations. *J Bone Joint Dis* A57:1, 1957.

McLeod R, Dahlin DC, Beabout JW: The spectrum of osteoblastoma. *AJR* 126:321, 1976.

McLeod RA, Beabout JW: The roentgenographic features of chondroblastoma. *Am J Roentgenol* 118:464, 1973.

Mirra JM: *Bone Tumors: Clinical Radiologic, and Pathologic Correlations.* Philadelphia, Lea & Febiger, 1989.

Mirra JM, Gold RH, et al: A new histologic approach to the differentiation of enchondroma and chondrosarcoma of the bones. *Clin Orthop* 201:214, 1985.

Montesano PX, McLain RF, Benson DR: Spinal instrumentation in the management of vertebral column tumors. *Sem Orthopaedics* 6:237, 1991.

Moser RP: Cartilaginous tumors of the skeleton. St. Louis, Mosby Year Book, 1990.

Norman A: Persistence or recurrence of pain: A sign of surgical failure in osteoid osteoma. *Clin Orthop* 130:263, 1978.

Norman A, Sissons HA: Radiographic hallmarks of peripheral chondrosarcoma. *Radiology* 151:589, 1984.

Parker BR, Pinckney L, Etcubanas E: Relative efficacy of radiographic and radionuclide bone surveys in the detection of the skeletal lesions of histiocytosis X. *Radiology* 134:377, 1980.

Pettine KA, Klasen RA: Osteoid osteoma and osteoblastoma of the spine. *J Bone Joint Surg* 68A:354, 1986.

Schajowicz F, Lemos C: Osteoid osteoma and osteoblastoma: Closely related entities of osteoblastic derivation. *Acta Orthop Scand* 41:272, 1970.

Schecter MS, Collins JD: Epidural lipoma: An unusual cause of a sclerotic vertebral body. *Spine* 8:804, 1983.

Szajowicz F, Lemos C: Osteoid osteoma and osteoblastoma. *Acta Orthop Scand* 41:272, 1970.

Unni KK, Dahlin DC: Premalignant tumors and conditions of bone. *Am J Surg Pathol* 3:47, 1979.

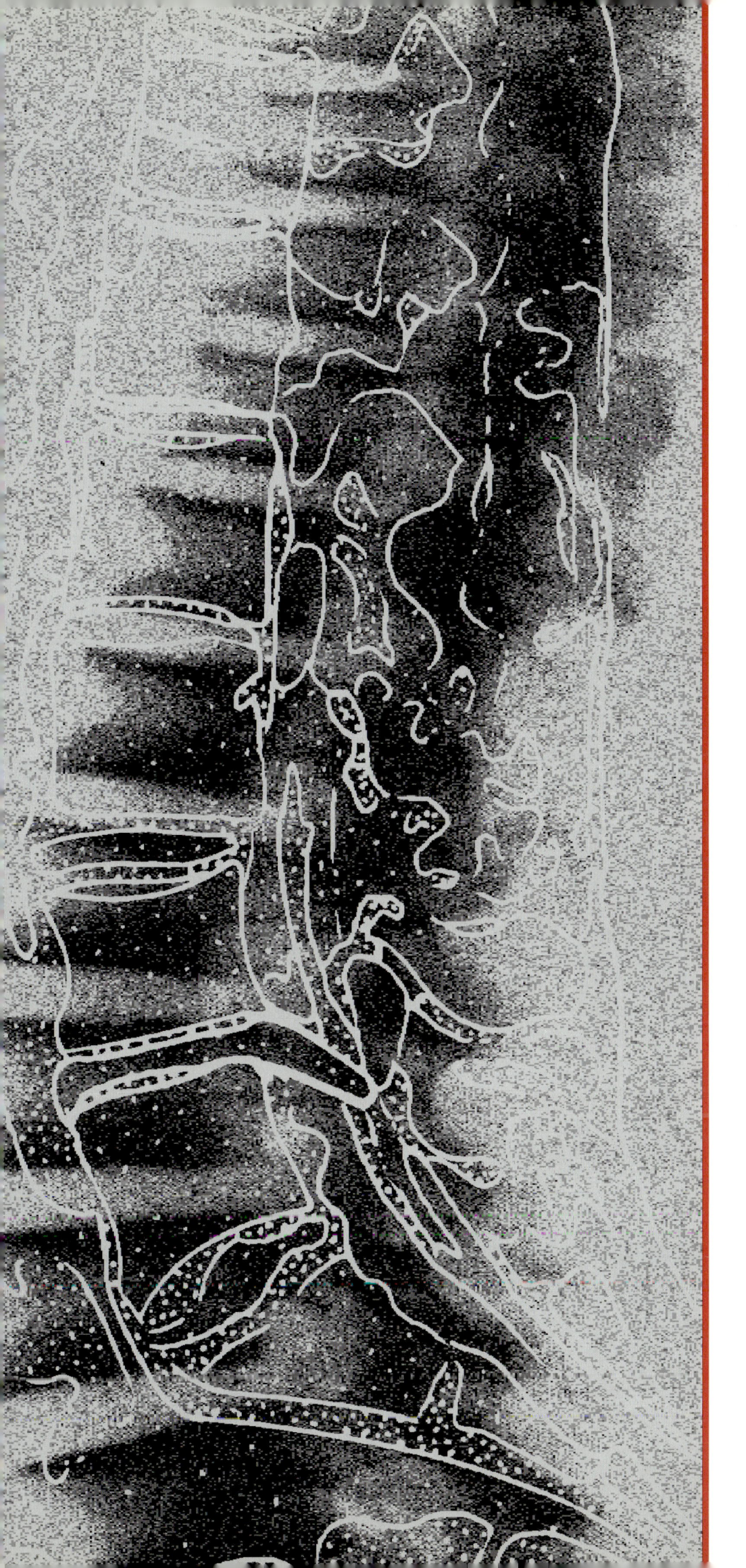

Malignant Tumors of the Vertebral Column

10

OSTEOSARCOMA

Osteosarcoma (osteogenic sarcoma) is one of the most common primary malignant tumors of bone. There are several types of osteosarcoma (Fig. 10.1), each having distinctive clinical, radiographic, and histologic characteristics. The common feature of all types is that the osteoid and bone matrix are formed by malignant cells of connective tissue. The vast majority of osteosarcomas are of unknown cause and can therefore be considered as idiopathic or *primary*. A smaller number of tumors can be related to known factors that predispose to malignancy, such as Paget disease, fibrous dysplasia, external ionizing irradiation, and ingestion of radioactive substances. These lesions are classified as *secondary* osteosarcomas. All types of osteosarcoma can be further subdivided, according to their anatomic site, into lesions of the appendicular skeleton and axial skeleton. Furthermore, they can be classified on the basis of their location in bone as central or juxtacortical. A separate group consists of primary osteosarcoma originating in the soft tissues (so-called extraskeletal or soft tissue osteosarcomas).

Histopathologically, osteosarcomas can be graded on the basis of their cellularity, nuclear pleomorphism, and degree of mitotic activity. Generally speaking, central osteosarcomas are much more common than juxtacortical tumors and tend to have a higher histologic grade. Although pul-

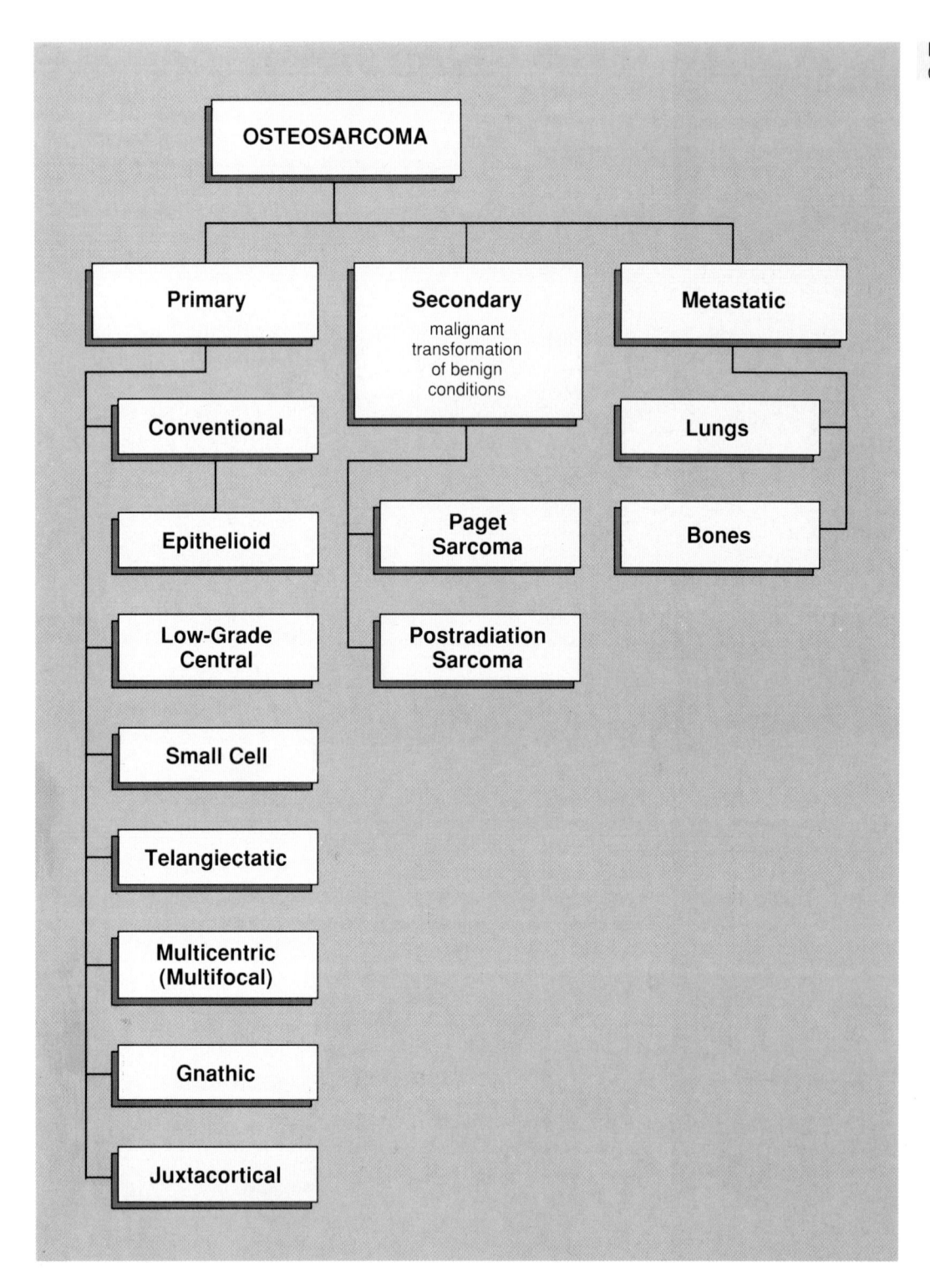

FIGURE 10.1 Classification of the types of osteosarcoma.

monary metastasis is the most common and most significant complication in most high-grade osteosarcomas, it is rare in osteosarcomas of the jaw and is a late complication in multicentric osteosarcomas.

Primary Osteosarcomas

Conventional Osteosarcoma

Conventional osteosarcoma is the most frequent type of osteosarcoma. Its incidence is highest during the second decade of life, and males are affected slightly more often than females. It has a predilection for the knee region (distal femur and proximal tibia), the second most common site being the proximal humerus. Primary osteosarcoma of the spine, in the absence of previous irradiation of Paget disease, is extremely rare and only a handful of cases have been reported (Marsh, 1970; Fielding, 1976). Patients usually present with bone pain, occasionally accompanied by a soft tissue mass or swelling. In some cases the presenting symptoms are related to pathologic fracture.

The distinctive radiologic features of conventional osteosarcoma, as demonstrated by plain film radiography, are medullary and cortical bone destruction, an aggressive periosteal reaction, a soft tissue mass, and tumor bone either within the destructive lesion or at its periphery, as well as in the soft tissue mass (Figs. 10.2, 10.3). In some instances the type of bone destruction is not so obvious, but patchy densities representing tumor bone, and an aggressive periosteal reaction on the conventional studies, are clues to the diagnosis. The most common types of periosteal response encountered with the tumor are the sunburst type and the Codman triangle; the lamellated (onion-skin) type of reaction is less frequently seen. Computed tomography (CT) (Fig. 10.4) and magnetic resonance imaging (MRI) are indispensable techniques for evaluation of these

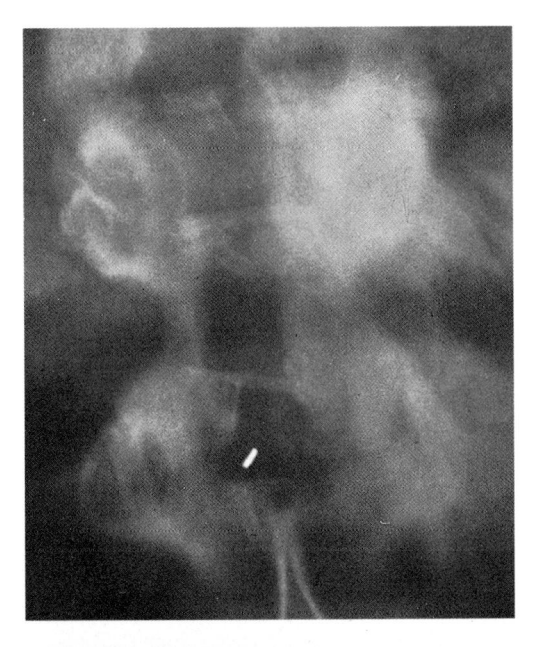

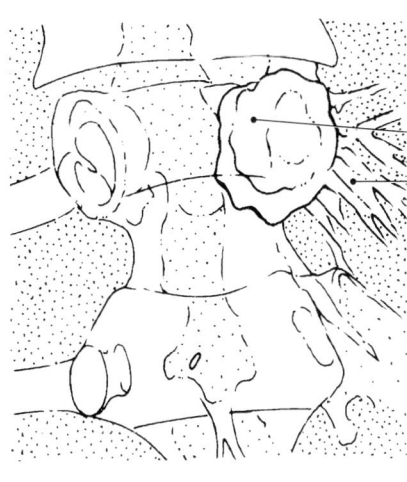

FIGURE 10.2 Anteroposterior tomogram of the thoracolumbar junction shows a sclerotic lesion affecting the left pedicle and lamina of T12 in this 20-year-old man who presented with paraplegia. The tumor, an osteosarcoma, is associated with a sunburst periosteal reaction and a soft tissue mass with the foci of a tumor bone. (Reproduced with permission from Bullough PG, Boachie-Adjei O: *Atlas of Spinal Diseases*. New York, Gower, 1988)

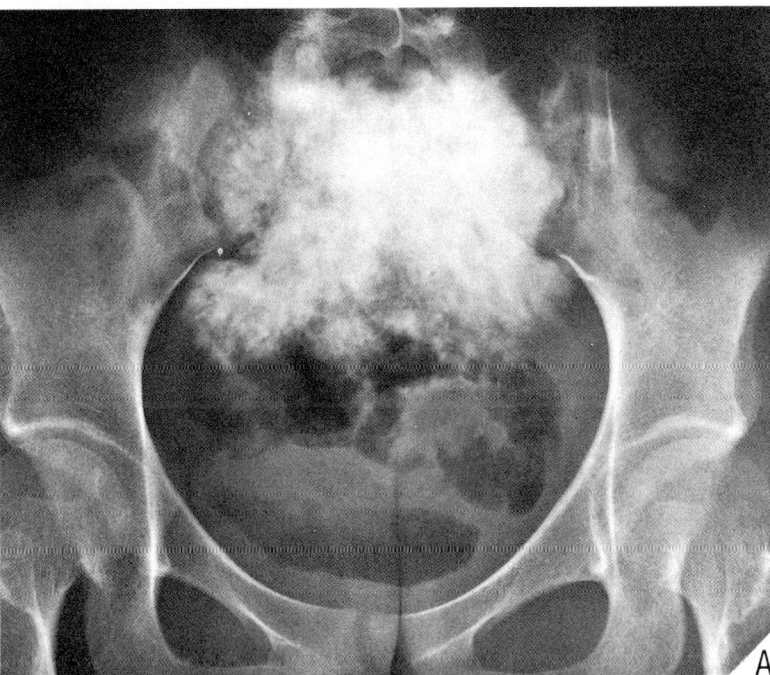

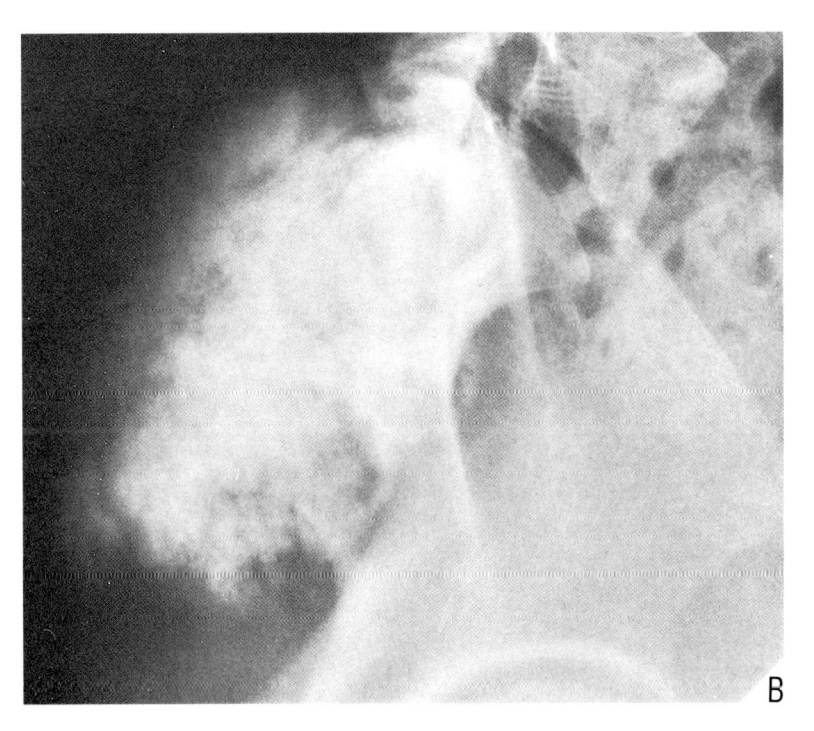

FIGURE 10.3 A 17-year-old girl presented with a tumor affecting the sacrum. The anteroposterior **(A)** and lateral **(B)** radiographs demonstrate the typical appearance of osteosarcoma: massive tumor bone formation with aggressive, sunburst type of periosteal reaction, and a large soft tissue mass.

tumors. Both techniques are also essential in monitoring the results of treatment. MRI is particularly effective for evaluation of intraosseous tumor extension and soft tissue involvement. On T1-weighted images, the solid, nonmineralized portions of osteosarcoma usually appear as areas of low to intermediate signal intensity. On T2-weighted images, the tumor demonstrates a high signal intensity. Osteosclerotic tumors demonstrate low signal intensity on all imaging sequences. MRI also may effectively demonstrate peritumoral edema. The soft tissues surrounding the tumor exhibit intermediate intensity signal on T1- and high intensity on T2-weighted images.

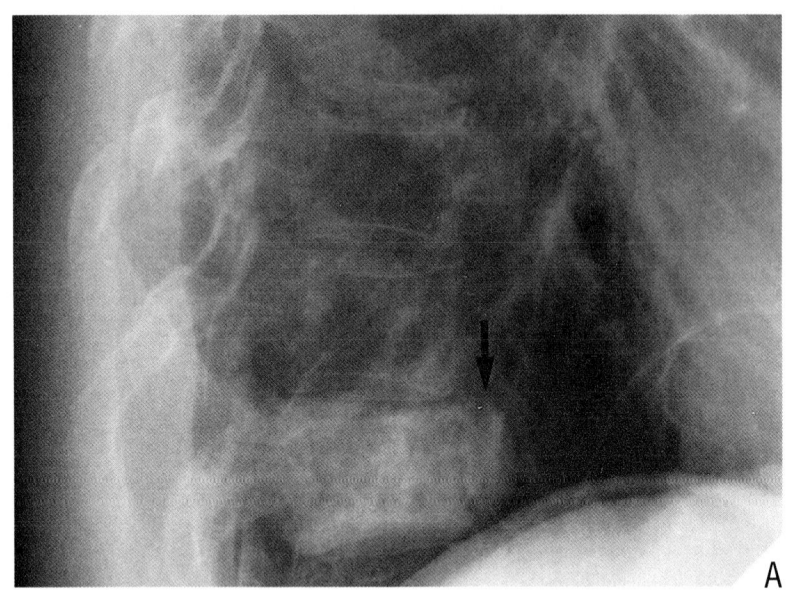

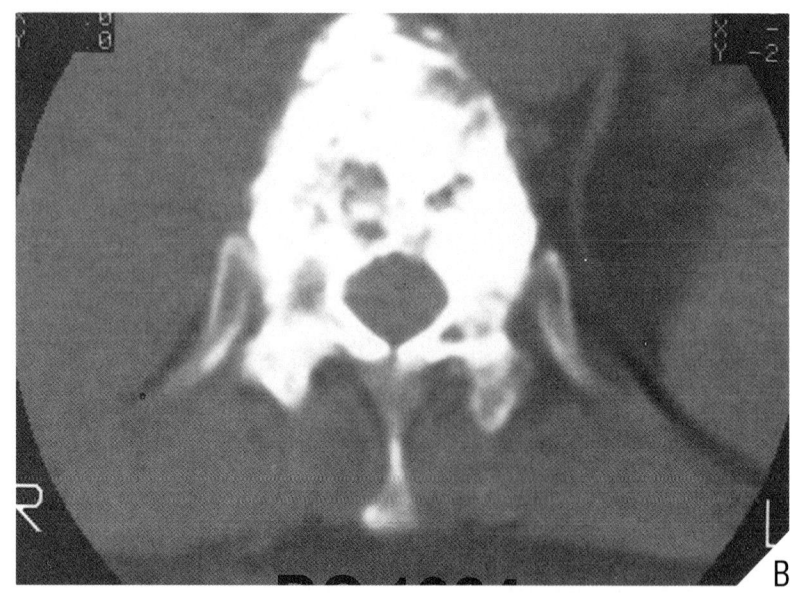

FIGURE 10.4 (A) Osteosarcoma affecting vertebral body of T9. Note the soft tissue extension anteriorly with tumor bone formation. **(B)** CT clearly shows lack of invasion of the spinal canal, and confirms the cortical breakthrough anteriorly associated with a soft tissue mass.

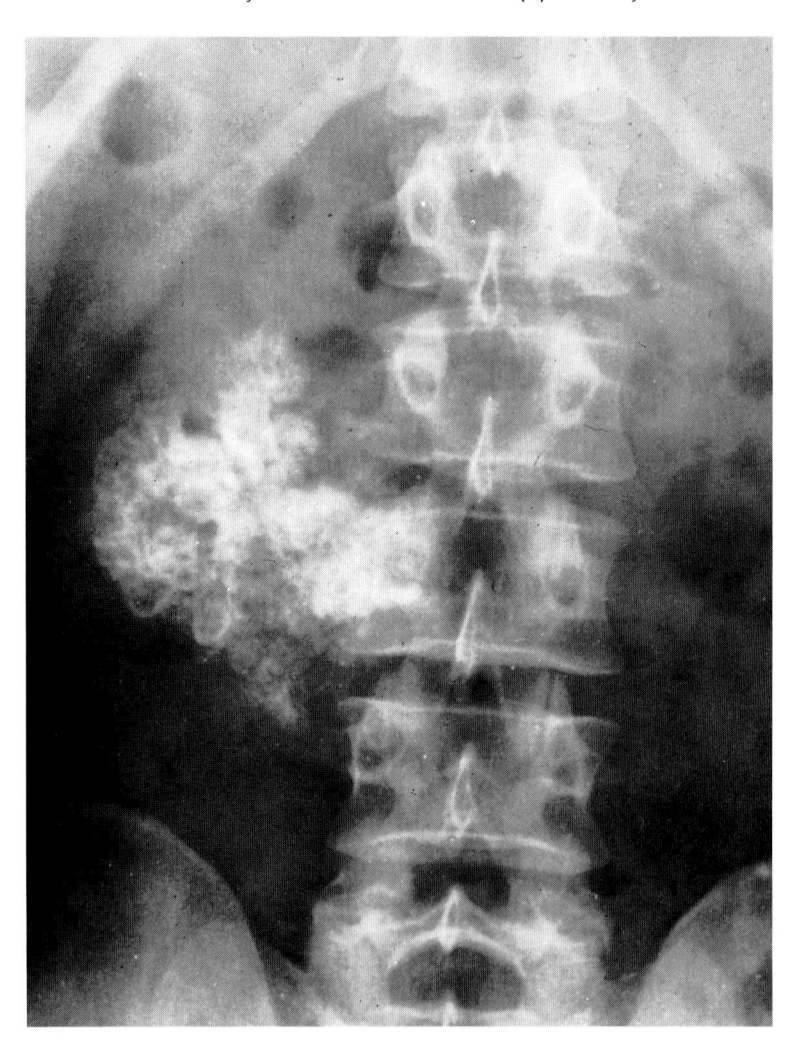

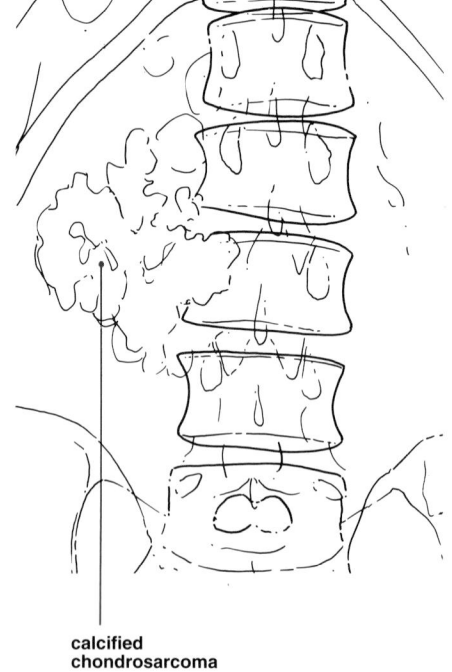

FIGURE 10.5 Anteroposterior view of the lumbar spine shows a large calcified mass arising from the vertebral body L3. This lesion was proved on biopsy to represent a malignant transformation of osteochondroma to chondrosarcoma. (Reproduced with permission from Bullough PG, Boachie-Adjei O: *Atlas of Spinal Diseases*. New York, Gower, 1988)

Imaging of the Spine in Clinical Practice

On the basis of the dominant histologic features, conventional osteosarcoma can be subdivided into three histologic subtypes: osteoblastic, chondroblastic, and fibroblastic.

Complications and Treatment. The most frequent complications of conventional osteosarcoma are pathologic fracture and the development of pulmonary metastases.

Treatment of osteosarcoma of the spine employs a course of multidrug chemotherapy, followed by wide resection of the bone and insertion of an allograft or a methymethacrylate construct, depending on the life expectancy. At present, the 5-year survival rate after adequate therapy exceeds 50% for lesions of the appendicular skeleton; however, the survival rate for lesions of the axial skeleton is much lower.

Multicentric Osteosarcoma

Simultaneous development of foci of osteosarcoma in multiple bones occurs very rarely. This type of osteosarcoma is usually characterized as having two variants: synchronous and metachronous. The multicentric form of osteosarcoma must be differentiated from primary osteosarcoma that has metastasized to other bones.

Secondary Osteosarcomas

In contrast to primary osteosarcomas, secondary lesions predominantly affect an older population. A large proportion of these tumors arise as a complication of Paget disease (osteitis deformans), and characteristically develop in pagetic bone. The typical radiographic changes observed in malignant transformation of Paget disease include a destructive lesion in the affected bone, the presence of tumor bone in the lesion, and an associated soft tissue mass. Osteosarcoma in these patients must be differentiated from metastases to pagetic bone from primary carcinomas elsewhere in the body, most commonly the prostate, breast, and kidney. Secondary osteosarcoma may also develop spontaneously in fibrous dysplasia and after radiation therapy for either benign bone lesions (eg, fibrous dysplasia and giant-cell tumor) or malignant processes in the soft tissues (eg, breast carcinoma and lymphoma).

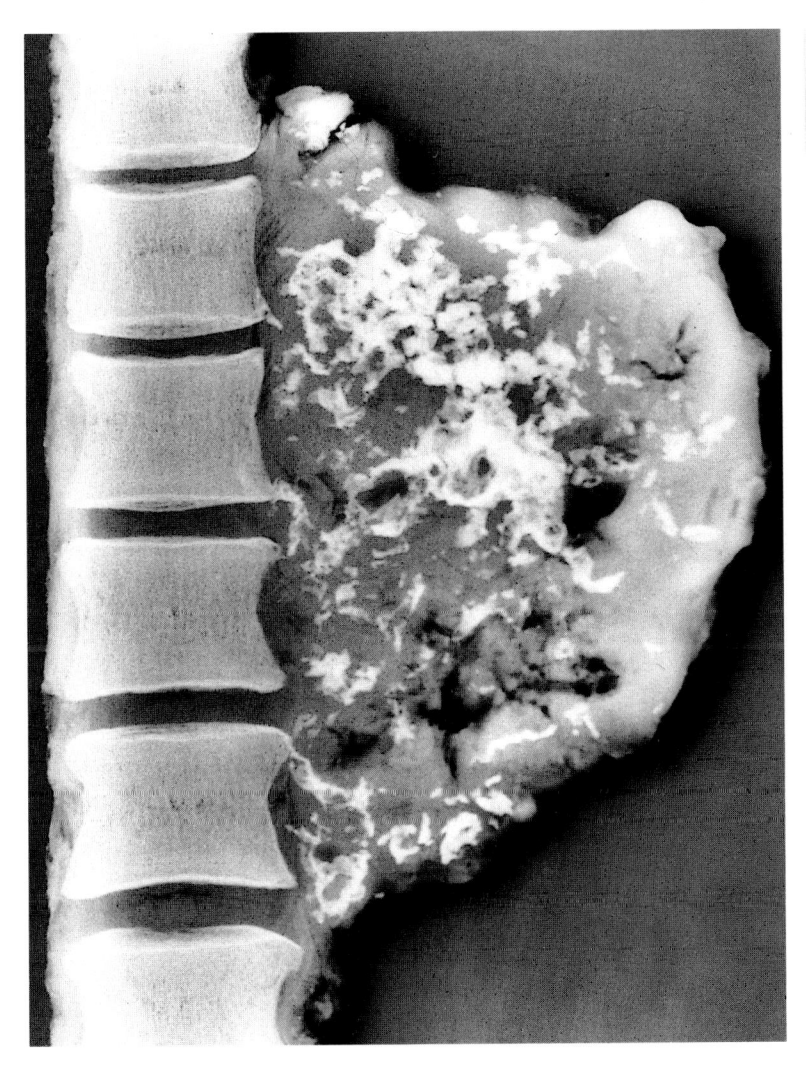

Chondrosarcoma

Chondrosarcoma is a malignant bone tumor characterized by the formation of cartilage by tumor cells. Chondrosarcoma of the spine constitutes about 15% of all cases. These lesions may be either central or peripheral and may occur either in vertebral body or the neural arch; occasionally, both sites are involved. It is not uncommon for more than one vertebra to be affected. As with osteosarcoma, there are several types, each with characteristic clinical, radiographic, and pathologic features.

Peripheral chondrosarcomas may develop from preexisting osteochondromas (Fig. 10.5) or may be of the periosteal type (Fig. 10.6).

Primary Chondrosarcomas

Conventional Chondrosarcoma

Also known as *central* or *medullary* chondrosarcoma, this tumor is twice as common in males as in females and usually affects adults, particulary those past the third decade of life. The sites most frequently involved are the pelvis and long bones, particularly the femur and humerus. Rarely,

FIGURE 10.6 Radiograph of the resected specimen of peripheral (juxtacortical, periosteal) chondrosarcoma demonstrates the lesion extending over five vertebral bodies. Foci of calcifications are characteristic of cartilage matrix. (Reproduced with permission from Bullough PG, Boachie-Adjei O: *Atlas of Spinal Diseases*. NewYork, Gower 1988)

this tumor may arise in the spine. Most conventional chondrosarcomas are slow-growing tumors, often discovered incidentally. Occasionally, local pain and tenderness are present.

On radiographic studies, conventional chondrosarcoma appears as an expansile lesion in the medulla, characterized by thickening of the cortex and characteristic endosteal scalloping; annular, popcorn-like or comma-shaped calcifications are seen in the medullary portion of the bone. A soft tissue mass is sometimes present. In typical cases, plain film radiography is sufficient for diagnosis, whereas CT and MRI help to delineate the extent of soft tissue involvement.

Histologically, chondrosarcoma is typified by the formation of cartilage by tumor cells. The tissue appears more cellular and pleomorphic than enchondroma, and contains an appreciable number of plump cells with large or double nuclei. Mitotic figures are infrequent. The histologic distinction among low-, intermediate-, and high-grade lesions is based on the cellularity of the tumor tissue, the degree of pleomorphism of the cells and nuclei, and the number of mitoses present. Some investigators (eg, Unni, 1976) disregard the last feature in grading these tumors.

Differential Diagnosis, Complications, and Treatment. In exceptional cases, particularly during the early stage of development, this lesion is indistinguishable from an enchondroma. Pathologic fractures through conventional chondrosarcomas are rare. Moreover, conventional chondrosarcomas are slow-growing tumors, and only rarely do they metastasize to distant organs. Because these lesions are unresponsive to radiation and chemotherapy, wide surgical resection is the therapy of choice.

DEDIFFERENTIATED CHONDROSARCOMA

Dedifferentiated chondrosarcoma is the most malignant of all chondrosarcomas and consequently carries a very poor prognosis; most patients succumb to the disease within 2 years of diagnosis. Out of 102 dedifferentiated chondrosarcomas studied by Mirra (1989), 2 were in the lumbar spine. Although on radiographic studies it sometimes resembles a conventional chondrosarcoma, its histologic composition is different. The microscopic appearance of dedifferentiated tissue is that of fibrosarcoma, malignant fibrous histiocytoma, or osteosarcoma. Radiographically, dedifferentiated chondrosarcomas exhibit calcific foci with aggressive bone destruction and are often associated with a large soft tissue mass.

Secondary Chondrosarcomas

Secondary chondrosarcomas, developing as a malignant transformation of osteochondroma (see Fig. 10.3) or endochondroma, are exceedingly rare in the spine.

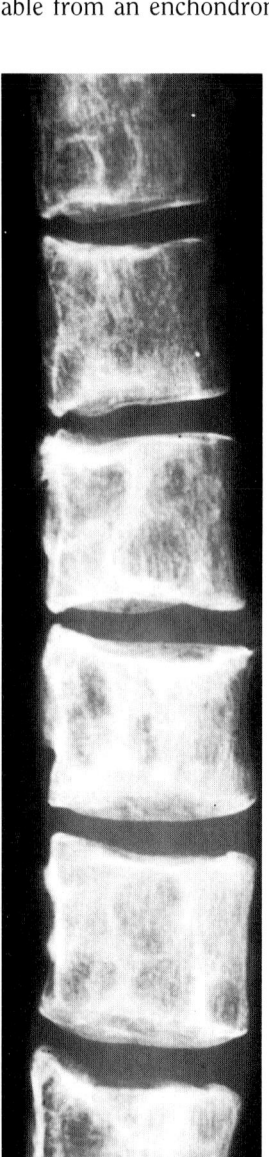

FIGURE 10.7 Specimen radiograph of the thoracolumbar spine affected by widespread metastatic Ewing sarcoma. Multiple lytic lesions are scattered throughout vertebral bodies. (Courtesy of Dr. Krishnan K. Unni. Reproduced with permission from Bullough PG, Boachie-Adjei O: *Atlas of Spinal Diseases.* New York, Gower, 1988)

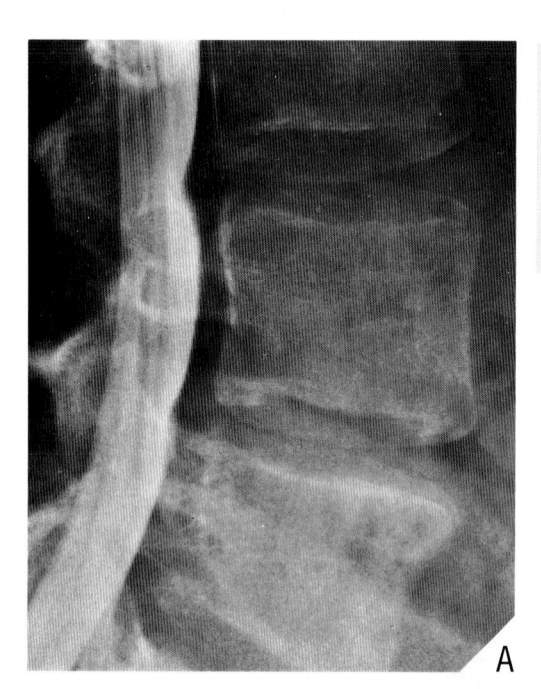

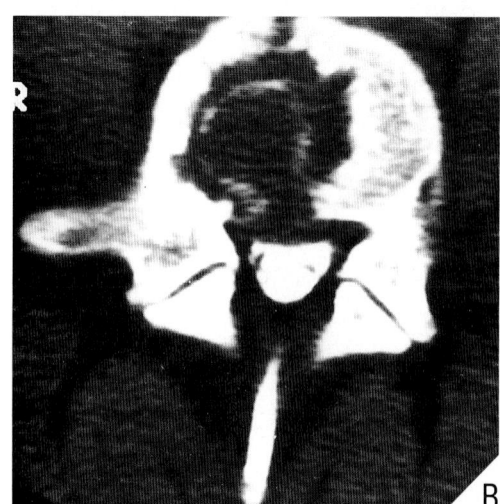

FIGURE 10.8 An 18-year-old woman presented with low back pain of several months' duration, which was attributed to the herniation of an intervertebral disk. **(A)** Myelogram shows that the disk is normal, but the body of L5 exhibits a mottled appearance and its posterior border is indistinct. **(B)** CT section demonstrates a large, osteolytic lesion extending from the anterior to the posterior margins of the vertebral body. Biopsy revealed a histiocytic lymphoma.

Ewing Sarcoma

Ewing sarcoma, a highly malignant neoplasm predominantly affecting children and adolescents, is representative of the so-called round cell tumors. Although its precise histogenesis is unknown, it is generally believed that Ewing sarcoma originates from bone marrow cells. About 90% of these tumors arise in persons under the age of 25, and the disease is extremely rare in African-Americans. Ewing sarcoma has a predilection for the diaphysis of long bones and for the ribs and flat bones such as the scapula and pelvis. Three percent of these tumors affect the spine. According to Huvos (1979), out of 167 cases of Ewing sarcoma studied at Memorial Hospital in New York, only 1 involved the lumbar spine and 1 the sacrum. In Mirra's (1989) experience, out of 871 cases, 4 involved the spine and 3 the sacrum. It has been reported that they occur more frequently in the sacrococcygeal region (Russin 1982). Extension into the paravertebral soft tissue is common, as is metastatic involvement of the vertebral column (Fig. 10.7).

The radiographic presentation of this malignancy is usually rather characteristic: the lesion is ill-defined, marked by a permeative or moth-eaten type of bone destruction, and is associated with an aggressive periosteal response and a large soft tissue mass. Occasionally the bone lesion itself is almost imperceptible, a soft tissue mass being the only prominent radiographic finding.

Histologically, Ewing sarcoma consists of a uniform array of small cells with round, hyperchromatic nuclei, scant cytoplasm, and ill-defined cell borders. The cytoplasm may contain a moderate amount of glycogen, demonstrable with the periodic acid–Schiff stain. The mitotic rate is high, and necrosis is often extensive. The demonstration of glycogen—which at one time was considered pathognomonic for Ewing sarcoma—has fallen into disfavor because it is now known that glycogen is not demonstrable in all of these tumors. Moreover, malignant lymphoma and the so-called primitive neuroectodermal tumors (PNET) contain glycogen. Since the advent of immunohistochemistry, lymphomas can usually be differentiated from Ewing sarcoma by the demonstration of leukocyte common antigen, which is a pathognomonic marker for the lymphomas.

Differential Diagnosis and Treatment

Ewing sarcoma often mimics metastatic neuroblastoma or osteomyelitis, and its radiographic distinction from the former is occasionally difficult or impossible.

Ewing sarcoma is usually treated with a preoperative course of chemotherapy, alone or combined with radiation therapy, to localize the tumor, followed by wide resection. Sometimes an affected vertebra can be reconstructed by means of an allograft.

Lymphoma of Bone

Once called *reticulum cell sarcoma, non-Hodgkin lymphoma,* or *lymphosarcoma,* lymphoma of bone is now known as *histiocytic lymphoma* or *large-cell lymphoma*. Primary lymphoma of bone is a rare tumor that occurs from the second to seventh decades of life, with a peak age of incidence from 45 to 75 years; it is slightly more prevalent in males. The lesion develops in the long bones, vertebrae, pelvis, or ribs.

On radiographic studies, histiocytic lymphoma exhibits a permeative or moth-eaten pattern of bone destruction or may appear as a purely osteolytic lesion, with or without a periosteal reaction (Figs. 10.8, 10.9). The affected bone can also present with an "ivory" appearance, as is commonly the case in lesions of the vertebrae (Fig. 10.10) or flat bones.

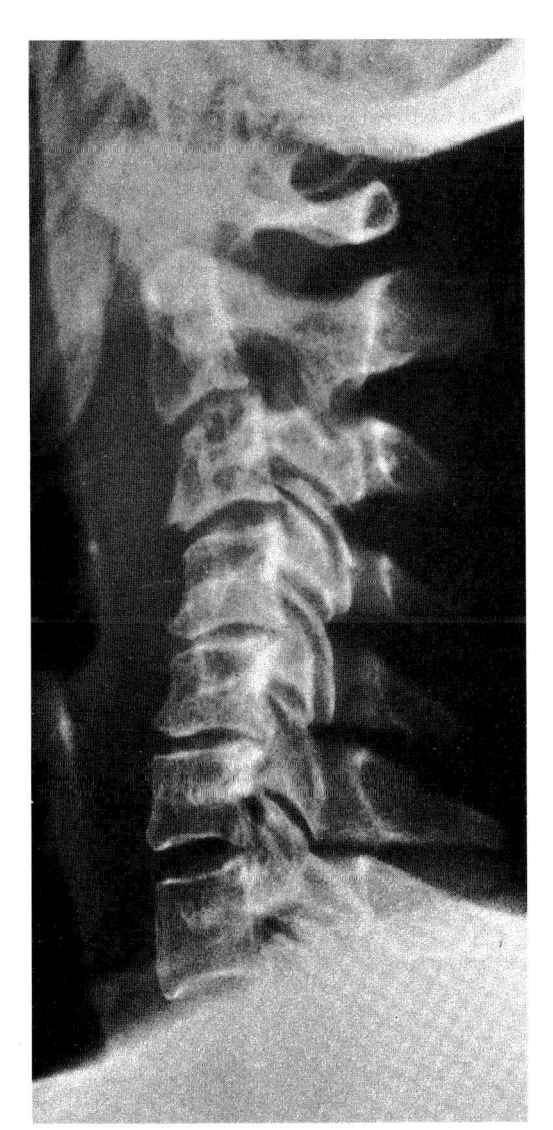

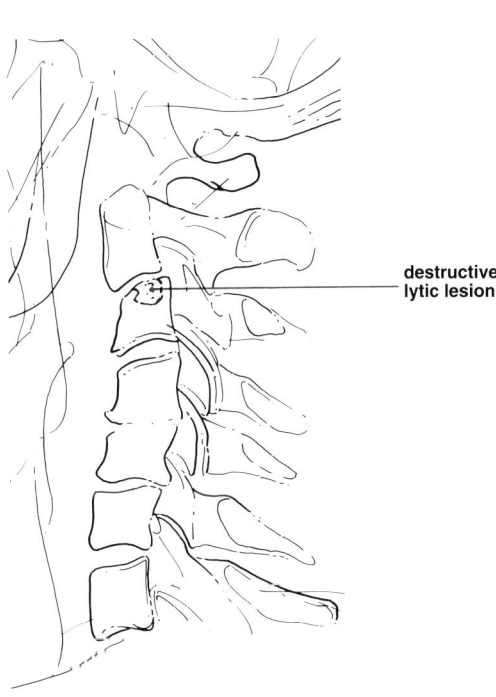

FIGURE 10.9 Lateral radiograph of the cervical spine of a middle-aged woman who presented with acute onset of pain in the upper part of cervical spine and rapidly progressive weakness of the lower limbs. Note a lytic lesion of the upper third of C3 with destruction of the vertebral endplate, associated with kyphotic deformity. Biopsy revealed a large-cell lymphoma.

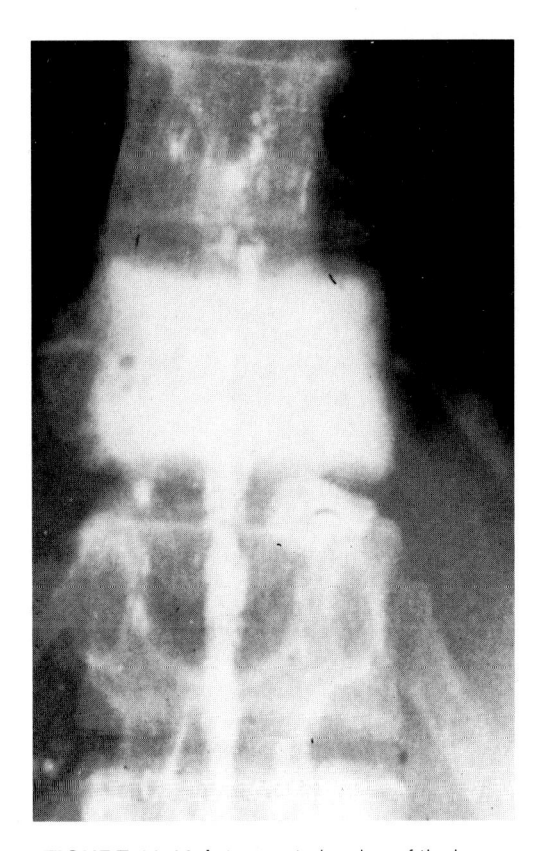

FIGURE 10.10 Anteroposterior view of the lower thoracic spine of a 35-year-old man who presented with vague back pain shows a sclerotic, ivory-like vertebra, which on biopsy proved to be Hodgkin lymphoma. (Reproduced with permission from Bullough PG, Boachie-Adjei O: *Atlas of Spinal Diseases.* New York, Gower, 1988)

Histologically, lymphomas are subdivided into non-Hodgkin lymphoma and Hodgkin lymphoma. Although secondary involvement of bones is relatively common in Hodgkin lymphoma, primary Hodgkin lymphoma of bone is extremely rare. Non-Hodgkin lymphomas are considered primary in bone only when a complete systemic workup reveals no evidence of extraosseous involvement. Viewed by microscopy, the tumor consists of aggregates of malignant lymphoid cells replacing marrow spaces and osseous trabeculae. As mentioned in the section on Ewing sarcoma, the most important single method of distinguishing lymphoma from all other round-cell tumors is the stain for leukocyte common antigen because lymphoid cells are the only cells that stain positively.

Differential Diagnosis

Histiocytic lymphoma must be distinguished from secondary involvement of the skeleton by systemic lymphoma. It may resemble Ewing sarcoma, particularly in younger patients, or Paget disease when there is a mixed sclerotic and osteolytic pattern.

Treatment

The treatment for primary lymphoma of bone consists of radiotherapy, since this tumor is radiosensitive. Some cases also require chemotherapy.

MYELOMA

Myeloma, also known as *multiple myeloma* or *plasma cell myeloma*, a tumor originating in bone marrow, is the most common primary malignant tumor of bone: it usually arises between the fifth and seventh decades and is more common in men than in women. The axial skeleton (skull, spine, ribs, and pelvis) are most commonly affected (Fig. 10.11), but no bone is exempt from involvement. Rarely, the presentation can take the form of a solitary lesion, in which case it is called a *solitary myeloma* or *plasmacytoma* (Fig. 10.12); far more often, however, it presents with widespread involvement, in which case the name *multiple myeloma* is applied. Mild and transient pain exacerbated by weightbearing and activity is present in about 75% of cases and may be the initial complaint. Because of this, early in its course and before establishment of the correct diagnosis, the disease may be mistaken for sciatica or intercostal neuralgia. Rarely, a pathologic fracture through the lesion is the first sign of disease. On laboratory studies, the urine contains Bence–Jones protein; the serum albumin:globulin ratio is reversed, and the total serum protein is elevated. Monoclonal gamma globulin with IgG and IgA peaks can be demonstrated on serum electrophoresis.

Histologically, the diagnosis is confirmed by the finding of sheets of atypical plasmacytoid cells replacing the normal marrow spaces. The neoplastic cells contain double or even multiple nuclei, usually hyperchromatic and enlarged, with prominent nucleoli.

Multiple myeloma can present in a variety of radiographic patterns (Fig. 10.13). Particularly in the spine, it may appear only as a diffuse osteoporosis with no clearly identifiable lesion; multiple compression fractures of the vertebral bodies may be evident. More commonly, multiple lytic lesions are scattered throughout the skeleton. In the skull, characteristic "punched-out" areas of bone destruction, usually uniform in size, are observed, while the ribs may contain lace-like areas of bone destruction and small osteolytic lesions sometimes accompanied by adjacent soft tissue masses. Areas of medullary bone destruction are present in the flat and long bones; when these areas abut the cortex, they are accompanied by scalloping of the inner cortical margin. There is usually no evidence of sclerosis or periosteal reaction. Fewer than 1% of myelomas are of a sclerosing type, in which case the entity is called *sclerosing myelomatosis*. Whereas in osteolytic myeloma only 3% of patients have polyneuropathy, the incidence of polyneuropathy in the osteosclerotic variant has been reported as 30% to 50%. Compared with classic myeloma, this variant usually occurs in younger individuals who have fewer plasma

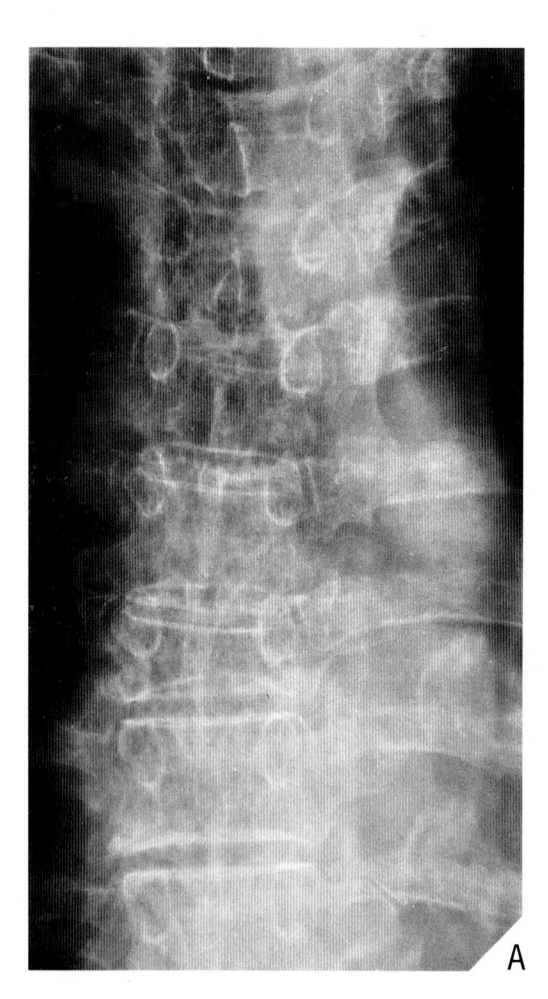

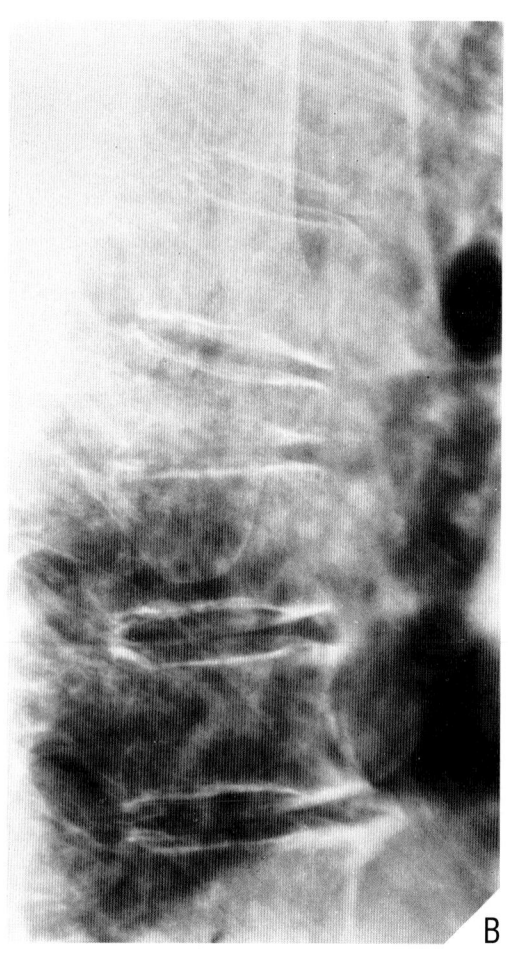

FIGURE 10.11 Anteroposterior (**A**) and lateral (**B**) radiographs of the spine in a 70-year-old man with multiple myeloma involving both the spine and appendicular skeleton show a compression fracture of the body of T8; several other vertebrae show only osteoporosis. The pedicles are preserved in contrast to metastatic disease of the spine, which usually also affects the pedicles.

cells in the bone marrow, lower levels of monoclonal protein, and a better prognosis.

An interesting variant of sclerosing myeloma is the so-called POEMS syndrome, first described in 1968 but gaining widespread acceptance only more recently. The syndrome consists of the following: polyneuropathy (P); organomegaly (O); particularly of the liver and the spleen; endocrine disturbances (E); such as amenorrhea and gynecomastia; monoclonal gammopathy (M); and skin changes (S), such as hyperpigmentation and hirsutism.

Differential Diagnosis

When the spine is involved, which is frequently the case, multiple myeloma must be differentiated from metastatic carcinoma. In this respect, the "vertebral pedicle sign" identified by Jacobson et al. (1958) may be helpful. These authors contend that in the early stage of myeloma, the pedicle, which does not contain as much red marrow as the vertebral body, is not involved, whereas in even an early stage of metastatic cancer the pedicle and vertebral body are both affected. In the late stages of multiple myeloma, however, both the pedicle and vertebral body may be destroyed. Radionuclide bone scanning can more reliably distinguish these two malignancies at this stage. Scintigraphy is invariably positive in cases of metastatic carcinoma, whereas in most cases of multiple myeloma there is no increased uptake of the radiopharmaceutical agent. This appears to reflect the purely lytic nature of most myelomatous lesions and the absence of significant reactive new bone formation in response to the tumor.

A solitary myeloma may create even greater diagnostic difficulty. If the lesion is entirely osteolytic, it may mimic other purely destructive processes such as giant-cell tumor, the "brown tumor" of hyperparathyroidism, fibrosarcoma, or a solitary metastatic focus of carcinoma from the kidney, thyroid, gastrointestinal tract, or lung.

Complications and Treatment

A common complication of myelomas of bone is pathologic fracture, especially in lesions of the long bones, ribs, sternum, and vertebrae. The development of amyloidosis has also been reported in about 15% of patients.

Treatment involves of radiotherapy and systemic chemotherapy. The 5-year survival rate is approximately 10%.

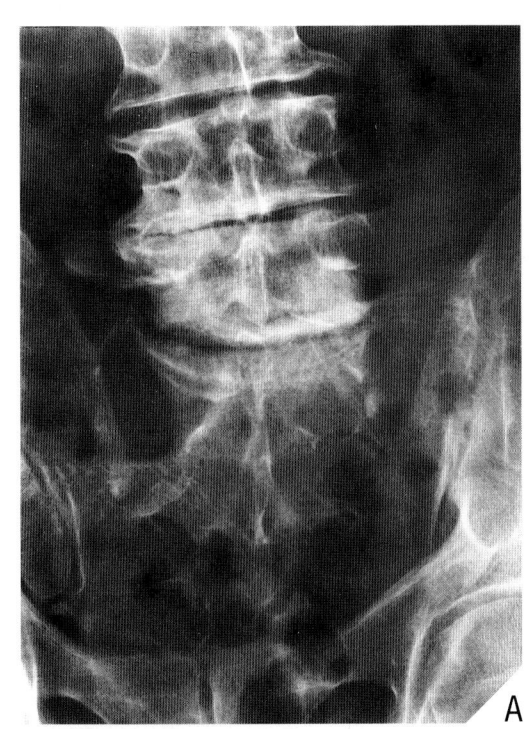

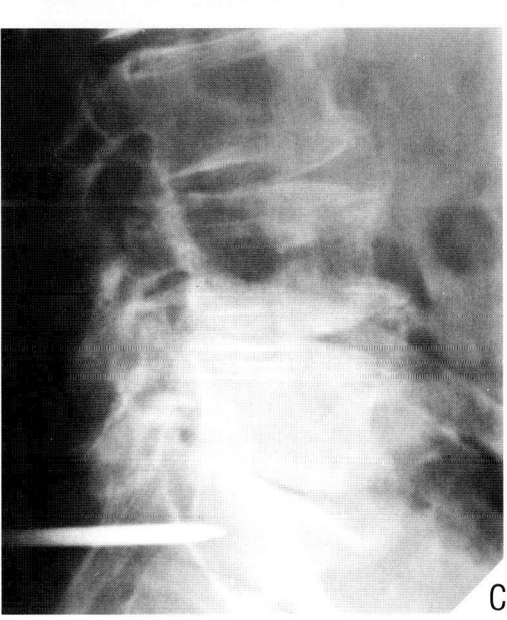

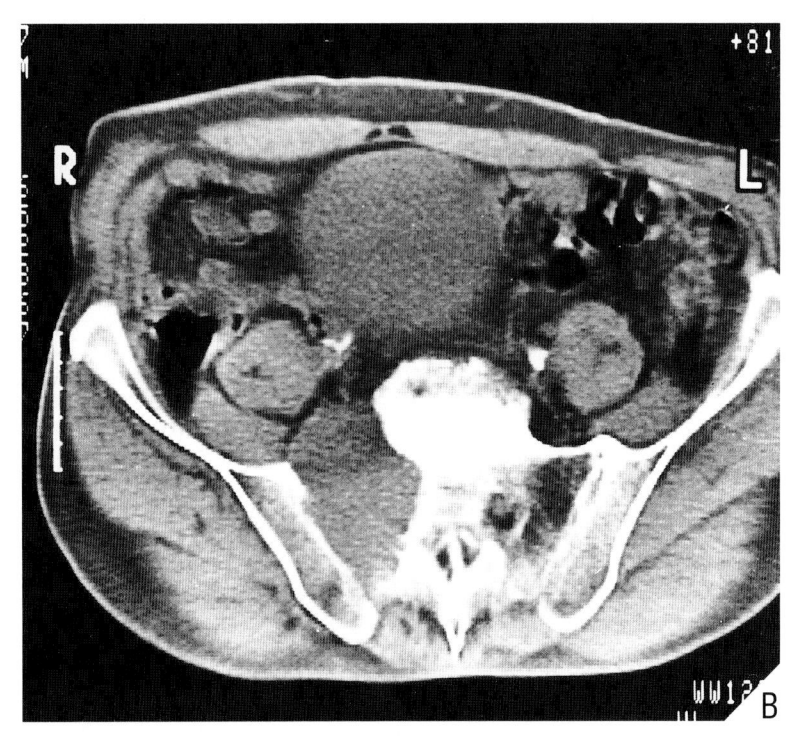

FIGURE 10.12 (A) Anteroposterior view of the lumbosacral spine in a 68-year-old man with low back pain shows a large lytic lesion in the right side of the sacrum, adjacent to the sacroiliac joint. **(B)** CT scan demonstrates an adjacent soft tissue mass. On the basis of these findings, a solitary myeloma, a metastatic lesion, malignant fibrous histiocytoma, and fibrosarcoma were considered in the differential diagnosis. **(C)** A fluoroscopy-guided biopsy yielded a diagnosis of plasmacytoma.

Fibrosarcoma

Fibrosarcoma is a malignant fibrogenic tumor that occurs in the patient's third to sixth decade and has a predilection for the femur, humerus, and tibia. The spine is only rarely affected: Mirra found that among 546 cases of fibrosarcoma, 1 affected the cervical spine, 2 the lumbar spine, and 2 were located in the sacrum. Secondary fibrosarcomas are a more common form in the spine, and they develop at sites of giant-cell tumor or Paget disease previously treated with irradiation.

Histologically, fibrosarcoma is characterized by tumor cells that produce collagen fibers. Characteristically, there is a "herring bone" pattern of fibrous growth with mild cellular pleomorphism. The tumor is not capable of producing osteoid matrix or bone, a factor distinguishing it from osteosarcoma.

Radiographically, fibrosarcoma is recognized by an osteolytic area of bone destruction and a wide zone of transition; the lesion is usually eccentrically located in the vertebral body. It exhibits little or no reactive sclerosis, and in most cases no periosteal reaction; a soft tissue mass, however, is frequently present. Fibrosarcoma may resemble a giant-cell tumor or a metastatic lesion.

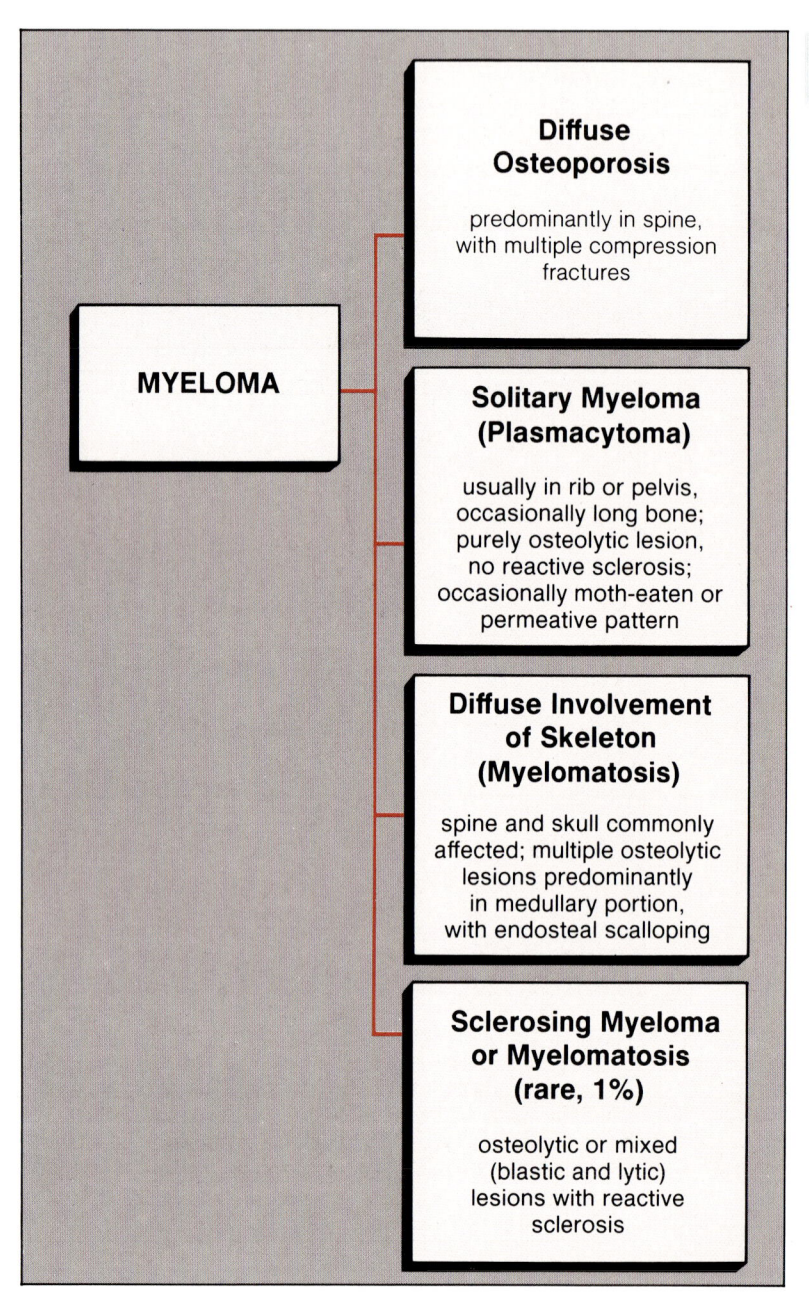

FIGURE 10.13 Variants in the radiographic presentation of myeloma.

MYELOMA

- **Diffuse Osteoporosis**
  predominantly in spine, with multiple compression fractures

- **Solitary Myeloma (Plasmacytoma)**
  usually in rib or pelvis, occasionally long bone; purely osteolytic lesion, no reactive sclerosis; occasionally moth-eaten or permeative pattern

- **Diffuse Involvement of Skeleton (Myelomatosis)**
  spine and skull commonly affected; multiple osteolytic lesions predominantly in medullary portion, with endosteal scalloping

- **Sclerosing Myeloma or Myelomatosis (rare, 1%)**
  osteolytic or mixed (blastic and lytic) lesions with reactive sclerosis

Treatment

Since these tumors do not respond satisfactorily to radiation or chemotherapy, surgical en bloc resection is the treatment of choice. The tumor has been reported to recur after local excision, and may spread to regional lymph nodes. The 5-year survival rate following treatment varies according to different studies from 29% to 67%.

CHORDOMA

A chordoma is a malignant bone tumor arising from developmental remnants of the notochord. Consequently, these tumors occur almost exclusively in the midline of the axial skeleton. Chordomas represent from 1% to 4% of all primary malignant bone tumors. They arise between the fourth and seventh decades, affecting men slightly more often than women. The three most common sites for chordoma are the sacrococcygeal area, the spheno-occipital area, and the C2 vertebra.

The radiographic appearance is that of a highly destructive lesion with irregular, scalloped borders; it is sometimes accompanied by calcifications in the matrix, probably resulting from extensive tumor necrosis (Fig. 10.14). Bone sclerosis has been reported in 65% of cases. Soft tissue masses are commonly associated with the lesion. Conventional radiography, including tomography, can usually delineate the tumor quite well (Fig. 10.15), but a CT scan or MRI are required to demonstrate soft tissue extension and invasion of the spinal canal.

Histologically, the tumor consists of bone aggregates of mucoid material separating cord-like arrays and lobules of large polyhedral cells with vacuolated cytoplasm and vesicular nuclei, referred to as *physaliphorous* cells.

Complications and Treatment

Invasion of the spinal canal by tumor may cause neurologic complications. Metastases are rare and usually occur late in the course of disease. The treatment for chordoma consists of complete resection, followed by radiation therapy. Cryosurgery with liquid nitrogen has been tried when complete surgical removal of the tumor was impossible.

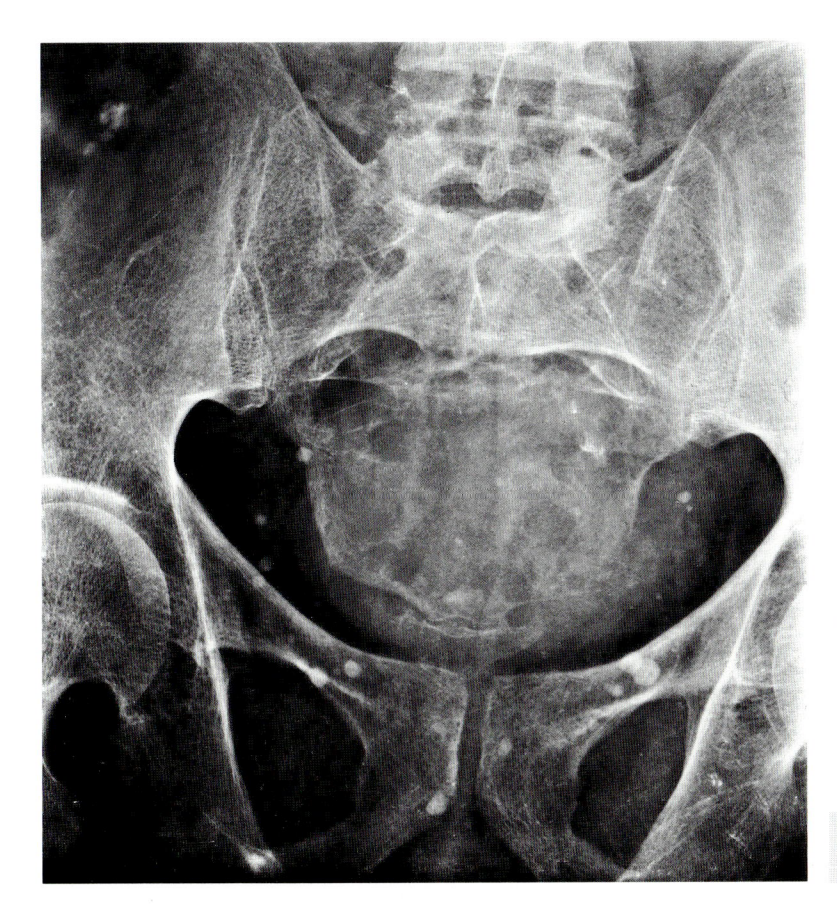

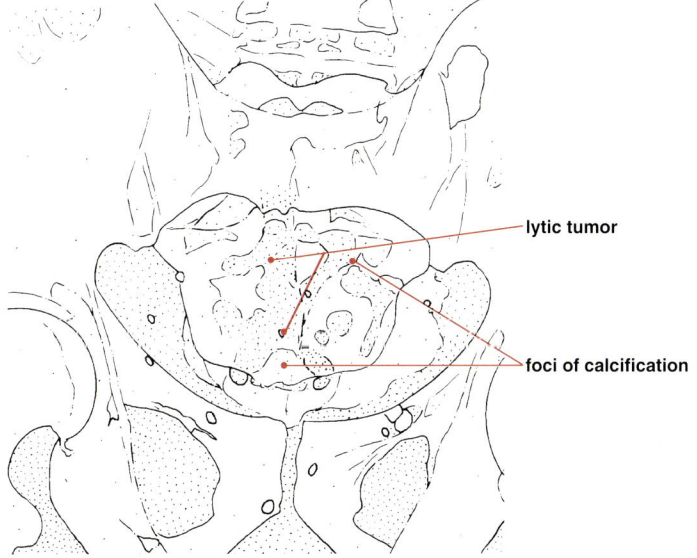

FIGURE 10.14 This destructive lesion in the sacrum of a 60-year-old woman proved to be a chordoma. Note its scalloped borders and the amorphous calcifications in the tumor matrix.

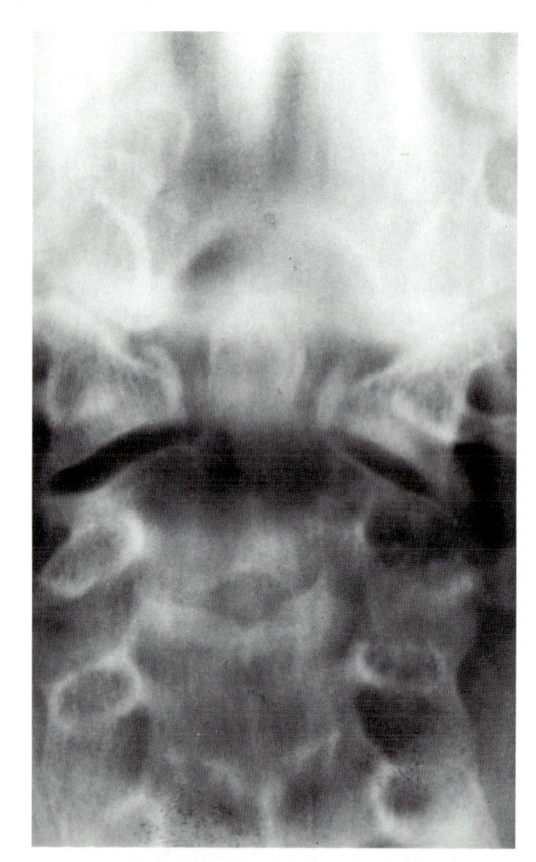

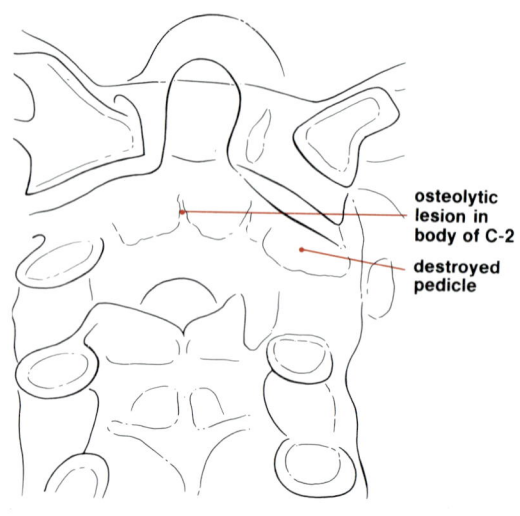

FIGURE 10.15 Open-mouth anteroposterior tomogram of the cervical spine of a 52-year-old man demonstrates an osteolytic lesion in the body of C2, which biopsy showed to be a chordoma.

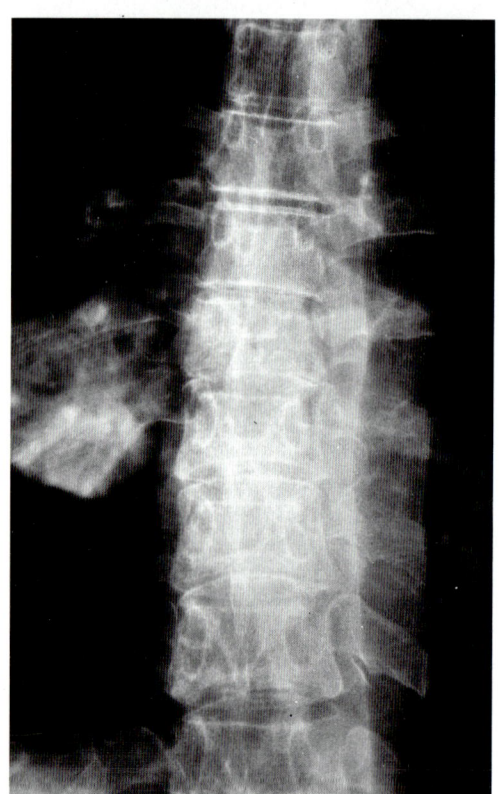

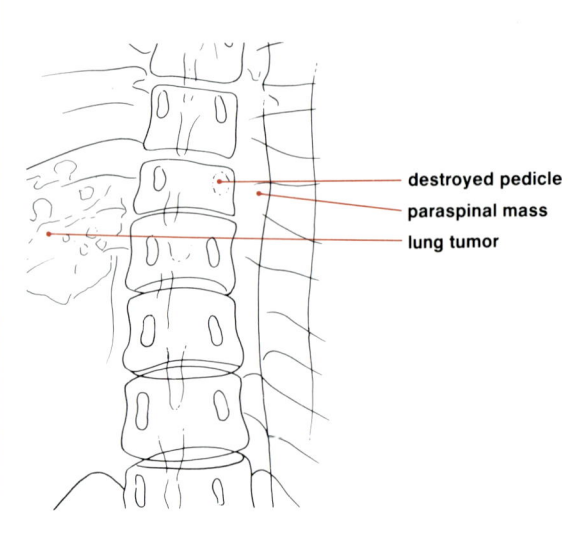

FIGURE 10.16 Anteroposterior view of the thoracolumbar spine in a 59-year-old woman with bronchogenic carcinoma shows a metastatic lesion in the body of T7. Note the destroyed left pedicle and associated paraspinal mass, features helpful in distinguishing this lesion from myeloma or neurofibroma. The lung tumor is obvious.

Imaging of the Spine in Clinical Practice

RADIATION-INDUCED SARCOMA

Radiation-induced sarcomas may arise in areas of normal bone included in radiation fields or after irradiation therapy for benign conditions, such as fibrous dysplasia and giant-cell tumor. In general, a sarcoma can develop only when at least 3000 rads are given within a 4-week span, although cases have been reported after exposure to only 800 rads. The latency period for radiation-induced tumors varies from 4 to 40 years, with an average of 11 years. The incidence of these lesions is very low, not exceeding 0.5%. The criteria for diagnosis of postirradiation sarcoma are as follows:

1. The initial lesion and the postirradiation sarcoma must not be of the same histologic type.
2. The site of the new tumor must be within the field of irradiation.
3. A minimum of 3 years must have elapsed since the previous radiation therapy.

Postirradiation osteosarcoma may also develop after ingestion and intraosseous accumulation of radioisotopes, as has been described in painters of radium watchdials. Regardless of the source of radiation, the most common histologic type of such tumors is osteosarcoma, followed by fibrosarcoma and malignant fibrous histiocytoma.

SKELETAL METASTASES

Skeletal metastases are the most frequent malignant bone tumors, and consequently, should always be considered in the differential diagnosis of malignant lesions, particularly in older patients. Most metastatic lesions involve the axial skeleton (the skull, spine, and pelvis) and the proximal segments of the long bones. Only very rarely does metastasis occur distal to the elbows or knees. These lesions result from the usual mechanism of hematogenous spread of a malignancy, by which a primary neoplasm erodes regional blood vessels, seeding malignant cells to the capillary beds of the lung and liver. The resultant tumor emboli reach the axial skeleton via communication with the vertebral venous plexus.

The incidence of metastases to bone varies according to the type of primary neoplasm and the duration of disease. Some malignant tumors have a far greater propensity for osseous metastatic involvement than do others. Because of their frequency, cancers of the breast, lung, and prostate are responsible for the majority of bone metastases, although primary tumors of the kidney, small and large intestines, stomach, and thyroid may also metastasize to bone. Carcinoma of the prostate has been reported to underlie nearly 60% of all bone metastases in men, whereas in women, carcinoma of the breast is responsible for nearly 70% of metastatic skeletal lesions.

Most skeletal metastases are "silent." In those that are not, pain is the major clinical symptom, with a pathologic fracture through a lesion only occasionally calling attention to the disease. Metastases to bone can be solitary or multiple, and can be further divided into purely lytic, purely osteoblastic, and mixed lesions. The primary tumors that give rise to purely lytic metastases are usually those of the kidney, lung, breast, thyroid, and gastrointestinal tract, although osteolytic lesions may become sclerotic after radiation therapy, chemotherapy, or hormonal therapy. Primary tumors responsible for purely blastic metastases are usually those of the prostate gland.

Detection of skeletal metastases is not always possible on routine radiography, since destruction of the bone may not be visible with this technique. Radionuclide bone scanning is the best means of screening for early metastatic lesions, whether they are lytic or blastic. Recently, however, several investigators have pointed out the usefulness of MRI in detecting metastases, particularly in the spine. The accuracy of MRI in identification of intramedullary lesions and assessment of spinal cord and soft tissue involvement has been well demonstrated.

In general terms, skeletal metastases may appear highly similar regardless of their primary source. However, in some instances the morphologic appearance, location, and distribution of metastatic lesions suggest their site of origin. Thus, for example, 50% of skeletal metastases are secondary to breast or bronchogenic carcinomas. Lesions that appear expanded and "blown-out" on plain films and highly vascular on arteriography are characteristic of metastatic renal carcinoma. Multiple round, dense foci or diffuse bone density are often seen in metastatic carcinoma of the prostate. In females, sclerotic metastases are usually from breast carcinoma.

Single metastatic lesions in a bone must be distinguished from primary malignant and benign bone tumors. A few characteristic features of metastatic lesions are helpful in making the distinction. Metastatic lesions usually present without or with only a small adjacent soft tissue mass, and usually lack a periosteal reaction unless they have broken through the cortex. The latter feature, however, is not invariably reliable, since in some series more than 30% of metastatic lesions—particularly metastases from carcinoma of the prostate—have been accompanied by a periosteal response. Metastatic lesions to the spine usually destroy the pedicle, a feature that is useful for distinguishing them from myeloma or neurofibroma invading the vertebra (Fig. 10.16).

Histologically, metastatic tumors are easier to diagnose than many primary tumors because of their essentially epithelial pattern. Although biopsies of suspected metastases are useful for diagnosis in patients with unknown primary tumors, only rarely are these procedures helpful in determining the exact site of an unknown primary tumor (Fig. 10.17).

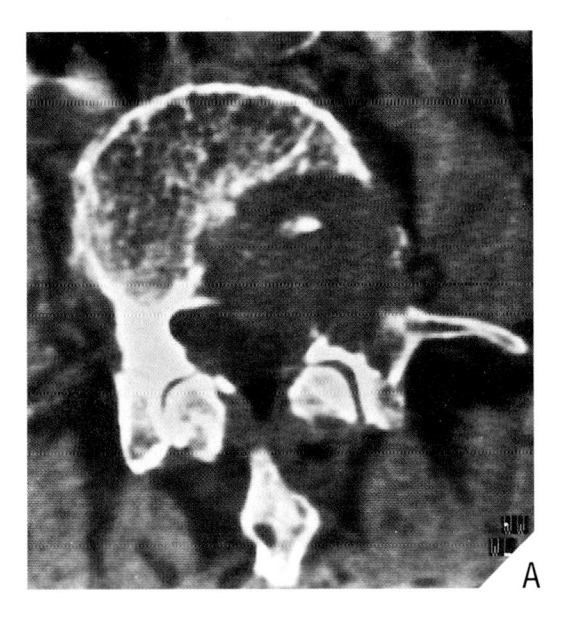

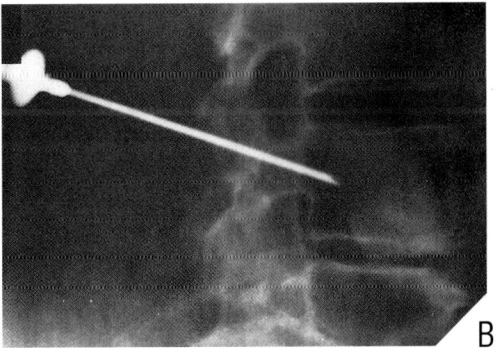

FIGURE 10.17 A 67-year-old woman who presented with low back pain and destructive lytic lesion of the body of L4 **(A)** was suspected of having either metastasis or myeloma. A needle-aspiration biopsy **(B)** yielded a tissue diagnosis of metastatic adenocarcinoma, although the site of the primary tumor was never determined.

Occasionally, if gland formation is present, a nonspecific diagnosis of meta-static adenocarcinoma can be made; however, the specific tumor type can rarely be detected. Exceptionally, a metastatic lesion may demonstrate a morphologic pattern that strongly suggests a primary tumor, such as the clear cells of renal carcinoma or the pigment production of melanoma.

Complications

Although metastases are themselves complications of a primary malignant process, it must be emphasized that they can cause secondary complications, such as pathologic fracture of the vertebra or compression of the thecal sac and spinal cord, thus producing neurologic symptoms (Fig. 10.18).

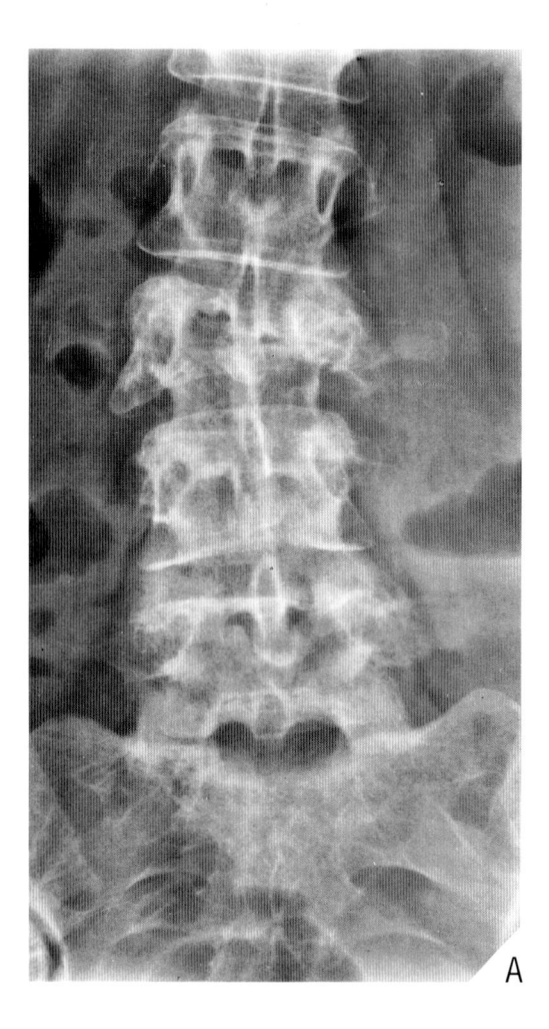

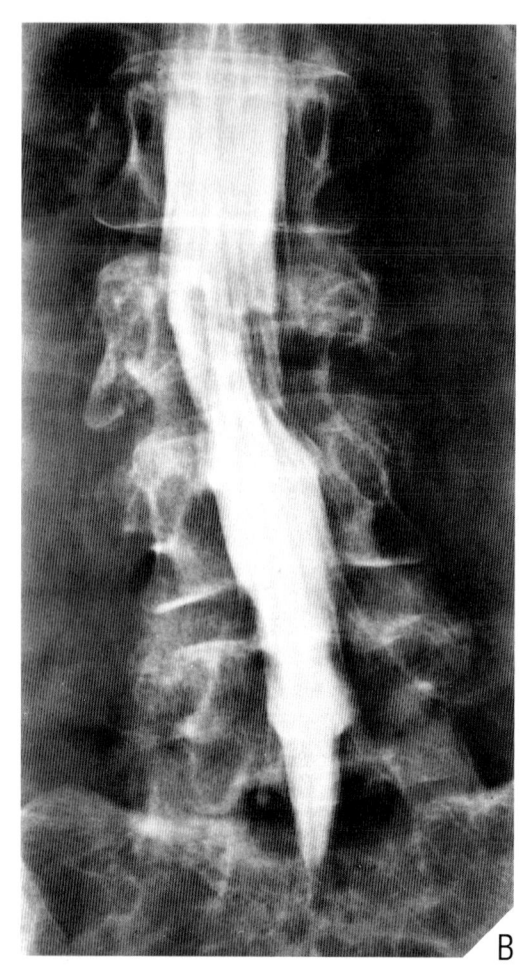

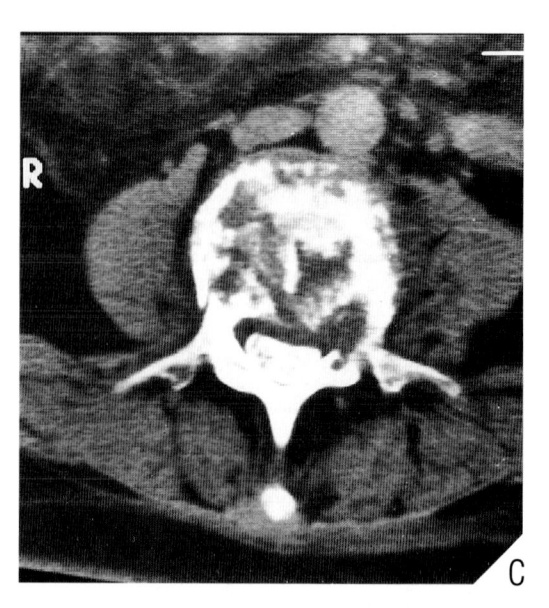

FIGURE 10.18 (A) Anteroposterior radiograph of the lumbar spine in a 47-year-old woman with breast carcinoma shows destruction of the body of L3 with a pathologic fracture. Note the involvement of the left pedicle. **(B)** A myelogram demonstrates compression of the thecal sac. **(C)** On CT scan a compression fracture of the vertebral body and involvement of the left pedicle are evident; the soft tissue extension of the tumor compresses the ventral aspect of the thecal sac.

Imaging of the Spine in Clinical Practice

Suggested Reading

Abrams HL: Skeletal metastases in carcinoma. *Radiology* 55:534, 1950.

Amstutz HC: Multiple osteogenic sarcomata—Metastatic or multicentric? *Cancer* 24:923, 1969.

Barnes R, Catto M: Chondrosarcoma of bone. *J Bone Joint Surg* 45B:729, 1966.

Bayrd ED, Bennett WA: Amyloidosis complicating myeloma. *Med Clin North Am* 34:1151, 1950.

Beltran J, Chandnani V, McGhee RA Jr, et al: Gadopentate dimeglumine-enhanced MR imaging of the musculoskeletal system. *Am J Roentgenol* 156:457, 1991.

Bergasgel DE: Plasma cell myeloma. *Cancer* 30:1588, 1972.

Bitter MA, Komaiko W, Franklin WA: Giant lymphnode hyperplasia with osteoblastic bone lesions and the POEMS (Takatsuki's) syndrome. *Cancer* 56:188, 1985.

Boston HC Jr, Dahlin DC, Ivins JC, et al: Malignant lymphoma (so-called reticulum cell sarcoma) of bone. *Cancer* 34:1131, 1974.

Brown TS, Paterson CR: Osteosclerosis in myeloma. *J Bone Joint Surg* 55B:621, 1973.

Campanacci M, Guernelli N, Leonessa C, et al: Chondrosarcoma: A study of 133 cases. *Ital J Orthop Traumatol* 1:387, 1975.

Castellino RA: The non-Hodgkin lymphomas: Practical concepts for the diagnostic radiologist. *Radiology* 178:315, 1991.

Daffner RH, Lupetin AR, Dash N, et al: MRI in the detection of malignant infiltration of bone marrow. *AJR* 146:353, 1986.

Dahlin DC, Beabout JW: Dedifferentiation of low-grade chondrosarcomas. *Cancer* 28:461, 1971.

Dahlin DC, Coventry MB: Osteogenic sarcoma: A study of six hundred cases. *J Bone Joint Surg* 49A:101, 1967.

deLange EE, Pope TL Jr, Fechner RE: Dedifferentiated chondrosarcoma: Radiographic features. *Radiology* 160:489, 1986.

Fielding JW, Fietti VG Jr, Hughes JEO, et al: Primary osteogenic sarcoma of the cervical spine. A case report. *J Bone Joint Surg* 58A:892, 1976.

Frouge C, Vanel D, Coffre C, et al: The role of magnetic resonance imaging in the evaluation of Ewing sarcoma. *Skel Radiol* 17:387, 1988.

Glicksman AS, Toker C: Osteogenic sarcoma following radiotherapy for bursitis. *Mt Sinai Med J* 43:163, 1976.

Hall FM, Gore SM: Osteosclerotic myeloma variants. *Skel Radiol* 17:101, 1988.

Healey JH, Lane JM: Chordoma: A critical review of diagnosis and treatment. *Orthop Clin North Am* 20:417, 1989.

Hermann G, Leviton M, Mendelson D, et al: Osteosarcoma: Relation between extent of marrow infiltration on CT and frequency of lung metastases. *Am J Roentgenol* 149:1203, 1987.

Hopper KD, Moser RP, Haseman DB, et al: Osteosarcomatosis. *Radiology* 175:233, 1990.

Huvous AG: *Bone Tumors—Diagnosis, Treatment and Prognosis,* 2nd ed. Philadelphia, W B Saunders, 1991.

Jacobson HG, Poppel MH, Shapiro JH, et al: The vertebral pedicle sign. A roentgen finding to differentiate metastatic carcinoma from multiple myeloma. *Am J Roentgenol* 80:817, 1958.

Klein MJ, Kenan S, Lewis MM: Osteosarcoma. Clinical and pathological considerations. *Orthop Clin North Am* 20:327, 1989.

Krishnamurthy GT, Tubis M, Hiss J, et al: Distribution pattern of metastatic bone disease. A need for total body skeletal image. *JAMA* 237:2504, 1977.

Levine E, De Smet AA, Huntrakoon M: Juxtacortical osteosarcoma: A radiologic and histologic spectrum. *Skel Radiol* 14:38, 1985.

Lichtenstein L, Jaffe HL: Ewing's sarcoma of bone. *Am J Pathol* 23:43, 1947.

Malcolm AJ: Osteosarcoma: Classification, pathology, and differential diagnosis. *Semin Orthop* 3:1, 1988.

Marsh HO, Choi C-B: Primary osteogenic sarcoma of the cervical spine originally mistaken for benign osteoblastoma. A case report. *J Bone Joint Surg* 52A:1467, 1970.

McKenna RJ, Schwinn CP, Soong KY, et al: Osteogenic sarcoma arising in Paget's disease. *Cancer* 17:42, 1964.

Mirra JM: *Bone Tumors. Clinical, Radiologic, and Pathologic Correlations.* Philadelphia, Lea & Febiger, 1989.

Mulvey RB: Peripheral bone metastases. *Am J Roentgenol* 91:155, 1964.

Pan G, Raymond AK, Carrasco CH, et al: Osteosarcoma: MR imaging after preoperative chemotherapy. *Radiology* 174:517, 1990.

Pear BL: Skeletal manifestations of the lymphomas and leukemias. *Semin Roentgenol* 9:229, 1974.

Schajowicz F: Ewing's sarcoma and reticulum cell sarcoma of bone: With special reference to the histochemical demonstration of glycogen as an aid to differential diagnosis. *J Bone Joint Surg* 41A:394, 1959.

Smith J, Ludwig RL, Marcove RC: Sacrococcygeal chordoma. A clinicoradiological study of 60 patients. *Skel Radiol* 16:37, 1987.

Sundaram M, McGuire MH, Herbold DR: Magnetic resonance imaging of osteosarcoma. *Skel Radiol* 16:23, 1987.

Tanaka O, Ohsawa T: The POEMS syndrome: Report of three cases with radiographic abnormalities. *Radiology* 24:472, 1984.

Thrall JH, Ellis BI: Skeletal metastases. *Radiol Clin North Am* 25:1155, 1987.

Unni KK, Dahlin DC, Beabout JW, et al: Parosteal osteogenic sarcoma. *Cancer* 37:2466, 1976.

Wetzel LH, Levine E, Murphey MD: A comparison of MR imaging and CT in the evaluation of musculoskeletal masses. *RadioGraphics* 7:851, 1987.

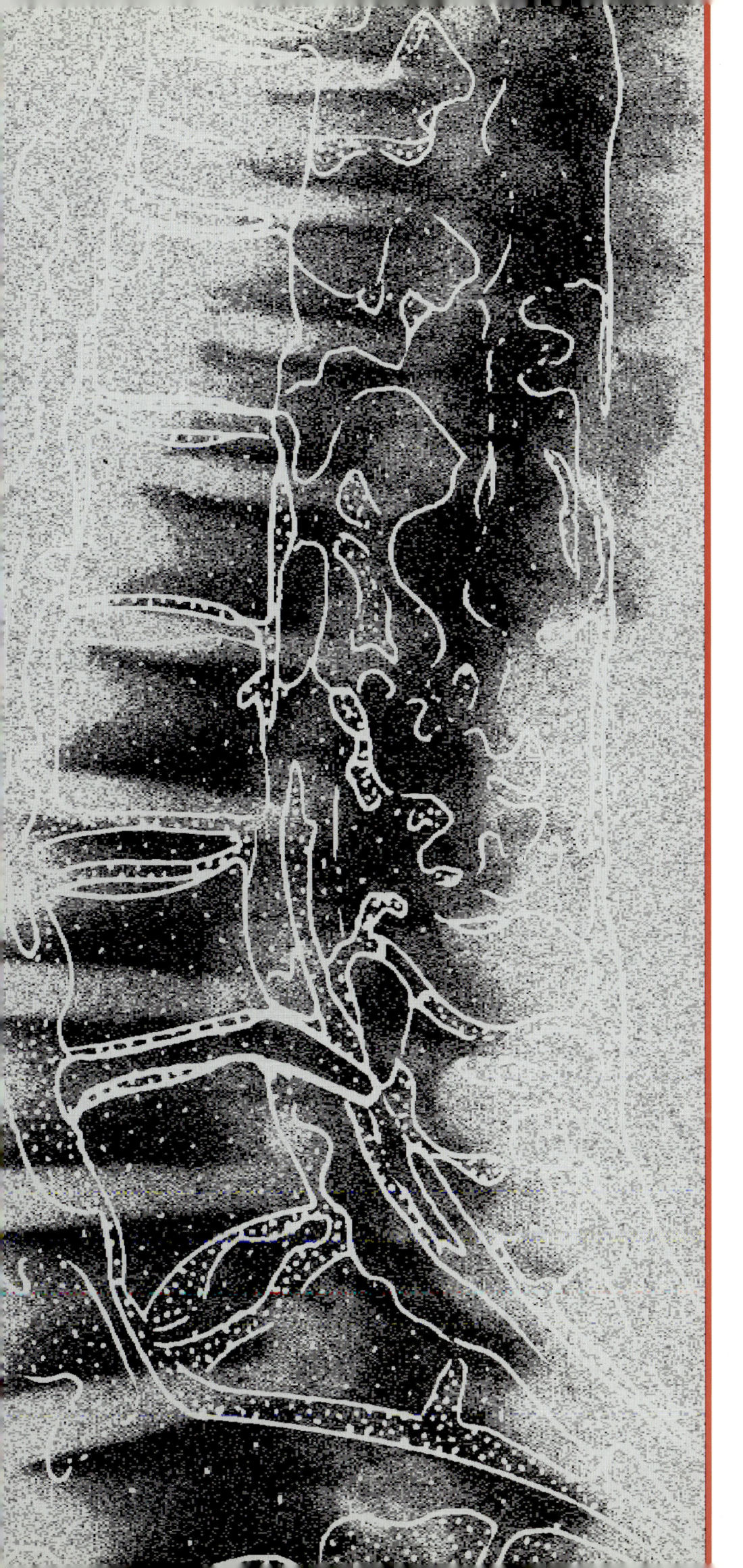

Diagnostic Workup and Treatment of Spinal Tumors

11

Differential Diagnosis of Back Pain

Ninety percent of all adults suffer from back pain at some time in their lives, with 50% of those recovering in 6 weeks and 90% recovering by 12 weeks. Because recovery in these patients is influenced primarily by patient education and aerobic conditioning, it appears that one of the roles of the treating physician is to exclude the presence of a spinal tumor or spinal infection in patients with persistent or atypical back pain.

The issue of how aggressive a patient's workup should be is based primarily on the patient's history and age. For example, a more aggressive workup is indicated when the history reveals previous treatment for neoplasia, family history of neoplasia, pain progressive for more than 12 weeks, or a history of night pain. Age should also influence the workup. Patients under the age of 20 are less likely to suffer from "idiopathic" back pain. The presence of a primary neoplasm should therefore be considered in this group of patients. The majority of spinal tumors in younger patients are benign (70%) and may include the lesions common to this age group, such as osteoid osteoma, osteoblastoma, aneurysmal bone cyst, and eosinophilic granuloma; however, malignant lesions of youth such as osteosarcoma and Ewing sarcoma must also be considered. Leukemia should also be included in the differential diagnosis, since the leukemic child may initially present with back pain and vertebral collapse, and a number of constitutional symptoms may lead to a misdiagnosis of infection. A good rule of thumb is to consider any adolescent with painful scoliosis or pain at rest as having a tumor until proven otherwise.

In patients who present over the age of 50 years, the likelihood of a metastatic lesion is significantly increased (Fig. 11.1). This may warrant a more aggressive workup at an earlier stage. In general, the most important aspect of working up a patient with back pain is to obtain a thorough history and physical examination. Plain radiographs are diagnostic of the neoplasm in more than 90% of cases, but occasionally a tumor in an early stage of development cannot be detected by this modality. If back pain persists, or if it increases over the next 6 to 12 weeks, a radionuclide bone scan and an erythrocyte sedimentation rate should be obtained. It is important to remember that some lesions, such as multiple myeloma, may be "cold" on scintigraphy. Therefore, in patients with persistent back pain and/or increasing neurologic findings despite a "normal" radionuclide bone scan, a serum protein electrophoresis study should be performed.

Diagnostic Imaging

The diagnostic approach to spinal tumors is similar to that for tumors elsewhere in the body. After a thorough history and physical examination, staging studies are performed, including plain radiography, total body scintigraphy, and cross-sectional imaging studies (CT or MRI). Reviewing the results of these studies can be quite useful in determining whether one is dealing with a solitary versus a multifocal lesion. Multifocal lesions are more apt to be metastatic.

The neuroradiologic tests include conventional tomography, myelography, CT (sometimes combined with myelography), and MRI. In general, CT provides a clearer picture of bone detail, whereas MRI allows a sharper delineation of the soft tissues, extension of the soft tissue components of the tumor, and the extent of neural element compromise. The superior soft tissue imaging by MRI, in addition to its multiplanar imaging capabilities, considerably enhances the surgeon's ability to plan treatment. Observation of soft tissue tumor extension and invasion of critical paravertebral structures is crucial to preoperative planning, and can eliminate many surprises at the time of surgery.

Once staging has been completed, a histologic diagnosis must be made. Tissue can be obtained by either needle biopsy or open biopsy. Although the needle biopsy is less invasive, samples may be difficult to interpret or may not show representative tissue. When adequate tissue cannot be obtained by needle biopsy, an open biopsy must be performed. In some instances it is more practical to perform a vertebrectomy instead of a simple biopsy, eg, in radiologically aggressive lesions of the cervical spine where the dissection required for biopsy (anterior medial retropharyngeal) is similar to that required for excision. Chondrosarcomas or giant-cell tumors can occasionally be treated by excisional biopsy, as their tendency towards local recurrence makes incisional biopsy somewhat more risky. In many cases, a rational treatment plan depends entirely on an unequivocal histologic diagnosis. The differential diagnosis of vertebral plana includes eosinophilic granuloma, Ewing sarcoma, and occasionally metastatic carcinoma; for a lytic lesion of a vertebral body the considerations are solitary plasmacytoma, metastasis, and chordoma. Treatment of these lesions differs so radically that no reasonable approach can be undertaken before a histologic diagnosis has been made. Likewise, without an adequate tissue sample obtained from a representative region of the tumor, the surgeon and the pathologist may be unable to reliably distinguish between benign but occasionally aggressive lesions, such as osteoblastoma or aneurysmal bone cyst, and frankly malignant tumors, such as osteosarcoma.

Treatment of Spinal Tumors

General Guidance

The treatment of most spinal tumors is palliative at best. Only a minority of these tumors (osteoid osteoma or osteoblastoma) can be reliably cured. Even aneurysmal bone cysts and giant-cell tumors, although histologically benign, can run a malignant clinical course. The surgeon must consider the

FIGURE 11.1 TUMORS METASTASIZING MOST FREQUENTLY TO THE VERTEBRAL COLUMN*

PRIMARY TUMOR	NO. CASES	%
Breast	576	37.7
Lung	377	24.7
Prostate	211	13.8
Kidney	154	10.2
Gastrointestinal	134	8.8
Thyroid	73	4.8
Total	1525	100.0

*Data obtained from 14 previously published series of metastatic spinal tumors are summarized (see Suggested Reading). (Reproduced with permission from Montesano PX, McLain RF, Benson DR: Spinal instrumentation in the management of vertebral column tumors. Semin Orthop 6:237, 1991)

natural history of the tumor, the patient's prospects for survival, and the risks of an extensive surgical procedure, and must then devise a plan that will provide the best quality of survival. In the case of metastatic lesions, quality of life is the primary consideration, and surgical treatment should aim at relief of pain and maintenance of neurologic function. The same holds true for most primary malignancies. Even in the latter lesions, however, therapeutic nihilism is inappropriate. Several authors have demonstrated improved survival, and occasional cure, with aggressive surgical treatment of spinal osteosarcomas, chondrosarcomas, and chordomas.

Ironically, perhaps the most aggressive approach should be used with certain benign tumors. Although many benign lesions (eosinophilic granuloma, hemangioma, osteochondroma) almost never require treatment, certain other benign but aggressive tumors can be lethal when the spine is involved. In the case of locally aggressive tumors such as low-grade chondrosarcoma or giant-cell tumor, the surgeon may have only "one shot" at excision, as the first local recurrence may prove unresectable. Fatalities due to recurrent giant-cell tumors and benign osteoblastomas have been reported.

For the most part, primary bone tumors are treated surgically, whereas metastatic lesions may be amenable to a more conservative approach if the following criteria are met:

1. The tumor should be sensitive to radiation therapy or chemotherapy; if maximal irradiation has been given previously, surgical therapy is indicated.
2. The spinal column should be stable.
3. Significant bone compromise of the canal should not be present.

For tumors that are not sensitive to radiation therapy, or when instability or canal compromise is present, surgery is recommended (Fig. 11.2). However, one must keep in mind that the key issue is the preservation of the quality of life. If the patient's projected survival is very limited, the most humane approach may be bracing and intravenous analgesics.

When surgical treatment is indicated (eg, in the case of a primary osteosarcoma), preoperative planning usually includes angiographic embolization to decrease the vascularity of the tumor and/or preoperative radiotherapy. The surgeon may also consider the use of preoperative and postoperative chemotherapy.

Surgical Approach

Whether a spinal tumor should be managed nonoperatively or surgically depends on several issues, considering that the ultimate goal is to abolish as much of the tumor as possible. For metastatic lesions, the decision to operate is dependent on the presence or absence of a vertebral body fracture and neurologic complications (Fig. 11.3). The other important issue is the stability of the spine. The spine is considered to be unstable when there is a pathologic fracture with more than 20 degrees of angulation measured on either the frontal or lateral radiographs, or when there is absence of sufficient bone mass anteriorly such that angulation or collapse can be expected. If a fracture produces neurologic compromise it should be considered unstable. These factors, combined with the potential sensitivity of the tumor to radiotherapy, will dictate the surgical approach. In general, radiosensitive tumors not complicated by pathologic fracture are amenable to bracing and radiotherapy. Tumors associated with pathologic fractures and collapse require correction of the spinal deformity. The latter is best achieved via a posterior approach, and correction should be followed by either vertebrectomy or radiotherapy, depending upon the tumor's sensitivity to radiation. Tumors that result in spinal instability and are accompanied by neurologic involvement are best managed by anterior vertebrectomy to ensure complete spinal canal decompression.

Posterior decompression is usually contraindicated, except in cases where tumors affect posterior elements of the vertebrae. Laminectomy provides no benefit over radiotherapy alone in patients with cord compression, and is associated with an unacceptably high incidence of severe complications. Anterior decompression and reconstruction have achieved neurologic recovery and satisfactory outcomes with fewer neurologic complications, less blood loss, and lower mortality. Finally, whenever possible, we favor the use of either autogenous bone grafts or allografts (Fig. 11.4). Although we do use methylmethacrylate constructs, we try to keep their use to a minimum in patients with an expected survival of 6 months or more.

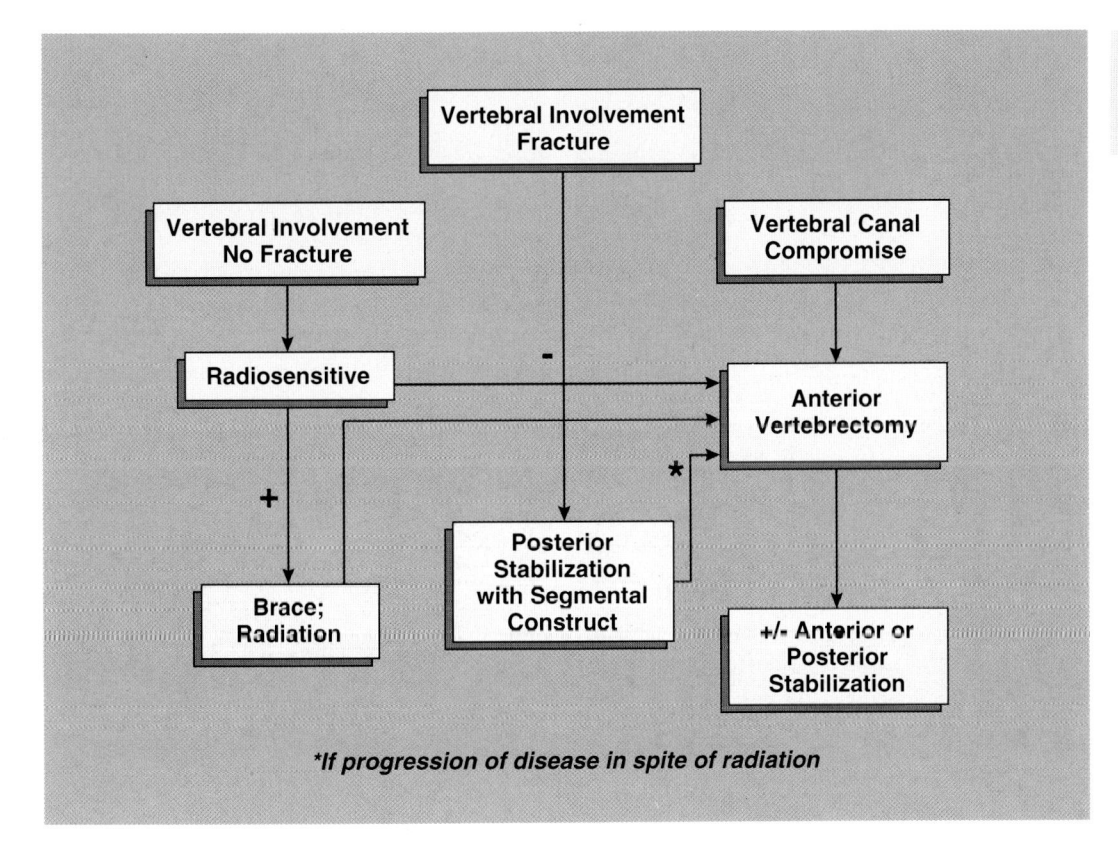

FIGURE 11.2 Management of metastatic tumors of vertebral column. (Reproduced with permission from Montesano PX, McLain RF, Benson DR: Spinal instrumentation in the management of vertebral column tumors. *Semin Orthop* 6:237, 1991)

*If progression of disease in spite of radiation

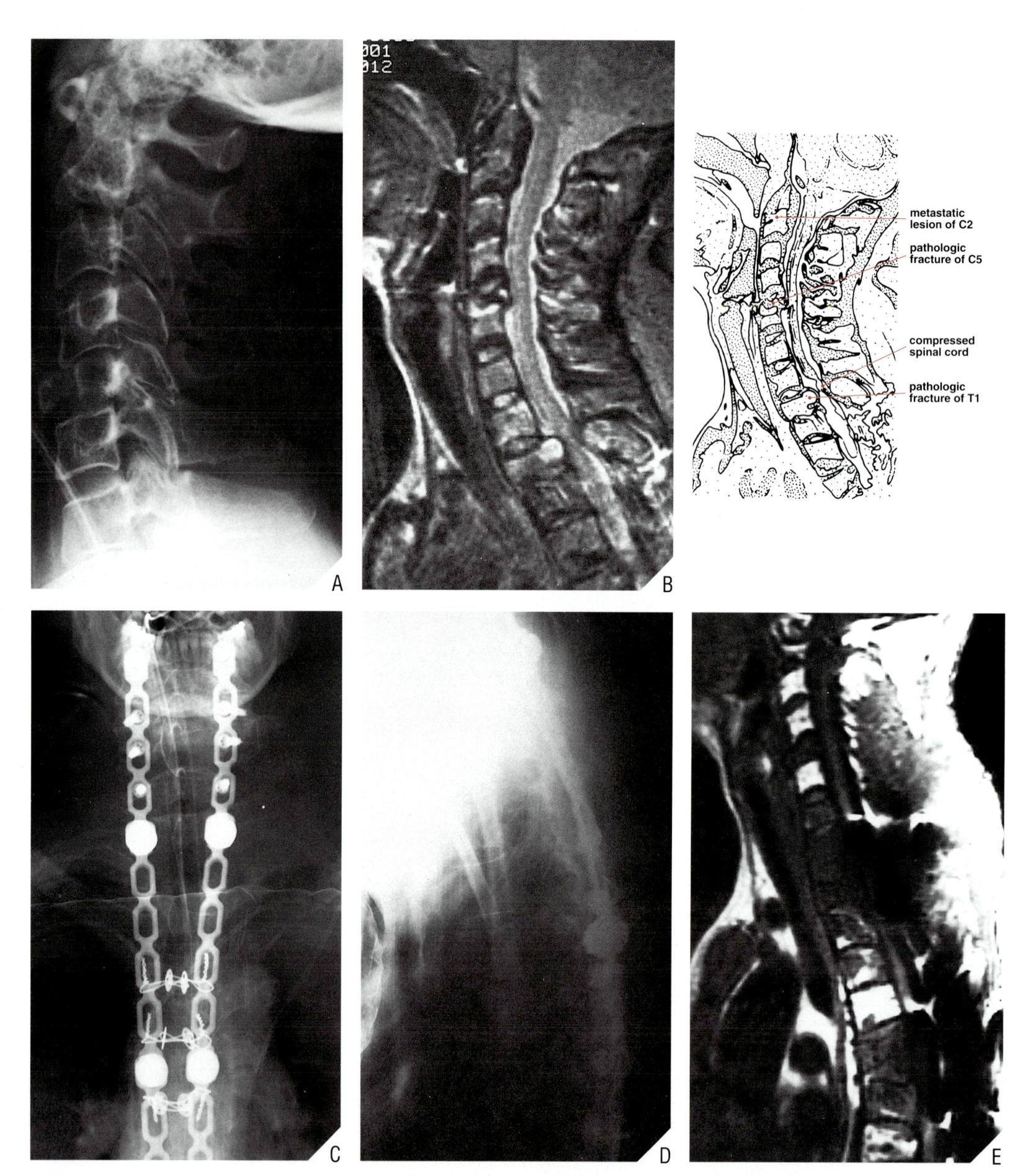

FIGURE 11.3 A 34-year-old female presented with metastatic breast carcinoma involving the axial skeleton. **(A)** Lateral radiograph demonstrates destructive lesions of C2 and C5. **(B)** Sagittal T2-weighted MR image shows extensive metastatic disease of cervical and upper thoracic spine. Bone marrow replacement by tumor is demonstrated by areas of high signal intensity. The pathologic fracture of T1 resulted in compression of the spinal cord. **(C,D)** Posterior reconstruction was performed using the Alta titanium reconstruction plates. **(E)** Postoperative sagittal T1-weighted MR image demonstrates the hardware in place (imaged as areas of signal void posterior to the spine). Vertebrae affected by metastatic disease demonstrate low signal intensity, whereas unaffected vertebrae are imaged with high signal intensity. (Reproduced with permission from Montesano PX, McLain RF, Benson DR: Spinal instrumentation in the management of vertebral column tumors. *Semin Orthop* 6:237, 1991)

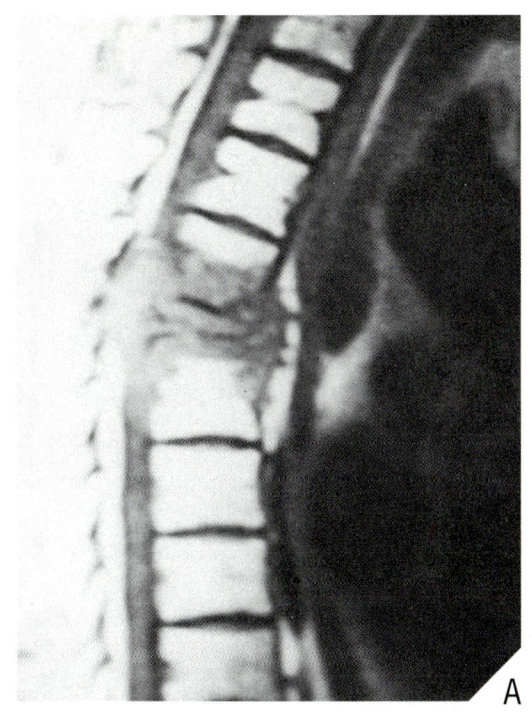

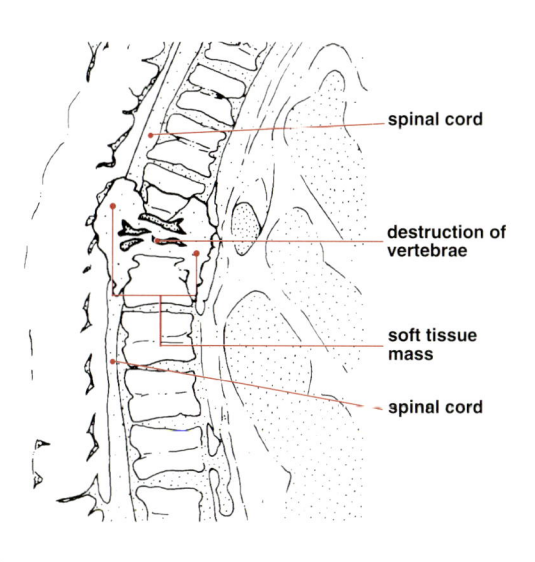

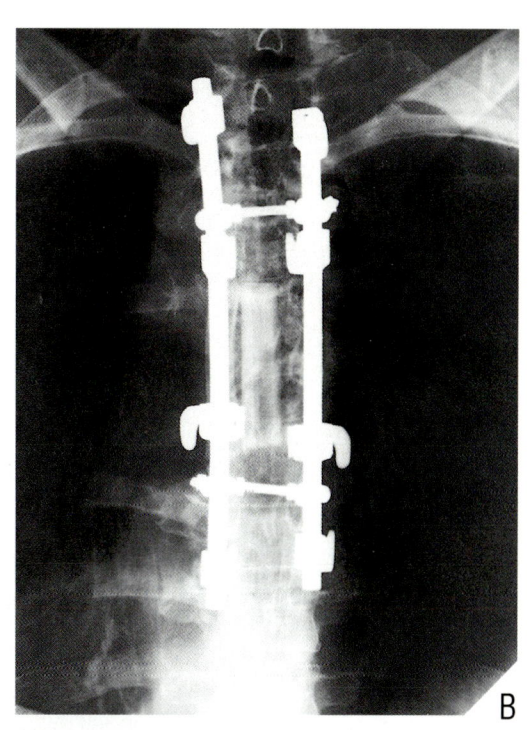

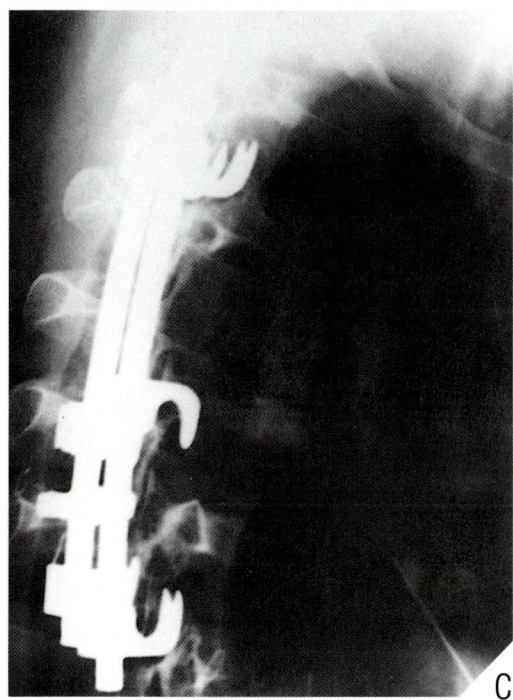

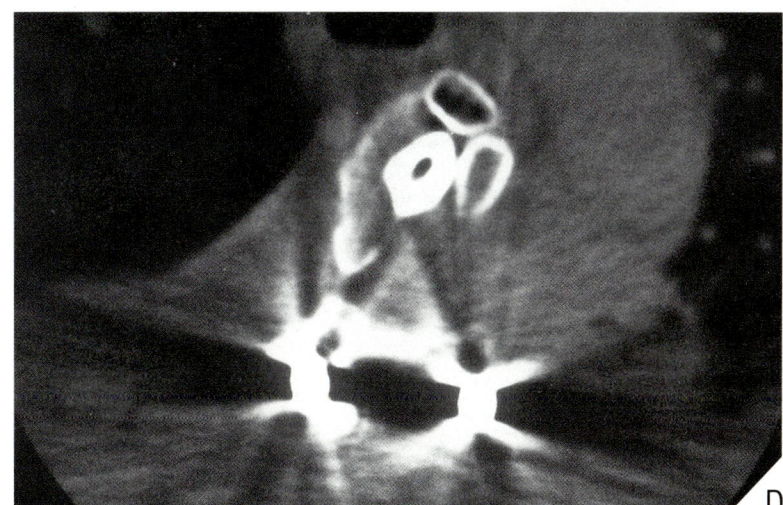

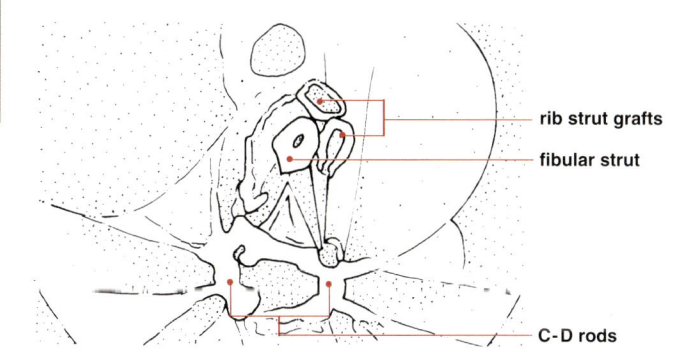

FIGURE 11.4 A 42-year-old male presented with metastatic prostate carcinoma affecting the T5, T6, and T7 vertebral bodies. **(A)** Sagittal T1-weighted MRI shows destruction of the vertebrae and a large soft tissue mass projecting anteriorly and posteriorly, compressing the spinal cord. **(B,C)** Anteroposterior and lateral radiographs show status post anterior and posterior reconstruction with C–D rods and application of allograft. **(D)** CT section after spinal canal decompression shows position of the rib strut and fibular strut grafts. (Reproduced with permission from Montesano PX, McLain RF, Benson DR: Spinal instrumentation in the management of vertebral column tumors. *Semin Orthop* 6:237, 1991)

Diagnostic Workup and Treatment of Spinal Tumors

Suggested Reading

Azouz EM, Kozlowski K, Marton D, et al: Osteoid osteoma and osteoblastoma of the spine in children. *Pediatr Radiol* 16:25, 1986.

Barwick KW, Hurvos AG, Smith J: Primary osteogenic sarcoma of the vertebral column. *Cancer* 46:595, 1980.

Clain A: Secondary malignant diseases of bone. *Br J Cancer* 19:15, 1965.

Coldwell DM: Embolization of paraspinal masses. *Cardiovasc Intervent Radiol* 12:252, 1985.

Constans JP, Divitiis E, Donzelli R, et al: Spinal metastases with neurosurgical manifestations: Review of 600 cases. *J Neurosurg* 59:111, 1983.

Fidler MW: Anterior decompression and stabilization of metastatic spinal fractures. *J Bone Joint Surg* 68B:83, 1986.

Francis KC, Hutter RVP: Neoplasms of the spine in the aged. *Clin Orthop* 26:54, 1963.

Gilbert RW, Kim JH, Posner JB: Epidural spinal cord compression from metastatic tumor: Diagnosis and treatment. *Ann Neurol* 3:40, 1978.

Godersky JC, Smoker WRK, Knutzon R: Use of magnetic resonance imaging in the evaluation of metastatic spinal disease. *Neurosurgery* 21:676, 1987.

Hall AJ, MacKay NNS: The results of laminectomy for compression of the cord or cauda equina by extradural malignant tumor. *J Bone Joint Surg* 55B:497, 1973.

Harrington, KD: Anterior decompression and stabilization of the spine as a treatment for vertebral collapse and spinal cord compression from metastatic malignancy. *Clin Orthop* 233:177, 1988.

Keim HA, Reina EG: Osteoid osteoma as a cause of scoliosis. *J Bone Joint Surg* 57A:159, 1975.

Kostuik JP, Errico TJ, Gleason TF, et al: Spinal stabilization of vertebral column tumors. *Spine* 13:250, 1988.

Manabe S, Tateishi A, Abe M, et al: Surgical treatment of metastatic tumors of the spine. *Spine* 14:41, 1989.

Marsh BW, Bonfiglio M, Brady LP, et al: Benign osteoblastoma: Range of manifestations. *J Bone Joint Surg* 56A:1, 1975.

McAfee PC, Bohlman HH, Ducker T, et al: Failure of stabilization of the spine with methylmethacrylate. *J Bone Joint Surg* 68A:1145, 1986.

McLain RF, Kabins M, Weinstein JN: Pedicle screw fixation for lumbar neoplasms. *J Spinal Dis* (in press).

McLain RF, Weinstein JN: Tumors of the spine. *Semin Spine Surg* 2:157, 1990.

Montesano PX: Anterior approach to fractures and dislocations of the thoracolumbar spine. *Oper Orthopaed* 3:1905, 1988.

Montesano PX, McLain RF, Benson DR: Spinal instrumentation in the management of vertebral column tumors. *Semin Orthop* 6:237, 1991.

Rogalsky RJ, Black GB, Reed MH: Orthopaedic manifestation of leukemia in children. *J Bone Joint Surg* 68A:494, 1986.

Shives TC, Dahlin DC, Sim FH, et al: Osteosarcoma of the spine. *J Bone Joint Surg* 68A:660, 1986.

Siegal T: Surgical decompression of anterior and posterior malignant epidural tumors compressing the spinal cord: A prospective study. *Neurosurgery* 17:424, 1985.

Siegal T, Tiqva P, Siegal T: Vertebral body resection of epidural compression by malignant tumors. *J Bone Joint Surg* 67A:375, 1985.

Springfield DS, Enneking WF, Neff JR, et al: Principles of tumor management. In Murray JA (ed): *Instructional Course Lectures,* vol. 33. St. Louis, AAOS, 1984.

Stener B: Total spondylectomy in chondrosarcoma arising from the seventh thoracic vertebra. *J Bone Joint Surg* 53B:288, 1971.

Stener B, Johnsen OE: Complete removal of three vertebrae for giant cell tumor. *J Bone Joint Surg* 53B:278, 1971.

Sundaresan N, Rosen B, Huvos AG, et al: Combined treatment of osteosarcoma of the spine. *Neurosurgery* 23:714, 1988.

Weinstein JN, McLain RF: Primary tumors of the spine. *Spine* 12:843, 1987.

White WA, Patterson RH, Bergland RM: Role of surgery in the treatment of spinal cord compression by metastatic neoplasm. *Cancer* 27:558, 1971.

Wright RL: Malignant tumors in the spinal extradural space: Results of surgical treatment. *Ann Surg* 157:227, 1963.

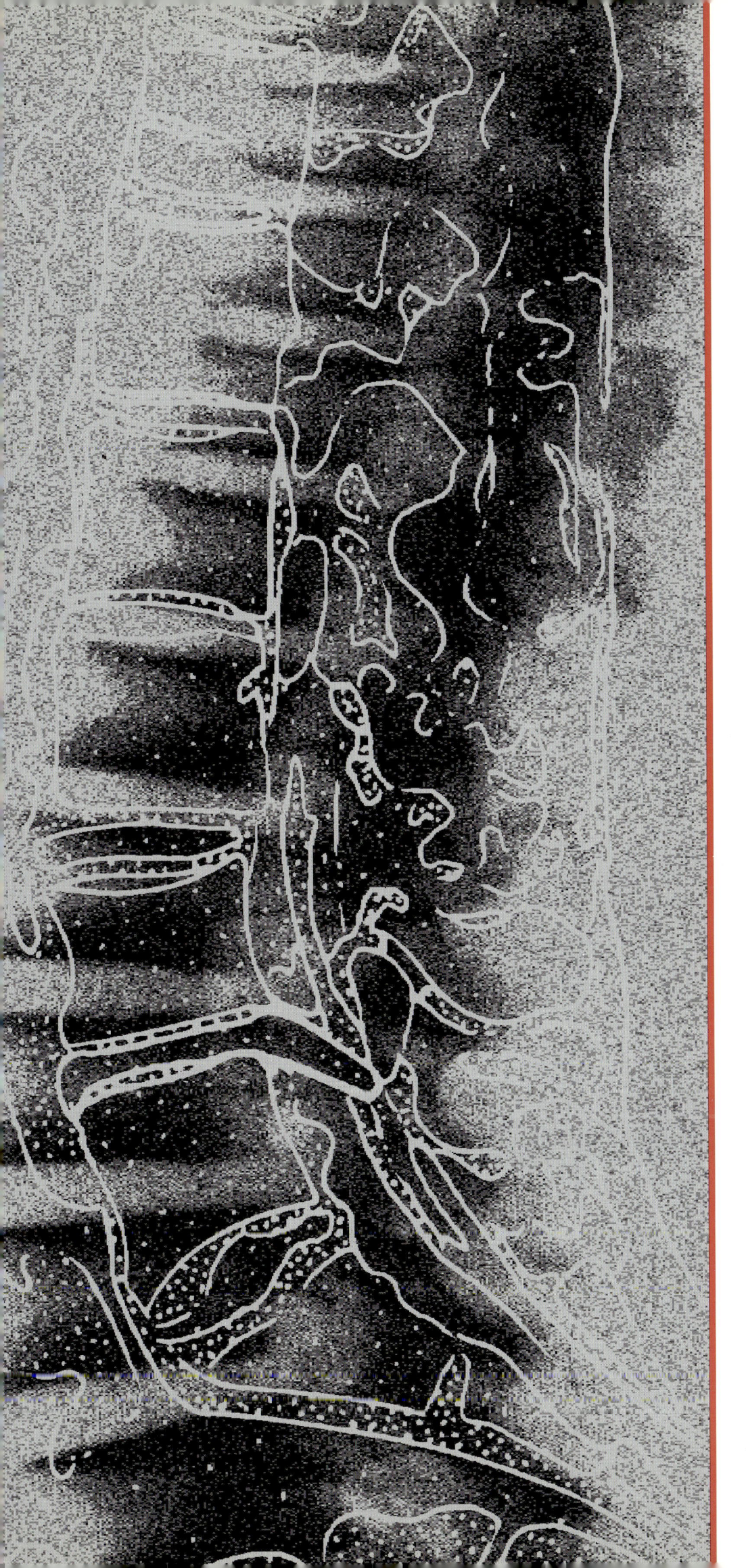

Radiologic Evaluation and Treatment of Infections of the Spine

12

Musculoskeletal Infections

Infections of the musculoskeletal system can be subdivided into three categories: those involving bones (osteomyelitis); those involving joints (infectious arthritis); and those involving the soft tissues (cellulitis).

Osteomyelitis

Three basic mechanisms allow an infectious organism—whether bacterium, virus, mycoplasma, rickettsia, or fungus—to reach the bone: spread via the bloodstream hematogenously from a remote site of infection, such as from the skin, tonsils, gallbladder, or urinary tract; spread from a contiguous source of infection, such as from the soft tissues, teeth, or sinuses; and direct implantation, such as through a puncture, a missile wound, or an operative procedure.

Hematogenous spread is common in children. The usual focus of infection develops in the metaphysis of a long bone, but only rarely in a vertebral disk (diskitis).

Contiguous spread and direct implantation are more common in adults. The sites of bone infection via either of these routes are directly related to the focus of soft tissue infection or the location of the wound resulting from trauma or surgery.

Infectious Arthritis

An infectious agent can enter the joint by the same basic routes as in osteomyelitis: direct invasion of the synovial membrane, either secondary to a penetrating wound or after surgery; spread from an infection of the adjacent soft tissues; and indirectly via a blood-borne infection. Infectious arthritis can also occur secondary to a focus of osteomyelitis in the adjacent bone.

Cellulitis

Soft tissue infections most commonly result from a break in the skin and direct introduction of an infectious agent. Some patients, such as those with diabetes, are particularly prone to cellulitis owing to a combination of factors, including skin breakdown and local ischemia.

Infections of the Spine

Infections in the spine can affect a vertebral body, an intervertebral disk, the paravertebral soft tissues, or the epidural compartment. Very rarely, an infection may involve the contents of the spinal canal and the spinal cord. The mechanisms of infection are the same as those of osteomyelitis and infectious arthritis elsewhere in the body (Fig. 12.1). An intervertebral disk infection, for example, may result from puncture of the canal or the disk itself during a procedure, or from a penetrating injury; it can also spread from a contiguous source of infection, such as a paraspinal abscess. Most common, however, infection develops after a surgical procedure such as laminectomy or spinal fusion, or during generalized bacteremia or sepsis. Regardless of the primary location of the infectious process, *Staphylococcus aureus* is responsible for over 90% of all infections of the spine.

Radiologic Evaluation of Infections of the Spine

The radiologic modalities used to evaluate infections of the spine include:

- plain film radiography (including magnification studies)
- conventional tomography
- computed tomography (CT)
- myelography and diskography
- fistulography (sinogram)
- radionuclide imaging (scintigraphy, bone scan)
- magnetic resonance imaging (MRI)
- percutaneous aspiration and biopsy (fluoroscopy- or CT-guided).

In most instances, plain film radiography is sufficient to demonstrate the pertinent features of spinal infection (Fig. 12.2). Magnification radiography is helpful in delineating subtle changes that represent cortical

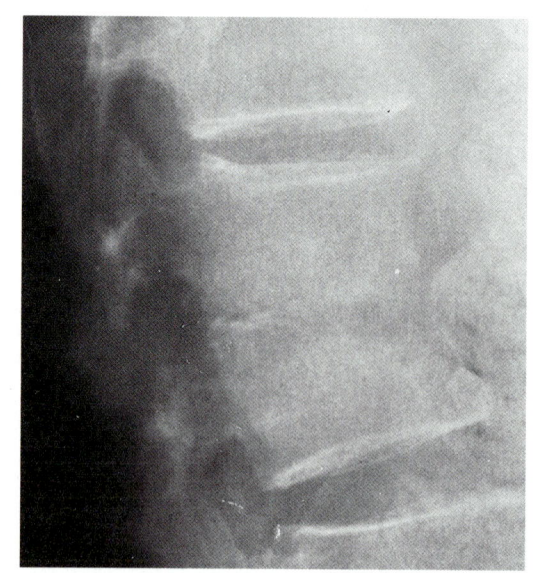

FIGURE 12.1 The potential routes of infection of a vertebra or an intervertebral disk are direct invasion, hematogenous spread, and extension from a focus of infection in the adjacent soft tissues.

FIGURE 12.2 A 48-year-old drug user developed spinal infection at L1–L2. The plain radiograph—lateral view of the lumbar spine—clearly demonstrates the characteristic features of disk space infection: disk space narrowing and loss of definition of the adjacent vertebral endplates.

Imaging of the Spine in Clinical Practice

destruction or periosteal new bone formation, and is occasionally required for differentiating osteoporosis from the early stages of infection, which may appear radiographically similar. Conventional tomography utilizing multidirectional motion (trispiral tomography) is particularly effective in demonstrating sequestra or subtle sinus tracts in the bone. CT plays a determining role in demonstrating the extent of infection in the vertebral body, intervertebral disk and soft tissues (Fig. 12.3), and at times can be very helpful in arriving at a specific diagnosis. CT is also an effective guidance modality for biopsy of the lesion (see Fig. 1.5).

Scintigraphy has a prominent role in the evaluation of infections. In suspected osteomyelitis, radionuclide bone scan using ^{99m}-technetium-labeled phosphonates is routinely used, since there is an accumulation of the tracer in the areas of infection (Fig. 12.4). A three-phase technique is particularly useful for distinguishing infected vertebra from infected perivertebral soft tissues when plain films are not diagnostic. However, once the bone has been violated by an insult that causes increased bone turnover, such as surgery or fracture, the routine bone scan with technetium labeled phosphonates becomes less specific for infection. Radionuclide studies using gallium (a ferric analogue) and indium are more specific in these instances. There is still no general agreement on the exact mechanism of gallium localization in infected tissues. After intravenous injections of gallium, more than 99% is bound to various plasma proteins, including transferrin, haptoglobin, lactoferrin, albumin, and ferritin. At least five mechanisms for the transfer of gallium from the plasma into inflammatory exudates and cells have been suggested. These include direct leukocyte uptake, direct bacterial uptake, protein-bound tissue uptake, increased vascularity, and increased bone turnover. Since gallium binds to the iron-binding molecule transferrin, the mechanism of gallium uptake in infectious processes is best explained by hyperemia and increased permeability, which increase delivery of the protein-bound tracer (transferrin) to the area of inflammation. Cells associated with the inflammatory response, particularly polymorphonuclear white cells in which lactoferrin is carried within intracytoplasmic granules, deposit iron-binding proteins extracellularly at the site of inflammation, serving to combat infection by sequestering needed iron from bacteria. The lactoferrin, which has a high binding affinity for iron, takes the gallium away from the transferrin.

Gallium can also be used to assess response to therapy. Particularly in vertebral osteomyelitis, gallium concentrations enhance the specificity of an abnormal bone scan and decreased gallium uptake closely follows a good response to therapy.

The other tracer used in infections is indium. Since indium-labeled white blood cells are usually not incorporated into areas of increased bone turnover, scintigraphy with ^{111}In-oxine-labeled leukocytes is used as a sensitive and specific test in the general diagnosis of infection of the musculoskeletal system, and in specific instances when infection complicates previous fracture or surgery. Like other imaging procedures in nuclear medicine, this test monitors the internal distribution of a tracer agent to provide diagnostic information. The inherent ability of white blood cells to localize at sites of inflammation makes their use in this test particularly effective in the diagnosis of infections. The sensitivity of indium scintigraphy in detecting infections is reported to be 83%, with a specificity of 94% and accuracy of 88%.

^{111}In-labeled leukocyte scintigraphy has also been reported to be highly specific and sensitive in the detection of paraspinal soft tissue abscesses. However, such studies are limited by poor spatial resolution. It may be dif-

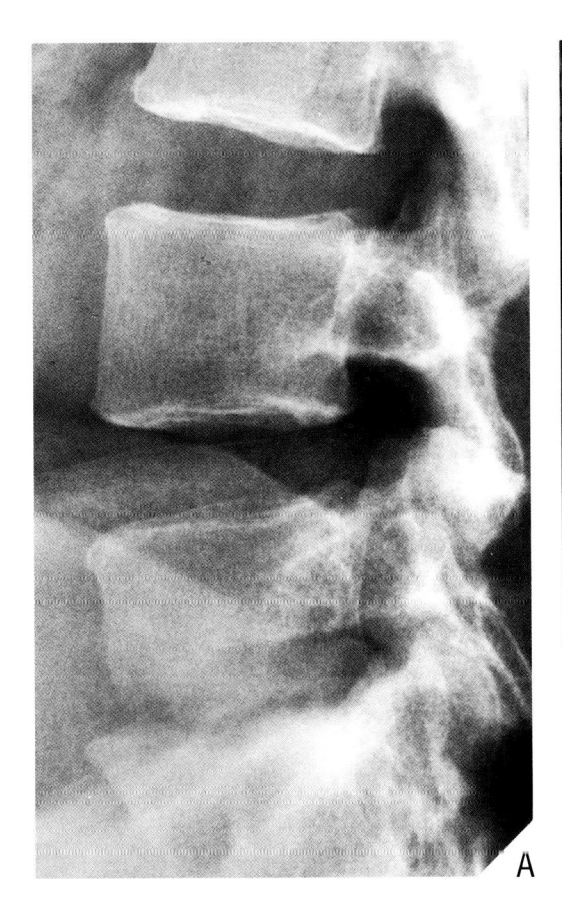

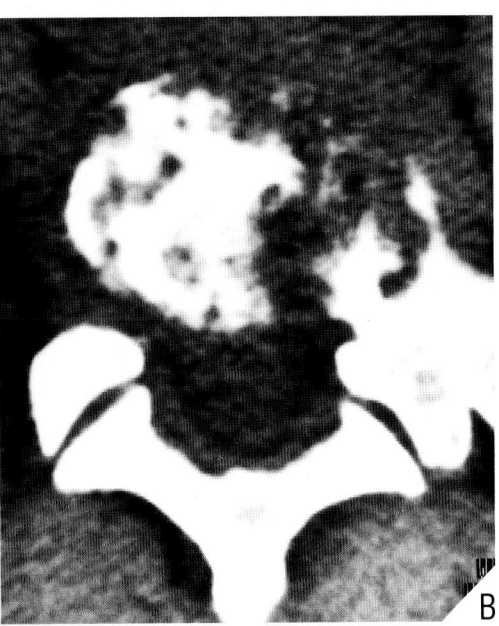

FIGURE 12.3 A 40-year-old man presented with lower back pain for 8 weeks, which he attributed to lifting a heavy object. **(A)** Lateral view of the lumbosacral spine shows narrowing of the L5–S1 disk space and fuzziness of the adjacent vertebral endplates. **(B)** CT section through the disk space clearly shows destruction of the disk and vertebral endplate characteristic of infection.

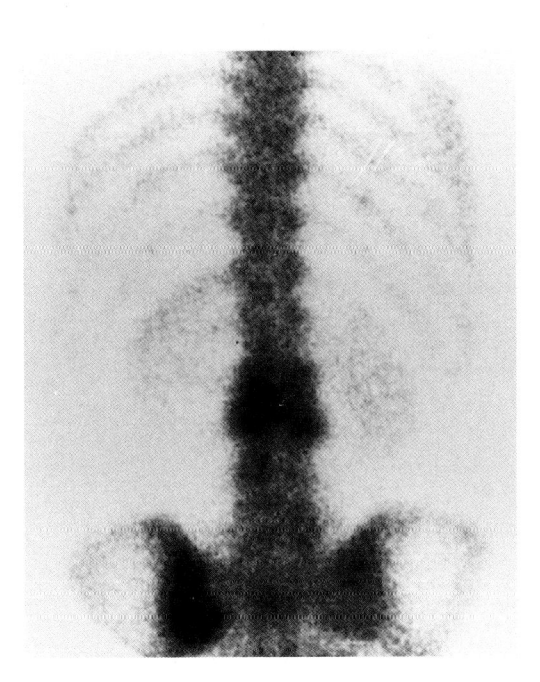

FIGURE 12.4 A 58-year-old woman presented with low back pain. After administration of 20 mCi (740 MBq) of Tc-99m MDP, there is increased activity at the level of L2–L3. Subsequent radiographs and needle-aspiration biopsy revealed infected intervertebral disk L2–L3 and vertebral osteomyelitis of L3. (Courtesy of Robert C. Stadalnik, M.D., Sacramento, CA)

ficult to differentiate between bone and soft tissue activity when the two are close together. In these instances, however, the study can be enhanced by sequential use of ^{99m}Tc-labeled phosphonates and indium.

Myelography is still useful for evaluating infections within the spinal canal, as well as vertebral osteomyelitis and disk infection (Fig. 12.5). Diskography is occasionally performed, mainly to obtain the tissue for bacteriologic examination; however, it may also reveal the extent of an infectious process in the disk and vertebra (Fig. 12.6). Fistulography (sinogram) is an important technique for outlining sinus tracts in the soft tissues and evaluating their extension into the bone.

Magnetic resonance imaging is also useful in the evaluation of bone and soft tissue infections. As recent studies have indicated, osteomyelitis, soft tissue abscesses, and various forms of cellulitis are well depicted by this modality (Beltram et al., 1987; Modic, 1986). MRI is as sensitive as ^{99m}Tc-MDP in demonstrating osteomyelitis, and is more specific and more sensitive than other scintigraphic techniques in demonstrating soft tissue infections, primarily because of its superior spatial resolution. The proper evaluation of spinal infections with MRI requires both T1- and T2-weighted images in at least two imaging planes. The diagnostic criteria for MRI in osteomyelitis are findings of decreased signal intensity in the

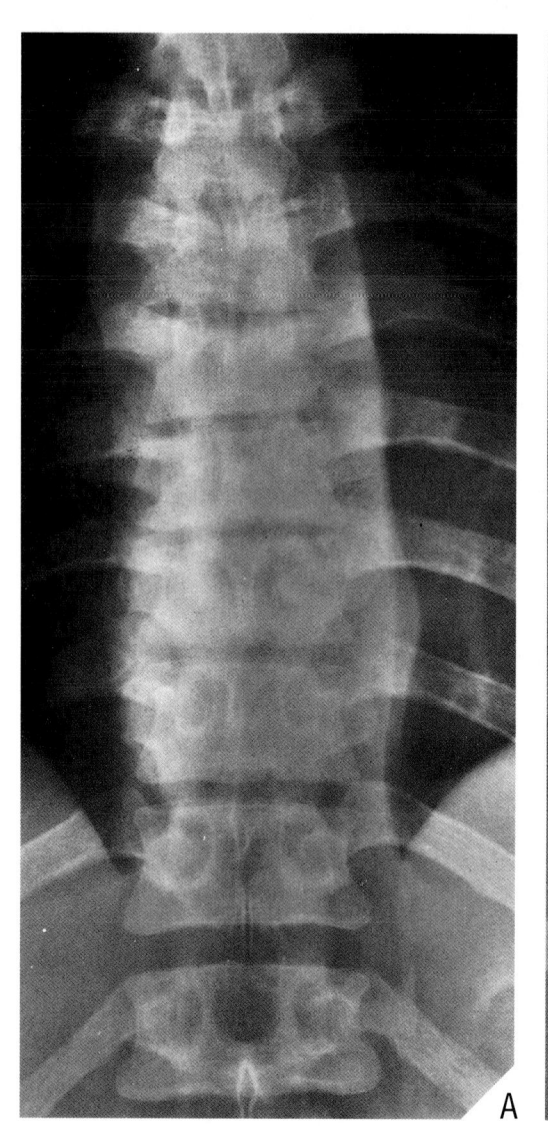

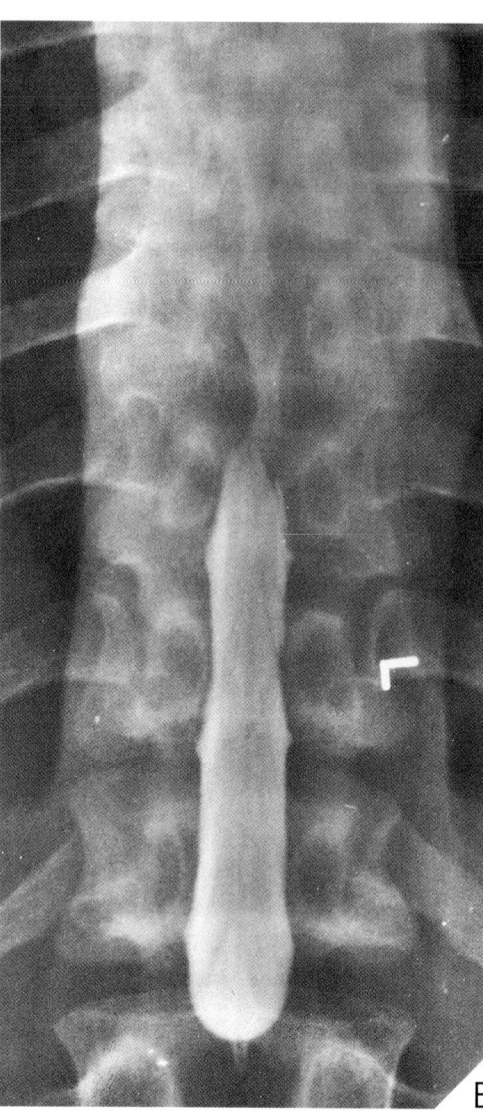

FIGURE 12.5 A 39-year-old man with a history of pulmonary tuberculosis developed neurologic symptoms of spinal cord compression. **(A)** Anteroposterior view of the thoracic spine shows minimal disk space narrowing at T9–T10 and a large left paraspinal mass. **(B)** A myelogram shows complete obstruction of the flow of contrast agent in the subarachnoid space at the level of the disk infection.

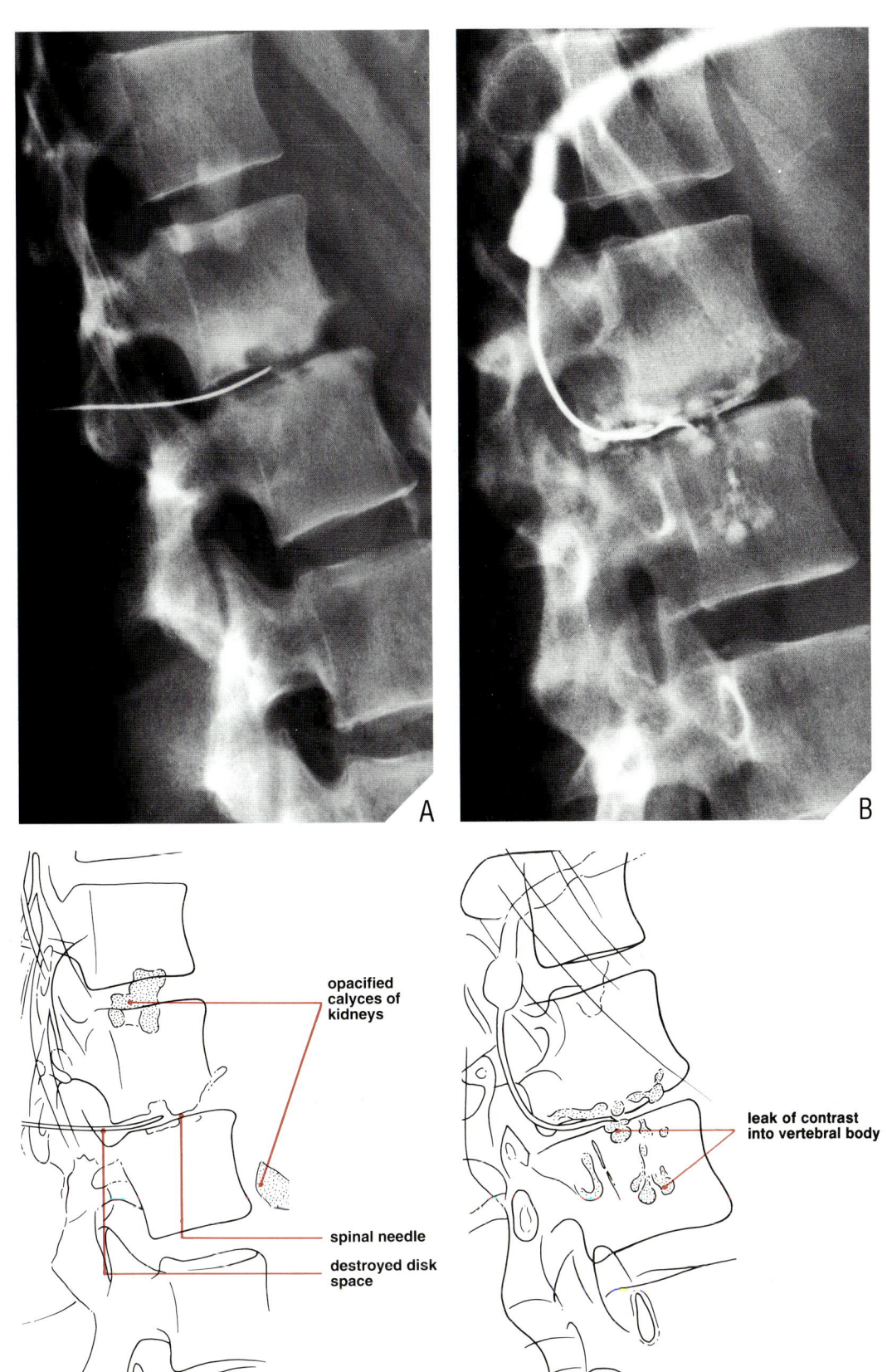

FIGURE 12.6 A 22-year-old heroin addict with back pain for 2 months developed an intervertebral disk infection. A diskogram was performed primarily to aspirate fluid for bacteriologic examination, which revealed *Pseudomonas aeruginosa*. Prior to the puncture, the patient received an intravenous injection of iodine contrast to visualize the kidneys, as a precautionary step before spine biopsy at that level. **(A)** Lateral radiograph of the lumbar spine shows narrowing of the disk space at L1–L2 and destruction of the adjacent vertebral endplates. The spinal needle is located in the center of the disk. **(B)** Lateral film obtained during the injection of metrizamide demonstrates extension of the contrast medium into the body of L2, indicating the presence of vertebral osteomyelitis.

Radiologic Evaluation and Treatment of Infections of the Spine   12.5

bone marrow on short TR/TE sequences (T1-weighting) and of increased signal intensity in the bone marrow on long TR/TE sequences (T2-weighting) (Fig. 12.7). Increased signal intensity of the soft tissues with ill-defined margins on long TR/TE sequences is considered indicative of edema and/or nonspecific inflammatory changes. Well-demarcated collections of increased signal intensity on T2-weighted sequences and decreased signal intensity on T1-weighted sequences, surrounded by a zone of decreased signal intensity, are considered indicative of soft tissue abscesses.

Percutaneous aspiration and CT- or fluoroscopy-guided biopsy of a suspected focus of infection can be done in the radiology suite; it can rapidly confirm a suspected diagnosis of infection, and can reveal the causative organism (see Fig. 1.5).

Treatment of Spinal Infections

After aspiration biopsy for culture and sensitivity, patients with disk space infection that is not accompanied by vertebral body destruction and collapse can be treated with intravenous antibiotics without surgical debridement. The selection of antibiotics is based on the findings of intervertebral disk aspiration or biopsy. If the cultures are negative, one should assume that the infectious agent is *Staphylococcus aureus,* and the patient should be treated accordingly. However, if the patient does not respond clinically and the sedimentation rate does not begin to fall within a couple of weeks, surgical intervention is indicated in the form of disk space debridement, often with the accompaniment of anterior fusion. Culture should then be repeated, and the patient should be given a broad-spectrum antibiotic.

Debridement and anterior fusion supplemented with posterior instrumentation and fusion are indicated in all cases of vertebral body collapse and instability (Figs. 12.8, 12.9).

Monitoring the Treatment and Complications of Spinal Infections

Radiography plays an indispensable role in monitoring the treatment of infectious disorders of the spine and adjacent soft tissues. Follow-up radiographs and radionuclide bone scan should be obtained at regular intervals to evaluate the disease state (acute, subacute, chronic, or inactive) and any complications that may arise. The differentiation of active from inactive osteomyelitis may, however, be extremely difficult on the basis of radiologic techniques alone. The extensive osteosclerotic changes of inactive infection may obscure small foci of osteolytic change that signify reactivation. Tomography is sometimes helpful in delineating fluffy periostitis, poorly marginated areas of osteolysis, and sequestra. Scintigraphy, particularly with gallium and indium-labeled white blood cells, and occasionally MRI, may be of further assistance in monitoring the progress of treatment.

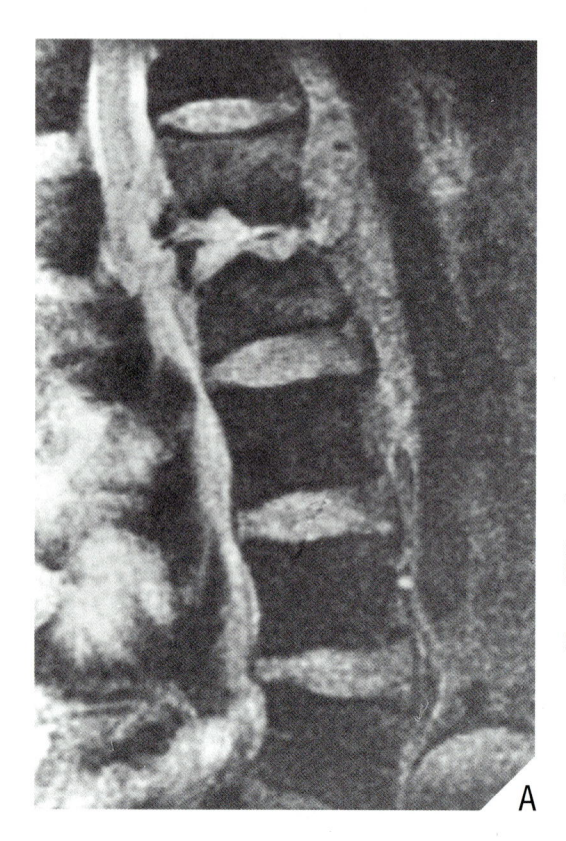

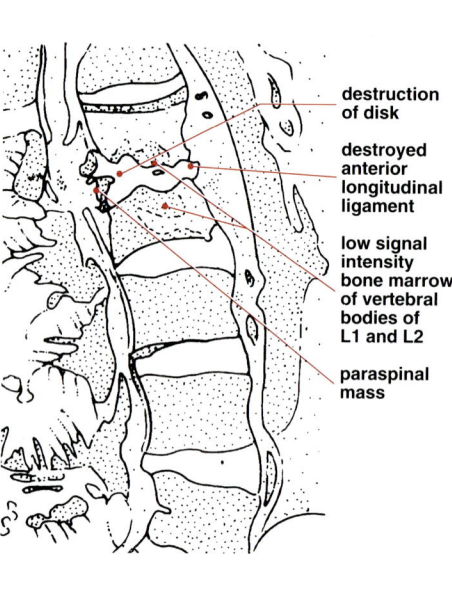

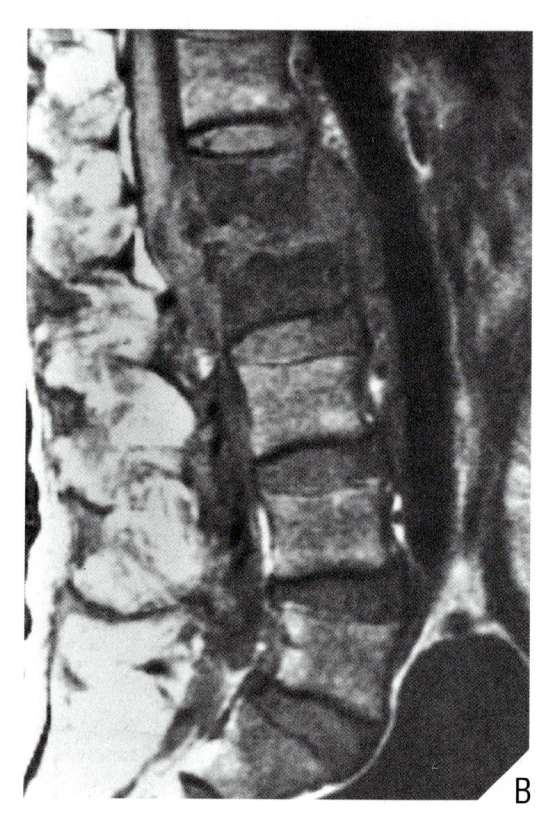

FIGURE 12.7 Vertebral osteomyelitis and disk space infection is well shown on MR images. **(A)** T1-weighted spin-echo sagittal MR demonstrates low signal intensity of the bone marrow of the vertebral bodies L1 and L2. Note destruction of the disk and a large paraspinal mass, posteriorly compressing thecal sac, and anteriorly destroying anterior longitudinal ligament. **(B)** Gradient-echo (MPGR) T2*-weighted sagittal MRI shows foci of high signal intensity in the affected vertebral bodies. The signal from the infected disk is also increased.

Imaging of the Spine in Clinical Practice

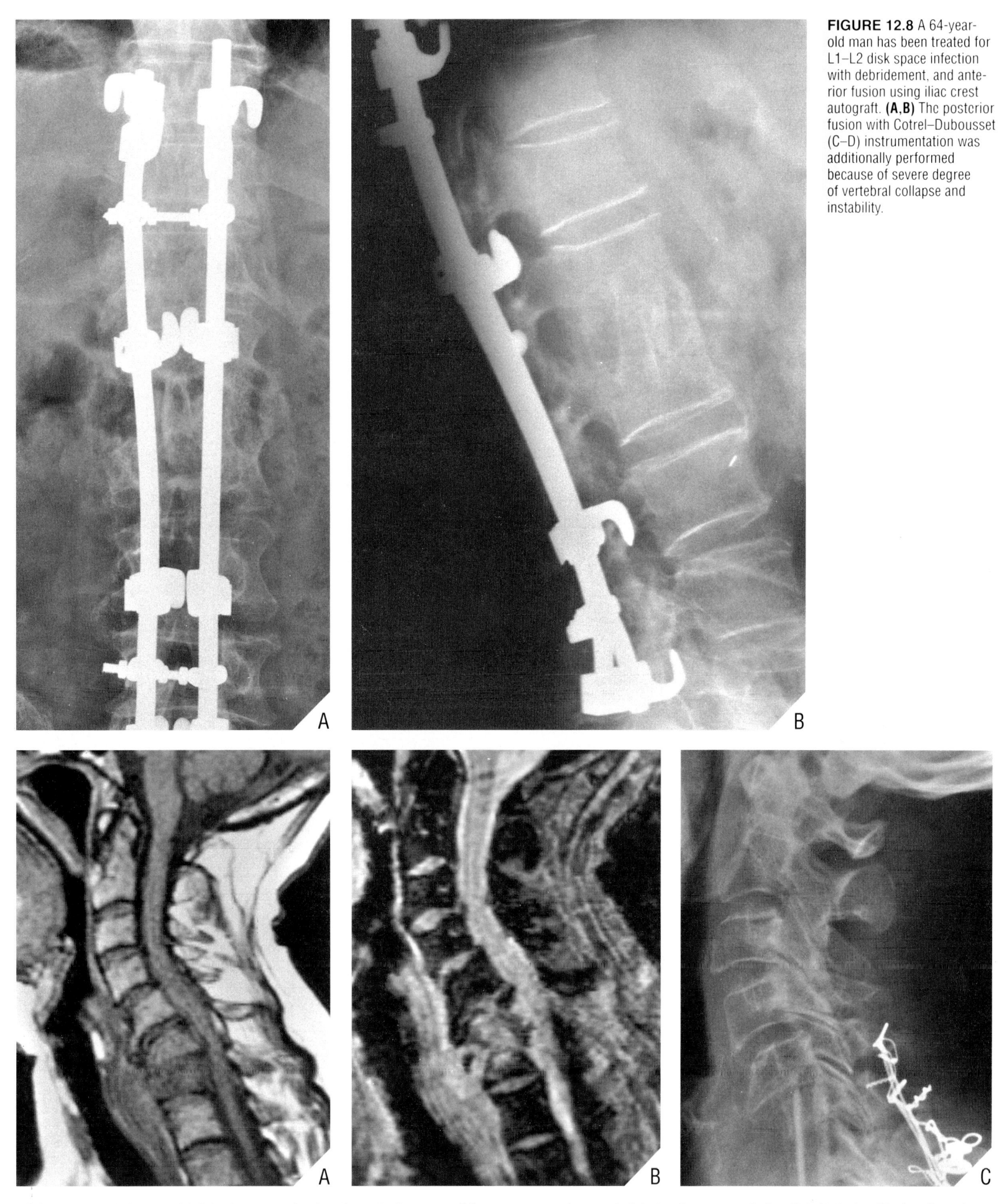

FIGURE 12.8 A 64-year-old man has been treated for L1–L2 disk space infection with debridement, and anterior fusion using iliac crest autograft. **(A,B)** The posterior fusion with Cotrel–Dubousset (C–D) instrumentation was additionally performed because of severe degree of vertebral collapse and instability.

FIGURE 12.9 A 64-year-old diabetic woman developed vertebral osteomyelitis and disk space infection at C6–C7. **(A)** Sagittal T1-weighted spin-echo MRI (TR600/TE20) shows decreased signal of the affected vertebrae, narrowing of the disk space C6–C7 associated with kyphotic deformity and a paravertebral soft tissue mass anteriorly. **(B)** Sagittal T2*-weighted gradient-echo (MPGR) MRI demonstrates the extent of destructive process better. Note high signal in the affected vertebral bodies, and impingement on the thecal sac and spinal cord by epidural abscess. **(C)** Treatment consisted of vertebrectomy, intravertebral fusion with allograft (fibular strut), and posterior fusion with the wires.

Radiologic Evaluation and Treatment of Infections of the Spine

Suggested Reading

Al-Sheikh W, Sfakianakis GN, Mnaymneh W, et al: Subacute and chronic bone infections: Diagnosis using In-111, Ga-67 and Tc-99m MDP bone scintigraphy, and radiography. *Radiology* 155:501, 1985.

Bassett LW, Gold RH, Webber MM: Radionuclide bone imaging. *Radiol Clin North Am* 19:675, 1981.

Beltran J, Noto AM, McGhee RB, et al: Infections of the musculoskeletal system: High-field-strength MR imaging. *Radiology* 164:449, 1987.

Bruno MS, Silverberg TN, Goldstein DH: Embolic osteomyelitis of the spine as a complication of infection of the urinary tract. *Am J Med* 29:865, 1960.

Butt WP: The radiology of infection. *Clin Orthop* 96:20, 1973.

David R, Barron BJ, Madewell JE: Osteomyelitis, acute and chronic. *Radiol Clin North Am* 25:1171, 1987.

Erdman WA, Tamburro F, Jayson HT, et al: Osteomyelitis: Characteristics and pitfalls of diagnosis with MR imaging. *Radiology* 180:533, 1991.

Fletcher BD, Scoles PV, Nelson AD: Osteomyelitis in children: Detection by magnetic resonance. *Radiology* 150:57, 1984.

Gilmour WM: Acute haematogenous osteomyelitis. *J Bone Joint Surg* 44B:841, 1962.

Graves VB, Schreiber MN: Tuberculous psoas muscle abscess. *J Can Assoc Radiol* 24:268, 1973.

Guyot DR, Manoli A II, King GA: Pyogenic sacroiliitis in IV drug users. *Am J Roentgenol* 149:1209, 1987.

Hoffer P: Gallium: Mechanisms. *J Nucl Med* 21:282, 1980.

Israel O, Gips S, Jerushalmi J, et al: Osteomyelitis and soft-tissue infection: Differential diagnosis with 24 hour/4 hour ratios of Tc-99m MDP uptake. *Radiology* 163:724, 1987.

Jacobson AF, Harley JD, Lipsky BA, et al: Diagnosis of osteomyelitis in the presence of soft-tissue infection and radiologic evidence of osseous abnormalities: Value of leukocyte scintigraphy. *Am J Roentgenol* 157:807, 1991.

Kido D, Bryan D, Halpren M: Hematogenous osteomyelitis in drug addicts. *Am J Roentgenol* 118:356, 1973.

Larcos G, Brown ML, Sutton RT: Diagnosis of osteomyelitis of the foot in diabetic patients: Value of ^{111}In-leukocyte scintigraphy. *Am J Roentgenol* 157:527, 1991.

Lewin JS, Rosenfield NS, Hoffer PB, et al: Acute osteomyelitis in children: Combined Tc-99m and Ga-67 imaging. *Radiology* 158:795, 1986.

Lisbona R, Rosenthal L: Observations on the sequential use of 99m Tc-phosphate complex and 67 Ga in osteomyelitis, cellulitis and septic arthritis. *Radiology* 123:123, 1977.

Merkel KD, Brown ML, Dewanjee MK, et al: Comparison of indium-labeled-leukocyte imaging with sequential technetium-gallium scanning in the diagnosis of low-grade musculoskeletal sepsis. A prospective study. *J Bone Joint Surg* 67A:465, 1985.

Modic MT, Feiglin DH, Piraino DW, et al: Vertebral osteomyelitis: Assessment using MR. *Radiology* 157:157, 1985.

Modic MT, Pflanze W, Feiglin DHI, et al: Magnetic resonance imaging of musculoskeletal infections. *Radiol Clin North Am* 24:247, 1986.

Renfrew DL, Whitten CG, Wiese JA, et al: CT-guided percutaneous transpedicular biopsy of the spine. *Radiology* 180:574, 1991.

Ruppert D, Barron BJ, Madewell JE: Osteomyelitis, acute and chronic. *Radiol Clin North Am* 1171, 1987.

Trueta J: The three types of acute, haematogenous osteomyelitis. *J Bone Joint Surg* 41B:671, 1959.

Schauwecker DS: Osteomyelitis: Diagnosis with In-111-labeled leukocytes. *Radiology* 171:141, 1989.

Tsan M: Mechanism of gallium-67 accumulation in inflammatory lesions. *J Nucl Med* 26:88, 1985.

Tumeh SS, Aliabadi PA, Weissmann BN, et al: Chronic osteomyelitis: Bone and gallium scan patterns associated with active disease. *Radiology* 158:685, 1986.

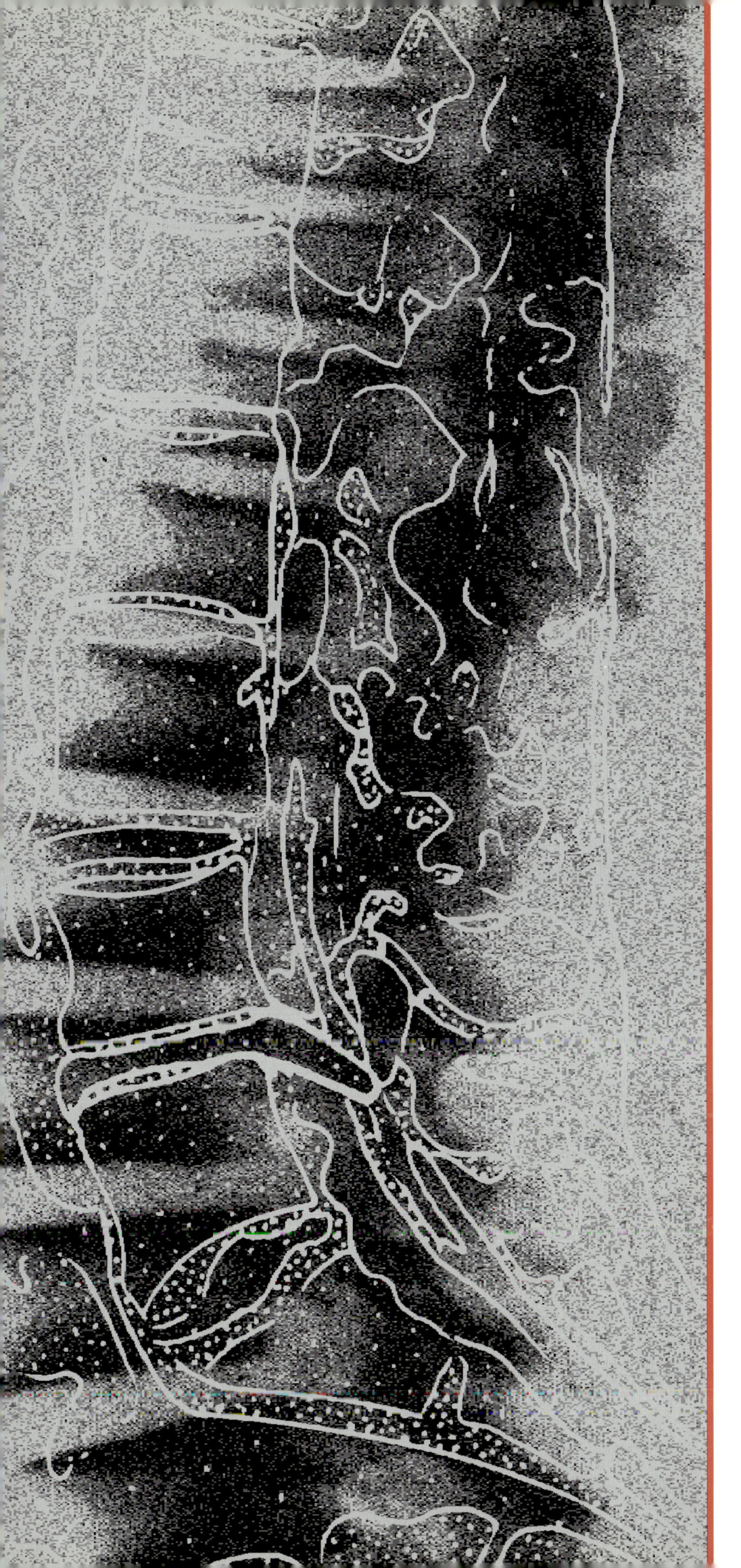

Pyogenic and Nonpyogenic Infections of the Spine

13

Pyogenic Infections

Infectious organisms can reach the spine by several routes. Hematogenous spread occurs via arterial and venous routes (Batson's paravertebral venous system) and the organism lodges in the vertebral body, commonly in the anterior subchondral region. This osteomyelitic focus can spread to the intervertebral disk through perforation of the vertebral endplate, causing disk space infection (diskitis) (Fig. 13.1). Disk space infection can also be induced directly by implantation of an organism through a puncture of the spinal canal, during spinal surgery or, rarely, by spread from a contiguous site of infection such as a paravertebral abscess (see Fig. 13.1). Disk infection can also occur in children via the hematogenous route, because there is still a blood supply to the disk.

Radiographically, disk infection is characterized by narrowing of the disk space, destruction of the adjacent vertebral endplates, and a paraspinal mass. Although most cases are obvious on standard anteroposterior and lateral films of the spine (Fig. 13.2; see also Figs. 12.2, 12.3A), conventional and computed tomography may yield additional information (Fig. 12.3B). Radionuclide bone scanning can detect early infection before any changes can be observed on radiograph (Fig. 13.3). Occasionally diskography is performed, but as with the use of arthrography in joint infections, the primary objective is to obtain a specimen for bacteriologic examination. A contrast study, however, may outline the extent of a disk infection (see Fig. 12.6).

Recently, MRI has become the a modality of choice for diagnosis and evaluation of infections of the spine. Characteristic findings of disk space narrowing, disk destruction, paraspinal soft tissue mass, and edematous changes in the paraspinal musculature are well demonstrated (Fig. 13.4). In addition, the involvement of the thecal sac and spinal cord may be more accurately shown than on CT (Fig. 13.5).

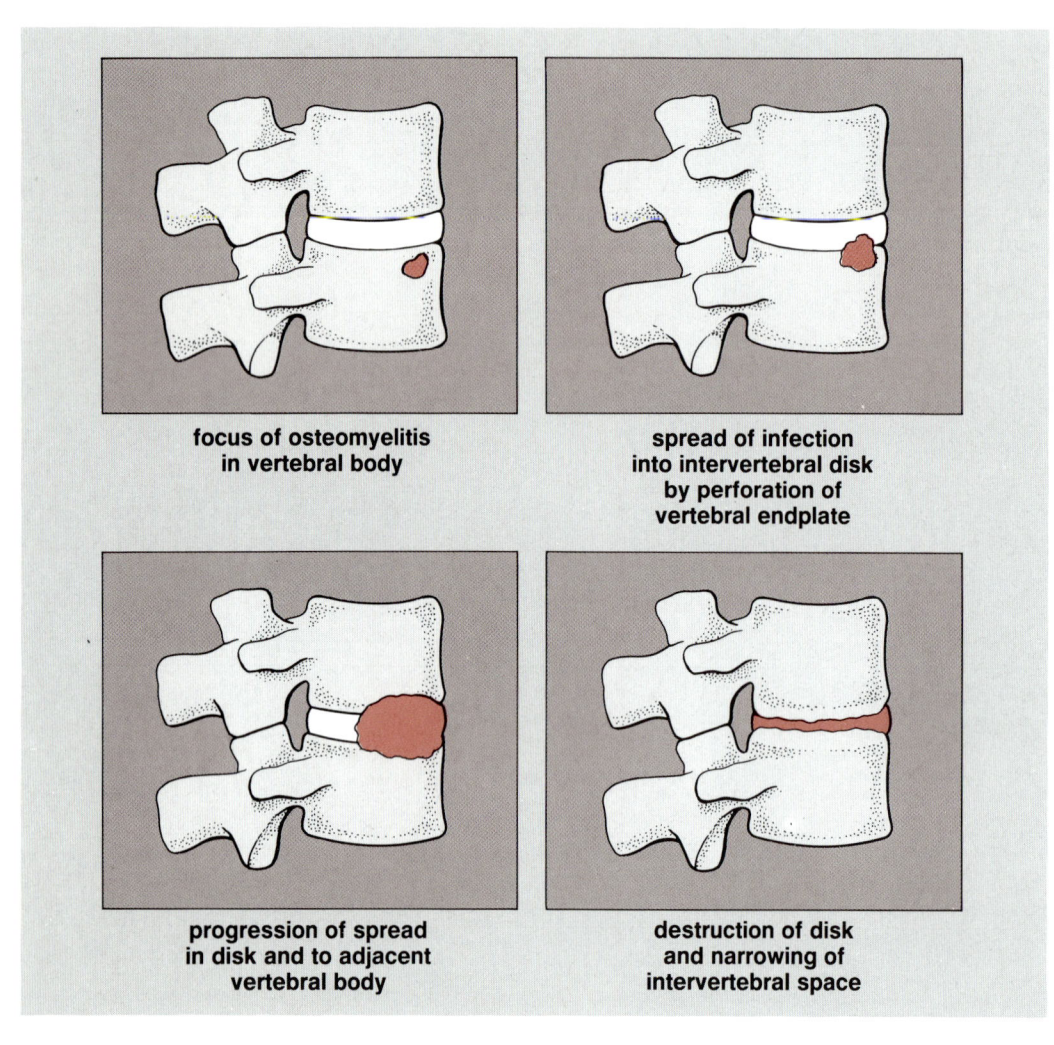

FIGURE 13.1 Sequential stages of involvement of a vertebral body and disk by an infectious process.

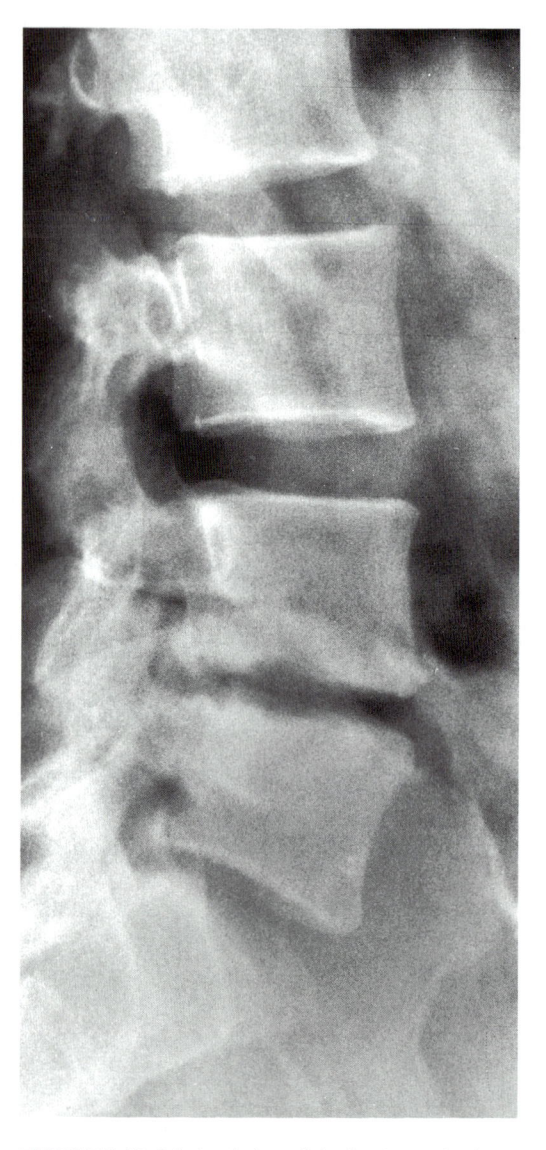

FIGURE 13.2 Lateral view of the lumbar spine in a 32-year-old man demonstrates the typical radiographic changes of disk infection. There is narrowing of the disk space at L4–L5, and the inferior endplate of L4 and superior endplate of L5 are indistinctly outlined. Note the normal endplates at the L3–L4 disk space.

Imaging of the Spine in Clinical Practice

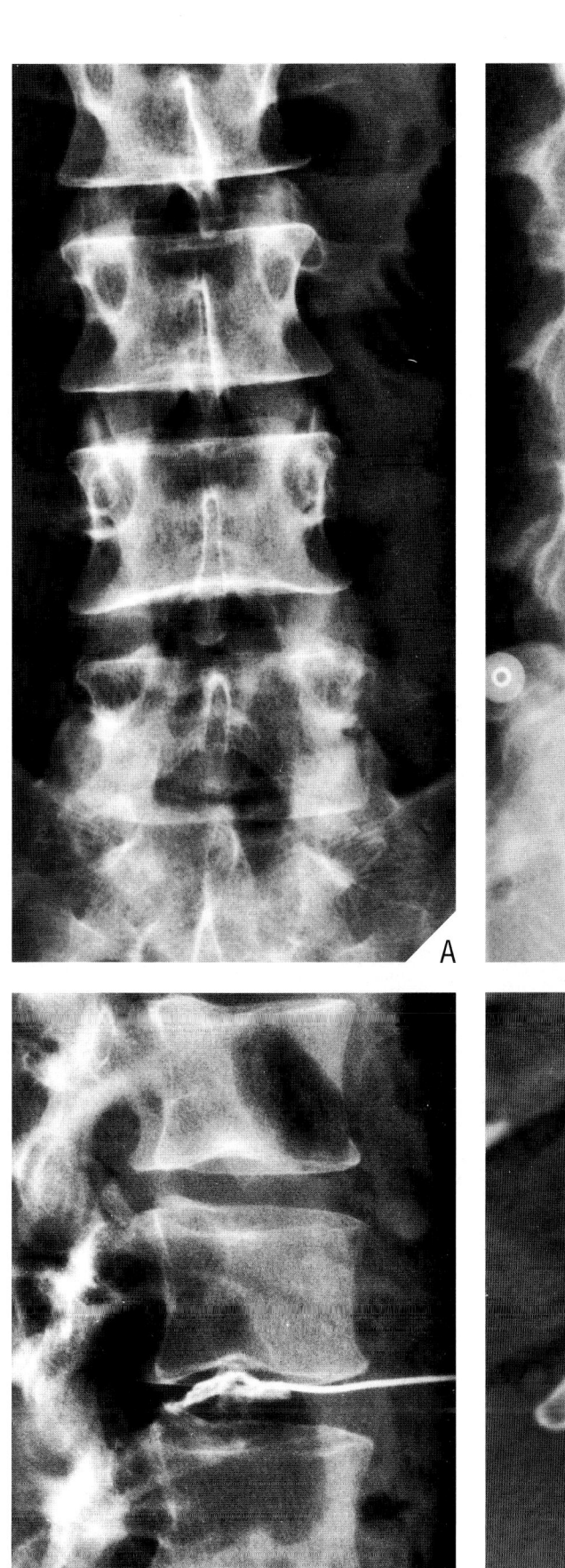

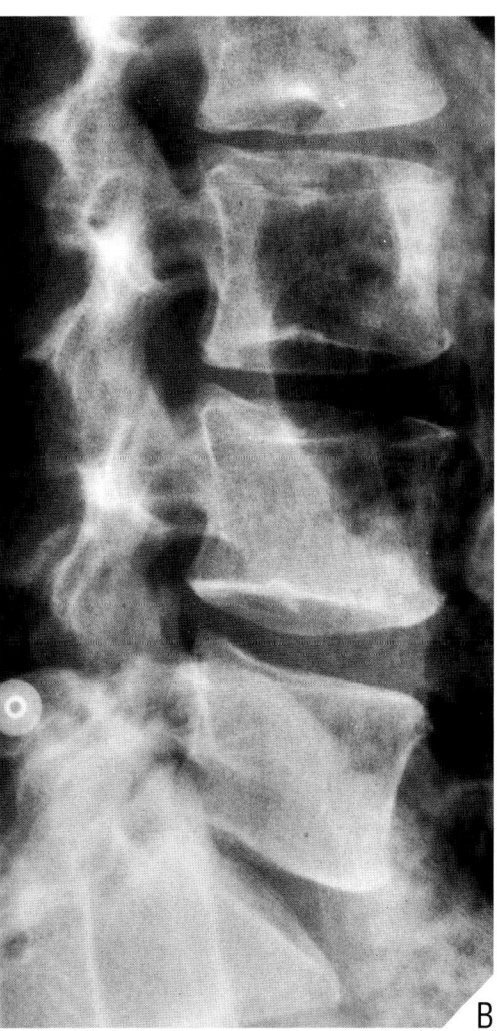

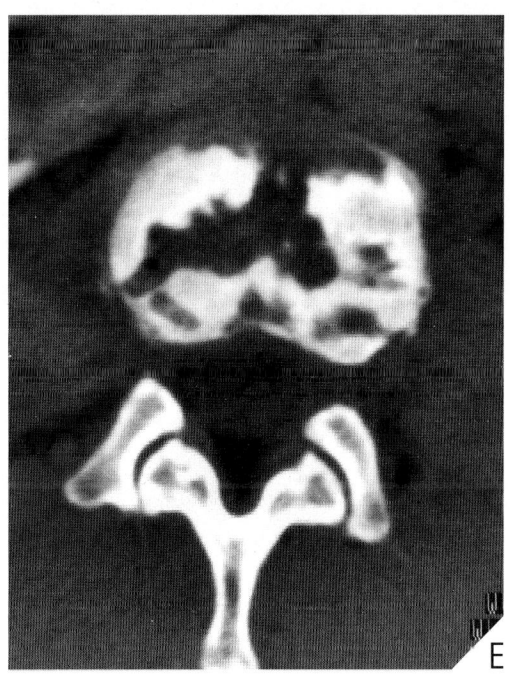

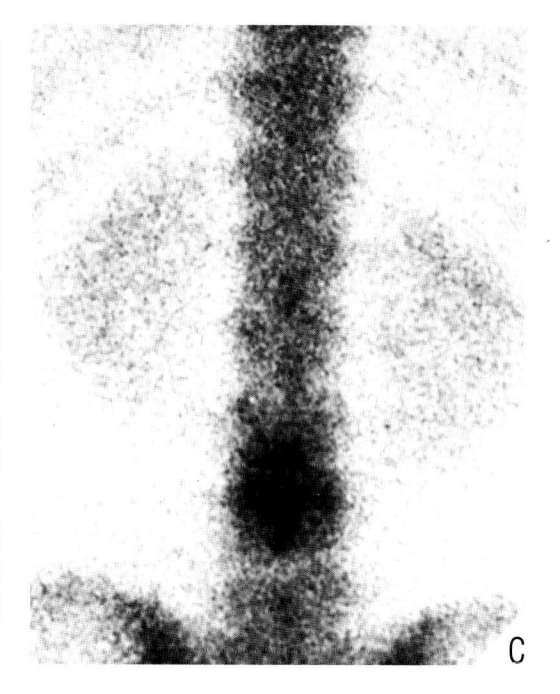

FIGURE 13.3 Standard anteroposterior **(A)** and lateral **(B)** radiographs of the lumbar spine of a 40-year-old man who complained of back pain for 4 weeks show no definite abnormalities. **(C)** Bone scan, however, reveals increased uptake of radio-pharmaceutical at the L3–L4 level. **(D)** On a subsequent diskogram, using the lateral approach, partial disk destruction is evident. **(E)** The extent of destruction is revealed by a CT scan. Bacteriologic examination of aspirated fluid yielded *Escherichia coli*.

Pyogenic and Nonpyogenic Infections of the Spine

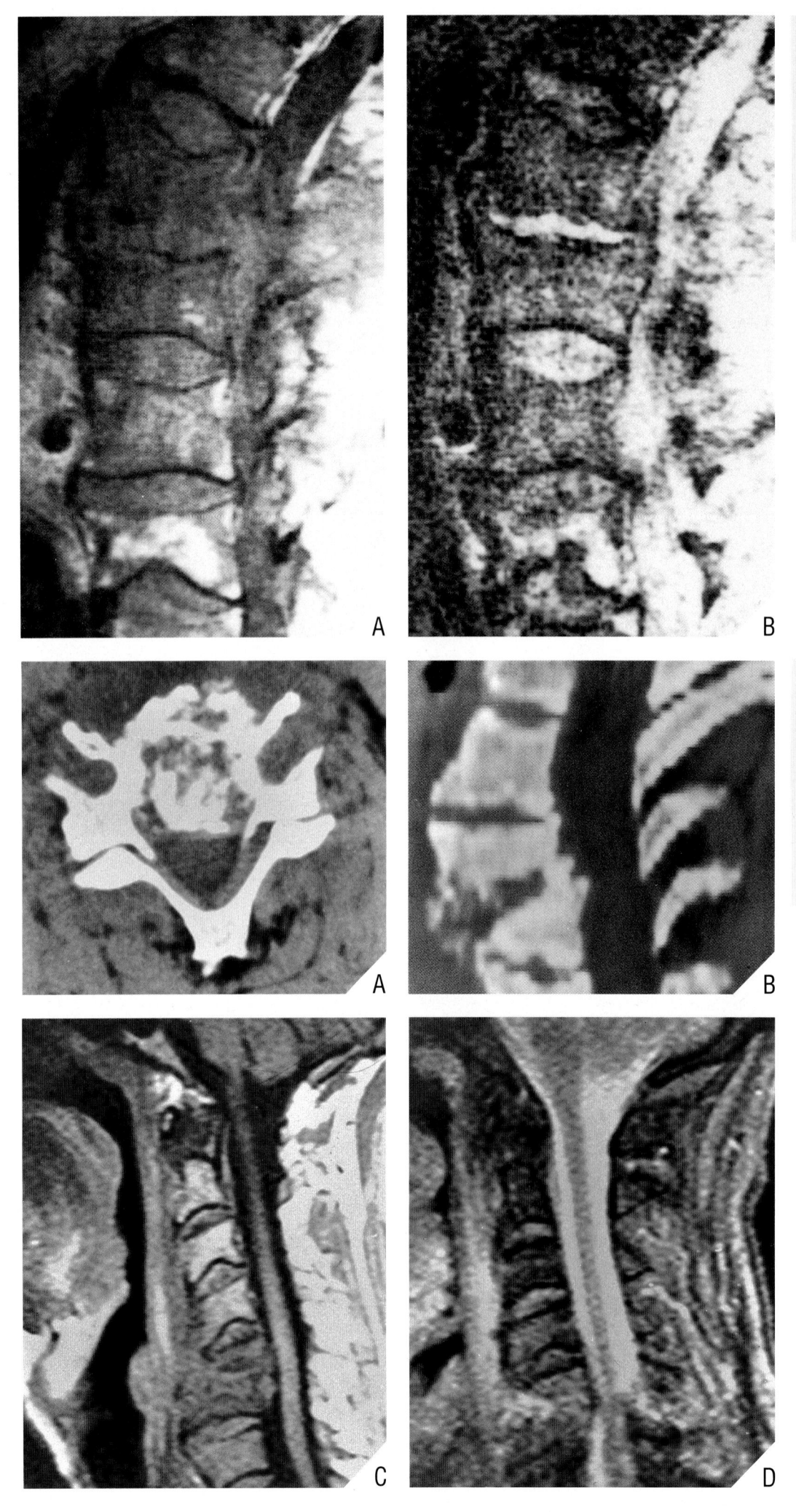

FIGURE 13.4 (A) Sagittal proton density-weighted spin-echo MR image (TR2000/TE20) in a patient who developed postsurgical disk space infection shows L4–L5 disk space narrowing, decreased signal intensity of adjacent vertebral bodies, indistinct vertebral endplates, and an extradural mass. **(B)** Sagittal T2-weighted spin-echo MR image (TR2000/TE80) demonstrates unusually bright signal of the infected disk L4–L5 and destruction of the posterior longitudinal ligament. (Reproduced with permission from Beltran J: *MRI: Musculoskeletal System.* New York, Gower, 1990)

FIGURE 13.5 A 43-year-old drug user developed disk space infection at C5–C6. A CT section through the disk space **(A)** and sagittal reformation image **(B)** show destruction of the disk and adjacent vertebral bodies; however, the involvement of the thecal sac cannot be accurately assessed. The parasagittal T1-weighted spin-echo MRI (TR400/TE20) shows not only the disk space and bony destruction, but also a soft tissue extension of infectious process with impingement on the ventral aspect of the thecal sac **(C)**. The midline sagittal T2-weighted spin-echo MRI (TR2000/TE20) in addition shows compression of the spinal cord by extradural mass **(D)**.

Imaging of the Spine in Clinical Practice

TUBERCULOSIS OF THE SPINE

Infection of the spine by the tubercle bacillus is known as *tuberculous spondylitis* or *Pott disease*. The vertebral body, intervertebral disk, or both, may be involved, the lower thoracic and upper lumbar vertebrae being the preferred sites of infection (Fig. 13.6). The disease constitutes 25% to 50% of all cases of skeletal tuberculosis.

The radiographic features of tuberculous infection of the spine are similar to those seen in pyogenic infections. There is disk space narrowing and the vertebral endplates adjacent to the involved disk show evidence of destruction. A paraspinal mass is common (Fig. 13.7). Rarely, the infectious process may destroy a single vertebra or part of a vertebra (pedicle) without invasion of the disk (Fig. 13.8).

Complications

Tuberculosis of the spine may cause the collapse of a partially or completely destroyed vertebra, leading to kyphosis and a gibbous formation (Fig. 13.9). Extension of infection to the adjacent ligaments and soft tissues is also rather common; the psoas muscles are often the site of secondary tuberculous infections, commonly called "cold" abscesses (Fig. 13.10). CT is an effective modality to demonstrate the presence and extent

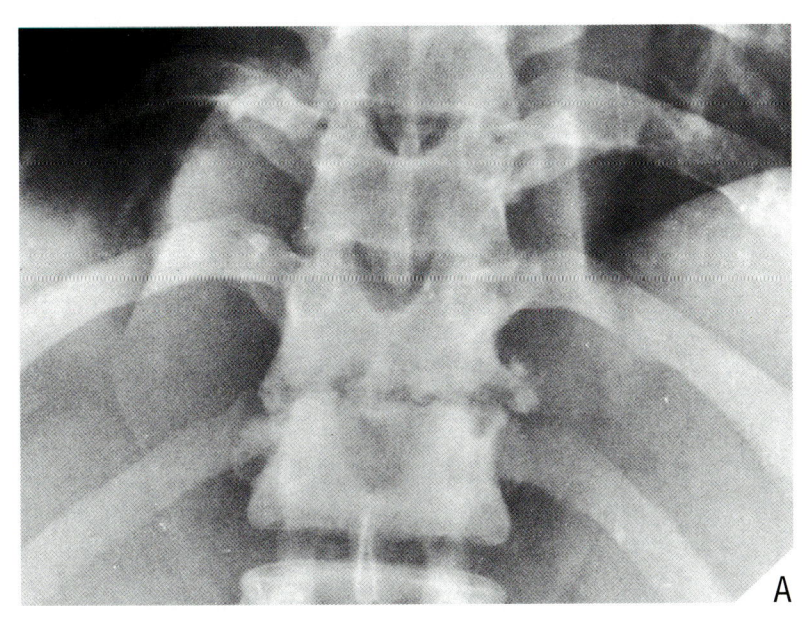

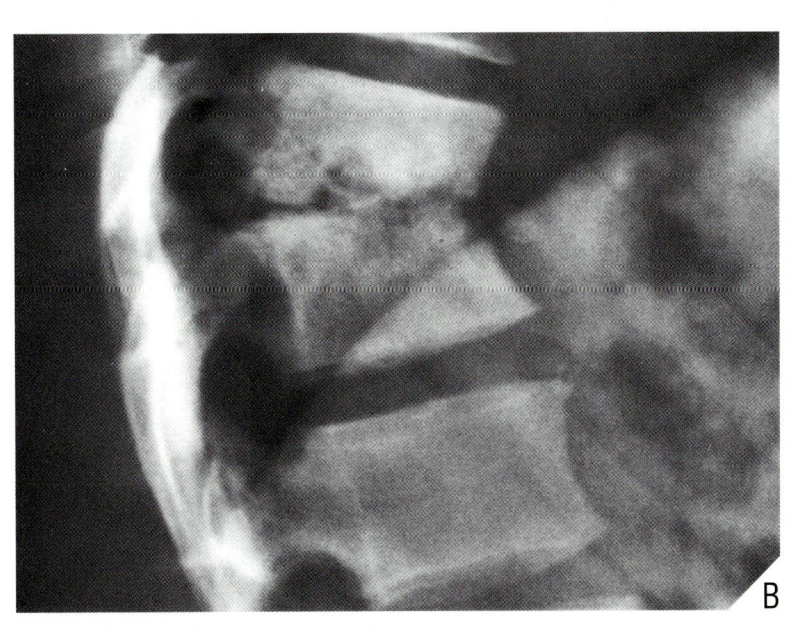

FIGURE 13.6 A 37-year-old man from India presented with pain in the lower thoracic spine. **(A)** Anteroposterior and **(B)** lateral-radiographs show characteristic features of spinal tuberculosis: involvement of T11–T12 disk space, destruction of adjacent vertebral bodies with gibbous formation, and a large, paraspinal mass with calcifications.

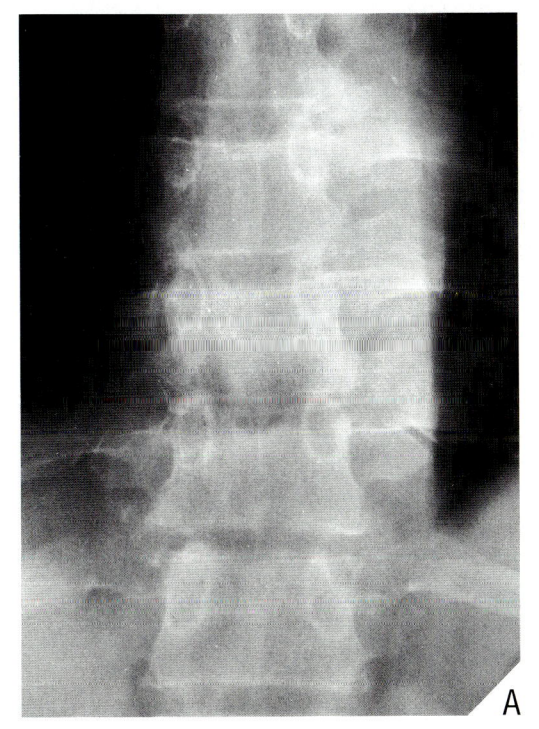

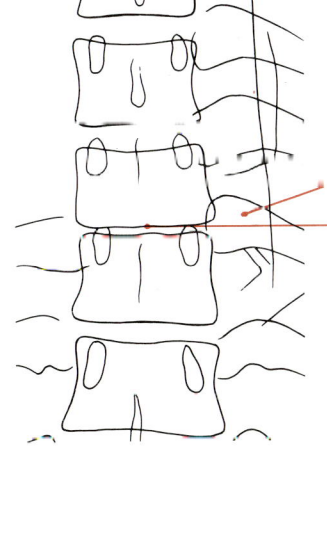

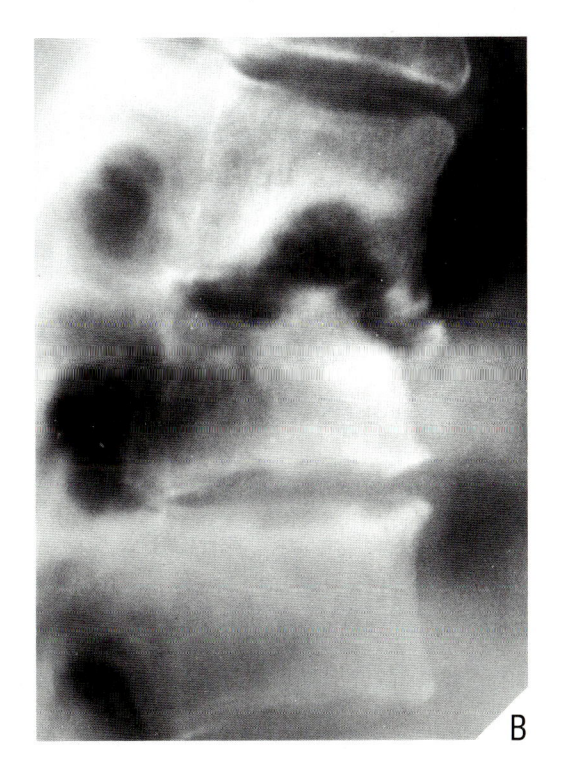

FIGURE 13.7 (A) Anteroposterior view of the thoracic spine in a 50-year-old man with tuberculosis spondylitis shows narrowing of the T8–T9 disk space, associated with a paraspinal mass on the left side. **(B)** Lateral tomogram shows destruction of the disk and extensive erosion of the inferior aspect of the body of T8.

Pyogenic and Nonpyogenic Infections of the Spine

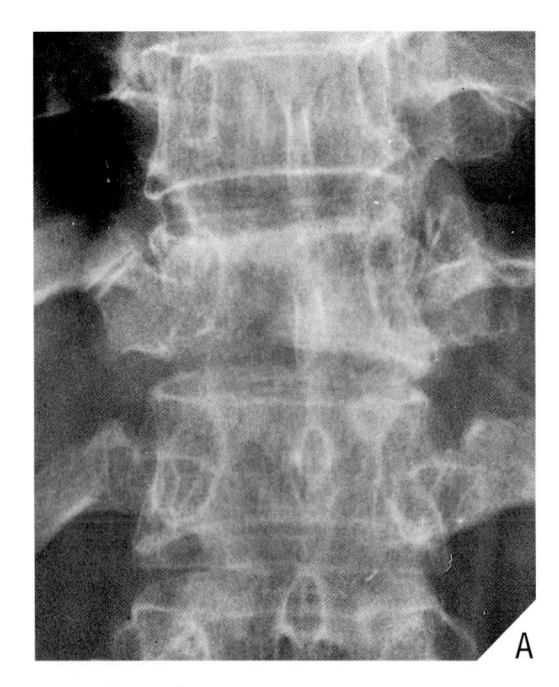

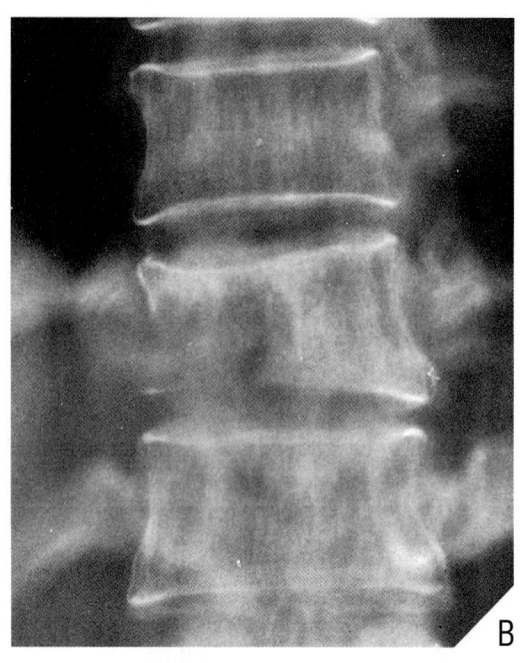

FIGURE 13.8 A 61-year-old woman, native of Puerto Rico, known to have pulmonary tuberculosis for many years, presented with a back pain of 3 months' duration. An anteroposterior film of the lower thoracic spine **(A)** and tomogram **(B)** show destructive changes of the vertebral body and pedicle of T10, without involvement of the disk space. This is an unusual presentation of spinal tuberculosis.

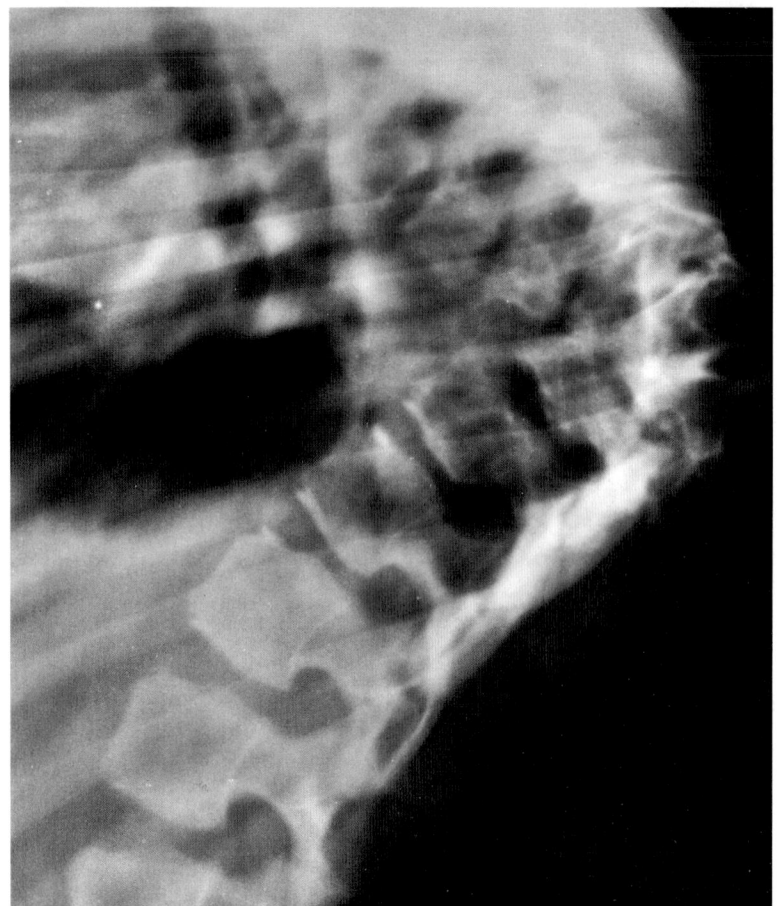

FIGURE 13.9 Lateral radiograph of the lower thoracic spine in a 12-year-old boy with longstanding pulmonary and spinal tuberculosis shows a gibbous formation at the site of a collapsed vertebra, a common complication of this condition. The severe kyphotic curve measures 110°.

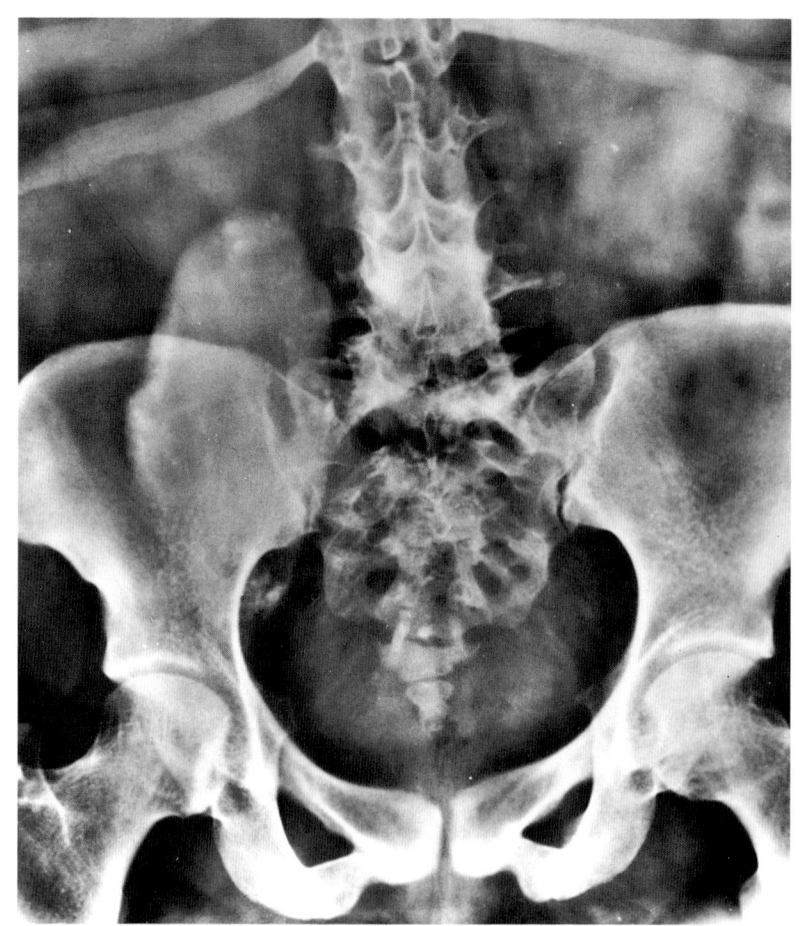

FIGURE 13.10 Anteroposterior film of the pelvis in a 35-year-old woman with spinal tuberculosis shows an oval radiodense mass with spotted calcifications overlapping the medial part of the ilium and right sacroiliac joint (right psoas muscle). This is the typical appearance of a "cold" abscess.

of this complication (Fig. 13.11). The most common complication of tuberculous spondylitis, however, is compression of the thecal sac and spinal cord, with resulting paraplegia. Myelography is very helpful in diagnosis when compression is suspected (Fig. 13.12).

Fungal Infections

Fungal infections of the spine are rare. The organism usually responsible for infections are *Cryptococcus neoformans,* causing cryptococcosis (torulosis), *Blastomyces dermatitidis* causing blastomycosis (North American), *Coccidioides immitis,* causing coccidioidomycosis, *Histoplasma capsulatum,* causing histoplasmosis, *Sporothrix schenckii,* causing sporotrichosis, and *Candida albicans,* causing candidiasis (moniliasis). In the United States, probably the most common spinal infection caused by the fungi is coccidioidomycosis.

Coccidioidomycosis is a systemic infection caused by the soil fungus *Coccidiodes immitis,* and is endemic in northern Mexico and the southwest part of the United States including Texas, New Mexico, Arizona, and California.

Skeletal coccidioidomycosis is the result of dissemination of the fungus from its primary pulmonary focus, or focus from elsewhere in the body. The reported incidence of disseminated coccidioidomycosis with bone involvement is 10% to 50%. The focus of coccidioidomycosis in bone is demonstrated radiographically as an osteolytic lesion with permeative or "moth-eaten" type of bone destruction. The next most common radiographic appearance is an osteolytic punch-out or well-circumscribed lesion without or, less frequently, with sclerotic borders. The spine is the

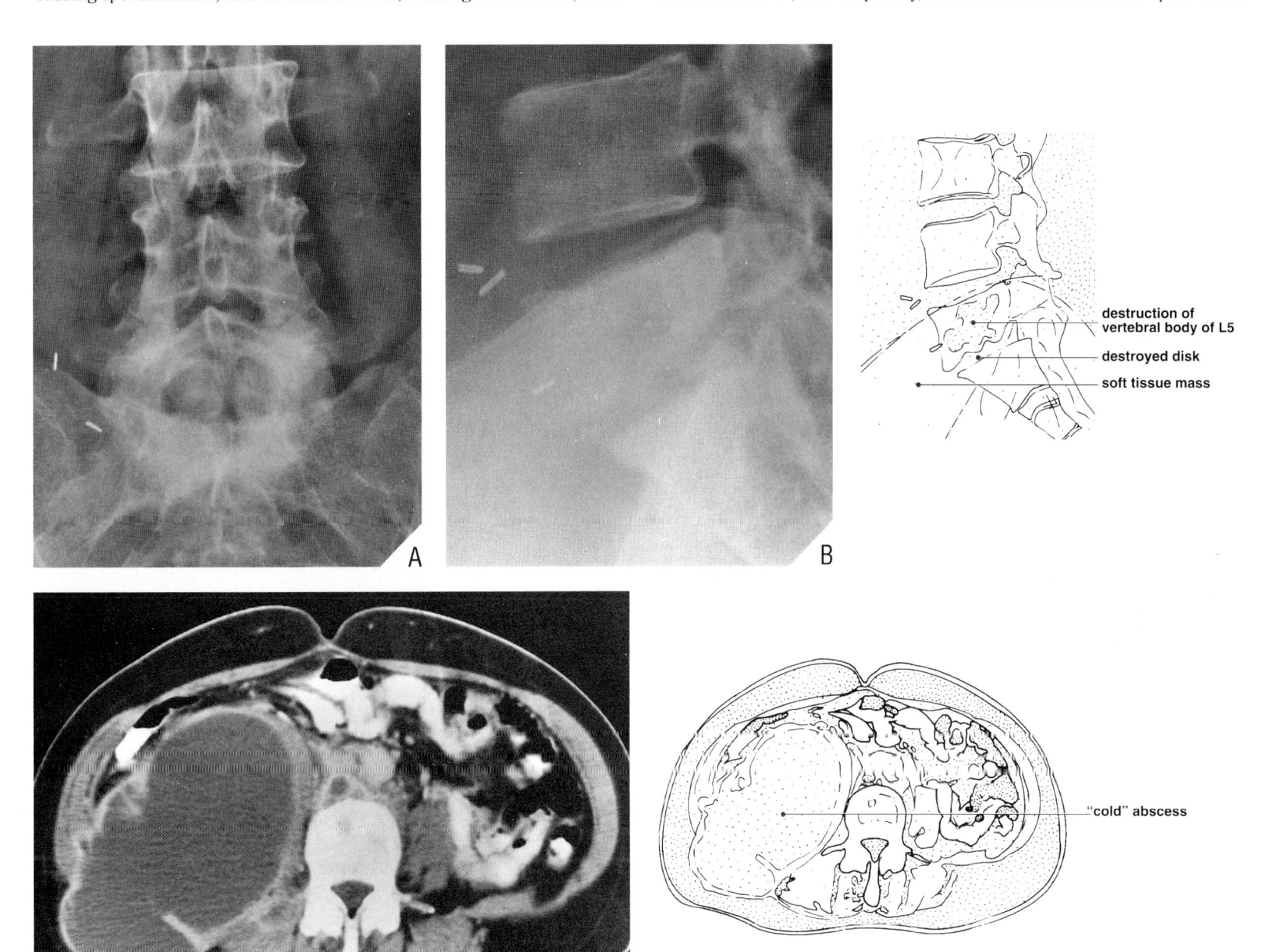

FIGURE 13.11 A 41-year-old Chinese woman with documented spinal tuberculosis developed secondary tuberculous infection of the right psoas muscle—a "cold" abscess. Anteroposterior **(A)** and lateral **(B)** views of the lower lumbar spine show infectious process destroying the vertebral body L5 and the disk L5–S1. The outline of the right psoas muscle is obscured and soft tissue prominence is seen anterolaterally. **(C)** Computed tomography section clearly shows the presence and extent of a "cold" abscess.

most common site of bone infection in disseminated coccidioidomycosis. Usually there are well-demarcated radiolucent lesions with or without evidence of endosteal new bone formation (Fig. 13.13). The pedicles may be involved, and a paraspinal soft tissue mass or abscess often forms. Indiscriminate destruction of adjoining vertebral bodies and their appendages is common, with relative disk space preservation, since the avascular intervertebral disk is a barrier to the organism, and the disk space is usually spared until the local bony disease has progressed. Unlike in spinal tuberculosis, gibbous formation in coccidioidomycotic spondylitis is rare.

Soft Tissue Infections

Soft tissue infections (cellulitis) usually result from direct introduction of organisms through a skin puncture; they are also seen as a complication of systemic disorders, such as diabetes. The most frequently encountered organisms are *Clostridium novyi* and *Clostridium perfringens*. These gas-forming organisms may cause an accumulation of gas in the soft tissues, which can easily be recognized on plain films as radiolucent bubbles or streaks in the subcutaneous tissues or muscles. This finding usually indi-

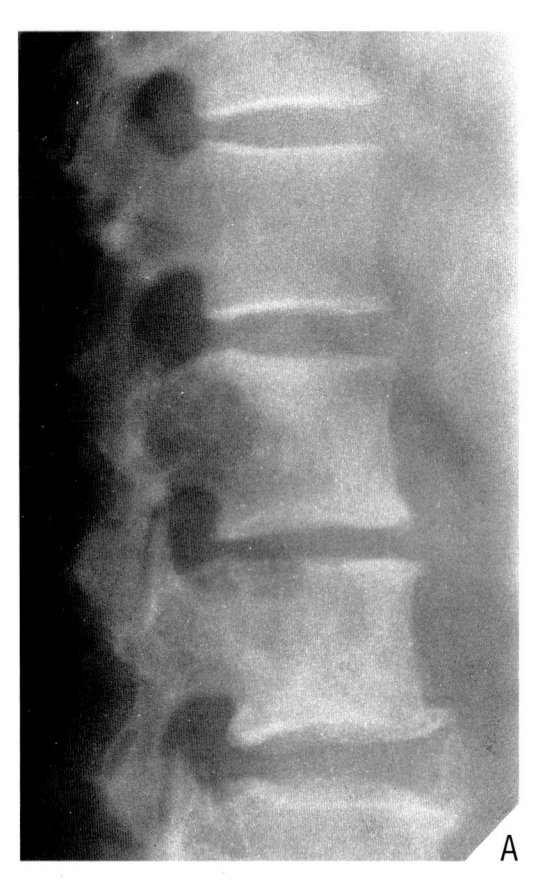

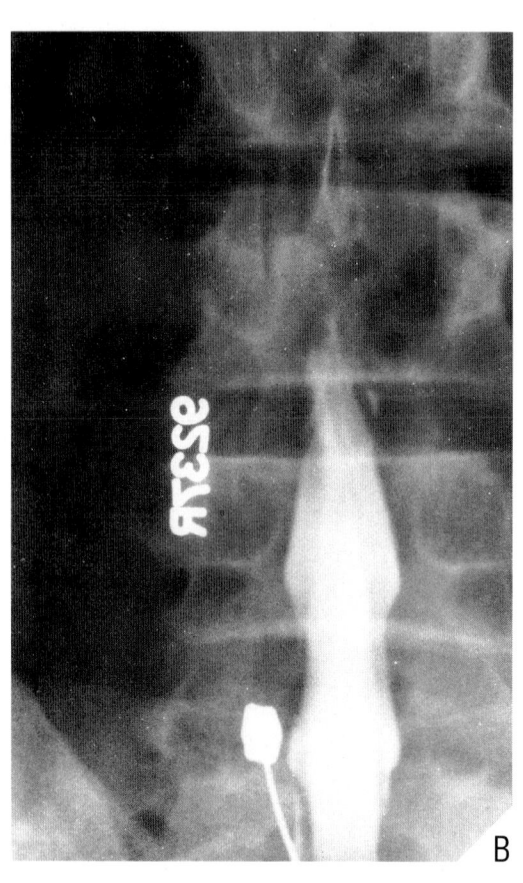

FIGURE 13.12 A 47-year-old man presented with back pain of 5 months' duration. Later, he developed numbing sensations in the lower extremities. Lateral radiograph **(A)** shows a lytic destruction of the posterior parts of vertebral bodies L2 and L3 and their respective pedicles. The disk space is narrowed. Anteroposterior radiograph obtained during myelographic examination **(B)** shows complete epidural block to the flow of contrast, due to compression of the thecal sac by tuberculous abscess.

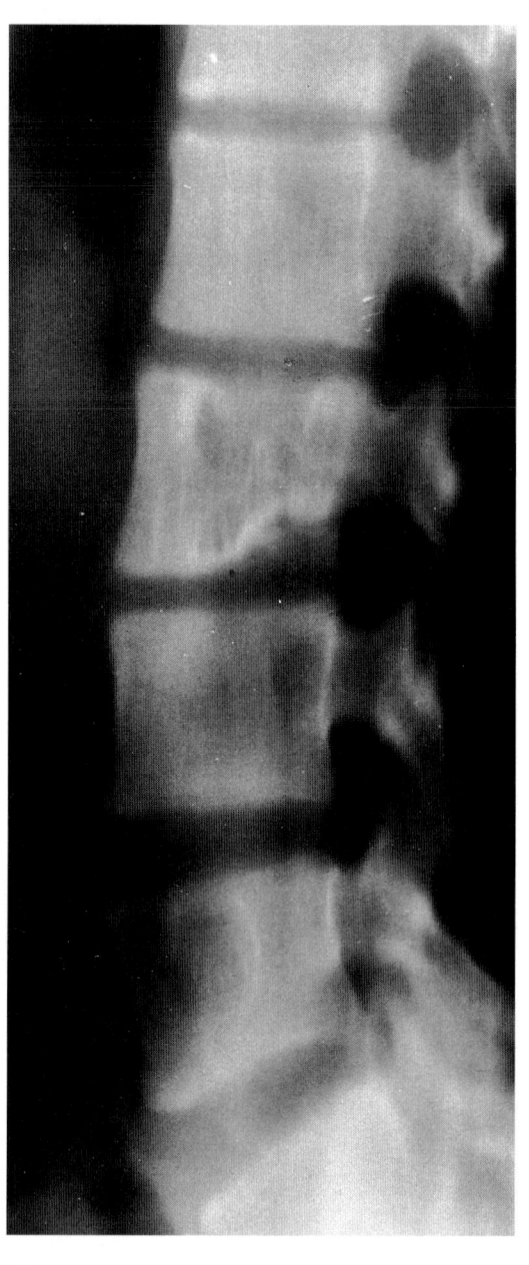

FIGURE 13.13 A 21-year-old man presented with increasing low back pain for a few months. The patient was previously diagnosed as having pulmonary coccidioidomycosis. The lateral tomogram of lumbar spine shows multiple, well-marginated osteolytic lesions affecting vertebral bodies of, L2, L3, L4, and L5. Some lesions show sclerotic border. The intervertebral disk spaces are relatively well preserved. (Courtesy of John P. McGahan, M.D., Sacramento, CA)

cates gangrene caused by anaerobic bacteria. Soft tissue edema and obliteration of fat and fascial planes are also evident on the standard examination.

Recently, MRI has been applied to evaluation of paraspinal soft tissue infection. In particular, soft tissue abscesses and involvement of muscles were accurately depicted with this modality. Soft tissue abscesses appear as rounded or elongated, well-demarcated areas showing decreased signal intensity on T1-weighted images, and increased signal intensity on T2-weighted images. Occasionally a peripheral band of decreased signal intensity is seen, which represents the fibrous capsule surrounding the abscess.

Suggested Reading

Bruno MS, Silverberg TN, Goldstein DH: Embolic osteomyelitis of the spine as a complication of infection of the urinary tract. *Am J Med* 29:865, 1960.

David R, Barron BJ, Madewell JE: Osteomyelitis, acute and chronic. *Radiol Clin North Am* 25:1171, 1987.

Fletcher BD, Scoles PV, Nelson AD: Osteomyelitis in children: Detection by magnetic resonance. *Radiology* 150:57, 1984.

Gilmour WM: Acute haematogenous osteomyelitis. *J Bone Joint Surg* 44B:841, 1962.

Graves VB, Schreiber MN: Tuberculous psoas muscle abscess. *J Can Assoc Radiol* 24:268, 1973.

Guyot DR, Manoli A II, King GA: Pyogenic sacroillitis in IV drug users. *AJR* 149:1209, 1987.

Kido D, Bryan D, Halpren M: Hematogenous osteomyelitis in drug addicts. *AJR* 118:356, 1973.

McGahan JP, Graves DS, Palmer PES: Coccidioidal spondylitis. Usual and unusual radiographic manifestations. *Radiology* 136:5, 1980.

McGahan JP, Graves DS, Palmer PES, et al: Classic and contemporary imaging of coccidioidomycosis.

Modic MT, Feiglin DH, Piraino DW, et al: Vertebral osteomyelitis: Assessment using MR. *Radiology* 157:157, 1985.

Ruppert D, Barron BJ, Madewell JE: Osteomyelitis, acute and chronic. *Radiol Clin North Am* 25:1171, 1987

Trueta J: The three types of acute, haematogenous osteomyelitis. *J Bone Joint Surg* 41B:671, 1987.

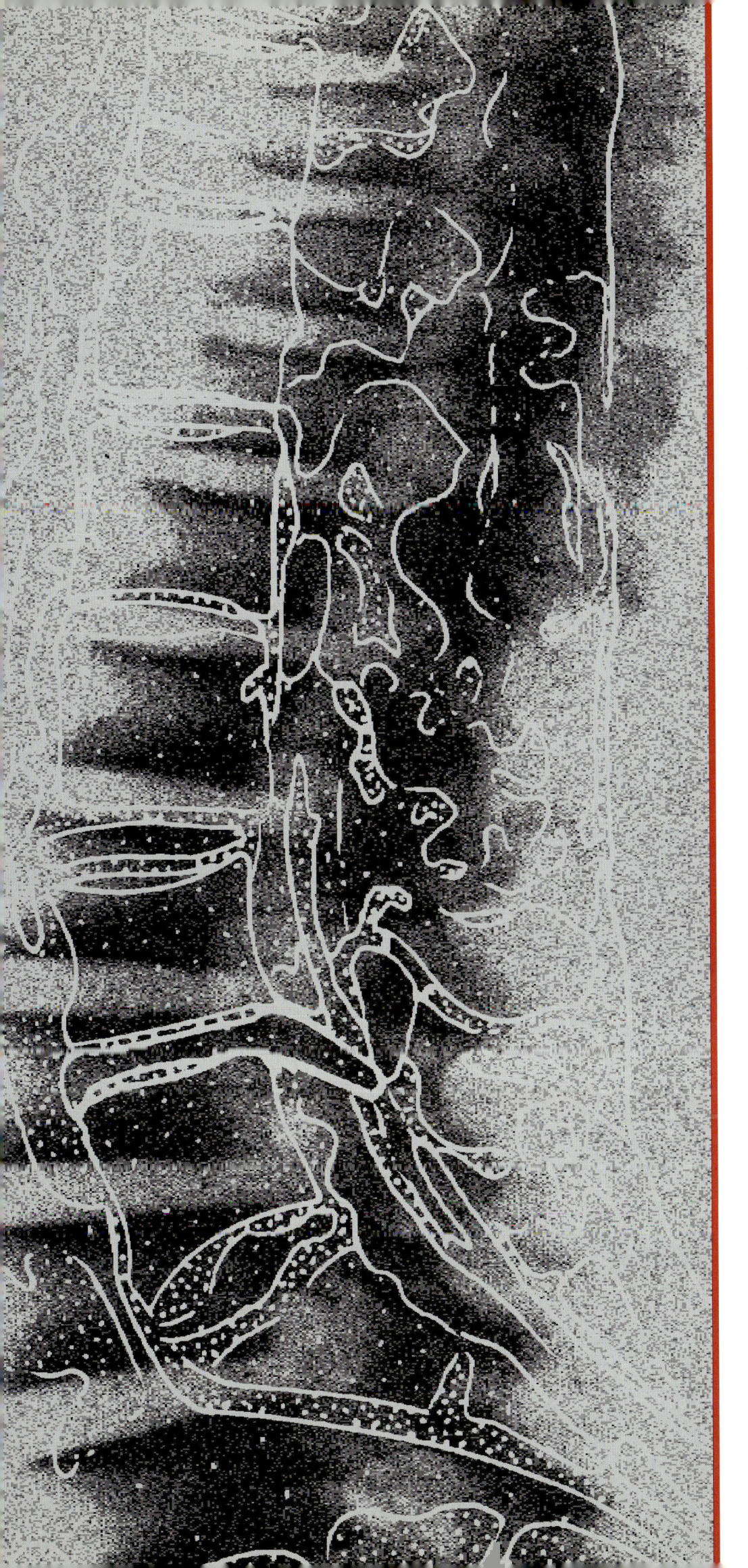

Radiologic Evaluation of Metabolic and Endocrine Disorders

14

Composition and Production of Bone

Bone tissue consists of two types of material: (1) an extracellular material, which includes *organic matrix* or *osteoid* tissue (collagen fibrils within a mucopolysaccharide ground substance) and an *inorganic crystalline component* (calcium phosphate or hydroxyapatite); and (2) a cellular material, which includes osteoblasts (cells that induce bone formation), osteoclasts (cells that induce bone resorption), and osteocytes (inactive cells).

Bone is a living, dynamic tissue: old bone is constantly being removed and replaced with new bone. Normally, this continuous process of bone resorption and formation is in balance (Fig. 14.1A), and the mineral content of the bones remains relatively constant. However, in some abnormal circumstances that disturb the metabolism of the bone, this balance may be upset. For example, when osteoblasts are more active than usual or osteoclasts less active, more bone is produced (a state known as "too much bone") (Fig. 14.1B). On the other hand, when osteoclasts are normal or overactive and osteoblasts underactive, less bone is produced ("too little bone") (Fig. 14.1C). A generalized reduction in bone mass may be caused by decreased mineralization of osteoid, with equilibrium in the rate of bone resorption and production (Fig. 14.1D).

The growth and mineralization of bone are influenced by a variety of factors, the most important of which are the amounts of growth hormone produced by the pituitary gland, calcitonin produced by the thyroid gland, and parathormone produced by the parathyroid glands, along with the dietary intake, intestinal absorption, and urinary excretion of vitamin D, calcium, and phosphorus. However, normal bone density changes with age, increasing from infancy to about age 40, and then progressively decreasing 8% per decade in women and 3% in men.

Evaluation of Metabolic and Endocrine Disorders

Most metabolic and endocrine disorders are characterized radiographically by abnormalities in bone density which are generally related to increased bone production, increased bone resorption, or inadequate bone mineralization. The bones affected by these conditions appear abnormally radiolucent (osteopenia) or abnormally radiodense (osteosclerosis) (Fig. 14.2).

Radiologic Imaging Modalities

The radiologic modalities most often used to evaluate metabolic and endocrine disorders of bone include the following:

1. Plain film radiography
2. Magnification radiography
3. Conventional tomography
4. Computed tomography (CT)
5. Radionuclide imaging (scintigraphy).

Plain film radiography is the simplest and most widely used method of evaluating bone density. This technique can usually detect even very small increases in bone density; however, it generally fails to detect decreases in overall skeletal mineralization unless the reduction reaches at least 30%. It must be pointed out that normal bone can acquire an abnormal radiographic appearance as a result of technical factors, such as improper settings for kilovoltage and milliamperage. Overexposure, for example, creates the appearance of increased bone radiolucency, whereas underexposure creates the appearance of increased bone radiodensity. For these reasons, inspection of a standard radiograph should focus less on apparent increases or decreases in bone density than on the thickness of the cortex of a bone. Cortical thickness is directly correlated with skeletal mineralization; it can be objectively measured and compared either with a normal standard or with subsequent studies in the same patient. The cortical thickness measurement is obtained by adding the width of the two cortices in the midpoint of a given bone, a sum that should be roughly one half the overall diameter of the bone; it can also be expressed as an index of bone mass, derived by dividing the combined cortical thickness by the total diameter of the bone (Fig. 14.3). The second or third metacarpal bone is frequently used to obtain these measurements (Fig. 14.4).

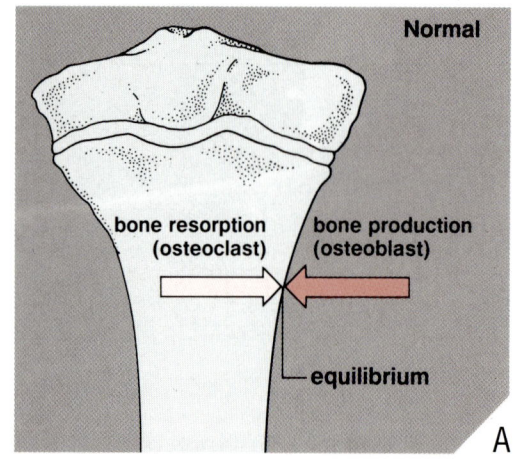

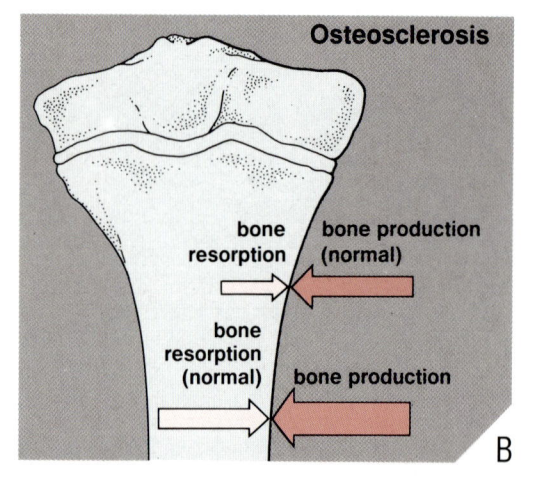

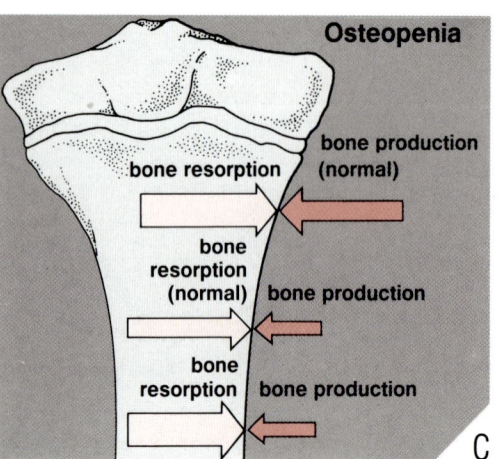

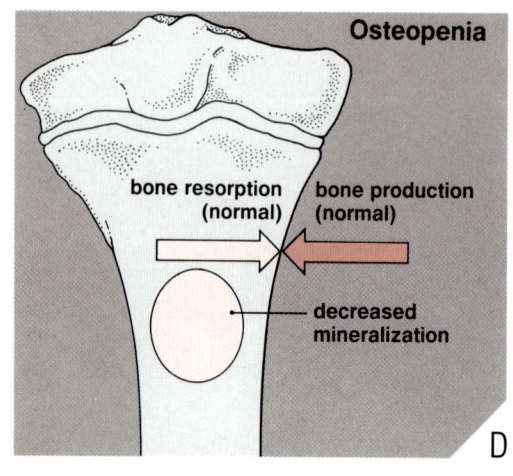

FIGURE 14.1 **(A)** In normal bone, the relationship between bone resorption and bone production is in balance. **(B)** One abnormal state ("too much bone") is characterized by decreased bone resorption and normal bone production, or by normal bone resorption and increased bone production. **(C)** The other abnormal state ("too little bone") is characterized by increased bone resorption and normal bone production, by normal bone resorption and decreased bone production, or by increased bone resorption and decreased bone production. **(D)** Too little bone may also be due to a decrease in bone mineralization, with bone resorption and production in balance.

FIGURE 14.2 METABOLIC AND ENDOCRINE DISORDERS CHARACTERIZED BY ABNORMALITIES IN BONE DENSITY

INCREASED RADIODENSITY	INCREASED RADIOLUCENCY
Secondary hyperparathyroidism	Osteoporosis
Renal osteodystrophy	Osteomalacia
Hyperphosphatasia	Rickets
Idiopathic hypercalcemia	Scurvy
Paget disease	Primary hyperparathyroidism
Osteopetrosis	Hypophosphatasia
Pycnodysostosis	Acromegaly
Melorheostosis	Gaucher disease
Hypothyroidism	Homocystinuria
Mastocytosis	Osteogenesis imperfecta
Myelofibrosis	Fibrogenesis imperfecta
Gaucher disease (reparative stage)	Cushing syndrome
Fluorine poisoning	Ochronosis (alkaptonuria)
Intoxication with lead, bismuth, or phosphorus	Wilson disease (hepatolenticular degeneration)

Cortical-Thickness Measurement

$ab + cd$ = combined cortical thickness

$\dfrac{ab + cd}{ad}$ = index of bone mass

$ab + cd \cong \dfrac{ad}{2}$

(the sum of the cortices approximates one-half the bone's diameter)

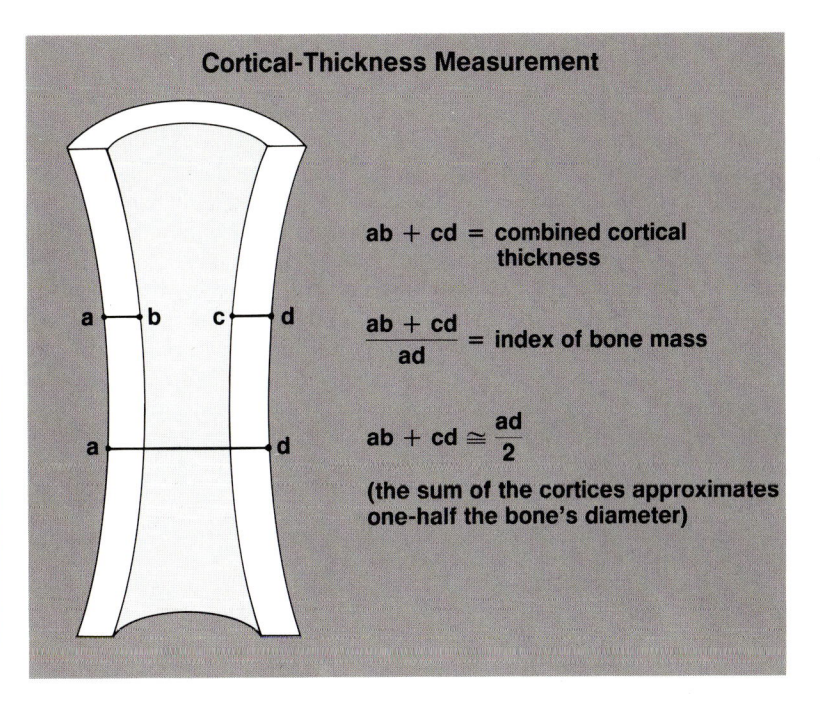

FIGURE 14.3 Determination of cortical thickness is based on the measurement of the cortices of the metacarpals (usually the second or third). It may be expressed either as the simple sum of the two cortices or as that sum divided by the total thickness of the bone, in which case it is considered an index of bony mass. Normally, the sum of the cortices should be roughly one half the overall diameter of the metacarpal bone.

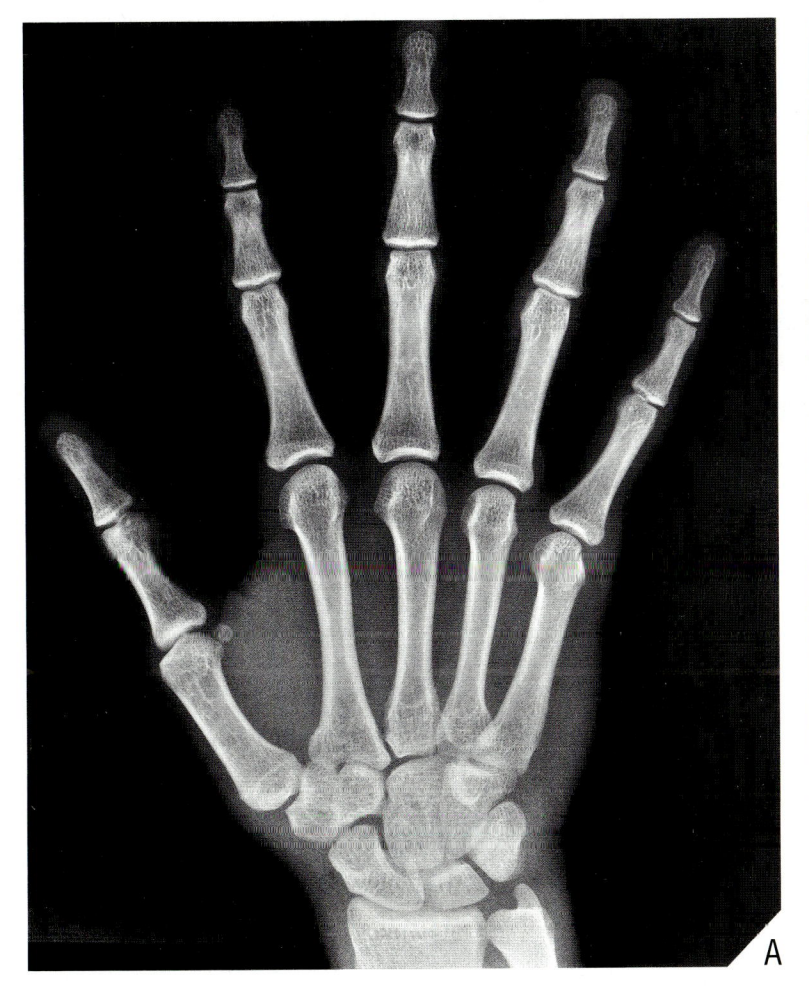

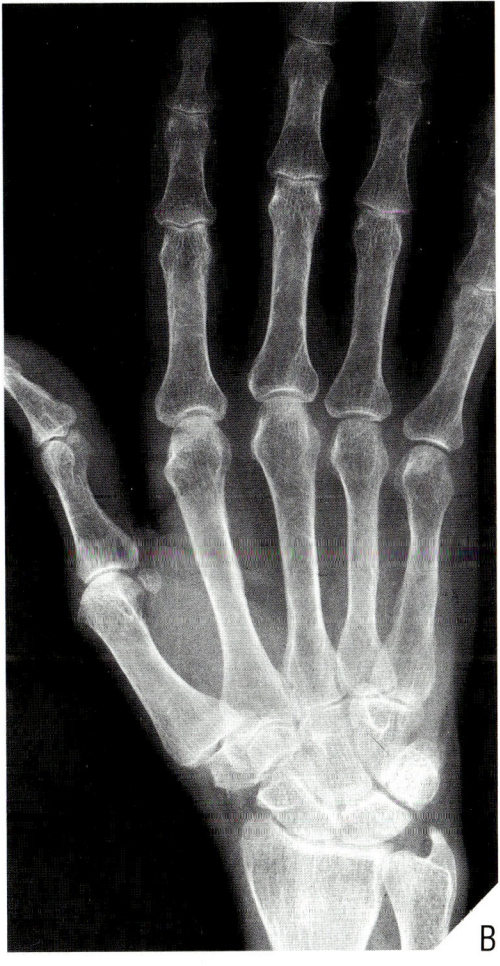

FIGURE 14.4 Dorsovolar views of the hand show normal **(A)** and abnormal **(B)** thickness of the cortex of the second and third metacarpal bones.

Radiologic Evaluation of Metabolic and Endocrine Disorders

A related method that also uses plain radiographs for assessing bone density is the photodensitometry technique. This technique is based on the observation that the photographic density of a bone on a radiographic film is proportional to its mass. Through the use of a photodensitometer, the photographic density of a given bone can be compared with that of known standard wedges for an accurate assessment of the degree of bone density.

The appearance of relative increased radiolucency of bone on standard radiographs should not be called osteoporosis, since such a finding is not specific for either osteoporosis, osteomalacia, or hyperparathyroidism. Most authorities agree that increased radiolucency is best termed *osteopenia* (poverty of bone). *Osteoporosis* refers specifically to a reduction in the amount of bone tissue (deficient bone matrix), and *osteomalacia* to a reduction in the amount of mineral in the matrix (deficient mineralization); both conditions are characterized by increased radiolucency of bone (Fig. 14.5). As Resnick (1981) pointed out, any condition in which bone resorption exceeds bone formation results in osteopenia, regardless of the specific pathogenesis of the condition. In fact, diffuse osteopenia is found in osteoporosis, osteomalacia, hyperparathyroidism, neoplastic conditions (such as multiple myeloma), and a wide variety of other disorders.

Although osteopenia is a nonspecific finding, plain film radiography can help detect other important radiographic features that can lead to a specific diagnosis. Among these are Looser zones, representing pseudofractures, which are characteristic of osteomalacia; widening of the growth plate and flaring of the metaphysis, which are typical findings in rickets; subperiosteal bone resorption, an identifying feature of hyperparathyroidism; or focal areas of osteolytic destruction and endosteal scalloping, which are characteristic of multiple myeloma.

Magnification radiography is useful in metabolic disorders for demonstrating the details of bone structure. The subperiosteal bone resorption characteristic of hyperparathyroidism or cortical tunneling, which may be seen in any process that causes increased bone resorption, can be well delineated on magnification studies. Cortical tunneling occurs very early in a pathologic process and may be found even in the absence of any other radiographic abnormalities.

Although conventional tomography is occasionally useful for demonstrating lesions that are not well visualized on conventional radiographs, it is CT that plays an important role in the evaluation of metabolic and endocrine disorders. The ability of CT to define a specific volume and to accurately measure the density of that volume makes it possible to perform quantitative analysis of bone mineral content. As Genant (1985) pointed out, CT also has the unique ability to measure the cancellous bone of the axial skeleton, particularly that of the vertebrae, a site that is especially sensitive to metabolic stimuli.

Several methods have been developed for assessing mineral content of the bones, including single-photon absorptiometry (SPA), dual-photon absorptiometry (DPA), dual x-ray absorptiometry (DXA) and, probably the most widely used, quantitative computed tomography (QCT). SPA is used to assess the status of peripheral long bones (distal radius, distal femur) and primarily measures cortical bone. These measurements are relatively insensitive to metabolic stimuli, and therefore are of limited value for monitoring changes in the individual patient. DPA and DXA are radiologic projection methods for measuring the bone mineral content of different skeletal areas, usually the lumbar spine and the proximal femur. Dual-photon absorptiometry uses a radioisotope that emits photons at two different energy levels and thus allows differentiation of yellow and red marrow from the mineral component of the trabecular bone. DPA is based on the contrast difference between low-energy and high-energy beam attenuation in both bone and soft tissue (bone yields a higher contrast at low energies than at high energies). QCT is a method for measuring the lumbar spine mineral content in which the average density values of a region are referenced to that of a calibration material scanned simultaneously with the patient. Measurements are performed on a CT scanner and use a mineral standard for simultaneous calibration, a computed radiogram (scout view) for localization, and either single- or dual-energy techniques. In quantitative CT scanning, a cross-sectional image of the vertebral body is obtained, allowing differentiation of cortical and trabecular bone. The attenuation referenced to a mineral equivalent phantom is expressed as a trabecular bone density in mg/cm^3 of calcium hydroxyap-

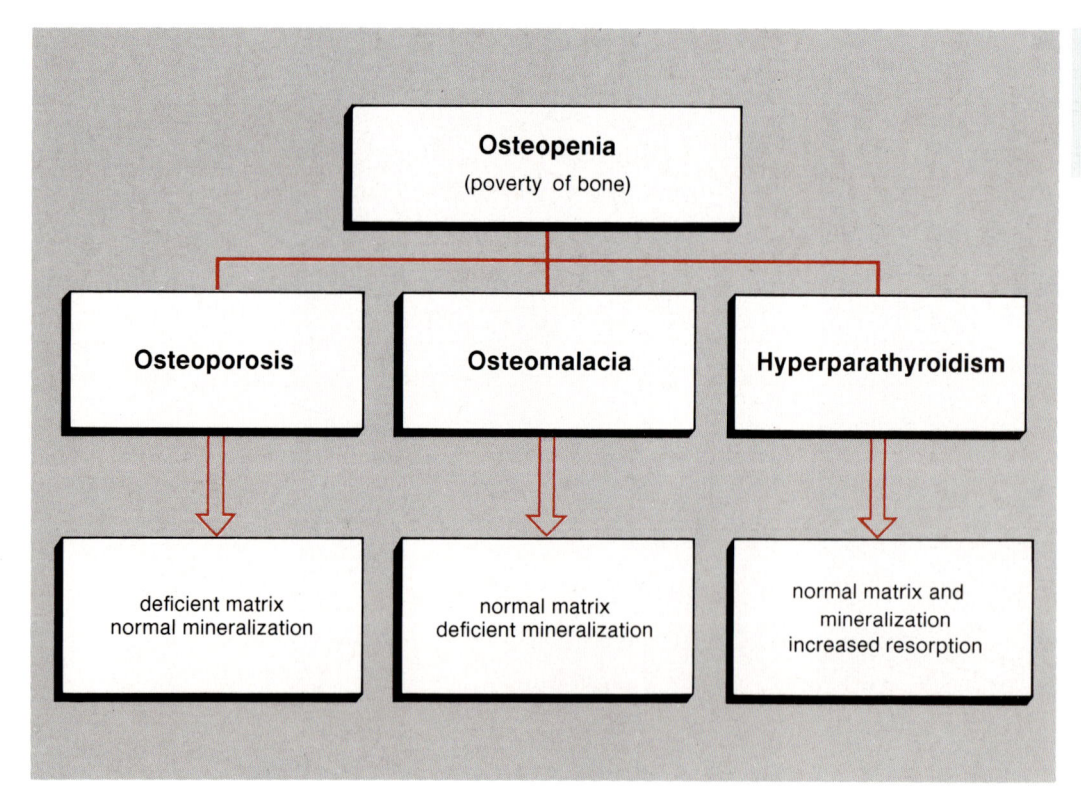

FIGURE 14.5 Increased radiolucency of bone on a standard radiograph is best termed osteopenia or bone rarefaction rather than osteoporosis, and it is a typical feature not only of osteoporosis but also of osteomalacia and hyperparathyroidism, which are clinically distinct conditions.

atite. The usual examination procedure consists of taking CT scans through the midplane line of three or four adjacent vertebral bodies (usually from T12 to L3 or L1 to L4). Axial images of the vertebral bodies are obtained by scanning of the midplane of vertebral bodies while the patient is lying supine on a standard phantom. The average density from all vertebrae is calculated. The patient's values are compared with the values of bone density calibrated in the phantom (Fig. 14.6). For measuring the spine, quantitative CT has advantages over other methods because of its great sensitivity and its precise three-dimensional anatomic localization, its ability to distinguish cancellous bone from cortical bone, and its ability to exclude extraosseous minerals from the measurement. All these methods are used in clinical practice to assess patients with metabolic disease affecting the skeleton, to establish a diagnosis of osteoporosis or assess its severity, and to monitor response to therapy. In general, the usefulness of CT for measurement of bone mineral lies in its ability to provide a measurement of trabecular, cortical, or integral bone, either of the axial or the appendicular skeleton. In particular, these methods are useful for measurement of spinal bone mineral density in postmenopausal women, in patients with existing osteoporosis, and in patients being treated with corticosteroids.

Finally, radionuclide imaging is occasionally employed in the evaluation of metabolic disorders. It is a nonspecific modality but is very sensi-

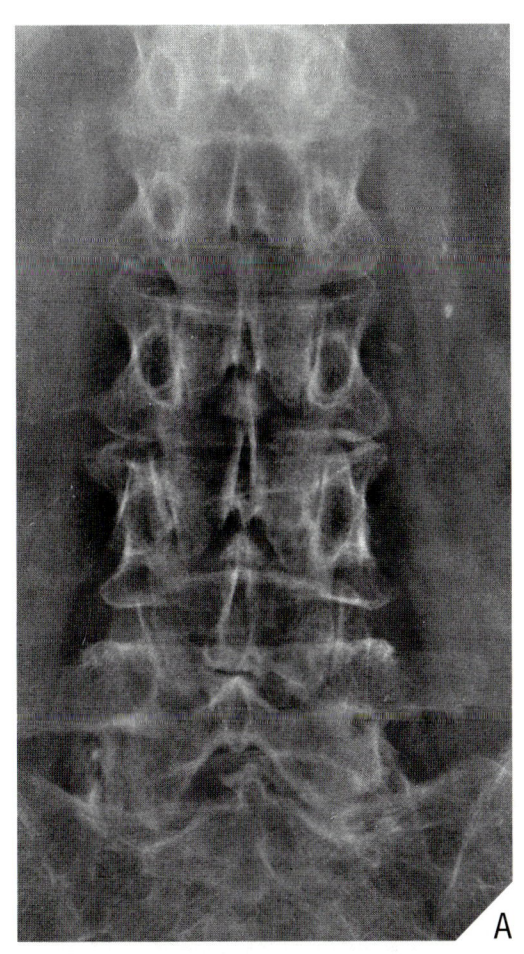

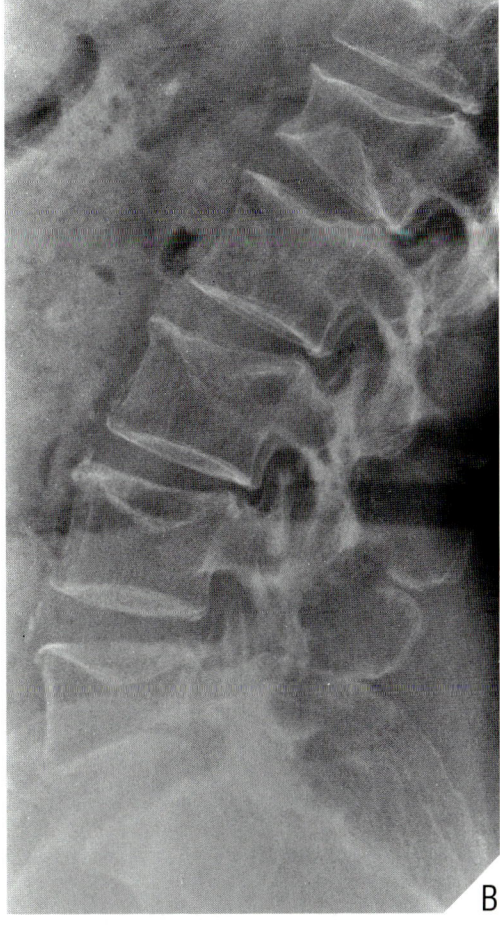

FIGURE 14.6 A 62-year-old woman was evaluated for degree of osteoporosis. The anteroposterior **(A)** and lateral **(B)** views of the lumbar spine show diffuse osteopenia with multiple compression fractures. Quantitative computed tomography (QCT) measurements were obtained with the patient supine on a standard bone mineral calibration phantom. Values were referenced to a translucent calibration phantom scanned with the patient, which contains tubes filled with standard solutions of potassium phosphate (representing minerals), ethanol (representing fat), and water (representing soft tissue). For each axial image, the regions of interest were positioned over the center portion of the phantom calibration compartments, as well as over the central portion of the vertebral body. Transverse (axial) CT scans were made through L1, L2, L3, and L4, with phantom included. Bone density values in mg/cm^3 were calculated for each vertebral body using the CT numbers (Hounsfield units) obtained from the calibrated density phantom **(C,D)**. Readings are averaged and compared with normal values for given age and sex. Average of readings for vertebral mineral content is also expressed in mg/cm^3. In this particular case, the average values of 77.4 mg of mineral/cm^3 are below the average values for the patient's age (97.5 mg/cm^3) as well as below the levels of fracture threshold (110 mg/cm^3).

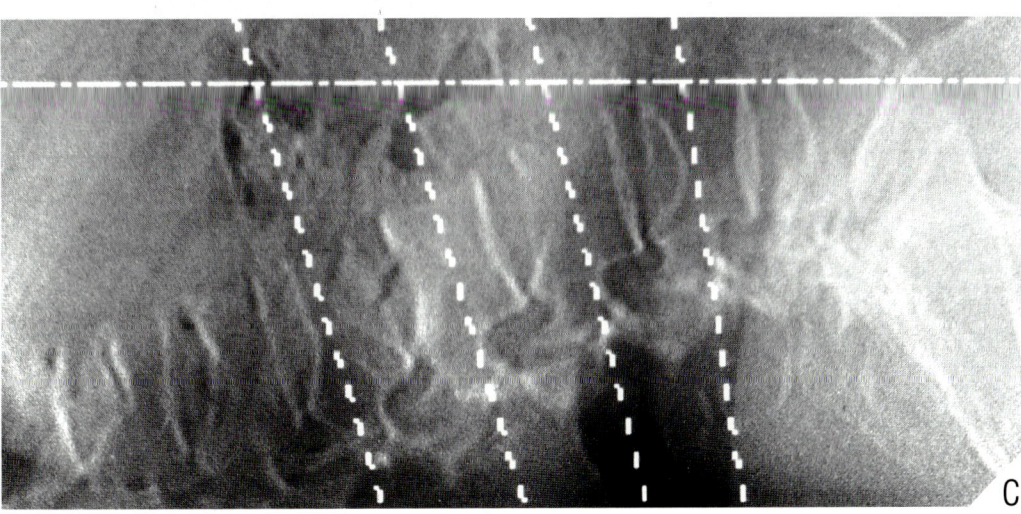

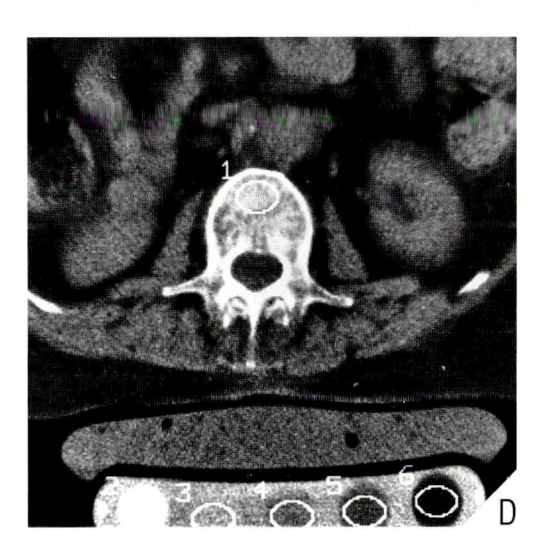

tive for detection of active bone turnover. It is particularly valuable for screening of patients with Paget disease to determine the distribution of the lesion and the activity of the disease (Fig. 14.7). It is also used to detect insufficiency-type stress fractures that are seen in osteomalacia and hyperparathyroidism. Monitoring the excretion and retention of technetium-labeled phosphate compounds is a sensitive way to determine abnormalities that accompany certain metabolic bone diseases. In renal osteodystrophy, radionuclide bone scan usually reveals absence of kidney images, reflecting poor renal function. Scintigraphic patterns in patients with osteoporosis at times may be characteristic. For instance, radionuclide bone scan may show increased uptake of a tracer in bones affected by disuse osteoporosis and reflex sympathetic dystrophy syndrome. Radionuclide bone scan can also be helpful in detecting the pathologic fractures in a variety of metabolic disorders.

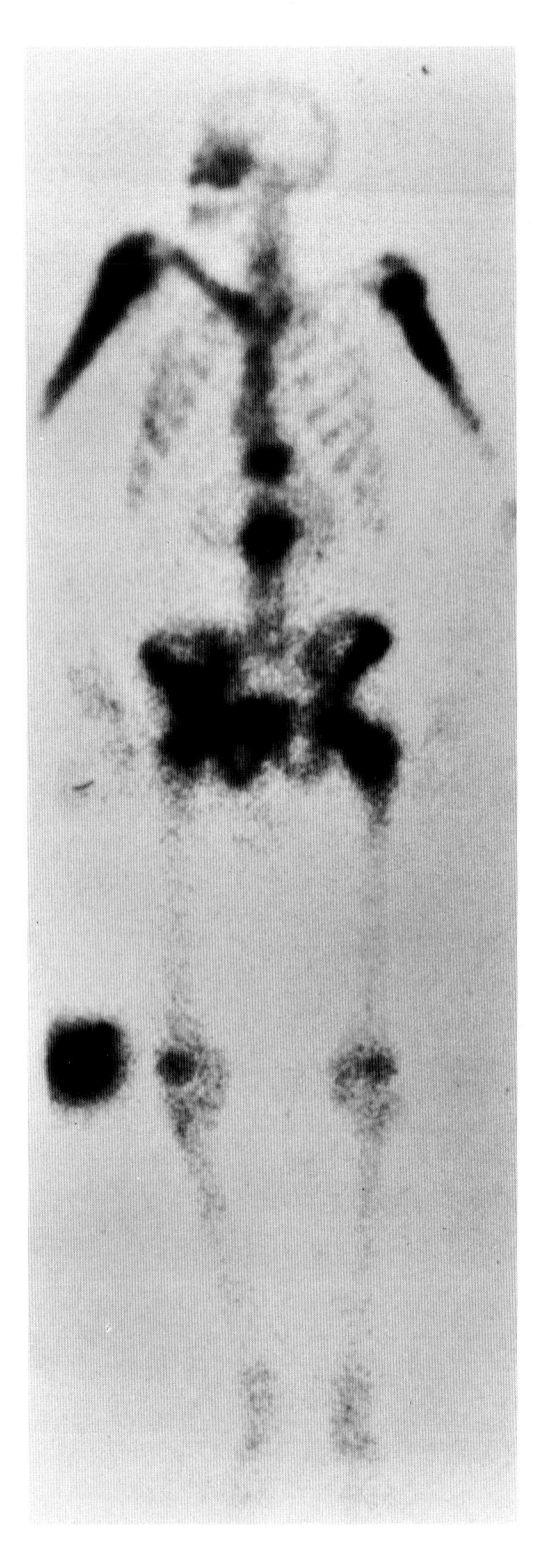

FIGURE 14.7 Radionuclide bone scan in this 72-year-old man with obvious clinical and radiographic evidence of Paget disease in the pelvis and proximal femora shows additional, silent sites of involvement in both patellae and humeri, as well as in several thoracic and lumbar vertebrae.

Suggested Reading

Cann CE: Quantitative CT for determination of bone mineral density: A review. *Radiology* 166:509, 1988.

Cann CE, Genant HK: Precise measurement of vertebral mineral content using computed tomography. *J Comput Assist Tomogr* 4:493, 1980.

Garn SM, Poznaski AK, Nagy JM: Bone measurement in the differential diagnosis of osteopenia and osteoporosis. *Radiology* 100:509, 1971.

Genant HK, Block JE, Steiger P, et al: Appropriate use of bone densitometry. *Radiology* 170:817, 1989.

Genant HK, Cann CE, Effinger B, et al: Quantitative computed tomography for spinal mineral assessment: current status. *J Comput Assist Tomogr* 9:602, 1985.

Griffith HJ, Zimmerman R, Baily G, et al: The use of photon absorptiometry in the diagnosis of renal osteodystrophy. *Radiology* 109:277, 1973.

Jensen PS, Orphanoudakis SC, Baron R, et al: Determination of bone mass by CT and correlation with quantitative histomorphometric analysis. *J Comput Assist Tomogr* 3:847, 1979.

Krolner B, Nielsen SP: Bone mineral content of the lumbar spine in normal and osteoporotic women: Cross-sectional and longitudinal studies. *Clin Sci* 62:329, 1982.

Krolner B, Nielsen SP: Measurement of bone mineral content (BMC) of the lumbar spine, part I: Theory and application of a new two-dimensional dual photon attenuation method. *Scand J Clin Lab Invest* 40:485, 1980.

Lang P, Steiger P, Faulkner K, et al: Osteoporosis. Current techniques and recent developments in quantitative bone densitometry. *Radiol Clin North Am* 29:49, 1991.

Mazess RB: Bone densitometry of the axial skeleton. *Orthop Clin North Am* 21:51, 1990.

Mazess RB, Barden HS: Measurement of bone by dual-photon absorptiometry (DPA) and dual-energy x-ray absorptiometry (DEXA). *Ann Chir Gynaecol* 77:197, 1988.

Pullan BR, Roberts TE: Bone mineral measurement using an EMI scanner and standard methods: A comparative study. *Br J Radiol* 51:24, 1978.

Resnick D, Niwayama G: Osteoporosis. In: *Diagnosis of Bone and Joint Disorders*, Vol 2. Philadelphia, W B Saunders, 1981, p 1638.

Reynolds WA, Karo JJ: Radiographic diagnosis of metabolic bone disease. *Orthop Clin North Am* 3:521, 1972.

Rupich R, Pacifici R, Delabar C, et al: Lateral and dual energy radiography: New technique for the measurement of L3 bone mineral density. *J Bone Miner Res* 4:S194, 1989.

Sartoris DJ, Resnick D: Dual energy radiographic absorptiometry for bone densitometry: Current status and prospective. *AJR* 152:241, 1989.

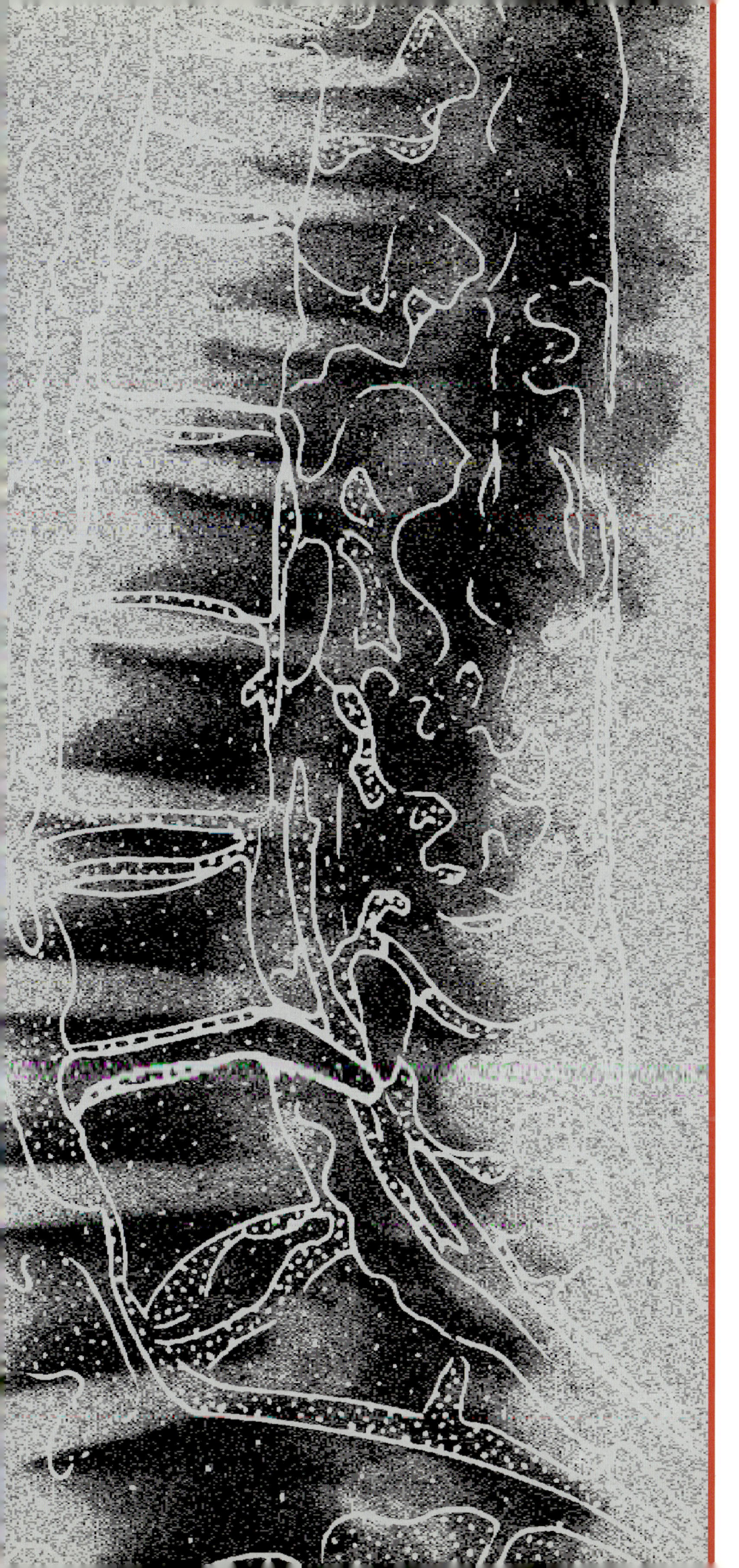

Osteoporosis, Osteomalacia, Rickets, and Hyperparathyroidism

15

OSTEOPOROSIS

Osteoporosis is a generalized metabolic bone disease characterized by insufficient formation or increased resorption of bone matrix, resulting in decreased bone mass. Although there is a reduction in the amount of bone tissue, whatever bone tissue is present is fully mineralized. In other words, the bone is quantitatively deficient but qualitatively normal.

Osteoporosis has a variety of possible causes, and consequently manifests in a number of different forms (Fig. 15.1). The basic distinction between forms of osteoporosis is between those types that are *generalized* or *diffuse*, involving the entire skeleton, and those that are *localized* to a single region or bone (*regional*); the basic distinction between possible causes is between those that are *congenital* and those that are *acquired*.

Generalized Osteoporosis

Certain radiologic features are common to virtually all forms of osteoporosis, regardless of their specific cause. There is always some diminution of cortical thickness and a decrease in the number and thickness of the trabeculae of spongy bone. These changes are more prominent in nonweightbearing segments and those not subject to stress. The first sites affected by osteoporosis, and which are best demonstrated radiographically, are the periarticular regions, where the cortex is anatomically thinner. In the long bones, the thickness of the cortices decreases, the bones become brittle, and there is increased clinical incidence of fractures, particularly fractures of the proximal femur, the proximal humerus, the distal radius, and the ribs.

The other major area in which osteoporotic changes are evaluated is the axial skeleton, the spine in particular. This is especially the case in osteoporosis associated with aging—*involutional* (*senescent* and *postmenopausal*) *osteoporosis*—in which the vertebral bodies are particularly vulnerable. Initially there is a relative increase in the density of the vertebral endplates caused by resorption of the spongy bone, rendering what is called an "empty-box" appearance (Fig. 15.2). Later, an overall decrease in density occurs with loss of trabecular pattern, creating a "ground glass" appearance. A typical feature of vertebral involvement in osteoporosis is

---

FIGURE 15.1 CAUSES OF OSTEOPOROSIS

GENERALIZED (DIFFUSE)

Genetic (Congenital)
Osteogenesis imperfecta
Gonadal dysgenesis
Turner syndrome (XO)
Klinefelter syndrome (XXY)
Hypophosphatasia
Homocystinuria
Mucopolysaccharidosis
Gaucher disease
Anemias:
    Sickle-cell syndromes
    Thalassemia
    Hemophilia
    Christmas disease

Endocrine
Hyperthyroidism
Hyperparathyroidism
Cushing syndrome
Acromegaly
Estrogen deficiency
Hypogonadism
Diabetes mellitus
Pregnancy

Deficiency States
Scurvy
Malnutrition
Anorexia nervosa
Protein deficiency
Alcoholism
Liver disease

Neoplastic
Myeloma
Leukemia
Lymphoma
Metastatic disease

Iatrogenic
Heparin-induced
Dilantin-induced
Steroid-induced

Miscellaneous
Involutional
    (senescent/postmenopausal)
Amyloidosis
Ochronosis
Paraplegia
Weightlessness
Idiopathic

LOCALIZED (REGIONAL)

Immobilization (cast)
Disuse
Pain
Infection
Reflex sympathetic dystrophy
    syndrome (Sudeck atrophy)
Transient regional
    osteoporosis
Transient osteoporosis of
    the the hip
Regional migratory
    osteoporosis
Idiopathic juvenile
    osteoporosis
Paget disease (hot phase)

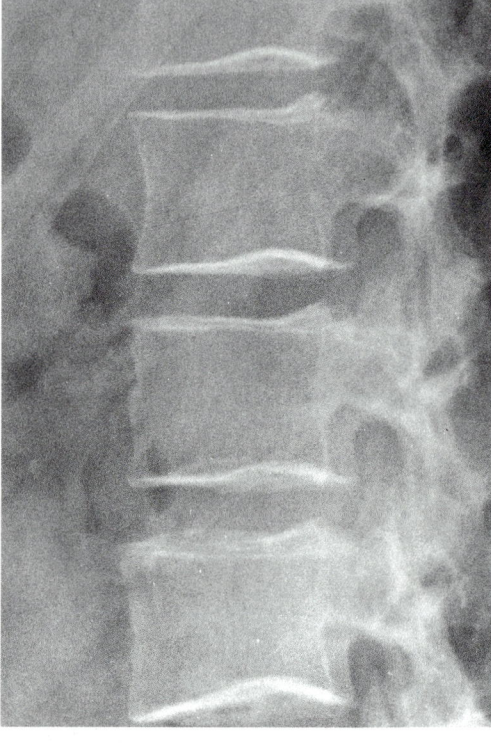

FIGURE 15.2 Lateral radiograph of the lumbar spine of an 89-year-old woman demonstrates a relative increase in the density of the vertebral endplates and resorption of the trabeculae of spongy bone, creating an "empty-box" appearance. This is commonly seen in involutional osteoporosis.

Imaging of the Spine in Clinical Practice

biconcavity of the vertebral body, which therefore exhibits a "fish-mouth" appearance ("codfish vertebrae") (Fig. 15.3). This presentation results from expansion of the disks, leading to arch-like indentations on both the superior and the inferior margins of the weakened vertebral bodies. Advanced stages are characterized by complete collapse of the vertebral body associated with a wedge-shaped deformity. In the thoracic spine this leads to increased kyphosis.

Of special interest in generalized osteoporosis are the three major varieties of *iatrogenic osteoporosis*. *Heparin-induced osteoporosis* may develop after long-term, high-dose (more than 10,000 units daily) heparin treatment. Precisely how this type of osteoporosis is initiated and develops is not clearly understood, although osteoclastic stimulation and osteoblastic inhibition with suppressed endochondral ossification have been implicated as potential causes. The changes may be reversible if the treatment is stopped. Spontaneous fractures of the vertebrae (Fig. 15.4), ribs, and femoral neck are noted on radiographic studies. *Dilantin-induced osteoporosis* occasionally develops after prolonged use of phenytoin (Dilantin). The vertebral columns and ribs are usually affected, and fractures are a common complication (Fig. 15.5).

Steroid-induced osteoporosis, arising either during the course of Cushing syndrome or during treatment with various corticosteroids (iatrogenic), is characterized by decreased bone formation and increased bone resorption. Although the axial skeleton is more often affected, the appendicular skeleton may also be involved. The spine undergoes a striking thickening and sclerosis of the vertebral endplates, without a concomitant change in the anterior and posterior vertebral margins.

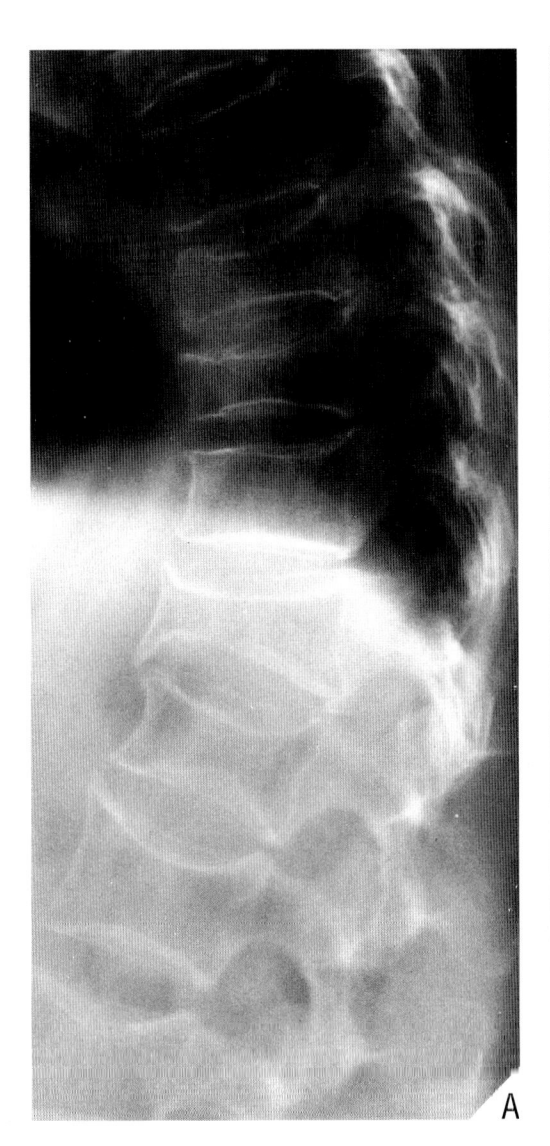

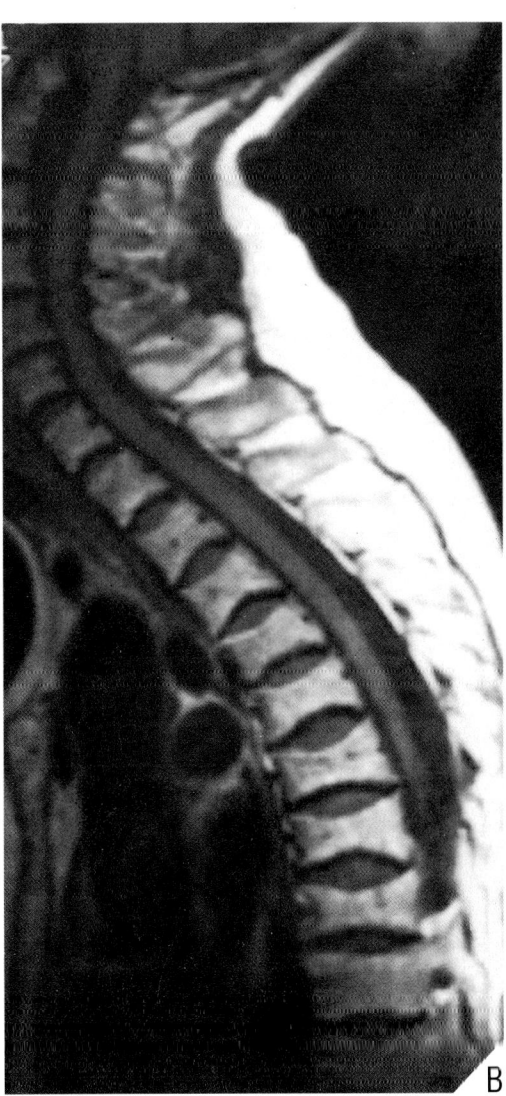

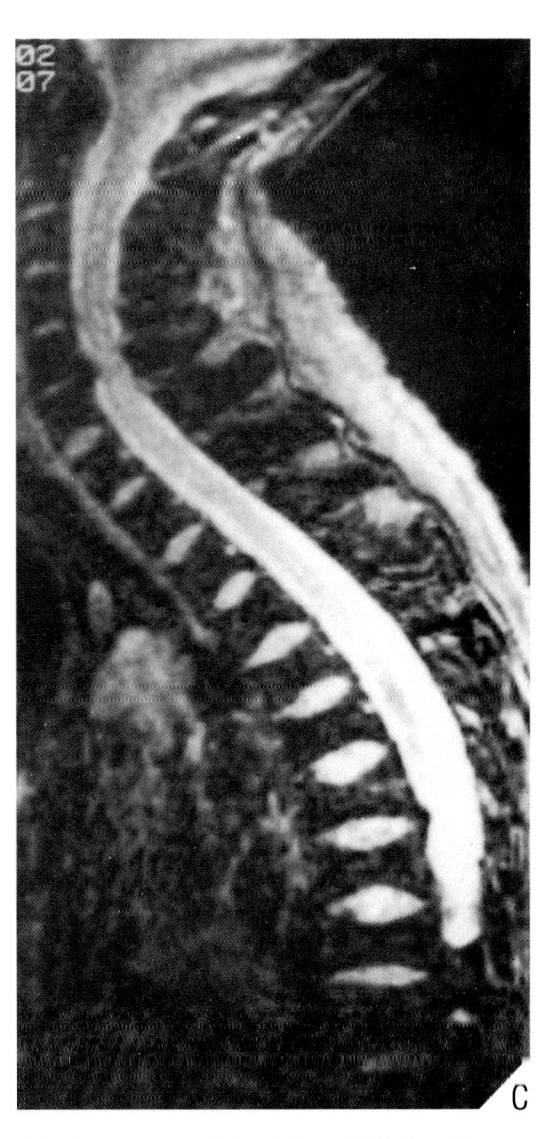

FIGURE 15.3 (A) Biconcavity of "codfish vertebrae," seen here on the lateral view of the thoracolumbar spine in an 80-year-old woman with osteoporosis, results from weakness of the vertebral endplates and intravertebral expansion of nuclei pulposi. **(B)** T1-weighted spin-echo sagittal MRI of the cervical and upper thoracic spine of another patient shows biconcave compression fractures of several thoracic vertebral bodies. The disks are expanded and show elliptical configuration. **(C)** Gradient-echo (GRASS) sagittal image demonstrates minimal alteration (mottling) of signal from the vertebral bodies. The intervertebral disks show normal high signal intensity for this sequence. (B,C reproduced with permission from Beltran J: *MRI Musculoskeletal System*. Gower, New York, 1990)

Rickets and Osteomalacia

Whereas in osteoporosis the fundamental change is decreased bone mass, in rickets, which occurs in children, and osteomalacia, which occurs in adults, the essential bone abnormality is failure of mineralization (calcification) of the bone matrix. Unless adequate amounts of calcium and phosphorus are available, proper calcification of osteoid tissue cannot occur.

In the past, the most common cause of rickets and osteomalacia was deficient intake of vitamin D, which is responsible for calcium and phosphorus homeostasis and for maintenance of proper bone mineralization. Now, however, the major causes include (1) *inadequate intestinal absorption*, resulting in loss of calcium and phosphorus through the gastrointestinal tract, in patients who have gastric, biliary, or enteric abnormalities or have undergone gastrectomy or other gastric surgery; (2) *renal tubular disorders* (proximal and/or distal tubular lesions frequently leading to renal tubular acidosis); and (3) *renal osteodystrophy* secondary to renal failure, which leads to loss of calcium through the kidneys. Several other conditions associated with osteomalacia have been identified, such as neurofibromatosis, fibrous dysplasia, and Wilson disease, but the exact relationship between the underlying disorder and osteomalacia is still unclear.

Osteomalacia, which results from the same pathologic mechanism that causes rickets, occurs only after bone growth has ceased. It is characterized by changes in the cortical and trabecular bone of the axial and appendicular skeleton. Osteomalacia is most often caused by faulty absorption of the fat-soluble vitamin D from the gastrointestinal tract secondary to malabsorption syndrome. It may also result from dysfunction of the proximal renal tubules—so-called renal osteomalacia. The most common clinical presentation of this condition is bone pain and muscle weakness.

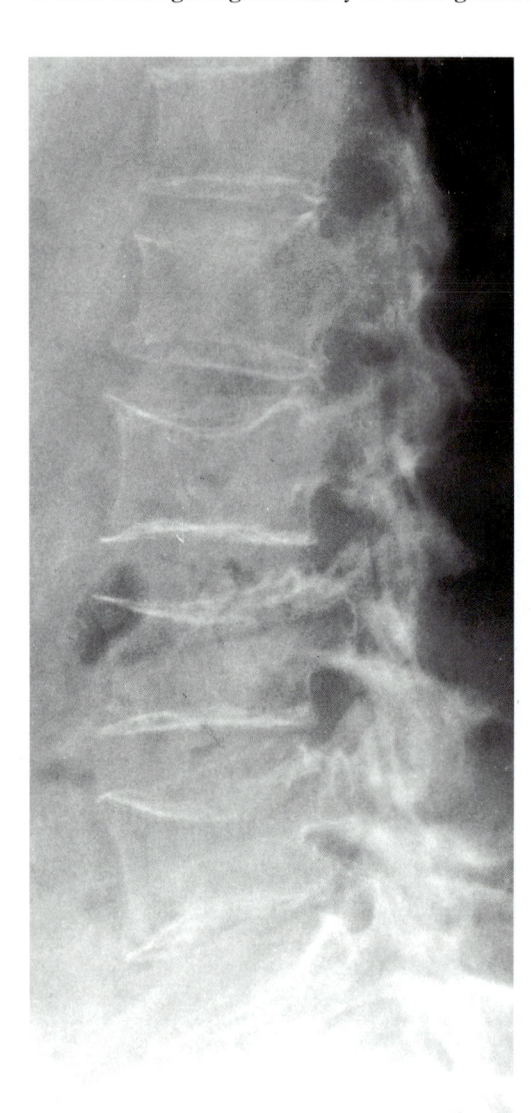

FIGURE 15.4 A 51-year-old woman with chronic leg ulcers and recurrent deep vein thrombosis was receiving large daily doses of heparin. Lateral view of the lumbar spine demonstrates severe osteoporosis and multiple compression fractures of the vertebral bodies.

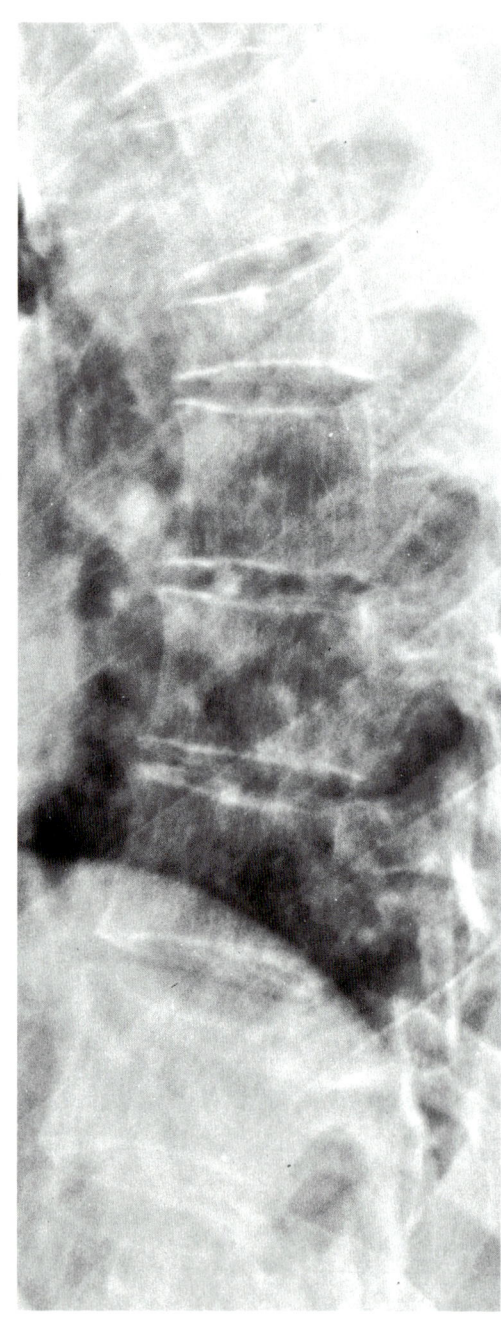

FIGURE 15.5 A 32-year-old man with a convulsive-seizure disorder of unknown etiology was undergoing prolonged treatment with phenytoin (Dilantin). Lateral view of the thoracic spine demonstrates severe osteoporosis with compression fracture of T6. There is marked accentuation of the vertical trabeculae in the vertebral bodies, a frequent finding in patients with osteoporosis.

Histologically, osteomalacia is characterized by excessive quantities of inadequately mineralized bone matrix (osteoid), which coats the surfaces of trabeculae in spongy bone and lines the Haversian canals in the cortex.

RENAL OSTEODYSTROPHY

A skeletal response to longstanding renal disease, renal osteodystrophy (also referred to as *uremic osteopathy*) is usually associated with chronic renal failure due to glomerulonephritis or pyelonephritis. The condition is also seen in patients who are on dialysis or who have undergone renal transplantation.

Two main mechanisms, acting in unison but varying in severity and proportion, are responsible for the bone changes associated with this condition: (1) secondary hyperparathyroidism; (2) abnormal vitamin D metabolism. The secondary hyperparathyroidism is provoked by phosphate retention and leads to depression of serum calcium, which in turn stimulates release of parathormone from the parathyroid glands. The abnormal vitamin D metabolism is affected by renal insufficiency, since the kidney is the source of an enzyme, 25-OH-D-1α-hydroxylase, which converts the inactive vitamin D from 25-hydroxyvitamin D (25-OH-D) to the active form, 1,25-dihydroxyvitamin D $(1,25(OH)_2D)$. Only this most potent, physiologically active form of vitamin D is responsible for calcium and phosphorus homeostasis and for maintenance of proper bone mineralization.

The major radiographic manifestations of renal osteodystrophy are those associated with rickets, osteomalacia, and secondary hyperparathyroidism. Osteomalacia secondary to renal osteodystrophy is seldom seen in its pure form; usually there are superimposed changes typical of secondary hyperparathyroidism. Increased bone radiolucency and cortical thinning may be present, but Looser zones are very uncommon. In most patients, some sclerotic changes develop in the spine (Fig. 15.6).

HYPERPARATHYROIDISM

Pathophysiology

Hyperparathyroidism, also known as *generalized osteitis fibrosa cystica* and *Recklinghausen disease of bone*, is caused by hypersecretion of parathormone from the parathyroid glands. Increased production of this hormone is secondary to either hyperplasia of these glands (in 9% of cases) or adenoma (90%); only in very rare instances (1%) does hyperparathyroidism occur secondary to parathyroid carcinoma. Excessive secretion of parathormone, which acts on the kidneys and bone, leads to disturbances in calcium and phosphorus metabolism, resulting in hypercalcemia, hyperphosphaturia, and hypophosphatemia. Renal excretion of calcium and phosphate is increased and serum levels of calcium are elevated, whereas those of phosphorus are reduced; serum levels of alkaline phosphatase are also elevated.

Hyperparathyroidism can be divided into primary, secondary, and tertiary forms. The classic form of the disorder, *primary hyperparathyroidism*, is marked by increased secretion of parathormone resulting from hyperplasia, adenoma, or carcinoma of the parathyroid glands. Primary hyperparathyroidism is usually associated with hypercalcemia. Women are about three times more frequently affected than men, and the condition is most often seen in the third to fifth decades of life. *Secondary hyperparathyroidism* is caused by increased secretion of parathyroid hormone in response to a sustained hypocalcemic state. The fundamental cause of parathyroid gland hyperfunction is usually impaired renal function. Hyperphosphatemia due to renal failure results in chronic hypocalcemia, which in turn promotes increased parathyroid secretion. Although secondary hyperparathyroidism is usually hypocalcemic, it may be normocalcemic, representing an adaptive response to the hypocalcemic state. *Tertiary hyperparathyroidism* represents a transformation from a hypocalcemic to a hypercalcemic state. The parathyroid glands "escape" from the regulatory effect of serum calcium levels. Patients in whom this escape occurs are usually receiving kidney hemodialysis; they are considered to have autonomous hyperparathyroidism.

Although primary hyperparathyroidism is traditionally synonymous with the hypercalcemic form of the disorder, some patients nonetheless may have normal or even reduced serum calcium levels. For this reason, Reiss and Canterbury (1974) proposed an alternative method of classifying hyperparathyroidism based on serum calcium levels. In this system, hyperparathyroidism is considered either hypercalcemic, normocalcemic, or hypocalcemic.

Physiology of Calcium Metabolism

To understand the clinical, pathologic, and radiologic manifestations of hyperparathyroidism, knowledge of the interrelated roles of parathyroid hormone and vitamin D in the metabolism of calcium is essential.

Serum concentrations of calcium are maintained within a narrow normal physiologic range (2.20–2.65 mmol/L or 8.8–10.6 mg/dL) by the intestines and kidneys, the major sites of classic negative feedback mechanisms that balance calcium intake and excretion. The bones also contribute to preservation of calcium homeostasis and, because they represent approximately 99% of elemental calcium in the human body, are considered to be a calcium reservoir. Essential to these mechanisms, involving a variety of hormones, is the action of parathyroid hormone (PTH), a polypeptide hormone whose secretion is induced by a decrease in the level of calcium in the extracellular fluid. In primary hyperparathyroidism, there is inappropriate oversecretion of PTH in the presence of elevated serum calcium levels, whereas secondary hyperparathyroidism is marked by appropriate PTH production in response to chronic hypocalcemia.

PTH works to increase serum calcium concentration by several means. Predominant among these is the action of PTH to conserve calcium in the kidneys by promoting increased reabsorption of calcium, as well as increased excretion of phophates, in the distal renal tubules. It also promotes release of calcium and phosphorus from bone by increasing the number and activity of osteoclasts, resulting in bone resorption, although the exact mechanism by which this occurs is not fully understood. Finally, although PTH has been shown to have no direct effect on intestinal calcium absorption, it plays a role in stimulating vitamin D metabolism, with subsequent increased absorption of calcium and phosphorus by the intestines.

Both forms of vitamin D in the human body—ergocalciferol (vitamin D_2), a synthetic compound and frequent food additive, and cholecalciferol (vitamin D_3), formed predominantly in the skin from 7-dehydrocholesterol by the action of ultraviolet light—are metabolized to 25-hydroxy vitamin D in the liver. The critical step in the metabolism of vitamin D occurs in the kidneys, where 25-hydroxy vitamin D undergoes hydroxylation to its most active form, 1,25-dihydroxy vitamin D, and an inactive metabolite, 24,25-dihydroxy vitamin D. This step is catalyzed by the renal enzyme 1-α-hydroxylase, which is synthesized in the kidneys under the stimulation of PTH in the presence of decreased serum calcium and phosphate levels. This gives the kidneys a unique central role in the metabolism of vitamin D. 1,25-dihydroxy vitamin D is the primary mediator of calcium and phosphorus absorption in the small intestine. The kidneys have the ability to switch between producing the active and inactive forms of vitamin D, yielding a fine control of calcium metabolism.

The symptoms of hyperparathyroidism are related to hypercalcemia, skeletal abnormalities, and renal disease. Hypercalcemia produces weakness, muscle hypotonia, nausea, anorexia, constipation, polyuria, and polydipsia. The skeletal abnormalities most commonly seen are generalized osteopenia and foci of bone destruction, which are commonly referred to as *brown tumors*. These pseudotumors represent areas of fibrous scarring in which osteoclasts collect, blood decomposes, and cysts form. Kidney involvement leads to nephrocalcinosis, impairment of renal function, and uremia.

Radiographic Evaluation

In the skeletal system, the major target sites for hyperparathyroidism are the shoulders, the hands, the vertebrae, and the skull. Standard radiography is usually sufficient to demonstrate its characteristic features: generalized osteopenia (Fig. 15.7); subperiosteal, subchondral, and cortical bone resorption; "brown tumors"; and soft tissue and cartilage calcifications. Subperiosteal resorption is particularly well demonstrated on plain films of the hands, where it usually affects the radial aspect of the middle phalanges of the middle and index fingers.

In secondary hyperparathyroidism, other characteristic features may be present in addition to the radiographic abnormalities just discussed. A generalized increase in bone density occurs, particularly in younger patients. In the spine, this change is reflected in dense sclerotic bands seen adjacent to the vertebral endplates, giving the vertebrae a sandwich-like appearance. This phenomenon is termed "rugger-jersey" spine, because the sclerotic bands form horizontal stripes resembling those on the shirts worn by rugby (rugger) players (Fig. 15.8). However, it must be kept in mind in the evaluation of hyperparathyroidism that osteosclerotic changes may also occur as a manifestation of healing, either spontaneously or as a result of treatment. Deposition of calcium in fibrocartilage, articular cartilage, and soft tissue is common, and vascular calcifications are much more frequent in patients with secondary hyperparathyroidism.

Complications

Both primary and secondary hyperparathyroidism may be complicated by pathologic fractures, which usually occur in the ribs and vertebral bodies. Scintigraphy is useful in detecting these complications.

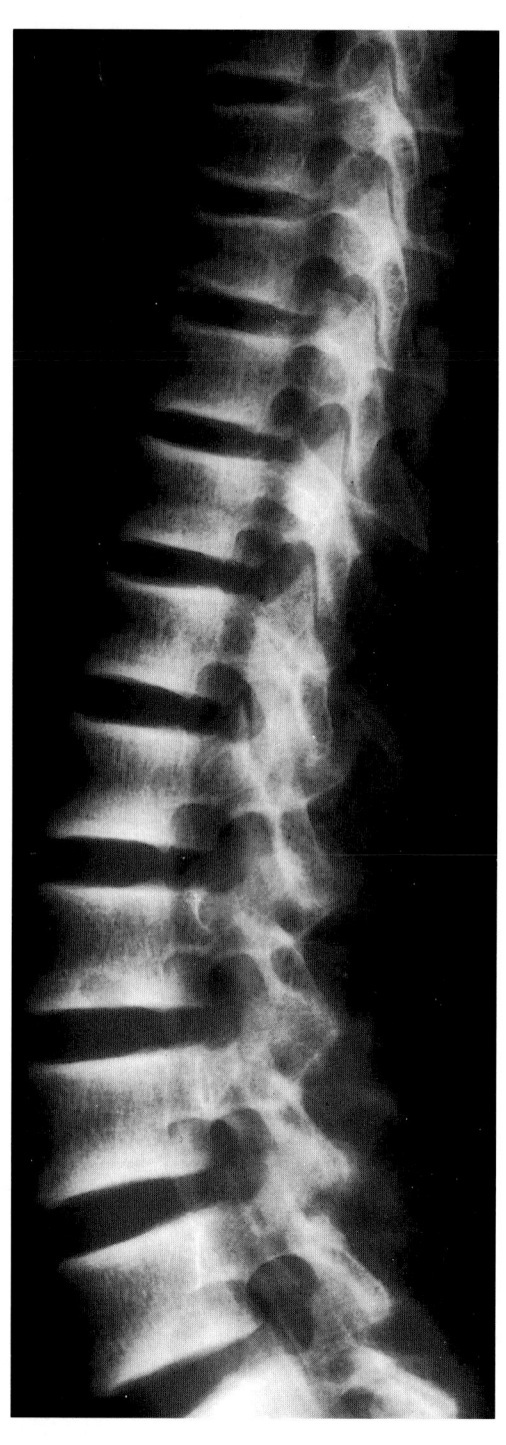

FIGURE 15.6 Specimen radiograph of the spine from a patient with renal osteodystrophy. The cancellous bone has a blurred pattern and there is irregular thickening of the endplates, giving the spine a "rugger-jersey" appearance (Reproduced with permission from Bullough PG, Boachie-Adjei O: *Atlas of Spinal Diseases.* New York, Gower, 1988)

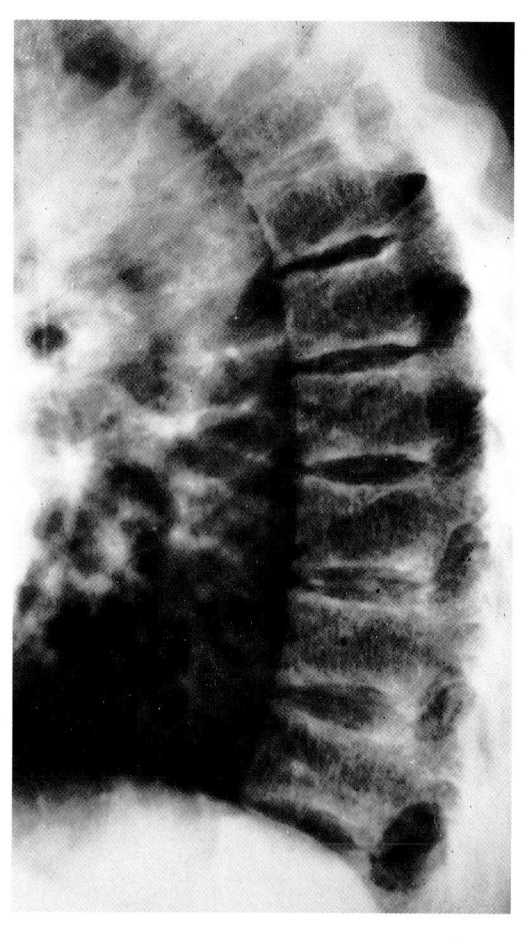

FIGURE 15.7 A 20-year-old woman presented with severe hypercalcemia due to a parathyroid adenoma. The lateral film of the thoracic spine demonstrates diffuse osteopenia associated with some irregularity of the vertebral endplates. Note the disk calcifications in the lower thoracic segment. (Reproduced with permission from Bullough PG, Boachie-Adjei O: *Atlas of Spinal Diseases.* New York, Gower, 1988)

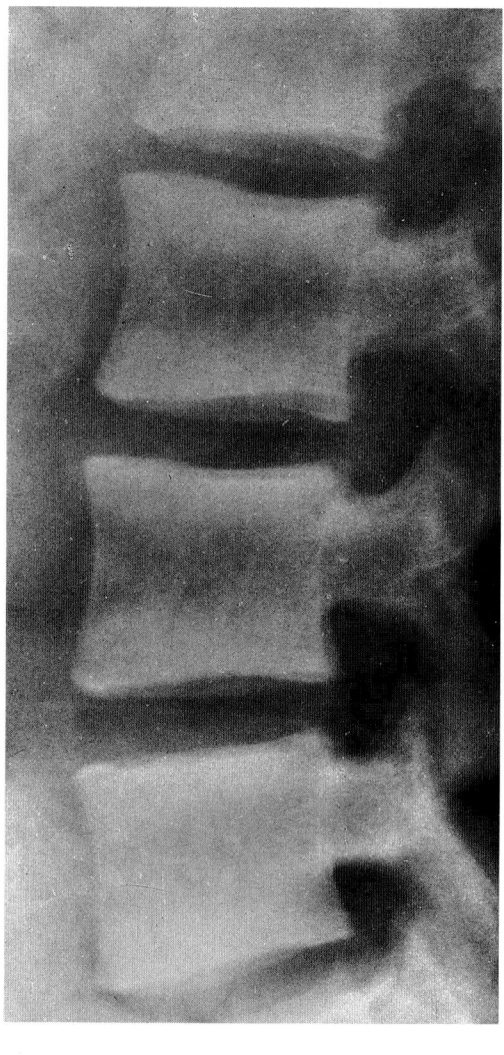

FIGURE 15.8 A 17-year-old boy with chronic renal failure developed secondary hyperparathyroidism. Lateral radiograph of the lumbar spine demonstrates sclerotic bands adjacent to the vertebral endplates—the so-called rugger-jersey spine.

Suggested Reading

Dunn AW: Senile osteoporosis. *Geriatrics* 22:175, 1989.

Genant HK, Heck LL, Lanzl LH, Rossmann K, Vander Horst J, Paloyan E: Primary hyperparathyroidism: A comprehensive study of clinical, biochemical and radiographic manifestations. *Radiology* 109:513, 1973.

Gillespy T III, Gillespy MP: Osteoporosis. *Radiol Clin North Am* 29:77, 1991.

Greenfield GB: Roentgen appearance of bone and soft tissue changes in chronic renal disease. *AJR* 116:749, 1972.

Griffith GC, Nichols G Jr, Asher JD, et al: Heparin osteoporosis. *JAMA* 193:91, 1965.

Hayes CW, Convay WF: Hyperparathyroidsim. *Radiol Clin North Am* 29:85, 1991.

Houang MTW, Brenton DP, Renton P, et al: Idiopathic juvenile osteoporosis. *Skel Radiol* 3:17, 1978.

Jensen PS, Kliger AS: Early radiographic manifestations of secondary hyperparathyroidism associated with chronic renal disease. *Radiology* 125:645, 1977.

Jones G: Radiological appearance of disuse osteoporosis. *Clin Radiol* 20:345, 1969.

Kaplan FS: Osteoporosis: Pathophysiology and prevention. *Clin Symp* 39:2, 1987.

Mankin HJ: Rickets, osteomalacia, and renal osteodystrophy—Part I. *J Bone Joint Surg* 56A:101, 1974.

Mankin HJ: Rickets, osteomalacia, and renal osteodystrophy—Part II. *J Bone Joint Surg* 56A:352, 1974.

Massry S, Ritz E: The pathogenesis of secondary hyperparathyroidism of renal failure. *Arch Intern Med* 138:853, 1978.

McCarthy JT, Kumar R: Behavior of the vitamin D endocrine system in the development of renal osteodystrophy. *Semin Nephrol* 6:21, 1986.

Parfitt AM: Renal osteodystrophy. *Orthop Clin North Am* 3:681, 1972.

Parfitt AM, Chir B: Hypophosphatemic vitamin D refractory rickets and osteomalacia. *Orthop Clin North Am* 3:681, 1972.

Pitt MJ: Rachitic and osteomalacic syndromes. *Radiol Clin North Am* 19:581, 1981.

Pitt MJ: Rickets and osteomalacia. In Resnick D (ed): *Bone and Joint Imaging*. Philadelphia, WB Saunders, 1989.

Reiss E, Canterbury JM: Spectrum of hyperparathyroidism. *Am J Med* 56:794, 1974.

Resnick D: The "rugger jersey" vertebral body. *Arthritis Rheum* 24:1191, 1981.

Resnick DL: Fish vertebrae. *Arthritis Rheum* 25:1073, 1982.

Richardson ML, Pozzi-Mucelli RS, Kanter AS, et al: Bone mineral changes in primary hyperparathyroidsim. *Skel Radiol* 15:85, 1986.

Rossi RL, ReMine SG, Clerkin EP: Hyperparathyroidism. *Surg Clin North Am* 65:187, 1985.

Sackler JP, Liu L: Case reports: Heparin-induced osteoporosis. *Br J Radiol* 46:548, 1973.

Shapiro R: Radiologic aspects of renal osteodystrophy. *Radiol Clin North Am* 10:557, 1972.

Weller M, Edelken J, Hodes PJ: Renal osteodystrophy. *Am J Roentgenol* 104:354, 1968.

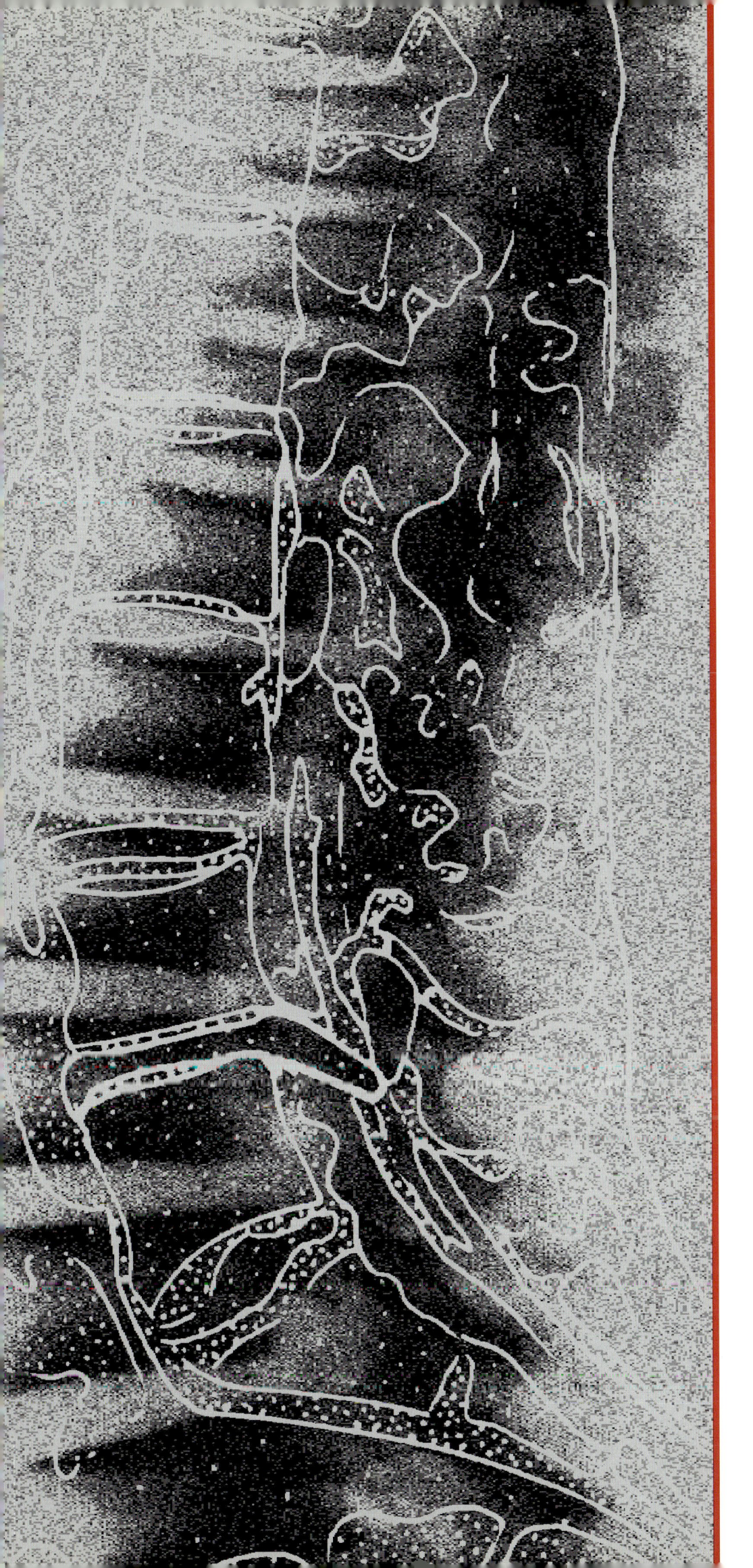

Paget Disease

16

PATHOPHYSIOLOGY

Paget disease, a relatively common disorder of bone, is a chronic, progressive disturbance in bone metabolism that primarily affects older persons. It is slightly more common in men than in women (3:2), with an average age of onset between 45 and 55 years, although the disease also has been known to occur in young adults. The prevalence of Paget disease varies considerably in different parts of the world, with the greatest incidence in the United Kingdom, Australia, and New Zealand.

The precise nature of Paget disease and its etiology are still unknown. Sir James Paget (1877) named the disease *osteitis deformans*, in the belief that the basic process was infectious in origin. Other etiologies have also been proposed, such as neoplastic, vascular, endocrinologic, immunologic, traumatic, and hereditary processes. Recent ultrastructural studies and the discovery of giant multinucleated osteoclasts containing microfilaments in the cytoplasm, as well as intranuclear inclusion bodies, suggest a viral etiology. Some investigators have obtained immunocytologic evidence identifying the particles as analogous to those from measles group virus materal. Other immunologic studies have demonstrated viral antigens in affected cells, identical to those from respiratory syncytial virus.

Whatever the fundamental cause of Paget disease, its basic pathologic process has to do with the interplay between bone resorption and formation of appositional new bone. There is disordered and extremely active bone remodeling secondary to osteoclastic bone resorption and osteoblastic bone formation in a characteristic mosaic pattern, which is the histologic hallmark of this condition. Biochemically, the increase in osteoblastic activity is reflected in elevated serum levels of alkaline phosphatase, which can rise to extremely high values. Similarly, the increase in osteoclastic resorption of bone is reflected in high urinary levels of hydroxyproline, which is formed as a result of the breakdown of collagen.

The skeletal abnormalities seen in Paget disease are frequently asymptomatic and may be an incidental finding on radiographic examination or at autopsy. When the changes are symptomatic, the clinical manifestations are often related to complications of the disease, such as deformity of the long bones, warmth in the involved extremity, periosteal tenderness and bone pain, fractures, secondary osteoarthritis, neural compression, and sarcomatous degeneration. The distribution of lesions varies from monostotic involvement to widespread disease. The following bones are those most often affected, in order of decreasing frequency: pelvis, femur, skull, tibia, vertebrae, clavicle, humerus, and ribs.

RADIOGRAPHIC EVALUATION

The radiographic features of Paget disease correspond to the pathologic processes in the bone and depend on the stage of the disorder. In the early phase, the *osteolytic* or *hot phase*, active bone resorption is evident as a radiolucent wedge or an elongated area with sharp borders that destroys the cortex and cancellous bone as it advances along the shaft. This phenomenon is frequently described as "advancing wedge," "candle flame," and

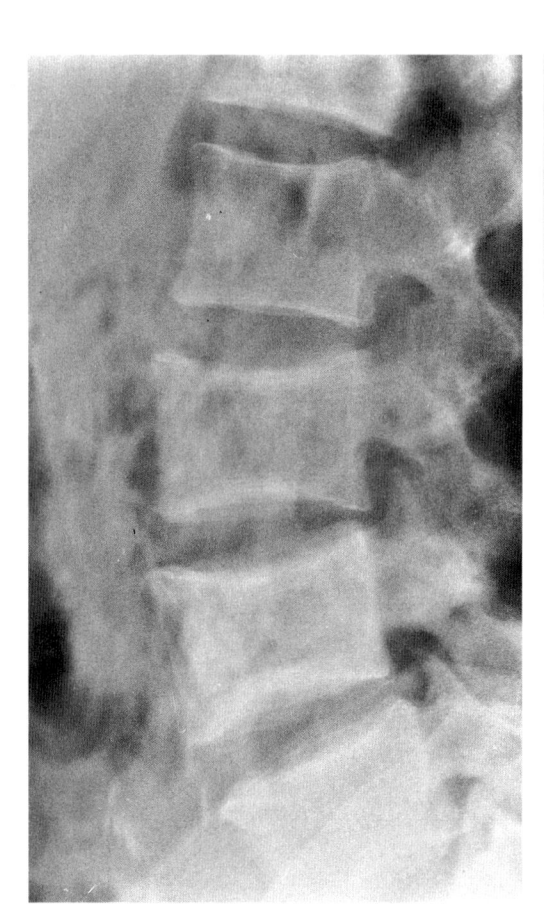

FIGURE 16.1 Involvement of the lumbar spine in the mixed phase of Paget disease can be recognized by the "picture-frame" appearance of the the vertebral bodies created by dense, sclerotic bone on the periphery and greater radiolucency in the center. Note the partial replacement of vertebral endplates by coarsely trabeculated bone. (Reproduced with permission from Sissons HA, Greenspan A: Paget's disease. In Taveras JM, Ferrucci JT (eds): *Radiology—Imaging, Diagnosis, Intervention.* Philadelphia, J B Lippincott, 1986)

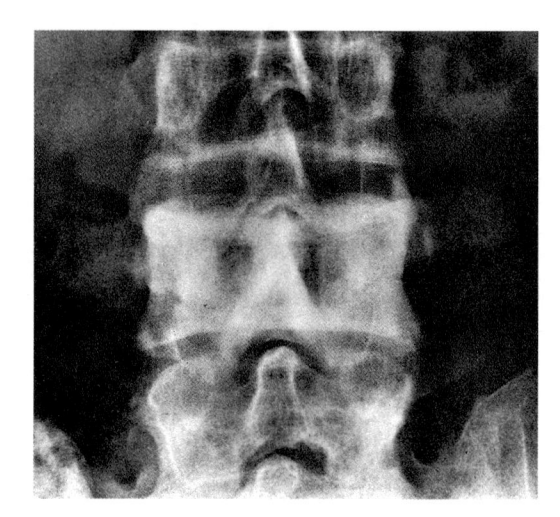

FIGURE 16.2 Anteroposterior film of the lumbar spine in a 54-year-old man with polyostotic Paget disease shows involvement of L3 vertebra. Note the lack of distinction between the endplates and cancellous bone of the vertebral body.

"blade of grass." In flat bones, such as the calvaria or the iliac bone, or in the vertebral body, an area of active bone destruction, known as *osteoporosis circumscripta*, appears as a purely osteolytic lesion.

In the *intermediate* or *mixed phase*, bone destruction is accompanied by new bone formation, with the latter process tending to predominate. Bone remodeling appears radiographically as thickening of the cortex and coarse trabeculation of cancellous bone. In the spine, the thin cortex of the vertebral body, which disappears in the hot phase, is later replaced by broad, coarsely trabeculated bone, forming what appears to be a "picture frame" around the body (Fig. 16.1). In the skull, focal, patchy densities with a "cotton-ball" appearance are characteristic.

In the *cool phase*, a diffuse increase of bone density occurs, together with enlargement and widening of the bone and marked cortical thickening, with blurring of the distinction between cortex and spongiosa. Bowing of the long bones may become a striking feature. Similar changes are observed in the skull, where obliteration of the diploic space is also a typical feature. In the spine, the vertebral body enlarges and the distinction between the endplates and cancellous bone disappears (Fig. 16.2).

DIFFERENTIAL DIAGNOSIS

Several conditions may mimic Paget disease. Paget disease itself may be mistaken for other pathologic processes. For example, a uniform increase in osseous density of the vertebrae may mimic lymphoma or metastatic cancer. The rugger-jersey appearance of the spine in secondary hyperparathyroidism may resemble Paget vertebrae. Vertebral hemangioma also looks very much like Paget vertebrae on a radiograph, except that the vertebral body is not enlarged and the vertebral endplates are well outlined. However, the condition that bears the most striking resemblance to Paget disease is familial idiopathic hypophosphatasia, also called *juvenile Paget disease*. In this condition, unlike Paget disease, the articular ends of the bone may not be affected.

COMPLICATIONS

Pathologic Fractures

Of the many complications that may be observed in patients with Paget disease, the most common are pathologic fractures. These are most often seen in long bones, but vertebrae may also be affected (Fig. 16.3). Fractures are more likely to occur during the osteolytic or hot phase and are frequently the main presenting manifestation of Paget disease.

Neurologic Complications

The neurologic complications of Paget disease are secondary to involvement of the vertebral column and skull. Collapse of a vertebral body, for example, causes extradural spinal canal block, which may lead to paraple-

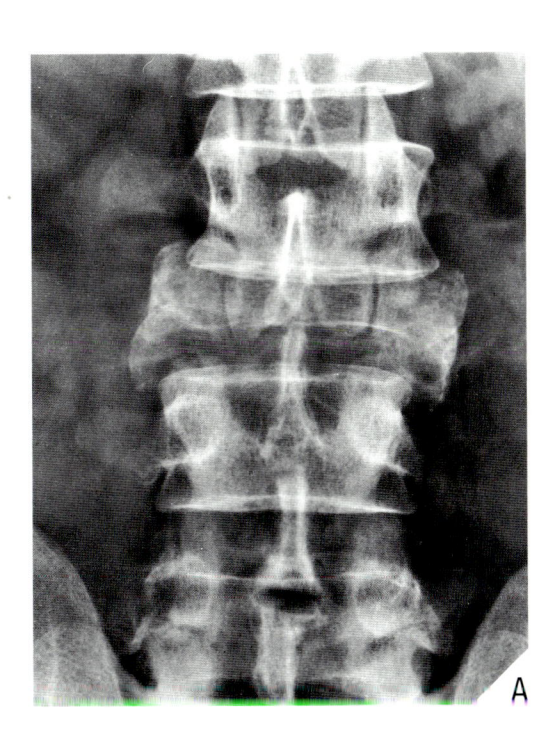

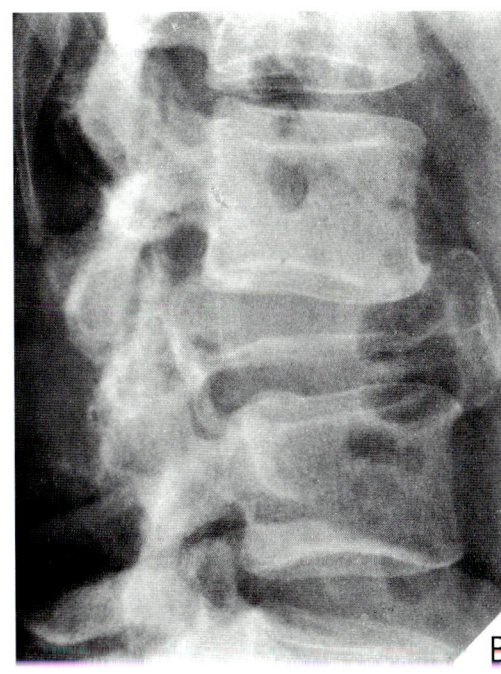

FIGURE 16.3 A 60-year-old man with Paget disease affecting the vertebrae presented with low back pain and neurologic symptoms. Anteroposterior **(A)** and lateral **(B)** radiographs of the lumbar spine show a pathologic compression fracture of L3 with encroachment on the spinal canal, which was the source of his symptoms. (Reproduced with permission from Sissons HA, Greenspan A: Paget's disease. In Taveras JM, Ferrucci JT (eds): *Radiology—Imaging, Diagnosis, Intervention*. Philadelphia, J B Lippincott, 1986)

gia. Severe involvement of the bony spinal canal may lead to spinal stenosis, the presence of which can be effectively demonstrated by CT or MRI (Figs. 16.4, 16.5). Basilar invagination cause by softening of the bone of the skull may lead to encroachment on the foramen magnum and ensuing neurologic deficit.

Neoplastic Complications

The coexistence of single or multiple giant cell tumors, which may be either benign or malignant, may complicate Paget disease. The usual site of these tumors is the calvaria or the iliac bone.

The development of a bone sarcoma is a major but rare complication of Paget disease (<1%). Osteosarcoma is by far the most common histologic type, followed by fibrosarcoma and chondrosarcoma, with the pelvis, femur, and humerus at highest risk for development of malignant transformation. The main radiographic features of this complication are development of a lytic lesion at the site of Paget disease, cortical breakthrough, and formation of a soft tissue mass; a periosteal reaction is rare. There is often a pathologic fracture as well. The radiographic appearance of Paget sarcoma must be distinguished from that of metastases from a primary carcinoma of the kidney, breast, or prostate. The metastatic deposit may be lodged in either unaffected or pagetic bone. The prognosis for patients

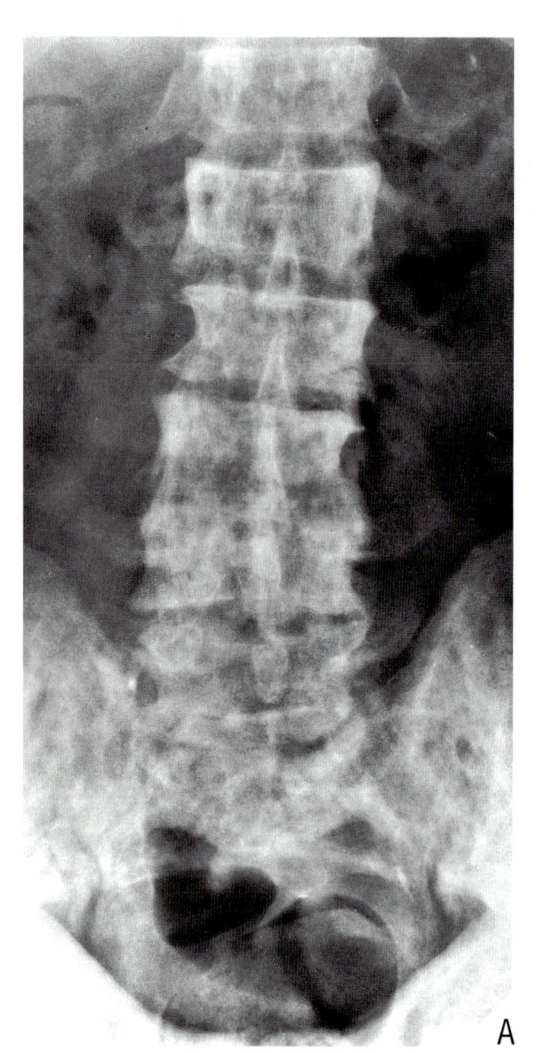

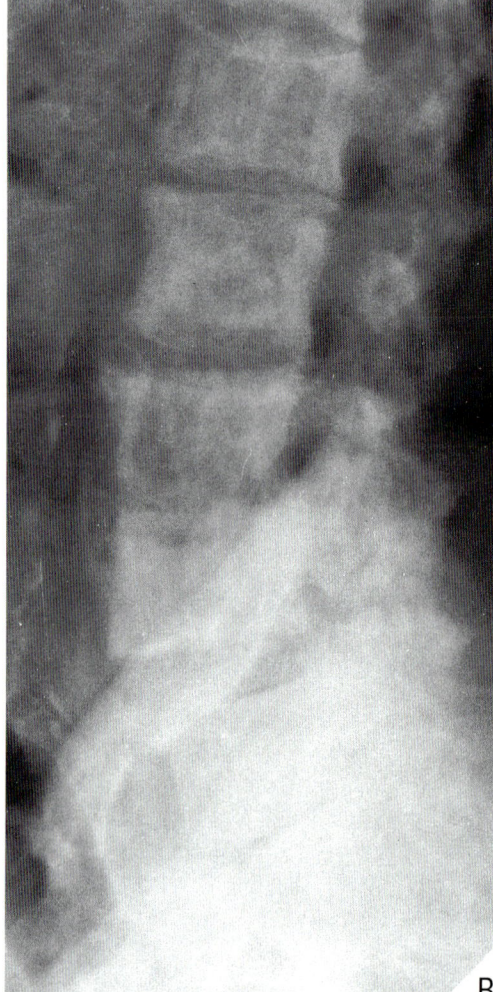

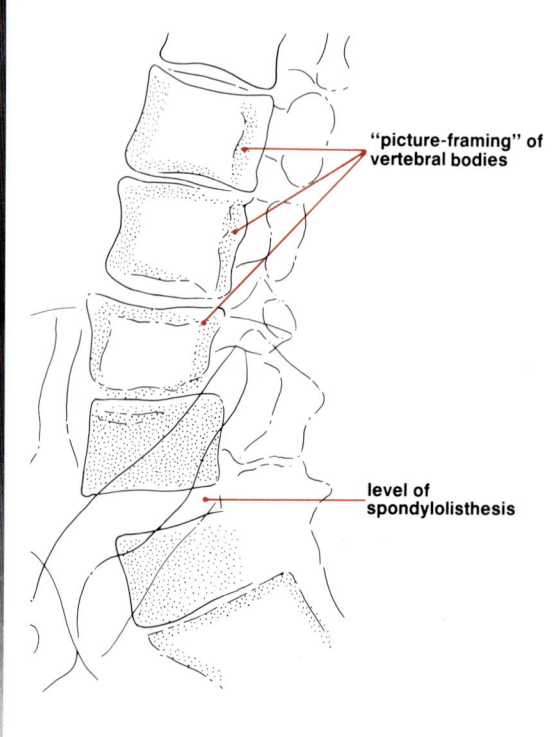

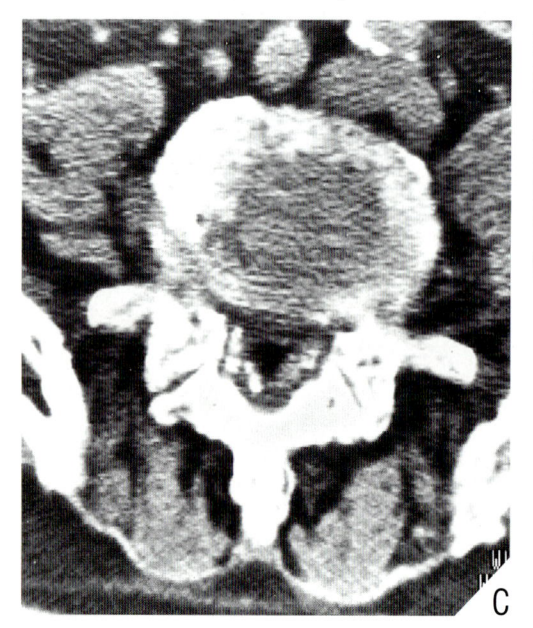

FIGURE 16.4 An 84-year-old man with extensive polyostotic Paget disease for many years developed degenerative spondylolisthesis and spinal stenosis. Anteroposterior **(A)** and lateral **(B)** views of the lumbar spine show Paget disease in the cool phase. Second-degree degenerative spondylolisthesis is seen at the L4–L5 level. **(C)** CT section through L5 demonstrates narrowing of the spinal canal characteristic of spinal stenosis, the major cause of most neurologic symptoms in Paget disease.

Imaging of the Spine in Clinical Practice

with sarcomatous degeneration of Paget disease is poor; the mean survival time usually does not exceed 6 to 8 months. Occasionally, an osteosarcoma in pagetic bone may metastasize to other bones and soft tissues; however, metastases to the lung, liver, and adrenals are considerably more likely.

ORTHOPEDIC MANAGEMENT

Because of the variety of clinical presentations of Paget disease, decisions regarding treatment must be based on the particular manifestations in the individual patient.

The role of the orthopedic surgeon in the management of Paget disease is to evaluate and treat the cause of pain, to assess and manage any deformities, and to provide therapy for pathologic fractures and tumors that develop in pagetic bone. The radiologist contributes to these aims by providing essential information. For example, CT is useful for demonstrating spinal stenosis, which frequently leads to neurologic symptoms in patients with Paget disease. Radionuclide imaging is also a valuable technique, particularly for determining the skeletal distribution of the disease.

Medical treatment consists of inhibition of osteoclastic activity by calcitonin and oral administration of diphosphonates, which bind to areas of high bone turnover, and thus decrease bone resorption. Administration of mithramycin inhibits RNA synthesis and has a potent cytotoxic effect on osteoclasts. The serum alkaline phosphatase determination and the 24-hour urinary hydroxyproline measurement are the main indicators of the response of the disease to medical treatment.

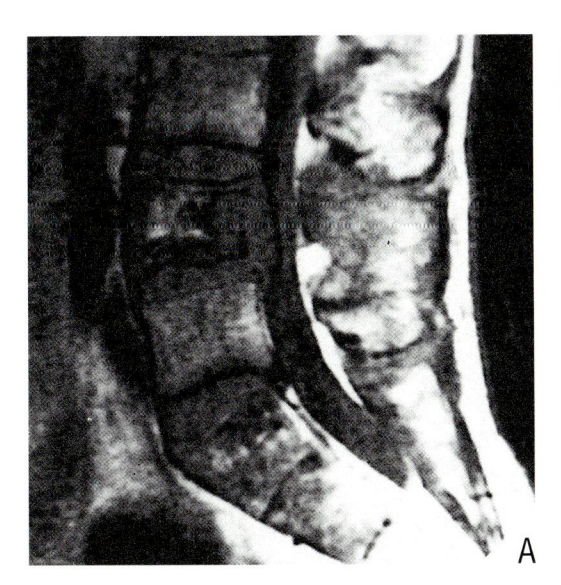

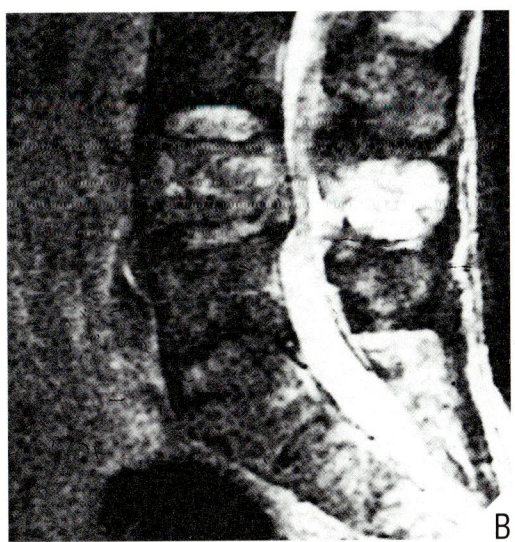

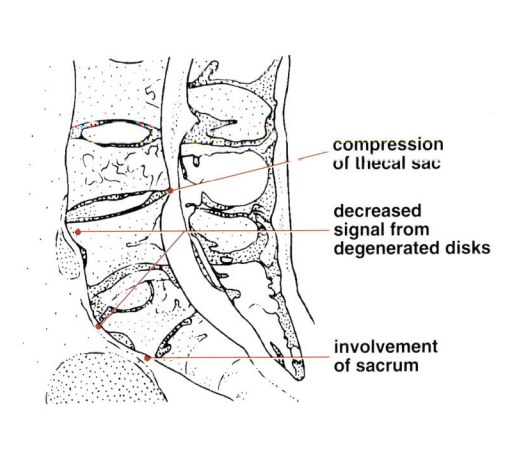

FIGURE 16.5 (A) T1-weighted spin-echo sagittal MRI of lower lumbar spine shows Paget disease affecting L4 and S1 vertebrae. The L4 vertebra is enlarged and its posterior cortex impinging on the thecal sac. **(B)** T2-weighted sagittal image better demonstrates the narrowing of the spinal canal and compression of the thecal sac. Note the alteration of the signal from the intervertebral disks L4–S1, indicating degenerative changes.

SUGGESTED READING

Barry HC: *Paget's Disease of Bone*. Edinburgh, Churchill-Livingstone, 1969.

Greenspan A, Norman A, Sterling AP: Precocious onset of Paget's disease—A report of three cases and review of the literature. *J Can Assoc Radiol* 28:69, 1977.

Hutter RVP, Foote FW Jr, Frazell EL, et al: Giant cell tumors complicating Paget's disease of bone. *Cancer* 16:1044, 1963.

Krane SM: Paget's disease of bone. *Clin Orthop* 127:24, 1977.

Lander PH, Hadjipavlou O: A dynamic classification of Paget's disease. *J Bone Joint Surg* 68B:431, 1986.

McKenna RJ, Schwinn CP, Soong KY, et al: Osteogenic sarcoma arising in Paget's disease. *Cancer* 17:42, 1964.

Milgram JW: Radiographical and pathological assessment of the activity of Paget's disease of bone. *Clin Orthop* 127:43, 1977.

Milgram JW: Orthopedic management of Paget's disease of bone. *Clin Orthop* 127:63, 1977.

Mirra JM: Pathogenesis of Paget's disease based on viral etiology. *Clin Orthop Relat Res* 217:162, 1987.

Mirra JM, Gold RM: Giant cell tumor containing viral-like intranuclear inclusions, in association with Paget's disease. Case report. *Skel Radiol* 8:67, 1982.

Paget J: On a form of chronic inflammation of bones (osteitis deformans). *Med Chir Trans* 60:37, 1877.

Roberts MC, Kressel HY, Fallon MD, et al: Paget's disease: MR imaging findings. *Radiology* 173:341, 1989.

Rosenbaum HD, Hanson DJ: Geographic variation in the prevalence of Paget's disease of bone. *Radiology* 92:959, 1969.

Sissons HA: Epidemiology of Paget's disease. *Clin Orthop* 45:73, 1966.

Sissons HA, Greenspan A: Paget's disease. In Taveras JM, Ferrucci JT (eds): *Radiology—Imaging, Diagnosis, Intervention*. Philadelphia, J B Lippincott, 1986.

Smith J, Botet JF, Yeh SDJ: Bone sarcomas in Paget's disease: A study of 85 patients. *Radiology* 152:583, 1984.

Wellman HN, Schauwecker D, Robb JA, et al: Skeletal scintimaging and radiography in the diagnosis and management of Paget's disease. *Clin Orthop* 127:55, 1977.

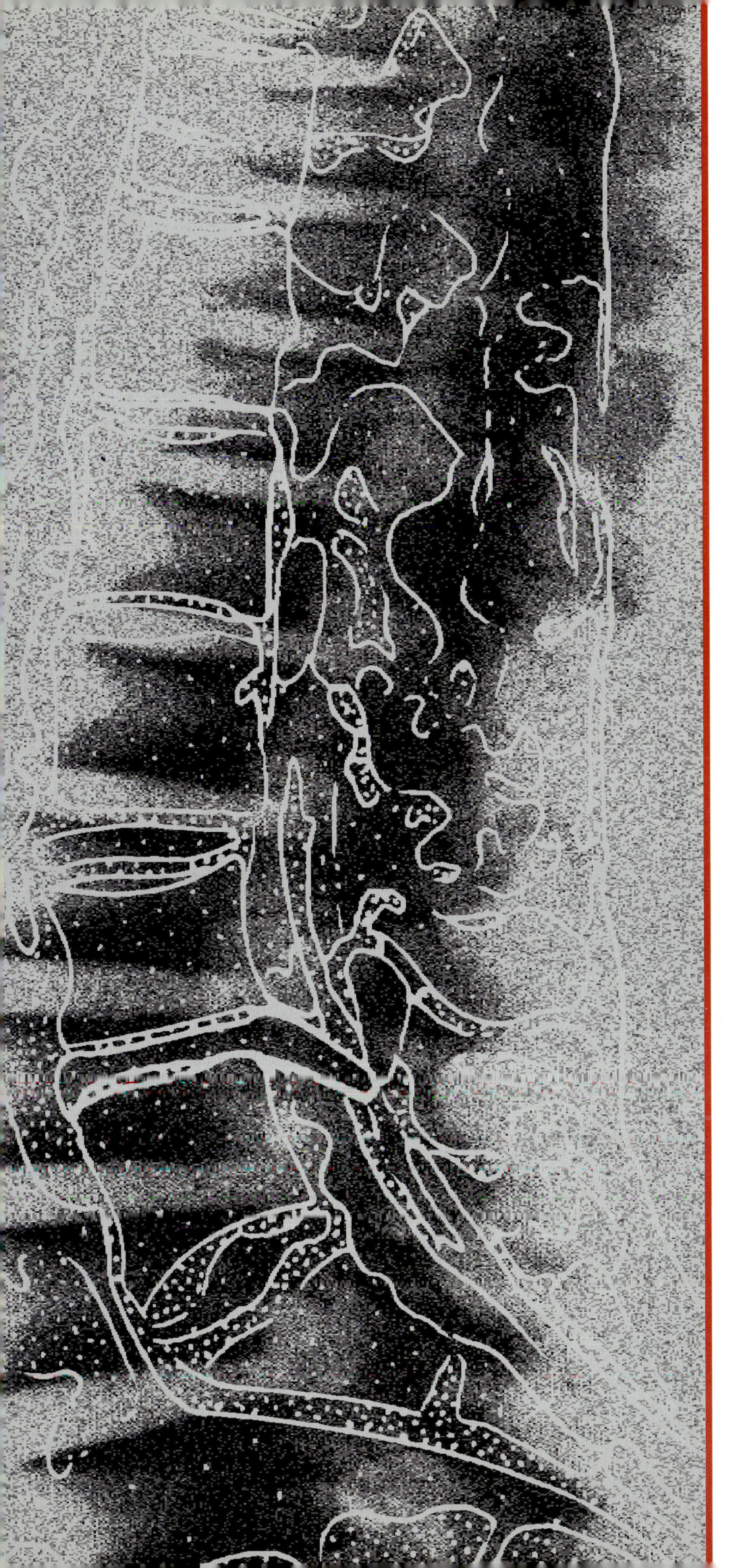

Miscellaneous Metabolic and Endocrine Disorders

17

Familial Idiopathic Hyperphosphatasia

Familial idiopathic hyperphosphatasia is a rare autosomal recessive disorder that affects young children, usually within the first 18 months of life, and exhibits a striking predilection for those of Puerto Rican descent. The condition is associated with progressive deformities of bones. Clinically, it is characterized by painful bowing of the limbs, muscle weakness and abnormal gait, pathologic fractures, spinal deformities, loss of vision and hearing, elevation of serum alkaline phosphatase, and an increase in the level of leucine aminopeptidase.

Radiographic Evaluation

Increased turnover of bone and skeletal collagen, demonstrable by radionuclide bone scan, is a characteristic finding in familial idiopathic hyperphosphatasia. Its radiographic features are typical. Although this disorder has no relationship to classic Paget disease, it is often referred to as *juvenile Paget disease* and it exhibits similar radiographic features (Fig. 17.1). The long bones are increased in size, showing thickening of the cortex and a coarse trabecular pattern. Similarly, bowing deformities are common, as are involvement of the spine, pelvis, and skull. However, unlike the patients with Paget disease, the epiphyses are usually not affected, and the vertebral bodies show a decrease in height (platyspondylisis) (Fig. 17.2).

Differential Diagnosis

There are a few conditions similar to familial idiopathic hyperphosphatasia that belong to the general group of endosteal hyperostoses or hyperostosis corticalis generalisata. In particular, an autosomal recessive form of these disorders, although classified as chronic hyperphosphatasia tarda (van Buchem disease) is, in fact, a distinct dysplasia; its onset is later than that of congenital hyperphosphatasia, and the age of patients ranges from 25 to 50 years. The major radiographic finding is a symmetrical thickening of the cortices of the long and short tubular bones. The femora are not bowed, and the articular ends are spared. The cranial bones show marked thickening of both the vault and the base. Serum alkaline phosphatase levels are elevated, and calcium and phosphorus levels are normal.

Acromegaly

Increased secretion of growth hormone (somatotropin) by the eosinophilic cells of the anterior lobe of the pituitary gland, as a result of either hyperplasia of the gland or a tumor, leads to acceleration of bone growth. If this condition develops before skeletal maturity (ie, while the growth plates are still open), it results in gigantism; development after skeletal maturity results in acromegaly. The onset of symptoms is usually insidious, and the involvement of certain target sites in the skeleton (eg, frontal sinuses, mandible, spine, hands, feet) is typical. Gradual enlargement of the hands and feet and exaggeration of facial features are the earliest manifestations. The characteristic facial changes result from overgrowth of the frontal sinuses, protrusion of the jaw (prognathism), accentuation of the orbital ridges, enlargement of the nose, lips, and tongue, and thickening and coarsening of the soft tissues of the face.

Radiographic Evaluation

Radiographic examination reveals a number of characteristic features of acromegaly. A lateral view of the skull demonstrates thickening of the cranial bones and increased density; the diploe may be obliterated. The sella turcica, which houses the pituitary gland, may or may not be enlarged.

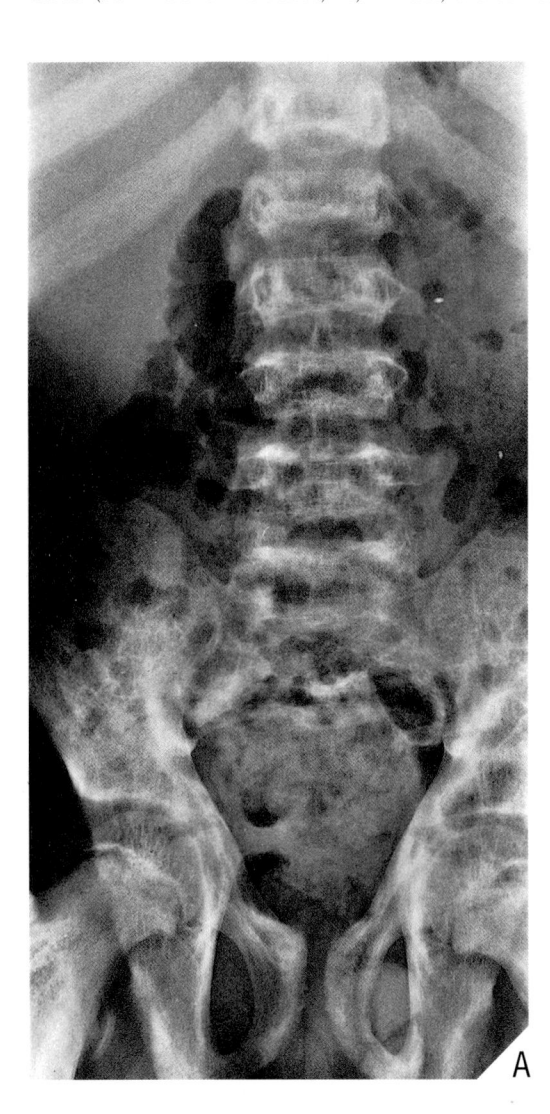

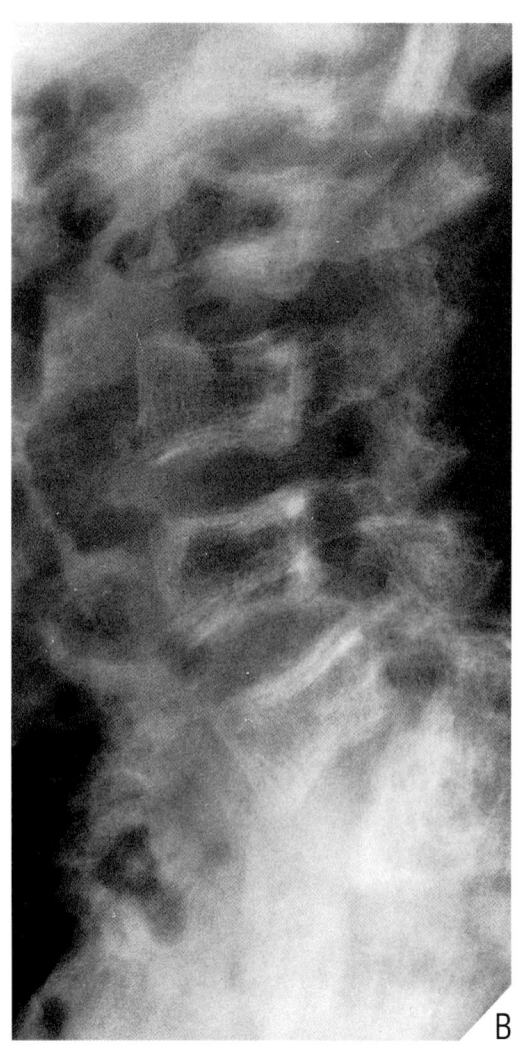

FIGURE 17.1 A 12-year-old Puerto Rican boy diagnosed with familial idiopathic hyperphosphatasia. **(A)** Anteroposterior view of the lumbosacral spine shows similar bony changes as seen in Paget disease—thickening of the cortices and coarse trabecular pattern. Note, however, the lack of involvement or articular ends of the femora. **(B)** Lateral radiograph shows "picture framing" of several vertebral bodies.

The paranasal sinuses become enlarged, and the mastoid cells are overpneumatized. The prognathous jaw, one of the obvious clinical features of this condition, is apparent on the lateral view of the facial bones.

The hands also exhibit revealing radiographic changes. The heads of the metacarpals are enlarged, and irregular bone thickening along the margins, simulating osteophytes, may be seen. Increase in size of the sesamoid at the metacarpophangeal joint of the thumb may be helpful in evaluating acromegaly. Values of the sesamoid index (determined by the height and width of this ossicle measured in millimeters) greater than 30 in women and greater than 40 in men suggest acromegaly, but in general the dividing line between normal and abnormal values is not sharp enough to allow individual borderline cases to be diagnosed on the basis of this index alone. Characteristic changes are also seen in the distal phalanges; their bases enlarge and the terminal tufts form spur-like projections. The joint spaces widen as a result of hypertrophy of articular cartilage, and hypertrophy of the soft tissues may also occur, leading to the development of square, spade-shaped fingers.

Evaluation of the foot on the lateral view allows an important measurement to be made, the heel-pad thickness. This index is determined by the distance from the posteroinferior surface of the os calcis to the nearest skin surface. In a normal 150-lb subject, the heel-pad thickness should not exceed 22 mm. For each additional 25 pounds of body weight, 1 mm can be added to the basic value; thus, 24 mm would be the highest normal value for a 200-lb person. If the heel-pad thickness is greater than the established normal value, acromegaly is a strong possibility and determination of growth hormone level by immunoassay is indicated.

The spine in acromegaly may also reveal identifying features. A lateral view of the spine may disclose an increase in the anteroposterior diameter of a vertebral body, as well as scalloping or increased concavity of the posterior vertebral margin (Fig. 17.3). Although the exact mechanism of this phenomenon is not known, bone resorption has been implicated as a potential cause. Other conditions have also been associated with posterior vertebral scalloping (Fig. 17.4). In addition, thoracic kyphosis is often increased in spinal acromegaly, and lumbar lordosis is accentuated. The

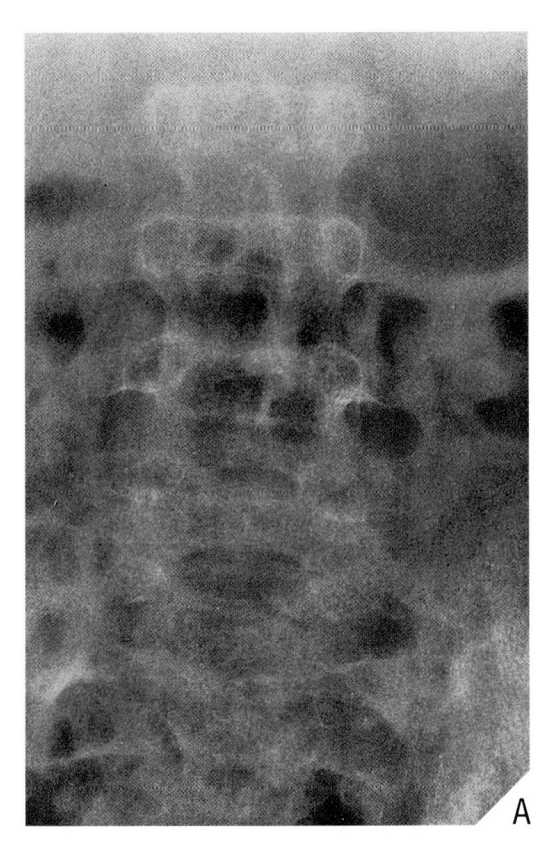

FIGURE 17.2 An anteroposterior (**A**) and lateral (**B**) radiograph of the lumbar spine in a 4½-year-old boy with *Familial Idiopathic Hyperphosphatasia* demonstrate characteristic platyspondylisis of the vertebral bodies.

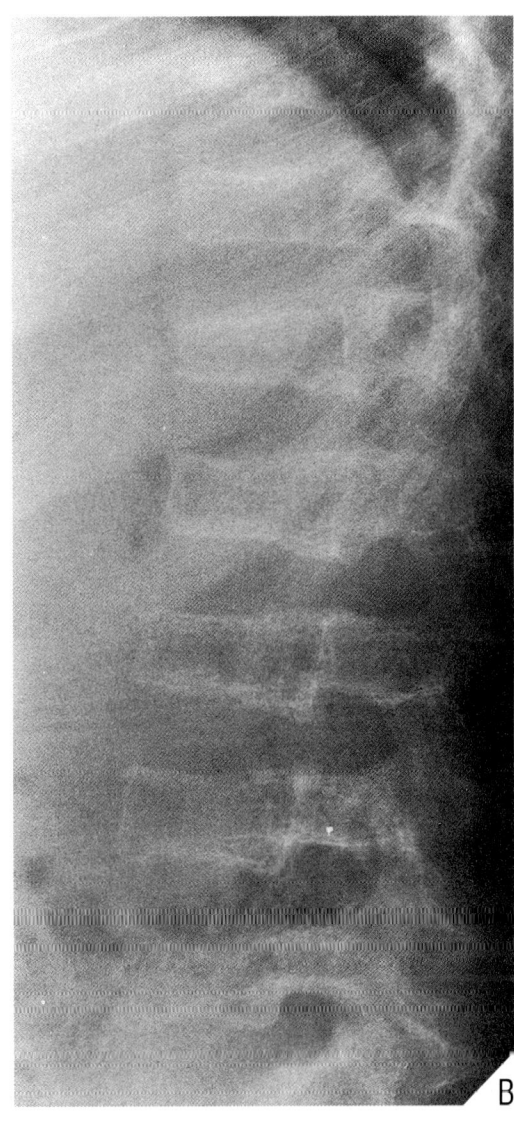

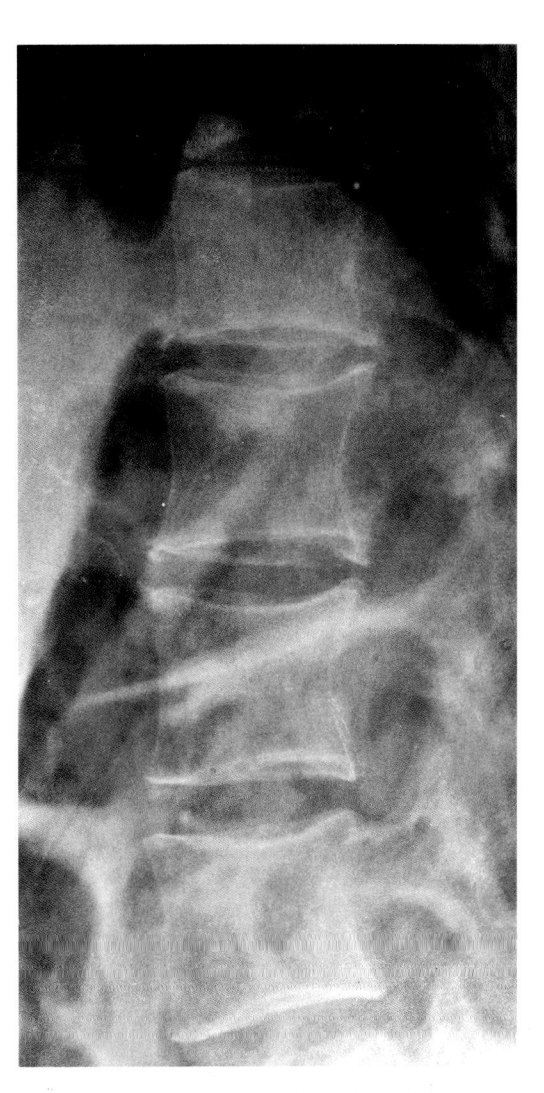

FIGURE 17.3 Lateral view of the thoracolumbar spine of a 49-year-old woman with acromegaly demonstrates posterior vertebral scalloping, a phenomenon apparently due to bone resorption.

intervertebral disk space may be wider than normal owing to overgrowth of the cartilaginous portion of the disk.

The articular abnormalities seen in acromegaly are the result of a frequent complication—degenerative joint disease. This, in turn, is caused by overgrowth of the articular cartilage and subsequent inadequate nourishment of abnormally thick cartilage. The combination of joint-space narrowing, osteophytes, subchondral sclerosis, and formation of cystlike lesions is similar to the primary osteoarthritic process.

GAUCHER DISEASE

Gaucher disease is a metabolic disorder characterized by the abnormal deposition of cerebrosides (glycolipids) in the reticuloendothelial cells of the spleen, liver, and bone marrow. These altered macrophages, called *Gaucher cells,* are the histologic hallmark of the disease.

Types

Gaucher disease is a familial disturbance of unknown etiology and is transmitted as an autosomal recessive trait. It is classified into three distinct categories:

Type I The nonneuronopathic or adult type is the most common form, occurring mainly in Ashkenazic Jews. Onset occurs in the first or second decade of life, and the patient usually lives a life of normal length. Bone abnormalities and hepatosplenomegaly characterize this form of disease.

Type II The acute neuronopathic form is lethal within the first year of life. This type apparently has no predilection for any specific ethnic groups.

Type III The subacute juvenile neuronopathic form begins in the latter part of the first year and follows a malignant course similar to that of type II. Patients suffer from mental retardation and seizures, and usually die by the end of the second decade of life.

The presenting clinical features depend on the type of disease. The adult form of the disorder (type I) is the most common, and typically presents with abdominal distension secondary to splenomegaly. Recurrent bone pain is a sign of skeletal involvement, and acute, severe bone pain, together with swelling and fever, suggests acute pyogenic osteomyelitis. This clinical complex, which is the result of ischemic necrosis of bone, has been called *aseptic osteomyelitis.* Pingueculae may be present in the eyes, and the skin may acquire a brown pigmentation. Epistaxis or other hemorrhages caused by thrombocytopenia may occur. The diagnosis is made by demonstrating characteristic Gaucher cells in bone marrow aspirate or in a biopsy specimen from the liver.

Radiographic Evaluation

The radiographic examination in Gaucher disease reveals characteristic findings. There is a diffuse osteoporosis, frequently associated with medullary expansion. In the ends of the long bones, this phenomenon is referred to as the "Erlenmeyer-flask" deformity. Localized bone destruction, assuming a honeycomb appearance, is also typically seen; gross osteolytic destruction is usually limited to the shafts of the long bones.

FIGURE 17.4 CAUSES OF SCALLOPING IN VERTEBRAL BODIES

INCREASED INTRASPINAL PRESSURE	DURAL ECTASIA	CONGENITAL DISORDERS	BONE RESORPTION
Intradural neoplasms	Marfan syndrome	Achondroplasia	Acromegaly
Intraspinal cysts	Ehlers–Danlos syndrome	Morquio disease	
Syringomyelia and hydromyelia	Neurofibromatosis	Hunter syndrome	PHYSIOLOGIC SCALLOPING
Communicating hydrocephalus		Osteogenesis imperfecta	

(Modified from Mitchell GE, Lourie H, Berne AS: The various causes of scalloped vertebrae and notes on their pathogenesis. Radiology 89:67, 1967)

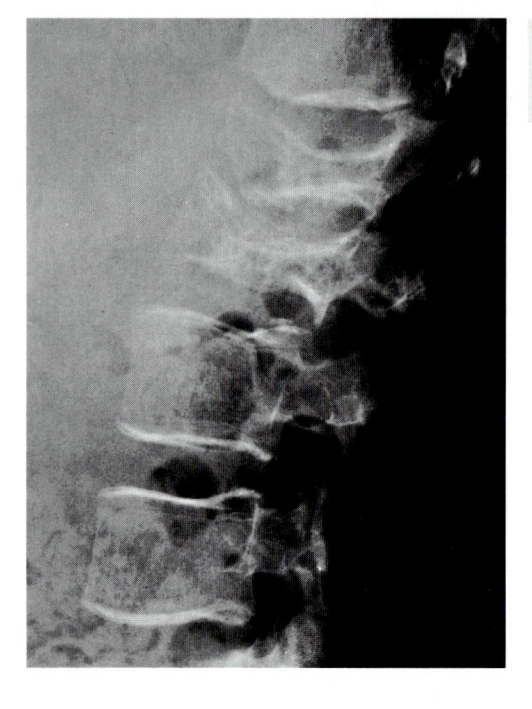

FIGURE 17.5 Lateral radiograph of the lumbar spine of a patient with Gaucher disease shows diffuse osteopenia and compression fractures of vertebral bodies L1 and L2. (Reproduced with permission from Bullough PG, Boachie-Adjei O: *Atlas of Spinal Diseases.* Philadelphia, J B Lippincott, 1988)

Imaging of the Spine in Clinical Practice

long bones. Moreover, sclerotic changes are common, occurring secondary to a repair process or bone infarctions. Medullary bone infarction and a periosteal reaction may lead to a bone-within-bone phenomenon, which may resemble osteomyelitis. In the spine, osteopenia is invariably present and compression fractures, similar to those encountered in other types of osteoporosis, are seen (Fig. 17.5). Less commonly, stepped deformities of the vertebral endplates, identical to the ones seen in sickle-cell disease, may be observed. Stepped deformity, also termed the "H" vertebra because it resembles this capital letter, is probably related to ischemia resulting from extrinsic compression of the vertebral vessels and intrinsic vascular abnormalities. Some investigators speculate that this deformity is caused by initial central collapse of the bone beneath the vertebral endplate, with subsequent peripheral growth recovery.

Complications

The most common complication of Gaucher disease is osteonecrosis of the femoral head. Superimposition of degenerative changes is also a frequent finding. Pathologic fractures are common and may involve the long bones as well as the spine. The most serious complication, fortunately a rare one, is malignant transformation at the site of bone infarcts into fibrosarcoma and malignant fibrous histiocytoma.

SUGGESTED READING

Desnick RJ: Gaucher disease (1882–1982): Centennial perspectives on the most prevalent Jewish genetic disease. *Mt Sinai J Med* 49:443, 1982.

Goldblatt J, Sachs S, Beighton P: The orthopedic aspects of Gaucher's disease. *Clin Orthop* 137:208, 1978.

Greenfield GB: Bone changes in chronic adult Gaucher's disease. *AJR* 110:800, 1970

Lang EK, Bessler WT: The roentgenologic features of acromegaly. *Am J Roentgenol* 86:321, 1961.

Lanir A, Hadar H, Cohen I, et al: Gaucher disease: Assessment with MR imaging. *Radiology* 161:239, 1986.

Levin B: Gaucher's disease: Clinical and roentgenologic manifestations. *AJR* 85:685, 1961.

McNulty JF, Pim P: Hyperphosphatasia. Report of a case with a 30-year follow-up. *AJR* 115:614, 1972.

Mitchell GE, Lourie H, Berne AS: The various causes of scalloped vertebrae and notes on their pathogenesis. *Radiology* 89:67, 1967.

Steinbach HL, Feldman R, Goldberg MB: Acromegaly. *Radiology* 72:535, 1959.

Stuber JL, Palacios E: Vertebral scalloping in acromegaly. *AJR* 112:397, 1971.

van Buchem FSP, Hadders HN, Hansen JF, et al: Hyperostosis corticalis generalisata. Report of seven cases. *Am J Med* 33:387, 1962.

van Buchem FSP, Hadders MN, Ubbens R: An uncommon familial systemic disease of the skeleton: Hyperostosis corticalis generalisata familiaris. *Acta Radiol* 44:109, 1955.

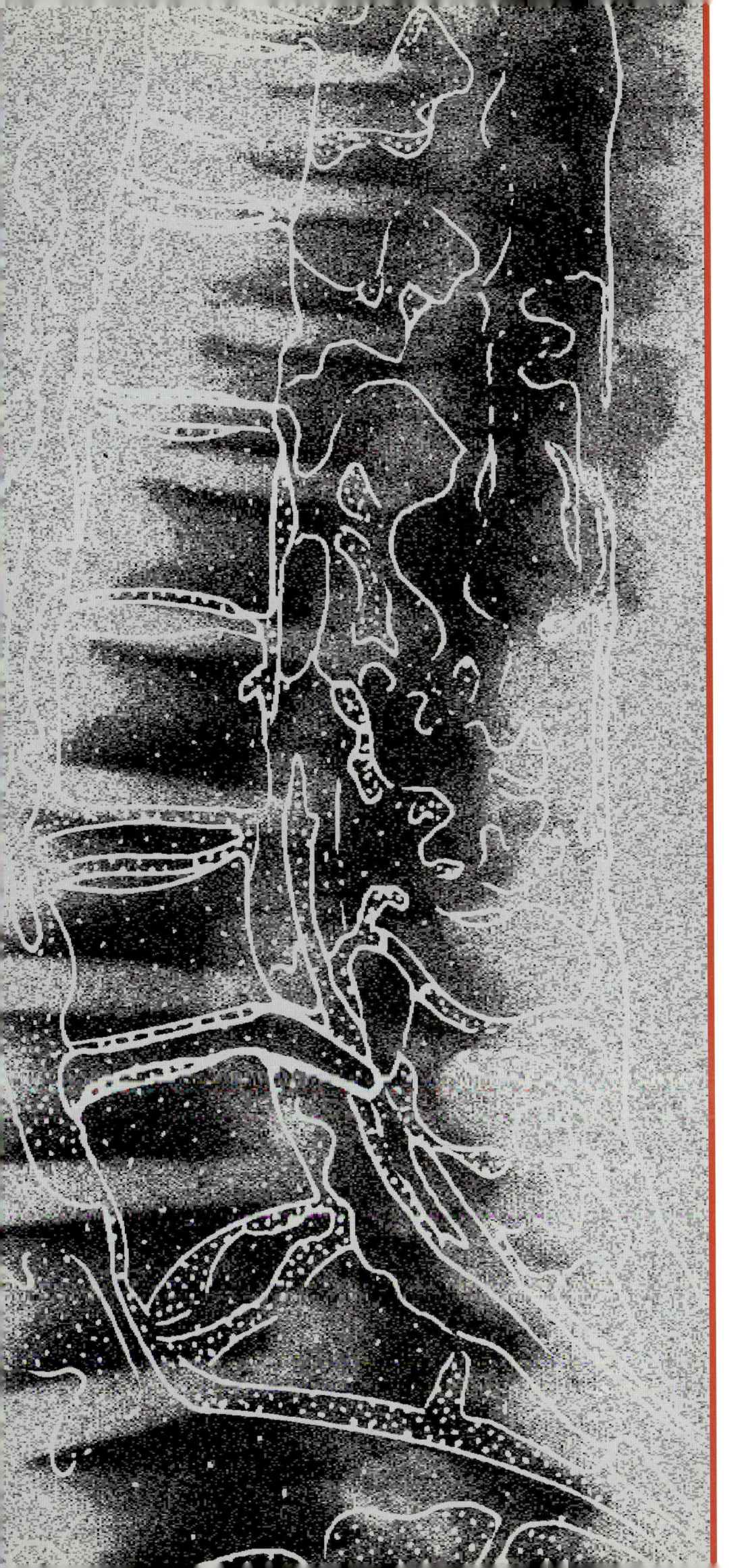

Radiologic Evaluation of Congenital and Developmental Anomalies

18

CLASSIFICATION

The conditions discussed in this and the following chapter comprise disturbances in skeletal development, growth, maturation, and modeling. Some of these anomalies arise during fetal development, such as congenital absence of a sacral bone (Fig. 18.1), block vertebrae, or hemivertebrae, and are obvious at the time the baby is born. Some may begin to develop during fetal life but become apparent later in childhood, such as mucopolysaccharidosis (see Fig. 19.35) or osteogenesis imperfecta tarda (see Fig. 19.29). Other anomalies, such as certain sclerosing dysplasias (see Fig. 19.41), develop after birth because of a genetic predisposition and become manifest later in life.

Congenital anomalies of the spine can be classified in various ways, but because of their complexity a full and detailed classification of these disorders is beyond the scope of this chapter.

RADIOLOGIC IMAGING MODALITIES

Radiologic examination is essential for the accurate diagnosis of many congenital and developmental spinal anomalies. It also plays an important part in monitoring the progress of treatment. In many instances the results of therapy, whether conservative or surgical, can be assessed only on the basis of the proper radiologic examination.

The radiologic imaging modalities most frequently used in diagnosing congenital malformations of the spine include the following:

1. Conventional radiography, including standard and special projections
2. Conventional tomography
3. Myelography
4. Computed tomography (CT)
5. Radionuclide imaging (scintigraphy, bone scan)
6. Magnetic resonance imaging (MRI).

In most instances, the diagnosis can be made on the standard radiographic projections specific for the anatomic site under investigation. As in most other orthopedic conditions, plain films of the spine should be obtained in at least two projections at 90° to one another. Supplemental views, however, particularly of complex structures, such as the sacrum, may occasionally be obtained.

Ancillary imaging techniques (eg, myelography) play an important role

FIGURE 18.1 Congenital anomalies related to disturbances in bone formation may be seen in the complete failure of a bone to form, as shown on this radiograph in a 1-year-old girl with sacral agenesis.

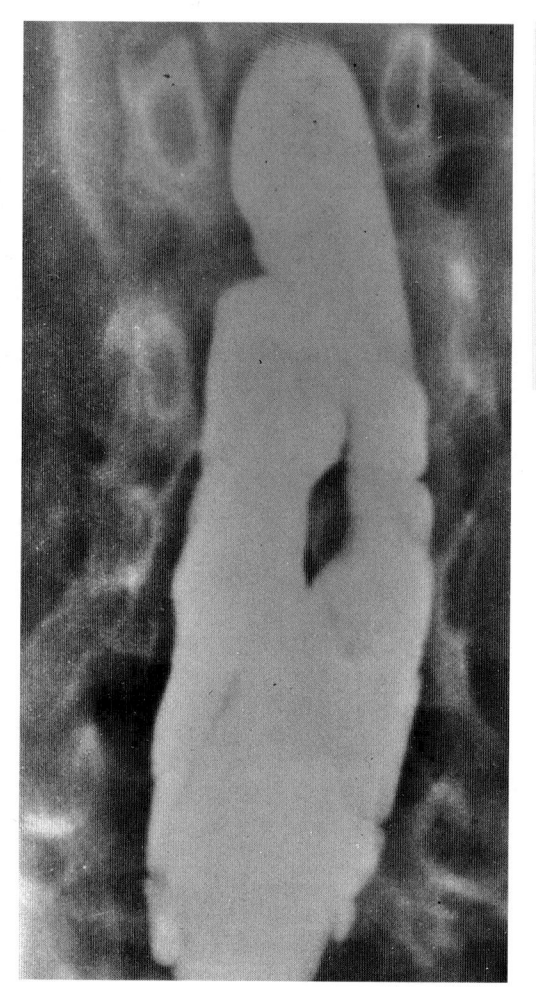

FIGURE 18.2 A myelogram of a 9-year-old girl demonstrates a filling defect in the center of the contrast-filled thecal sac, caused by a fibrous spur attached to the vertebral body. This finding is diagnostic of diastematomyelia, a rare congenital anomaly of the vertebrae and spinal cord. Note the associated finding of increase in the interpedicular distances.

Imaging of the Spine in Clinical Practice

in the evaluation of many congenital and developmental conditions of the spine (Fig. 18.2).

Magnetic resonance imaging is ideally suited for evaluating congenital and developmental anomalies of the spine since all components, including neural components, are imaged simultaneously (Fig. 18.3). Because MRI evaluation is mainly an assessment of neuroanatomic development, T1-weighted spin-echo images are usually the only images that are obtained (Fig. 18.4).

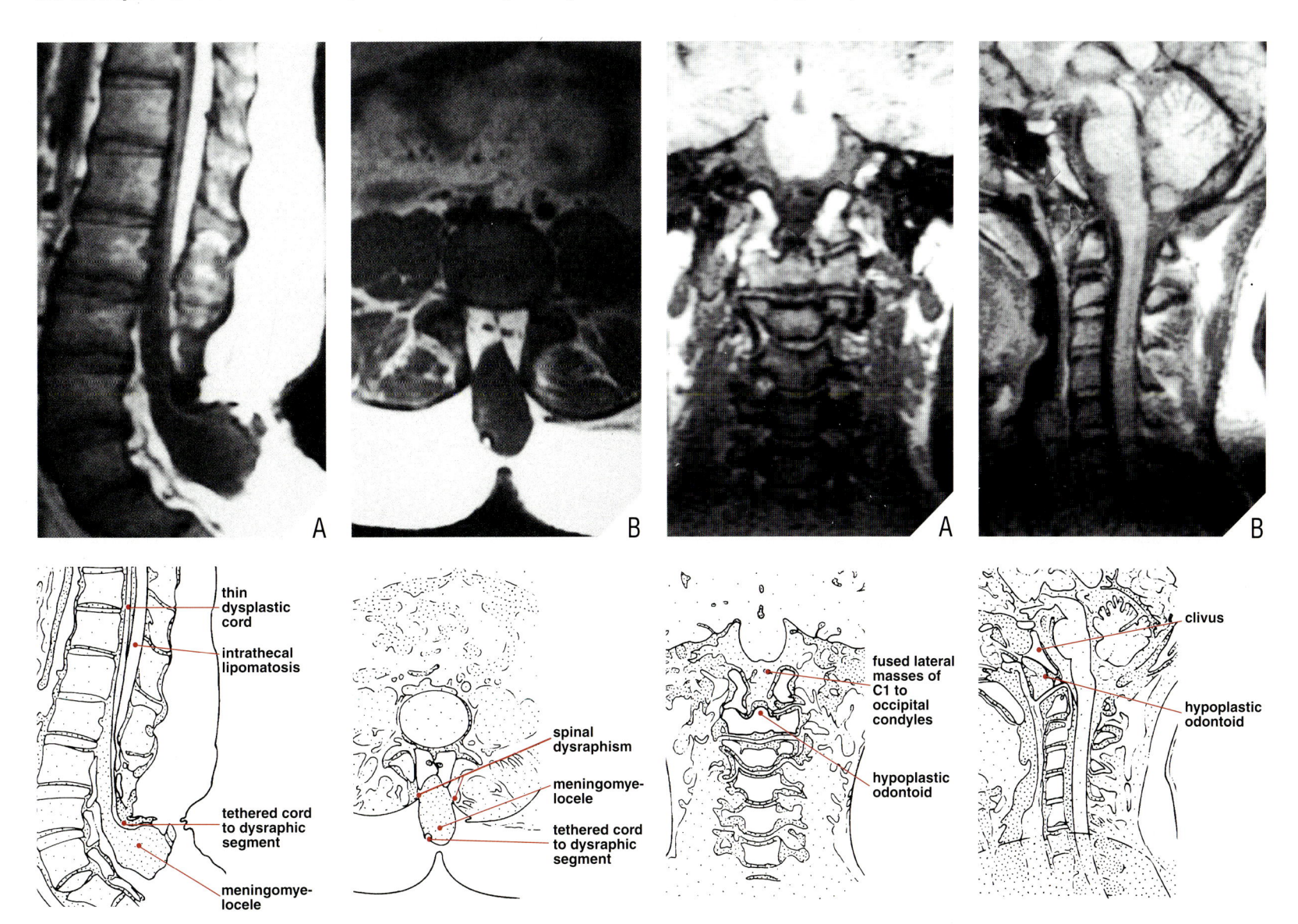

FIGURE 18.3 (A) On this T1-weighted spin-echo sagittal MRI of the thoracolumbar spine, a meningomyelocele is seen that demonstrates intermediate signal intensity due to the content of spinal fluid. A thin segment of tethered cord extends into the posterior aspect. The dysraphic segment (posterior elements defect) extends from the fourth lumbar vertebra through the sacrum. The widened lumbar canal and the large amount of epidural fat in the posterior thoracic canal are also part of this congenital anomaly. **(B)** On the axial section, the defect in the posterior elements is well demonstrated. The spinal canal is enlarged and contains epidural fat anteriorly to the meningomyelocele.

FIGURE 18.4 (A) T1-weighted spin-echo coronal MRI shows a normal developed body of second vertebra, but only rudimentary odontoid process. The atlas is fused with the occiput. **(B)** On the sagittal section, the relationship of the bony elements to the spinal canal can be well appreciated. Note the lack of any significant spinal stenosis. Rudimentary odontoid process again is well demostrated. The anterior arch of the atlas is not visualized because of fusion of first vertebra to the occiput.

Radiologic Evaluation of Congenital and Developmental Anomalies   **18.3**

Suggested Reading

Bailey JA: *Disproportionate Short Stature: Diagnosis and Management*. Philadelphia, W B Saunders, 1973.

Beighton P, Cremin B, Faure C, et al: International nomenclature of constitutional diseases of bone. *Ann Radiol* 27:275, 1984.

Holston S, Carthy H: Lumbosacral agenesis: A report of three new cases and a review of the literature. *Br J Radiol* 55:629, 1982.

International nomenclature of constitutional diseases of bone. *AJR* 131:352, 1978.

Page LK, Post MJD: Spinal dysraphism. In Post MJD (ed.): *Computed Tomography of the Spine*. Baltimore, Williams & Wilkins, 1984.

Rubin P: *Dynamic Classification of Bone Dysplasias*. Chicago, Year Book Medical Publishers, 1972.

Walker HS, Lufkin RB, Dietrich RB, et al: Magnetic resonance of the pediatric spine. *RadioGraphics* 7:1129, 1987.

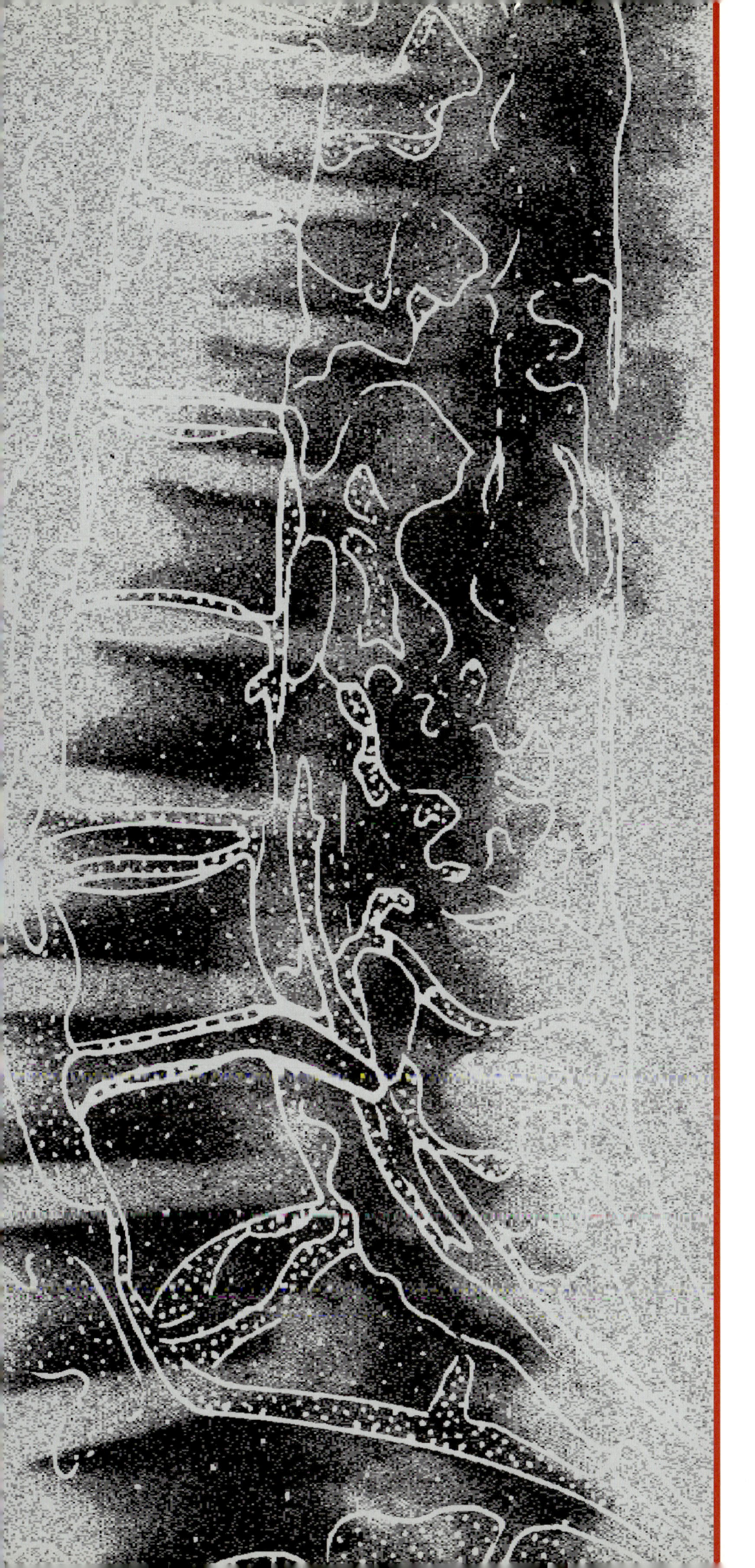

Scoliosis and Anomalies with General Effects on the Skeleton

19

SCOLIOSIS

Regardless of its etiology (Fig. 19.1), scoliosis is defined as a lateral curvature of the spine occurring in the coronal plane. This differentiates it from *kyphosis*, a posterior curvature of the spine in the sagittal plane, and *lordosis*, an anterior curvature of the spine, also in the sagittal plane (Fig. 19.2). When the curve occurs in both coronal and sagittal planes, the deformity is called *kyphoscoliosis*. Besides a lateral curvature, scoliosis frequently has a rotational component in which vertebrae rotate towards the convexity of the curve.

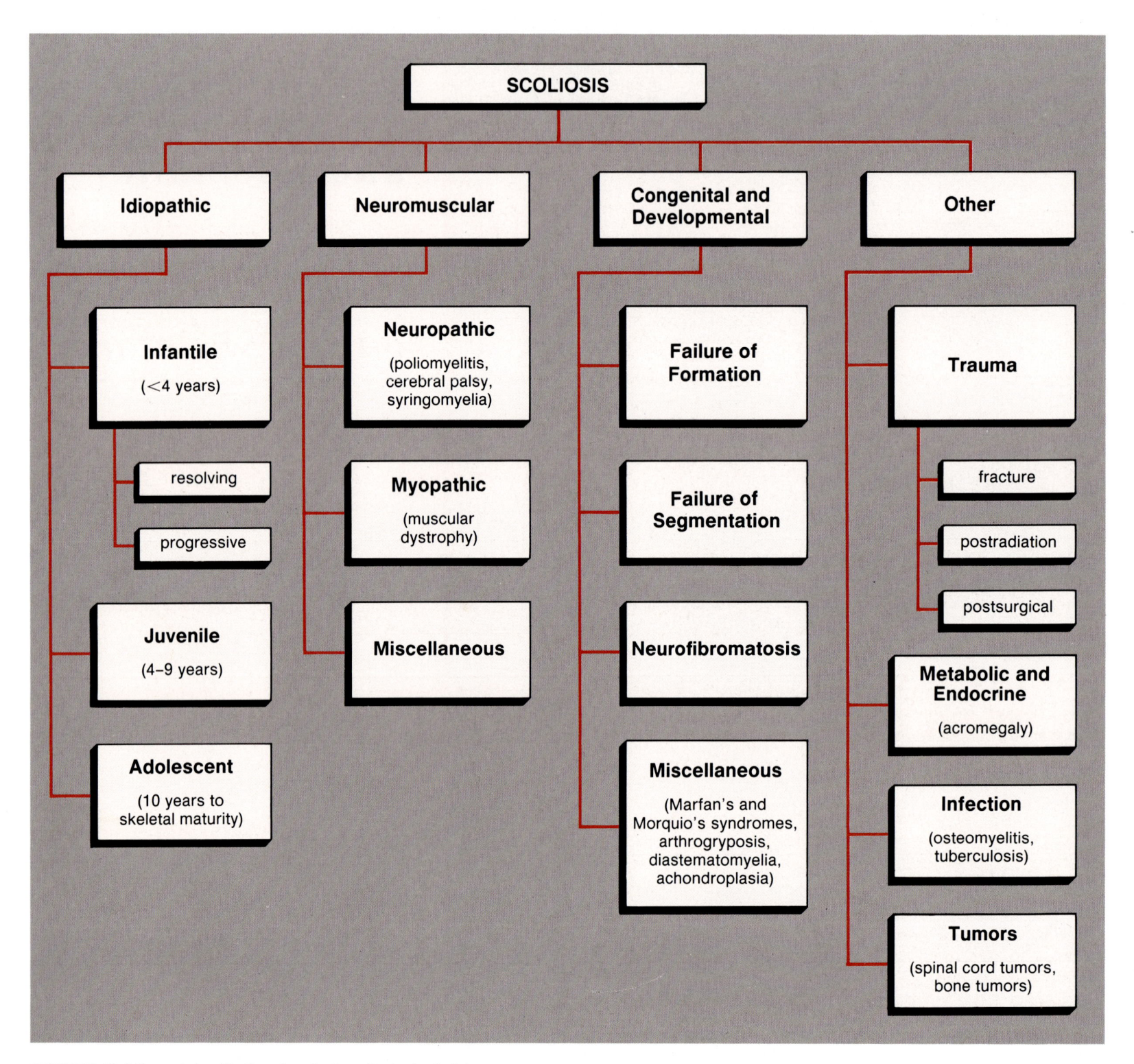

FIGURE 19.1 General classification of scoliosis on the basis of etiology.

Imaging of the Spine in Clinical Practice

Idiopathic Scoliosis

Idiopathic scoliosis, which constitutes almost 80% of all scoliotic abnormalities, can be classified into three groups: infantile; juvenile idiopathic; and adolescent.

The *infantile type*, of which there are two variants, occurs in children under 4 years of age; it is seen predominantly in boys, and the curvature usually occurs in the thoracic segment with its convexity to the left. In the *resolving* (benign) variant, the curve commonly does not increase beyond 30° and resolves spontaneously, requiring no treatment. The *progressive* variant carries a poor prognosis, with the potential for severe deformity unless aggressive treatment is initiated early in the process.

Juvenile idiopathic scoliosis occurs equally in boys and girls from the ages of 4 to 9 years. Patients with this type of scoliosis usually have a thoracic curve, convex to the right.

By far the most common type of idiopathic scoliosis, comprising 85% of cases, is the adolescent form, which is seen predominantly in girls from 10 years of age to the time of skeletal maturity. Small curves (<10°) have an equal incidence in boys and girls. However, larger curves (>10°) are four times more common in girls than in boys. The thoracic or thoracolumbar spine is most often involved, and the convexity of the curve is to the right (Fig. 19.3). Although the etiology of this type is unknown, it has been postulated that a genetic factor may be involved and that idiopathic scoliosis is a familial disorder. Recent studies of the etiology of adolescent idiopathic scoliosis are beginning to point to a concomitant decrease in proprioception of both the upper and lower extremities.

Curves progress most rapidly during the growth spurt, and usually cease to increase at the time of skeletal maturity. However, some curves (ie, those >50°) may go on to progress even after skeletal maturity. Curve progression has been found to be related to the type of curve (ie, thoracic and double major curves progress more than lumbar and thoracolumbar curves). In addition, it has been determined that curves of larger magnitude progress more than smaller curves do. The physiologic age of the child is also an important determinate to curve progression. The younger the child (as determined by Risser sign [see Fig. 19.18], lack of secondary sexual characteristics, and absence of menarche), the greater the curve progression.

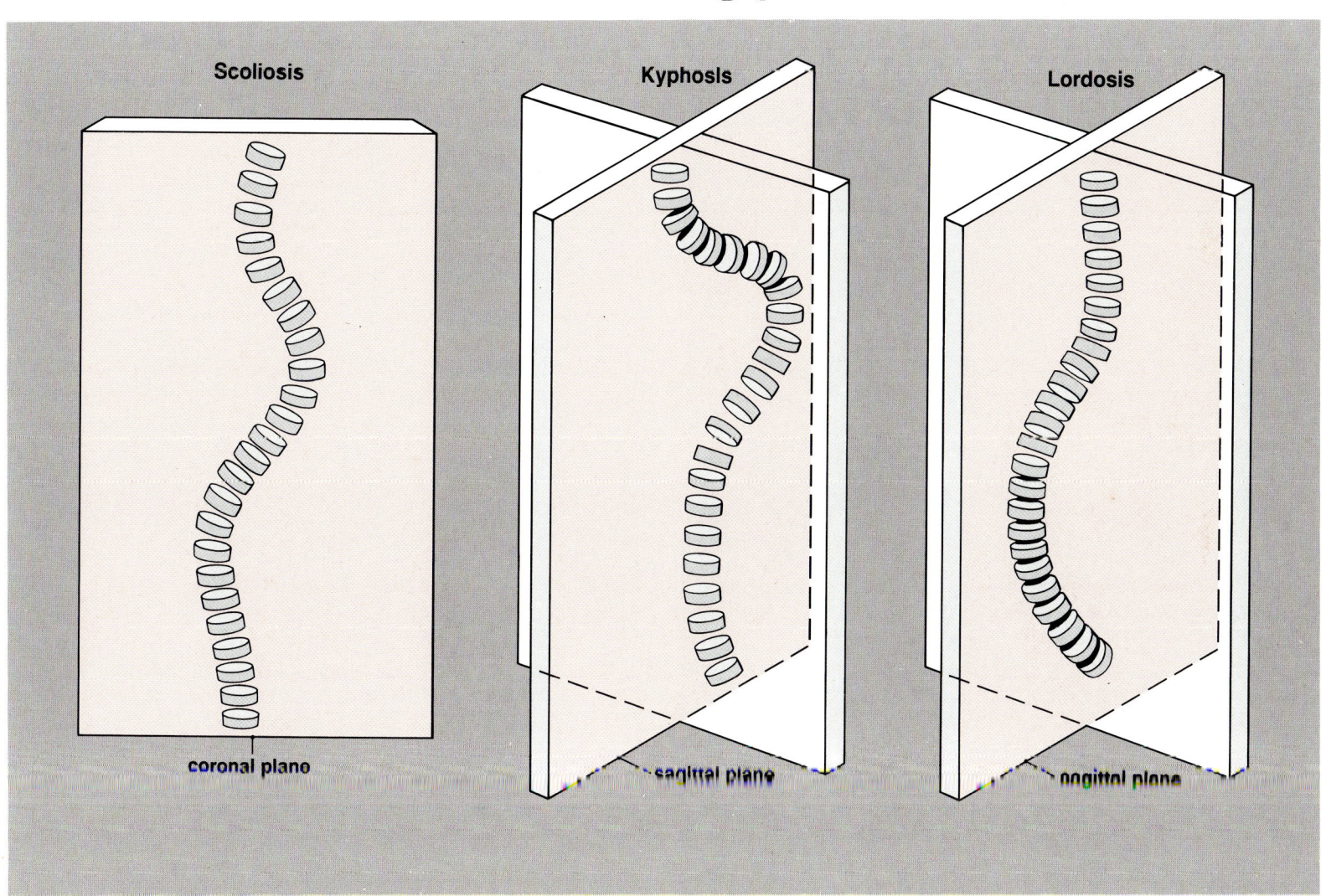

FIGURE 19.2 Scoliosis is a lateral curvature of the spine in the coronal (frontal) plane. Kyphosis is a posterior curvature of the spine and lordosis an anterior curvature, both occurring in the sagittal (lateral) plane.

Congenital Scoliosis

Congenital scoliosis is responsible for 10% of the cases of this deformity. According to MacEwen (1968), it can be classified into three general groups (Fig. 19.4): (1) those resulting from a *failure in vertebral formation*, which may be partial or complete (Fig. 19.5); (2) those caused by a *failure in vertebral segmentation*, which may be asymmetric and unilateral or symmetric and bilateral; and (3) those resulting from a *combination of the first two*. The effects of congenital scoliosis on balance and support result in faulty biomechanics throughout the skeletal system.

Congenital scoliosis and kyphosis is usually secondary to a defect that occurs between 1 and 2 months of gestation. It is also associated with other anomalies. In general, urinary tract anomalies are the most common, and are present in 20% of patients with congenital scoliosis. Typically, such anomalies lead to hydronephrosis. Pelvic kidneys have often been identified in patients with congenital scoliosis. Occasionally, lesions of the genitourinary tract can be lethal, therefore, in the work-up of a patient with congenital scoliosis, it is *always* necessary to perform an IVP (Fig. 19.6) or ultrasound. Other encountered anomalies include those

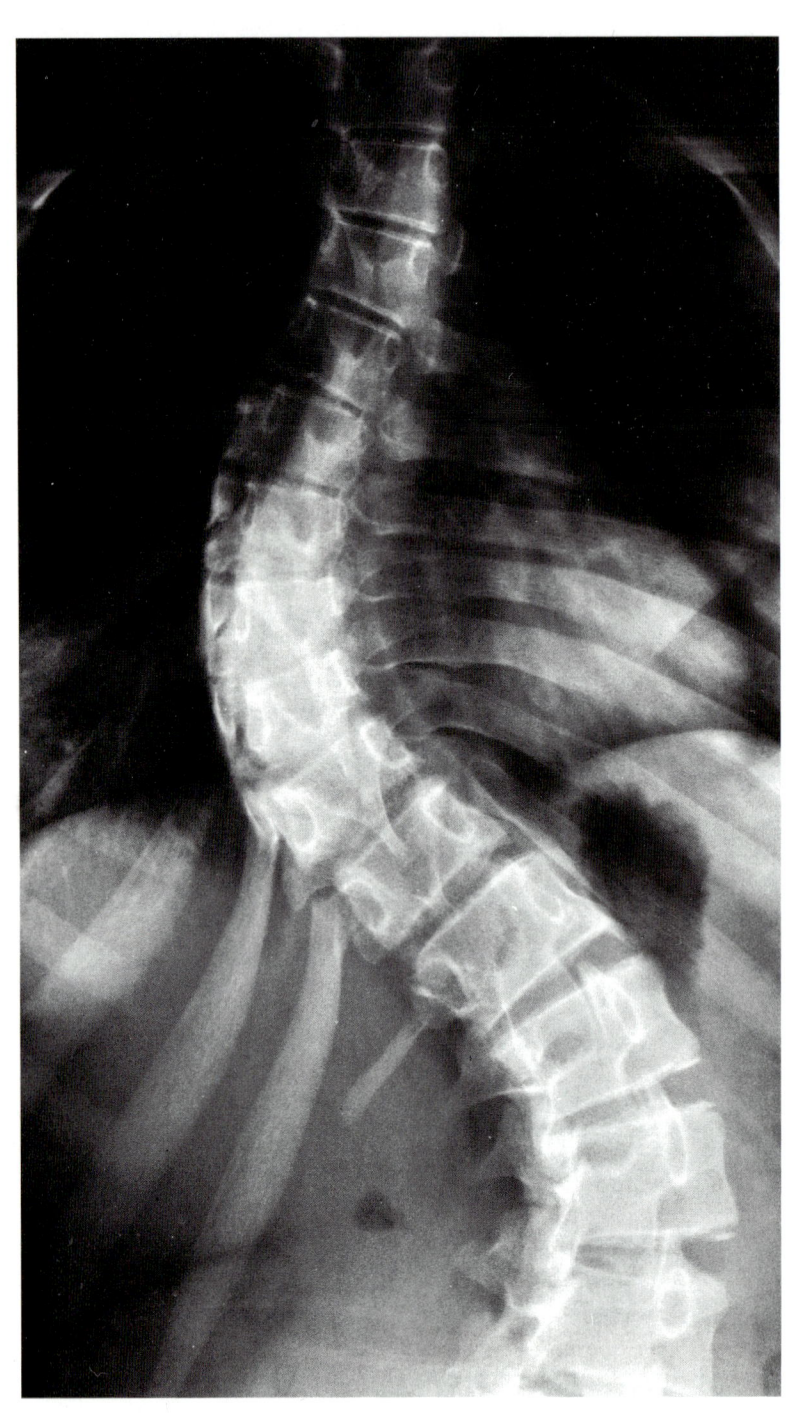

FIGURE 19.3 Anteroposterior view of the spine in a 15-year-old girl shows the typical features of idiopathic scoliosis involving the thoracolumbar segment. The convexity of the curve is the right; a compensatory curve in the lumbar segment has its convexity to the left.

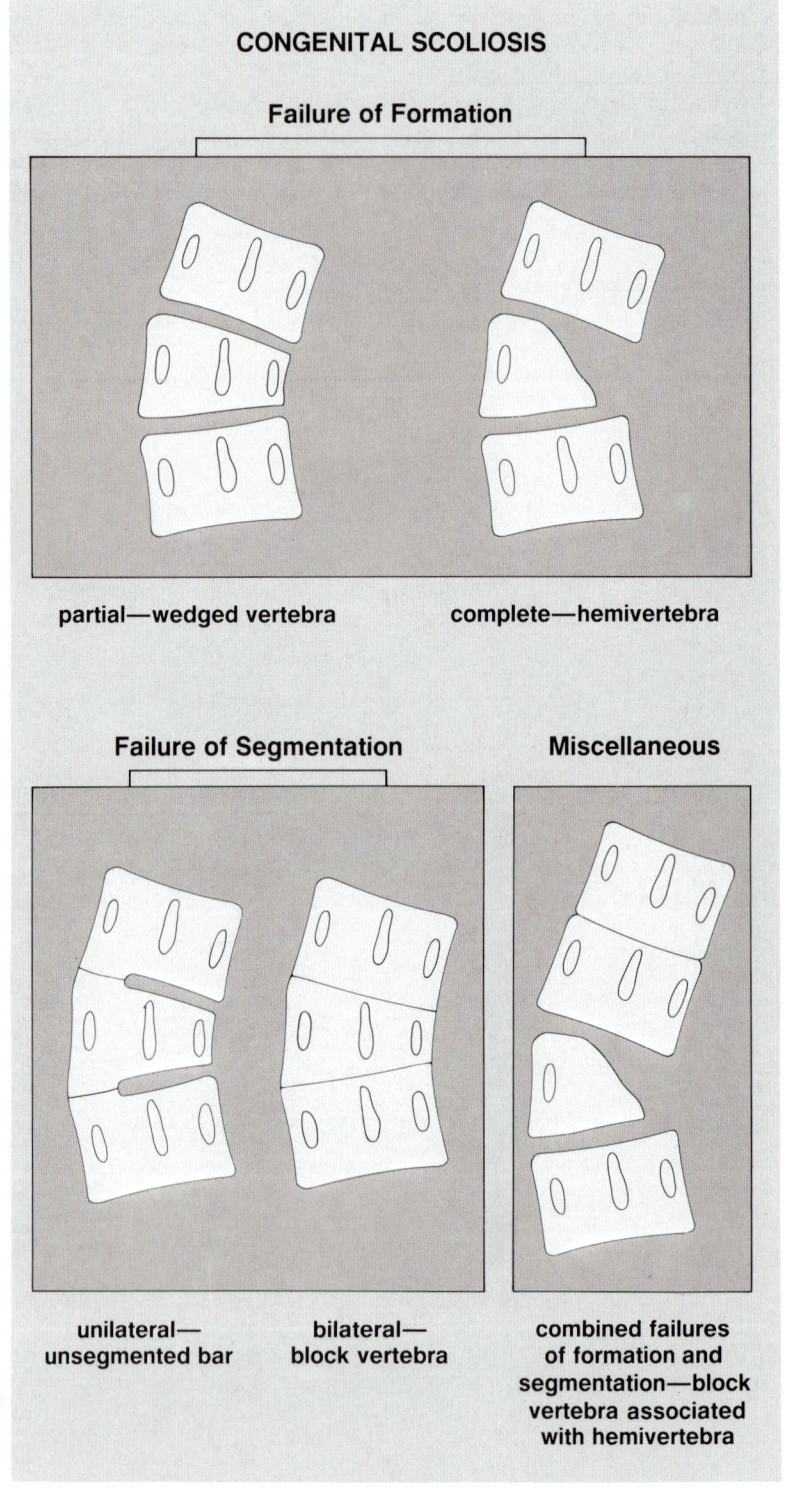

FIGURE 19.4 Classification of congenital scoliosis on the basis of etiology. (Adapted from MacEwen GD, Conway JJ, Miller WT: Congenital scoliosis with a unilateral bar. *Radiology* 90:711, 1968; and Winter RB, Moe JH, Eilers VE: Congenital scoliosis. A study of 234 patients treated and untreated. *J Bone Joint Surg* 50A:1, 1968)

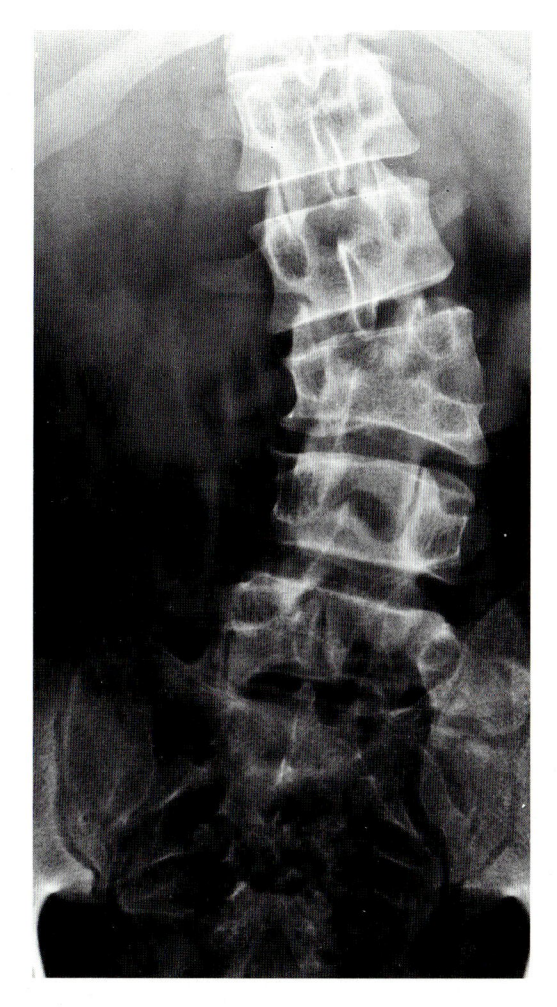

FIGURE 19.5 Anteroposterior view of the lumbosacral spine in a 22-year-old man demonstrates scoliosis due to hemivertebrae, a complete, unilateral failure of formation. Note the deformed L3 vertebra secondary to the faulty fusion of the hemivertebra on the left side, where two pedicles are evident. The resulting scoliosis has its convex border to the left. An associated anomaly is also apparent by the presence of the so-called transitional lumbosacral vertebra.

- fused hemivertebra
- transitional lumbosacral vertebra
- anomalous transverse process

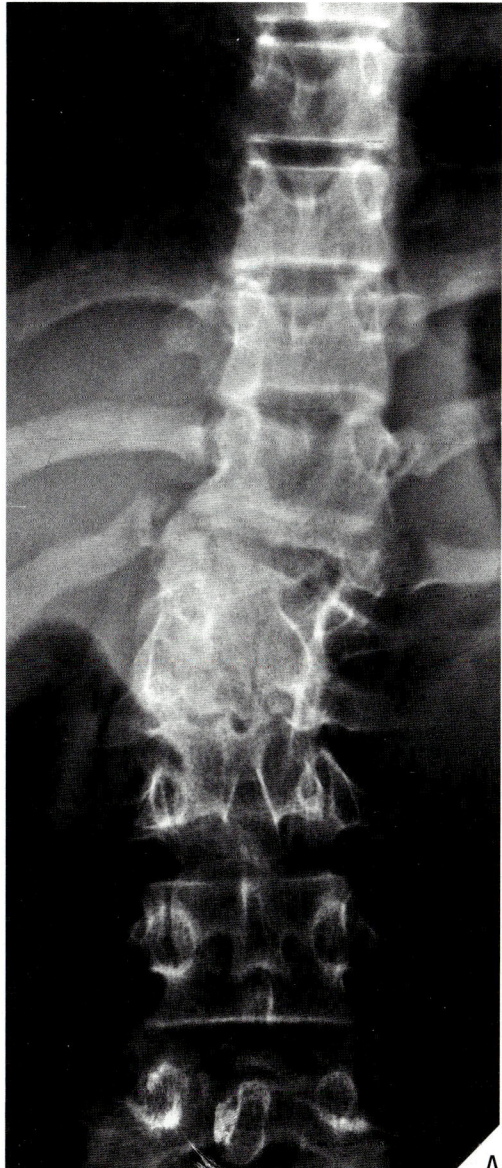

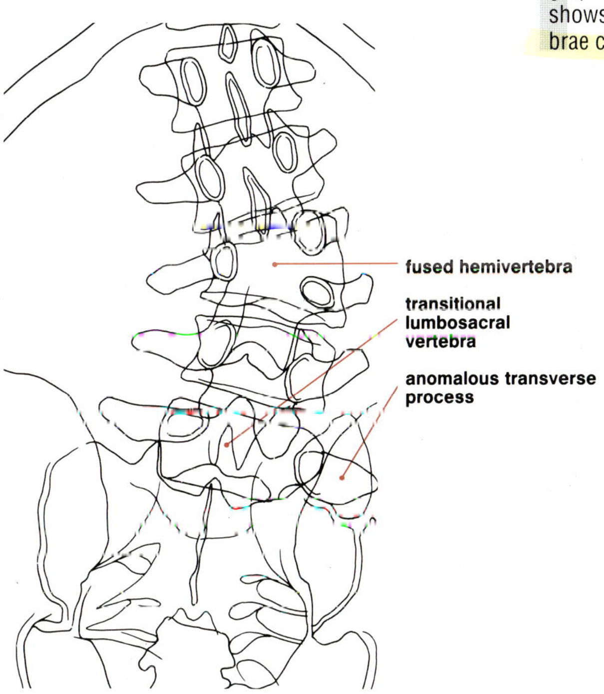

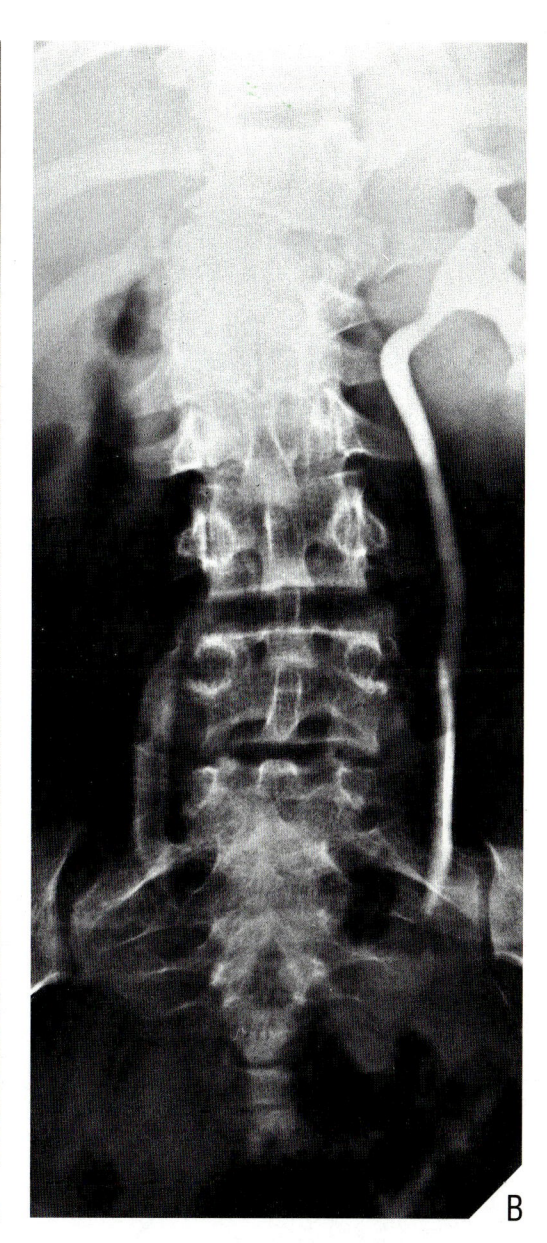

FIGURE 19.6 (A) Supine anteroposterior radiograph of the thoracolumbar spine in a 13-year-old girl shows congenital scoliosis secondary to block vertebrae consisting of a fusion of L1 to L3. **(B)** An IVP demonstrates only the left kidney, an example of renal agenesis. Congenital scoliosis is frequently associated with urinary tract anomalies.

Scoliosis and Anomalies with General Effects on the Skeleton

involving the central neural system (eg, diastematomyelia; see Fig. 18.2), the cardiovascular system, or extremities.

Congenital scoliosis progresses in about 75% of the patients. A unilateral, unsegmented bar opposed by a hemivertebra is the deformity that presents the greatest potential for progression, whereas a block vertebra is the deformity least likely to progress. In congenital kyphosis, a defect in formation presents the greatest risk of progression.

Miscellaneous Scolioses

Several other scolioses with specific etiologies may develop, including those secondary to neuromuscular, traumatic, infectious, metabolic, and tumor processes, among others.

Patients with spinal cord injury will often develop spinal deformity, and such deformity is almost inevitable when the lesion is complete and is above the level of T12.

FIGURE 19.7 STANDARD RADIOGRAPHIC PROJECTIONS AND RADIOLOGIC TECHNIQUES FOR EVALUATING SCOLIOSIS

PROJECTION/TECHNIQUE	DEMONSTRATION	PROJECTION/TECHNIQUE	DEMONSTRATION
Anteroposterior	Lateral deviation Angle of scoliosis (by Risser–Ferguson and Lippman–Cobb methods and scoliotic index) Vertebral rotation (by Cobb and Moe methods)	Lateral	Associated kyphosis and lordosis
		Conventional and computed tomography	Congenital fusion of vertebrae Hemivertebrae
		Myelography	Tethering of cord
Of vertebra	Ossification of ring apophysis as determinant of skeletal maturity	Magnetic resonance imaging	Abnormalities of nerve roots Compression and displacement of thecal sac Syringomyelia Diastematomyelia
Of pelvis	Ossification of iliac crest apophysis as determinant of skeletal maturity		
Lateral bending	Flexibility of curve Amount of reduction of curve	Intravenous urography	Associated anomalies of GU tract (in congenital scoliosis)

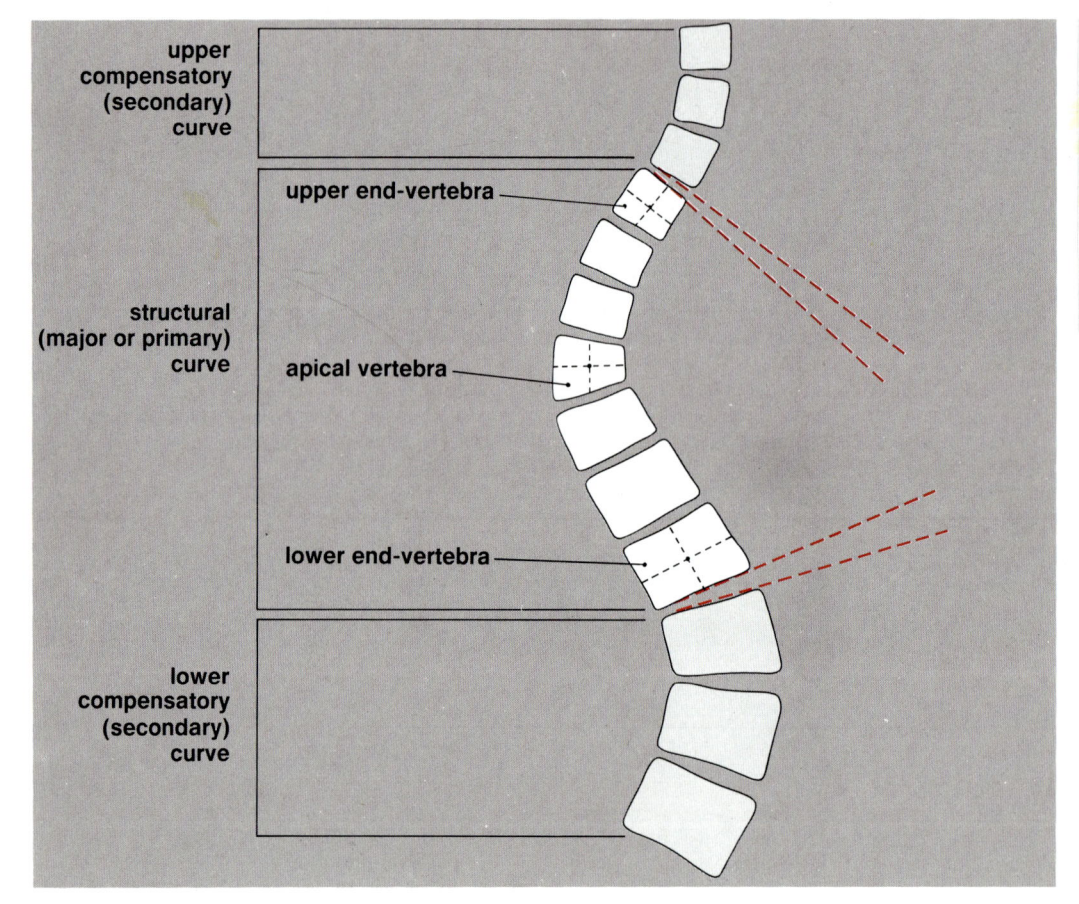

FIGURE 19.8 Terminology used in describing the scoliotic curve. The end-vertebrae of the curve are defined as those that tilt maximally into the concavity of the structural curve. The apical vertebra, which shows the most severe rotation and wedging, is the one whose center is most laterally displaced from the central line. The center of the apical vertebra is determined by the intersection of two lines, one drawn from the center of the upper and lower endplates and the other from the center of the lateral margins of the vertebral body; it should not be determined by diagonal lines through the corners of the vertebral body.

Imaging of the Spine in Clinical Practice

Neuromuscular scoliosis can occur secondary to cerebral palsy, myelodysplasia, spinal muscular atrophy, Duchenne muscular dystrophy, Friedreich ataxia, or quadriplegia. Their discussion is beyond the scope of this text.

Clinical Evaluation

It is important to obtain a thorough history. The age of the patient is recorded in both years and months. Note is also made of the age of the onset of menarche and the appearance of secondary sexual characteristics. A thorough family history of scoliosis is also obtained. It is important to determine when the curve was first seen, by whom it was first detected, whether it was associated with any previous injury to the spine or lower extremities, and whether there is associated pain. A thorough physical examination is then performed noting shoulder elevation, lateral thoracic shift, waistline asymmetry, or asymmetric elevation of the iliac crests. A note is also made of the presence or absence of cutaneous lesions (eg, café-au-lait spots), foot deformities, abnormalities of gait, and lower extremity weakness or lack of sensation. The patient is then examined in the forward-bending position for rib or flank comparisons and range of vertebral motion. The patient is also examined from the side to note the presence of thoracic kyphosis or lordosis.

Radiologic Evaluation

The radiographic examination of scoliosis includes standing anteroposterior and lateral films of the entire spine; a supine anteroposterior film centered over the scoliotic curve (see Fig. 19.3), which is used for the various measurements of spinal curvature and vertebral rotation (discussed below); and anteroposterior films obtained with the patient bending laterally to each side for evaluation of the flexible and structural components of the curve. Care should be taken to include the iliac crests in at least one of these radiograms for a determination of skeletal maturity (see Figs. 19.17, 19.18).

Ancillary techniques, such as conventional tomography and computed tomography (CT), may be required for evaluation of congenital lesions such as segmentation failures. MRI may be necessary to evaluate for possible intramedullary pathology (eg, syringomyelia) or spinal canal abnormalities (eg, diastematomyelia). Intravenous urography, also known as *intravenous pyelography* (IVP), is essential in congenital scoliosis for evaluating the presence of associated anomalies of the genitourinary tract (see Fig. 19.6).

An overview of the radiographic projections and radiologic techniques used in the evaluation of scoliosis is presented in Figure 19.7.

Measurements

To evaluate the various types of scoliosis, certain terms (Fig. 19.8) and measurements must be introduced. Measurement of the severity of a scoliotic curve has practical application not only in the selection of patients for surgical treatment but also in monitoring the results of corrective therapy. Two widely accepted methods of measuring the curve are the Lippman–Cobb (Fig. 19.9) and Risser–Ferguson techniques (Fig. 19.10). The measurements obtained by these methods, however, are not compa-

FIGURE 19.9 In the Lipman–Cobb method of measuring the degree of scoliotic curvature, two angles are formed by the intersection of two sets of lines. The first set of lines, one drawn tangent to the superior surface of the upper end-vertebra and the other tangent to the inferior surface of the lower end-vertebra, intersects to form angle (a). The intersection of the other set of lines, each drawn perpendicular to the tangential lines, forms angle (b). These angles are equal, and either may serve as the measurement of the degree of scoliosis.

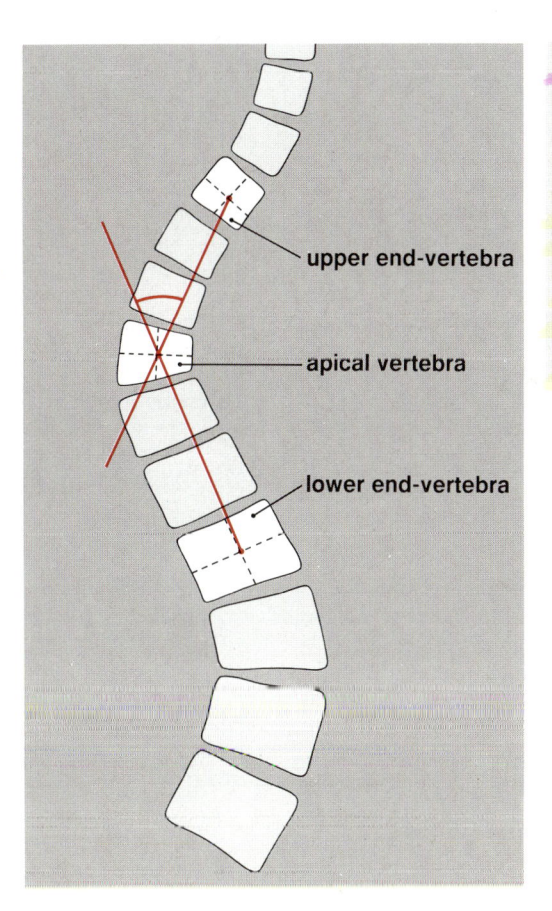

FIGURE 19.10 In the Risser–Ferguson method, the degree of scoliotic curvature is determined by the angle formed by the intersection of two lines at the center of the apical vertebra, the first line originating at the center of the upper end-vertebra and the other at the center of the lower end-vertebra.

rable. The values yielded by the Lippman–Cobb method, which determines the angle of curvature only by the ends of the scoliotic curve, depending solely on the inclination of the end vertebrae, are usually greater than those yielded by the Risser–Ferguson method. This also applies to the percentages of correction as determined by the two methods; the more favorable correction percentage is obtained by the Lippman–Cobb method. This method, which has been adopted and standardized by the Scoliosis Research Society, classifies the severity of scoliotic curvature into seven groups (Fig. 19.11). Another technique for measuring the degree of scoliosis, introduced by Greenspan and colleagues in 1978, uses a "scoliotic index." Designed to give a more accurate and comprehensive representation of the scoliotic curve, this technique measures the deviation of each involved vertebra from the vertical spinal line as determined by points at the center of the vertebra immediately above the upper end vertebra of the curve and at the center of the vertebra immediately below the lower end vertebra (Fig. 19.12). Its most valuable feature is that it minimizes the influence of overcorrection of the end-vertebrae in the measured angle, a frequent criticism of the Lippman–Cobb technique. Furthermore, short segments or minimal curvatures, often difficult to measure with the currently accepted methods, are easily measurable with this technique.

Recently, computerized methods for measuring and analyzing the scoliotic curve have been introduced. Although more accurate than the manual methods, they require more sophisticated equipment and are more time consuming than the methods described above.

In addition to the measurement of scoliotic curvature, the radiographic evaluation of scoliosis also requires the determination of other factors. Measurement of the degree of rotation of the vertebrae of the involved segment can be obtained by either of two methods presently in use. The Cobb technique for grading rotation uses the position of the spinous process as a point of reference (Fig. 19.13). On the normal anteroposterior radiograph of the spine, the spinous process appears at the center of the vertebral body if there is no rotation. As the degree of rotation increases, the spinous process migrates towards the convexity of the curve. The Nash–Moe method, also based on the measurement obtained on the anteroposterior projection of the spine, uses the symmetry of the pedicles as a point of reference, with the migration of the pedicles towards the convexity of the curve determining the degree of vertebral rotation (Fig. 19.14).

The final factor in the evaluation of scoliosis is the determination of *skeletal maturity*. This is important for both the prognosis and treatment of scoliosis, particularly the idiopathic type, since there is a potential for

FIGURE 19.11 LIPPMAN–COBB CLASSIFICATION OF SCOLIOTIC CURVATURE

GROUP	ANGLE OF CURVATURE
I	<20°
II	21°–30°
III	31°–50°
IV	51°–75°
V	76°–100°
VI	101°–125°
VII	>125°

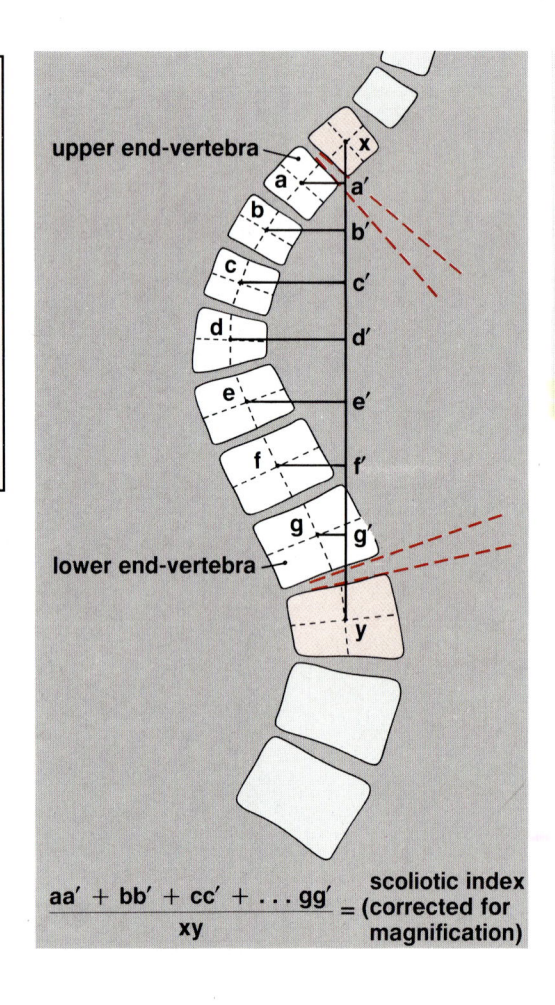

FIGURE 19.12 In the measurement of scoliosis using the scoliotic index, each vertebra (a–g) is considered an integral part of the curve. A vertical spinal line (xy) is first determined whose endpoints are the centers of the vertebrae immediately above and below the upper and lower end-vertebrae of the curve. Lines are then drawn from the center of each vertebral body perpendicular to the vertical spinal line (aa', bb',...,gg'). The values yielded by these lines represent the linear deviation of each vertebra; and their sum, divided by the length of the vertical line (xy) to correct for radiographic magnification, yields the scoliotic index. A value of zero denotes a straight spine; the higher the scoliotic index the more severe the scoliosis.

$$\frac{aa' + bb' + cc' + \ldots gg'}{xy} = \text{scoliotic index (corrected for magnification)}$$

COBB'S SPINOUS-PROCESS METHOD FOR DETERMINING VERTEBRAL ROTATION

Normal	+ Rotation	++ Rotation	+++ Rotation
spinous process in center	spinous process at b	spinous process at c	spinous process at d

FIGURE 19.13 In Cobb's spinous-process method for determining rotation, the vertebra is divided into six equal parts. Normally, the spinous process appears at the center. Its migration to certain points toward the convexity of the curve marks the degree of rotation.

MOE'S PEDICLE METHOD FOR DETERMINING VERTEBRAL ROTATION

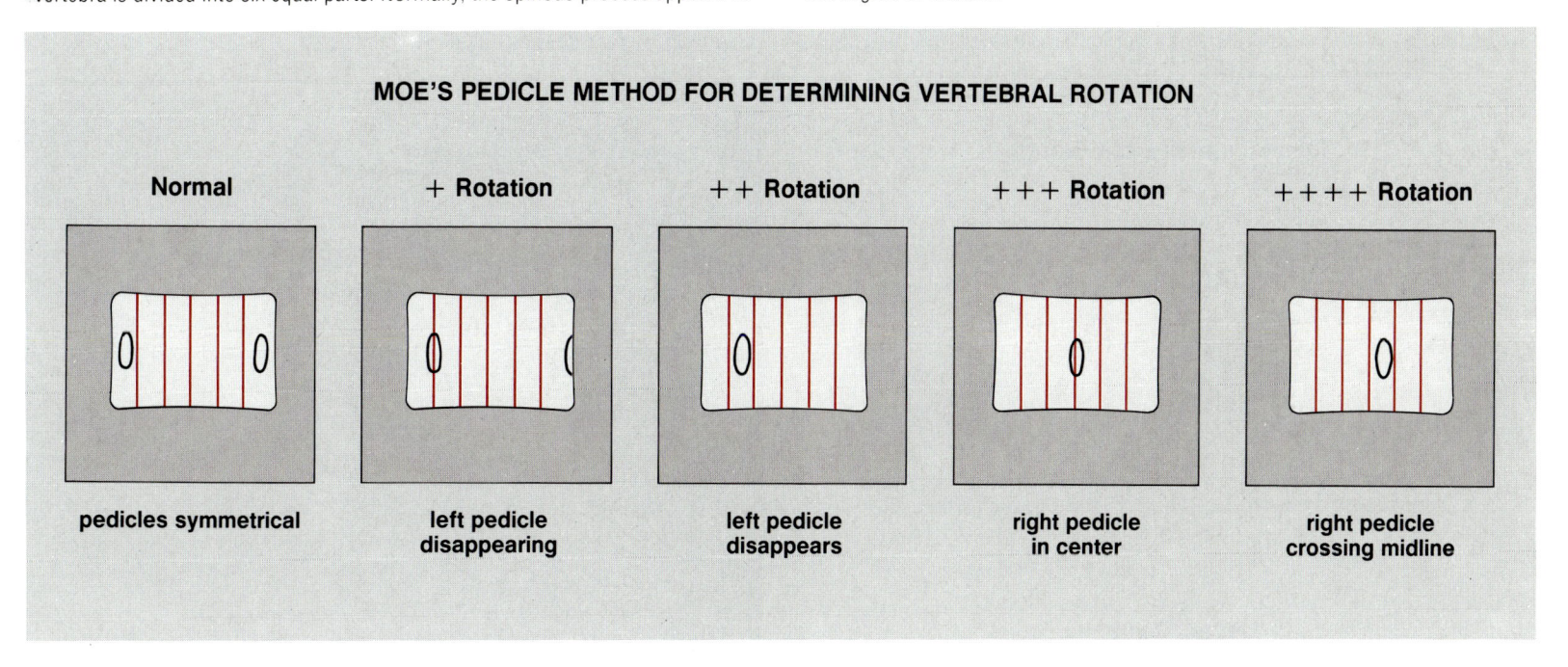

Normal	+ Rotation	++ Rotation	+++ Rotation	++++ Rotation
pedicles symmetrical	left pedicle disappearing	left pedicle disappears	right pedicle in center	right pedicle crossing midline

FIGURE 19.14 Nash–Moe pedicle method for determining rotation divides the vertebra into six equal parts. Normally, the pedicles appear in the outer parts. Migration of a pedicle to certain points toward the convexity of the curve determines the degree of rotation.

Scoliosis and Anomalies with General Effects on the Skeleton

significant progression of the degree of curvature as long as skeletal maturity has not been reached. Skeletal age can be determined by comparison of a radiograph of a patient's hand with the standards for different ages available in radiographic atlases. It can also be assessed by radiographic observation of the ossification of the apophysis of the vertebral ring (Fig. 19.15) or, as is most often done, from the ossification of the iliac apophysis (Fig. 19.16).

The vertebral ring apophyses lie at the upper and lower margins of the vertebral body, overlying the cartilaginous growth plate. These initially appear as separate secondary ossification centers, and form a complete ring that fuses to the vertebral body (see Fig. 19.15). They are best seen on lateral radiographs, but also can be identified on the frontal spine projection. Fusion of the apophysis with the vertebral endplate indicates cessation of all vertebral body potential for growth.

The ossification of the iliac apophysis is evaluated according to the description by Risser (1958). Ossification normally starts at the anterior superior iliac spine and progresses posteriorly to the posterior superior iliac spine. Once complete excursion of the ossification has occurred, fusion of the iliac crest follows. Risser divided the excursion into four quarters: 1 = 25% excursion; 2 = 50%; 3 = 75%; 4 = complete excursion; 5 = fusion to the ilium (Fig. 19.17.)

Treatment

Treatment of idiopathic scoliosis is dependent on curve magnitude, documentation of progression, and the physiologic age of the patient. Curves measuring 0° to 10° require no treatment; these patients are usually re-examined at yearly intervals. Curves measuring 11° to 20° are usually treated conservatively with observation. However, documentation of progression greater than 10° is an indication for brace treatment. Curves measuring 21° to 30° are also treated with observation with repeat radiographic examination at 6-month intervals. Documentation of 5° progression indicates the need for a brace. Curves measuring 31° or more at initial presentation warrant brace treatment. Surgery is reserved for curves that present with a magnitude of more than 45° to 50°, especially if they present at a relatively young age, before menarche and with a Risser stage of 0 or 1 (see Fig. 19.17). Once skeletal maturity is reached, the chance of progression is significantly diminished; however, curves initially measuring more than 50° have been shown to progress at 1° per year even after skeletal maturity.

Congenital scoliosis with documented high potential for progress is best treated early. The standard treatment for congenital scoliosis is early posterior fusion. However, simultaneous or subsequent anterior fusion should be considered to prevent the development of the crankshaft phenomenon. Crankshaft phenomenon is a three-dimensional torsional deformity caused by a posterior tether (posterior fusion) which is opposed by continued growth anteriorly of the vertebral bodies. (J. Dubousset, H. Shuffelbarger—personal communication). Congenital kyphosis can be treated with posterior fusion if treatment is undertaken before the age of 5 years, and usually leads to spontaneous improvement. However, combined anterior and posterior fusion may be necessary in older patients. Only patients with neurologic deficit secondary to a congenital hemivertebra are indicated for anterior spinal decompression, and only when the neurologic deficit does not abate with bed rest.

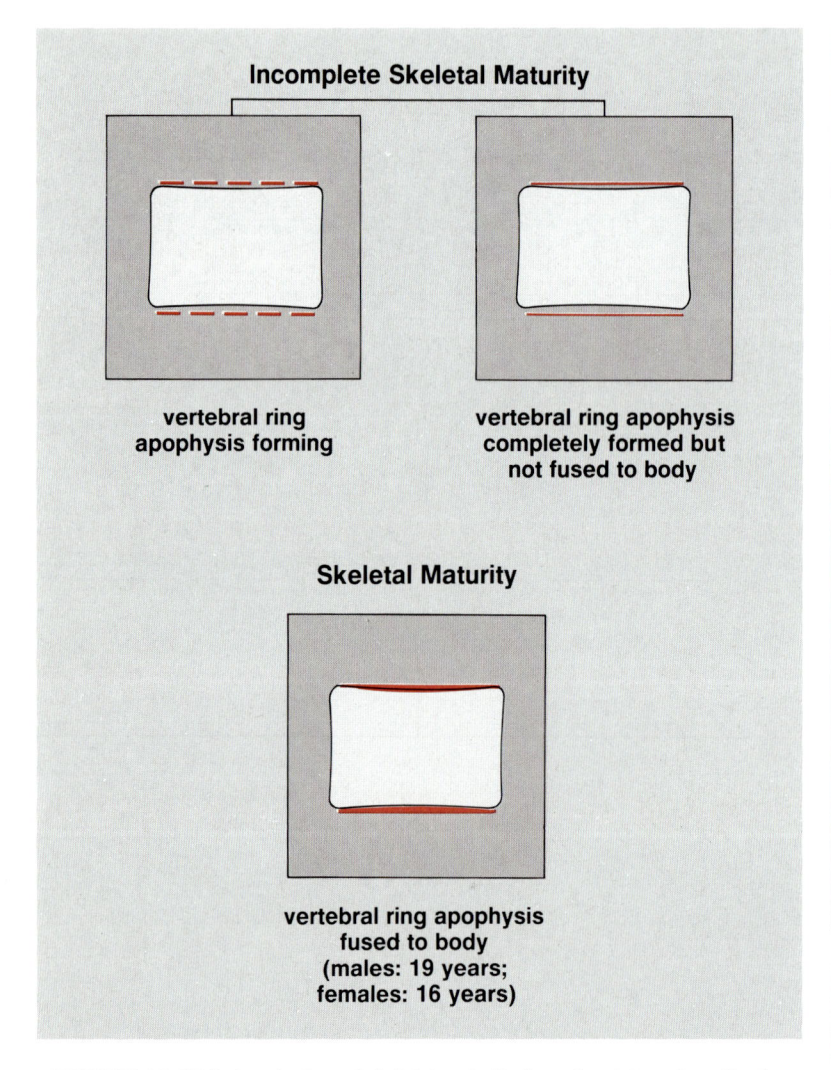

FIGURE 19.15 Determination of skeletal maturity from the status of ossification of the vertebral ring apophysis.

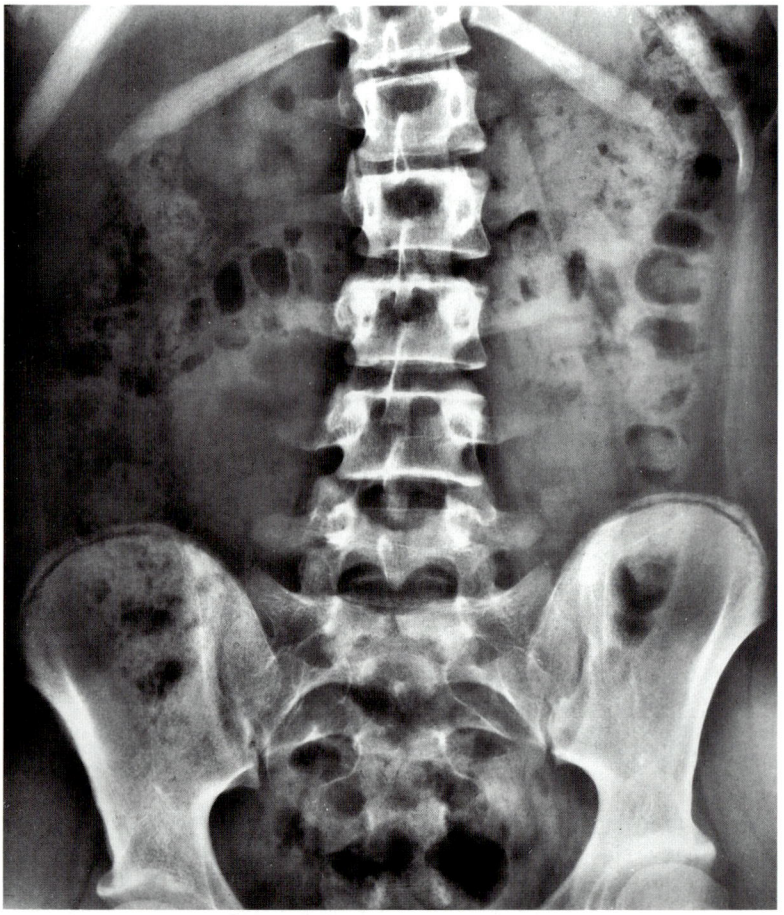

FIGURE 19.16 The status of ossification of the iliac apophysis is helpful in determining skeletal age. Progression of the apophysis in this 14-year-old girl with idiopathic scoliosis has been completed, but the lack of fusion with the iliac crest indicates continuing skeletal maturation (see Fig. 19.17).

In neuromuscular types of scoliosis, the degree of curvature is usually related to the severity of the neurologic deficit. Treatment is aimed at preserving the patient's functional ability. When the curve is so severe (>50°) that it threatens the patient's ability to sit (ie, the upper extremities must be used for support), surgical stabilization is indicated—usually, a combined anterior and posterior fusion with posterior instrumentation.

Patients with myelodysplasia present with an even more complex problem, as their spinal deformity may be secondary to their neurologic deficit or congenital deformity (ie, failure of formation or failure of segmentation). Treatment consists of anterior release and fusion combined with posterior instrumentation and fusion.

Spinal muscular atrophy is a progressive disease secondary to anterior horn-cell degeneration in the spinal cord. These patients usually develop progressive scoliosis in which bracing has not been shown to be effective. As with other neuromuscular curves, surgical treatment is indicated once the curve reaches approximately 50°. Once again, treatment is usually by multilevel anterior surgical diskectomy and fusion, followed by a posterior instrumentation and fusion.

Duchenne muscular dystrophy is an X-linked recessive disorder, and therefore predominantly affects boys. It is usually progressive, and affected children lose their ability to ambulate by age 13. Many of these patients develop a severe scoliosis which interferes with their ability to sit. Once again, bracing is not effective in these patients. Spinal fusion is usually indicated at an earlier stage in patients with Duchenne muscular dystrophy than with other paralytic spine deformities. Long posterior fusions at an early stage can usually be offered to the patients with spinal deformities secondary to Duchenne muscular dystrophy.

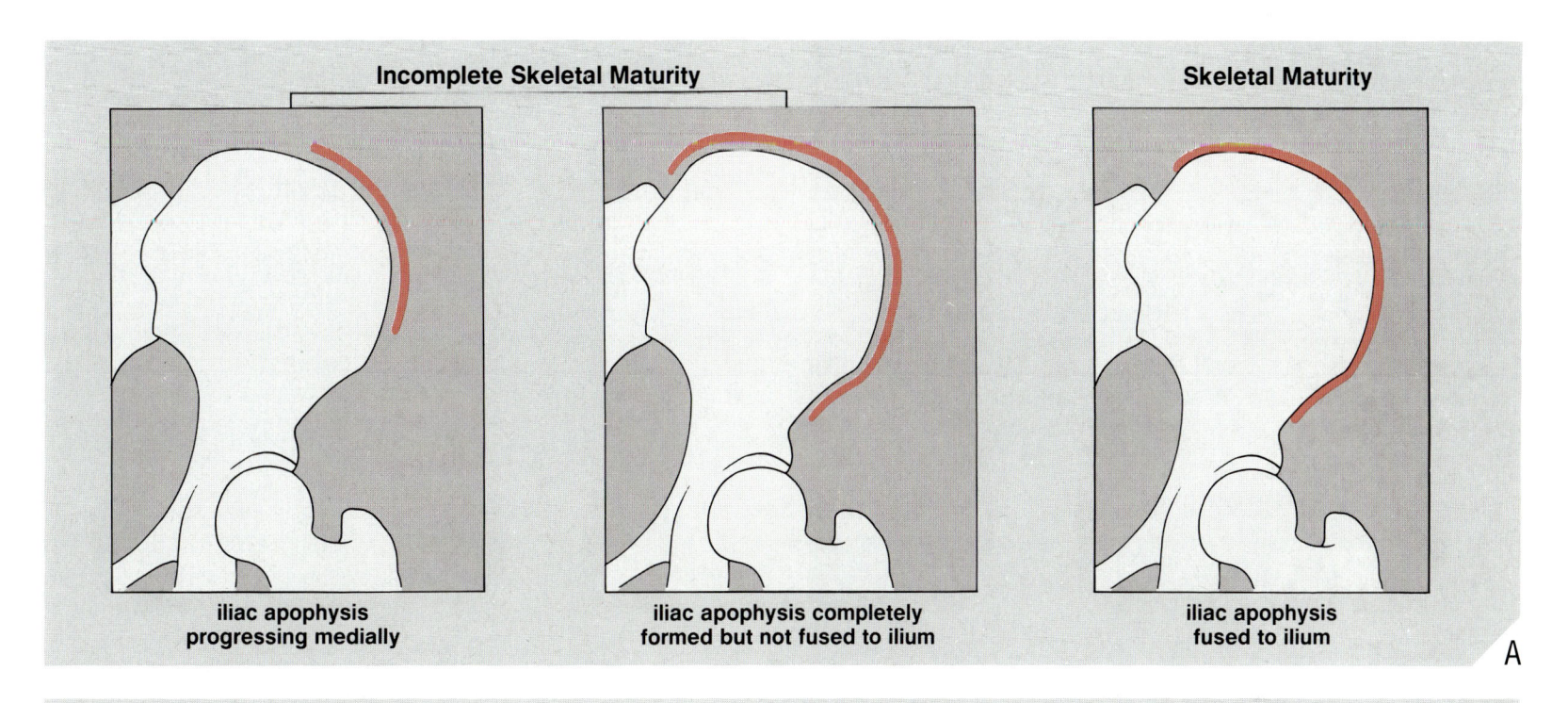

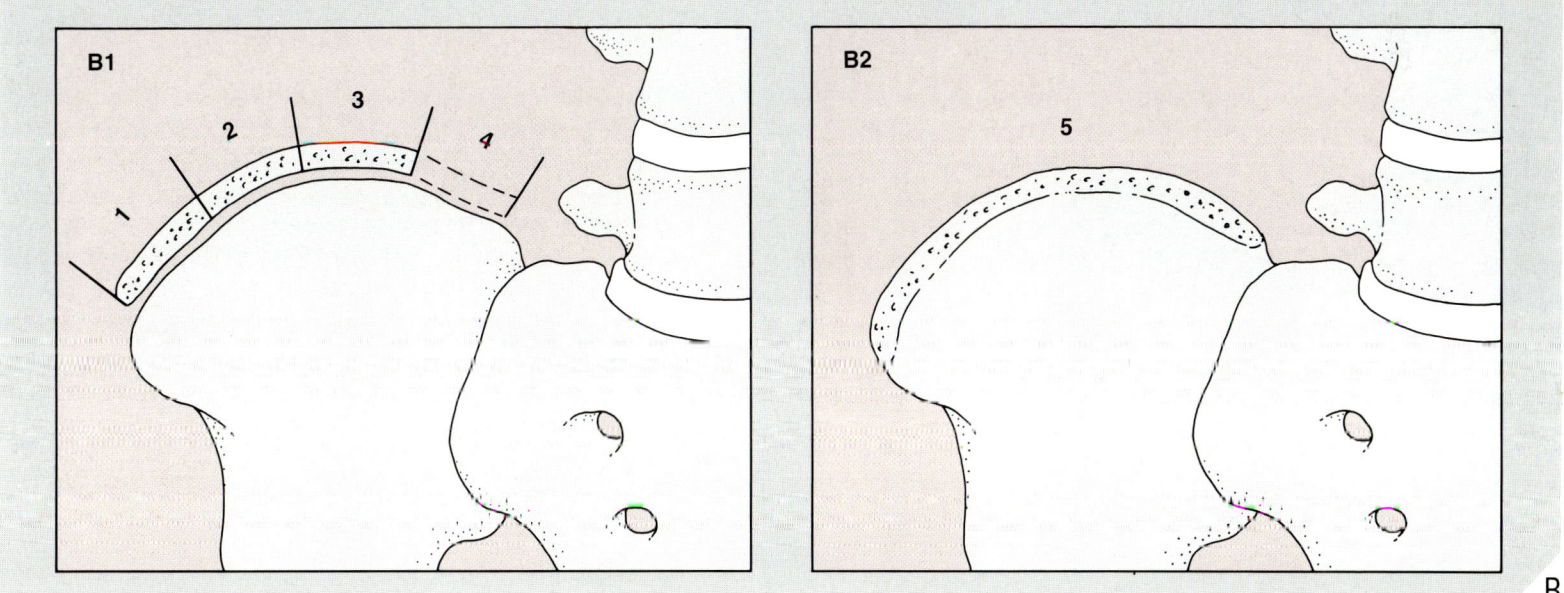

FIGURE 19.17 (A) Determination of skeletal maturity from the status of ossification of the iliac apophysis. **(B)** According to Risser, the iliac crest is divided into quarters, and the excursion or stage of maturity is designated as the amount of progression (1 = 25% excursion; 2 = 50%; 3 = 75%; 4 = complete excursion; 5 = fusion to the ilium). In the example shown in B1, the excursion is 75% complete, and the Risser sign is thus 3. In B2, the excursion has been completed and the apophysis has fused with the iliac crest—a Risser 5. (Modified from Lonstein JE. Patient evaluation. In Bradford DS, Lonstein JE, Moe JH, et al. (eds): *Moe's Textbook of Scoliosis and Other Spinal Deformities*, 2nd ed. Philadelphia, W B Saunders, 1987).

A variety of surgical procedures are available for the treatment of scoliosis. The main objective of surgery is to balance and fuse the spine and thus prevent the deformity from progressing; the secondary objective is to correct the scoliotic curve to the extent of its flexibility. Determining the level of fusion depends on several factors, including the etiology of the scoliosis and the age of the patient, as well as the pattern of the scoliotic curve and the extent of vertebral rotation as evaluated during the radiographic examination.

Spinal fusion is now usually accompanied by internal fixation of the spine to provide stability, correction of the curve, and increased fusion rate. One of the most popular methods for internal fixation is the Harrington–Luque technique, which uses square-ended Harrington distraction rods on the concave side of the curve and a Luque rod on the convex side of the curve. Wire loops are then inserted through the bases of the spinous processes and connected to two contoured paravertebral rods (Fig. 19.18). The most important part of the procedure involves

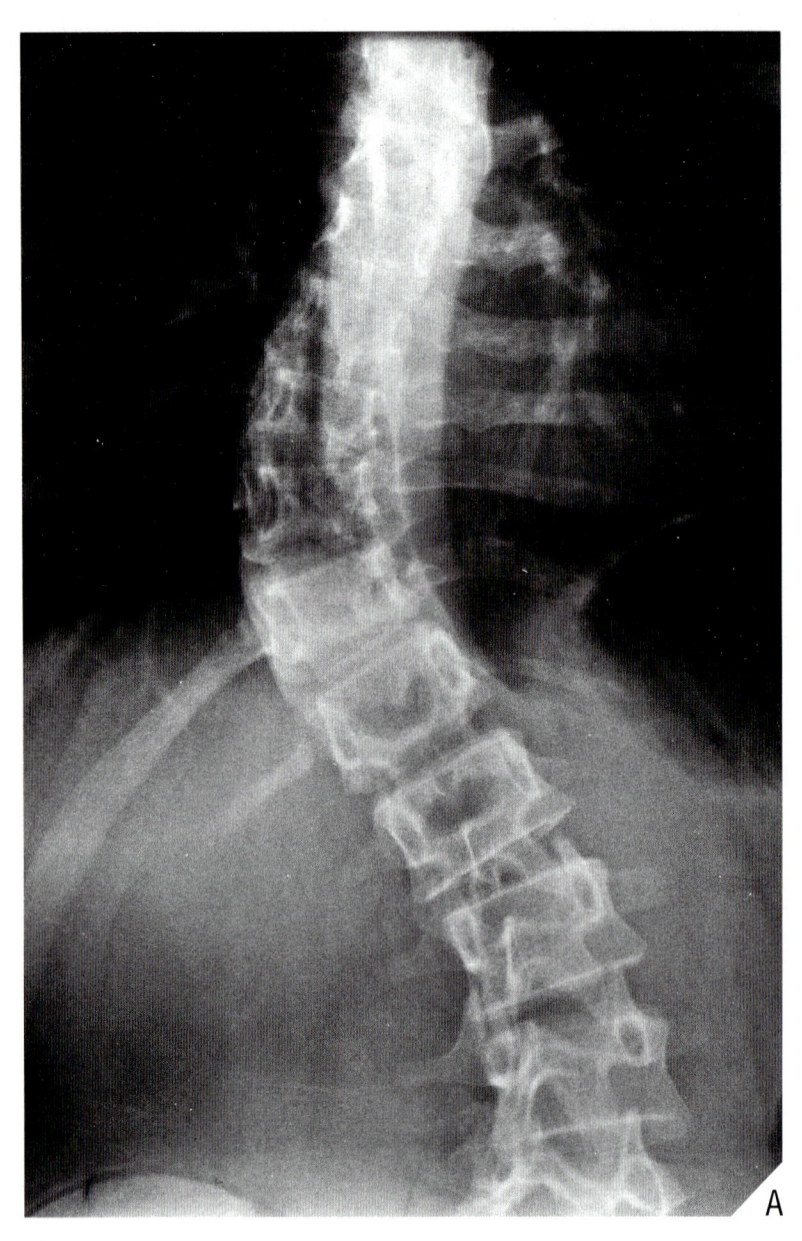

FIGURE 19.18 (A) Preoperative anteroposterior radiograph of the lumbar spine in a 15-year-old girl shows idiopathic dextroscoliosis. **(B)** Postoperative film shows the placement of the Harrington distractor and two Luque rods. Note the multiple wires fixed into the prebent L-rods.

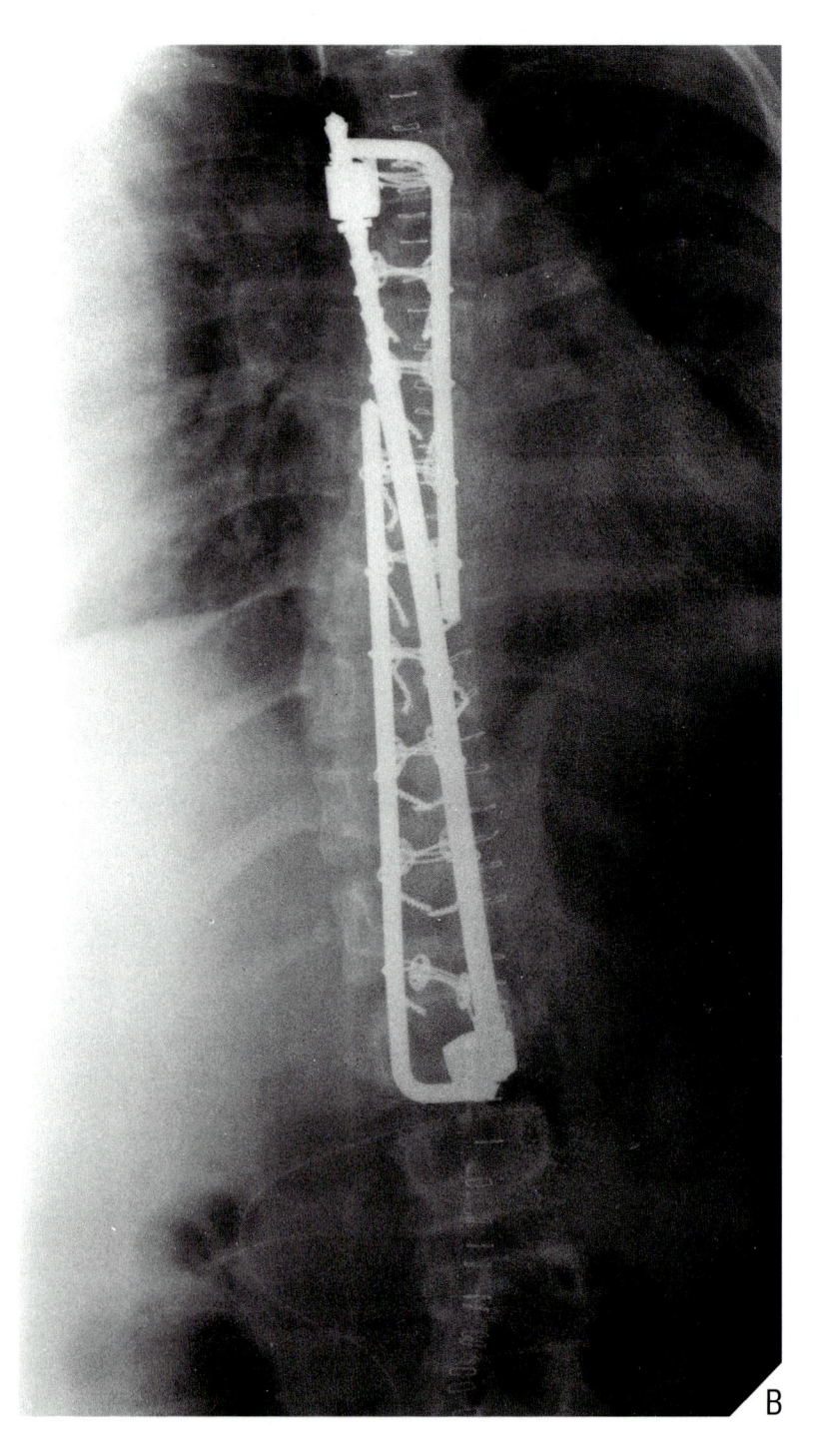

Imaging of the Spine in Clinical Practice

decortication of the laminae and spinous processes, obliteration of the posterior facet joints by removal of the cartilage, and the placement of an autogenous bone graft from the iliac crest along the concave side of the curve. Luque rods are often used in paralytic curve with pelvic obliquity. These rods are anchored to the pelvis by inserting them between the cortical tables of the ilium. They enter the ilium posterosuperiorly and are directed towards the anteroinferior iliac spines. Sublaminar wires are inserted at previously chosen levels and are then tightened around the rods (Fig. 19.19). Recently, Cotrel–Dubousset spinal instrumentation using knurled rods has gained popularity. Fixation is achieved via multiple hooks or screws which purchase the spine at several levels. The two knurled rods are additionally stabilized by at least two transverse traction devices (Figs. 19.20, 19.21). The Zielke technique, involving anterior fixation of the spine and obliteration of the intervertebral disks, is also used in the surgical treatment of scoliosis. This is especially true for curves involving the thoracolumbar and lumbar segments (Fig. 19.22).

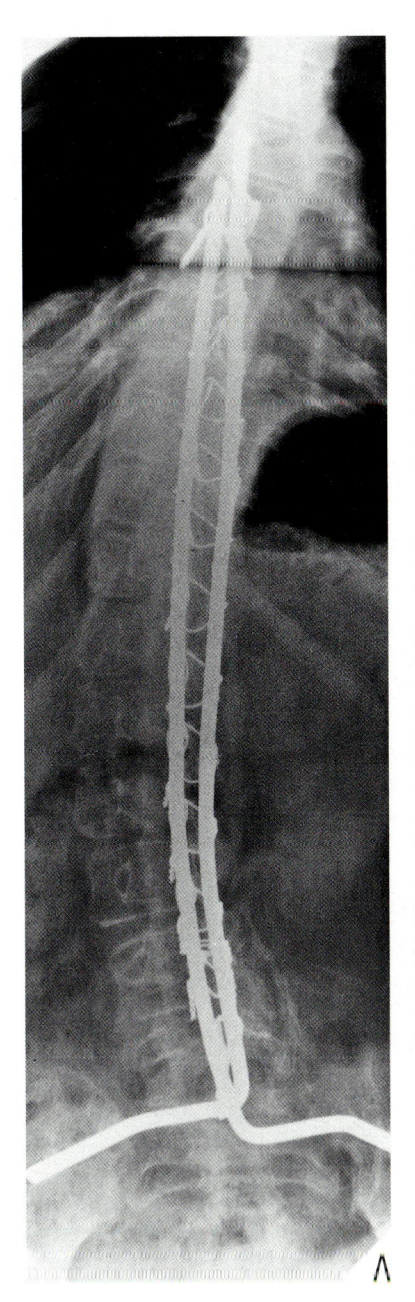

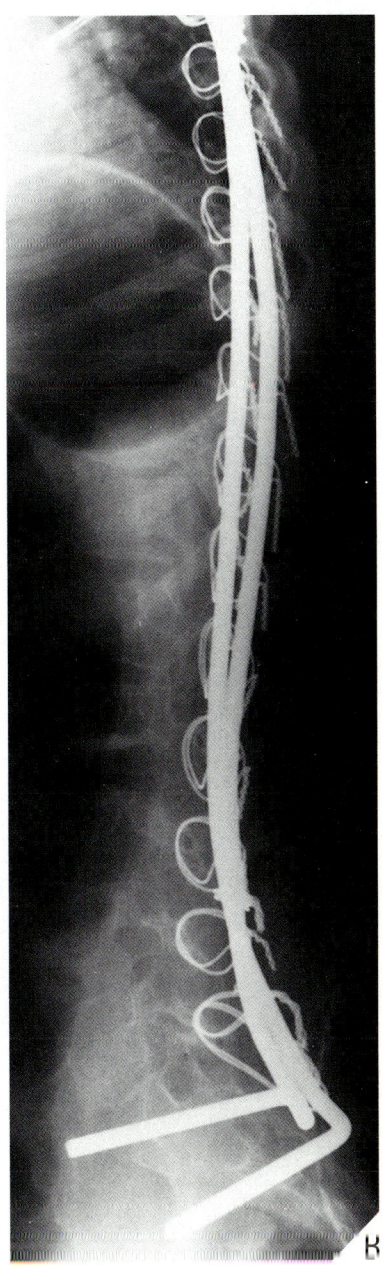

FIGURE 19.19 (A,B) A 12-year-old girl with progressive paralytic scoliosis of 49° (measured by Lippman–Cobb method) due to cerebral palsy has been treated with Luque rods instrumentation that included pelvic anchoring. Autogenous bone graft has been placed on the concave side of the curve. The procedure resulted in correction of the scoliotic curve to 31°.

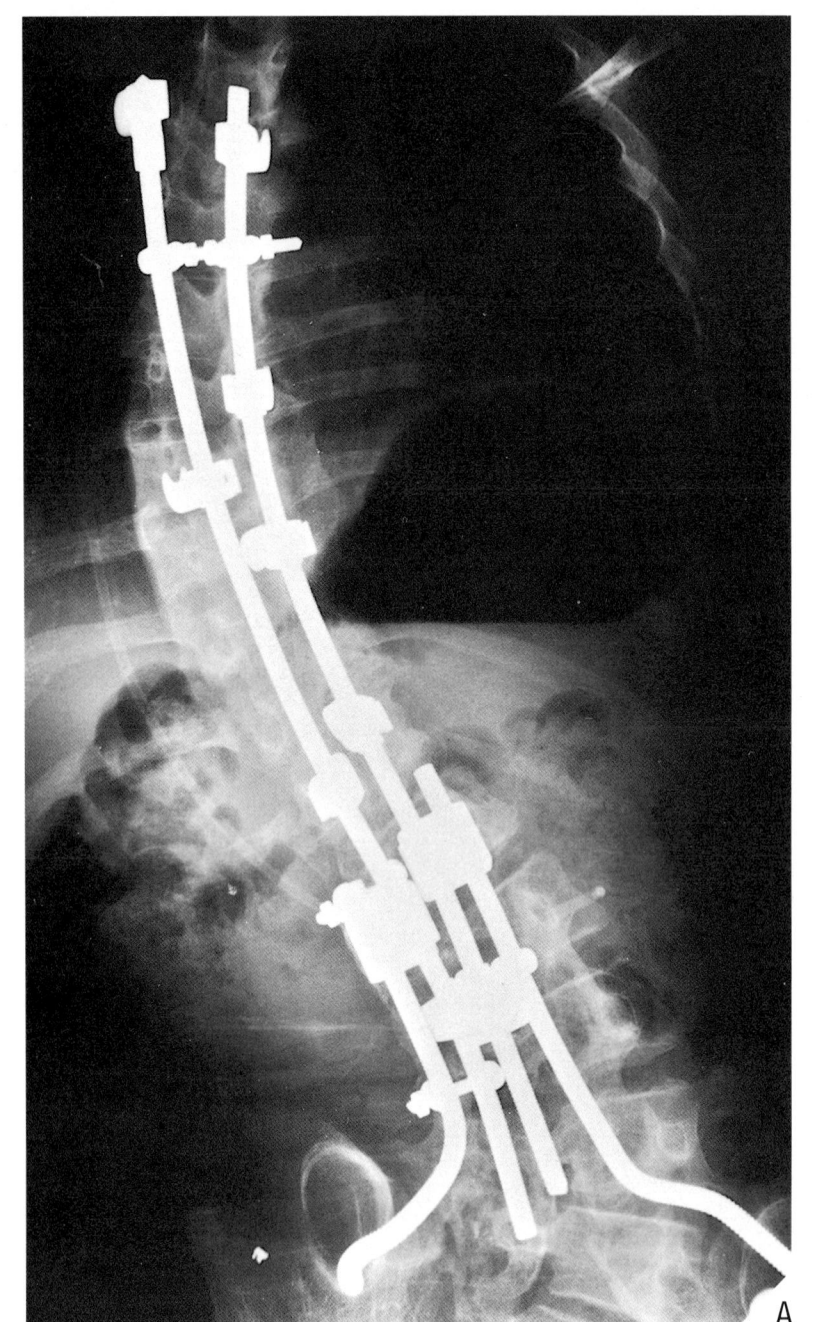

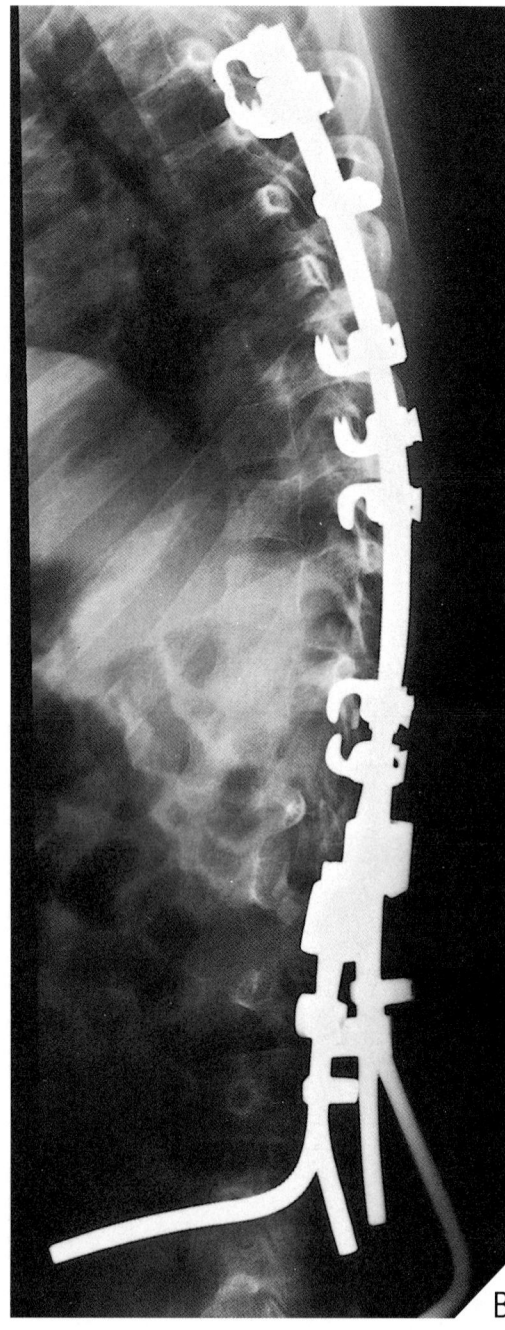

FIGURE 19.20
(A,B) A 17-year-old boy with progressive paralytic thoracolumbar scoliosis of 45° secondary to myelomeningocele has been treated with Cotrel–Dubousset spinal instrumentation using knurled rods. Surgery reduced his primary curve to 30°.

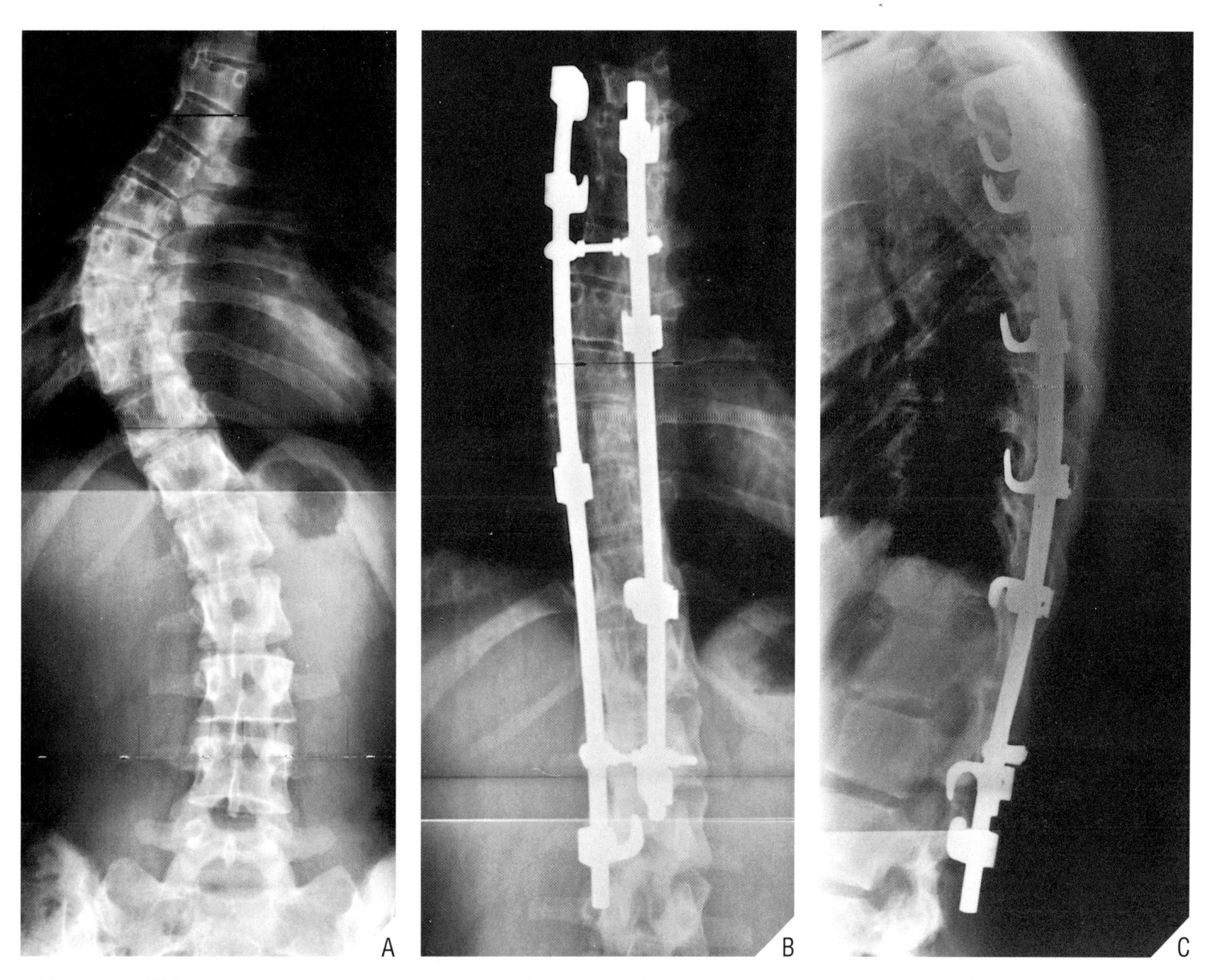

FIGURE 19.21 (A) A 14-year-old girl presented with progressive type of idiopathic scoliosis in thoracolumbar segment that measured 55°. The compensatory curve in the lumbar segment measured 35°. **(B,C)** After treatment with Cotrel–Dubousset spinal instrumentation, her primary scoliotic curve has been corrected to 12°, and her lumbar curve to 10°.

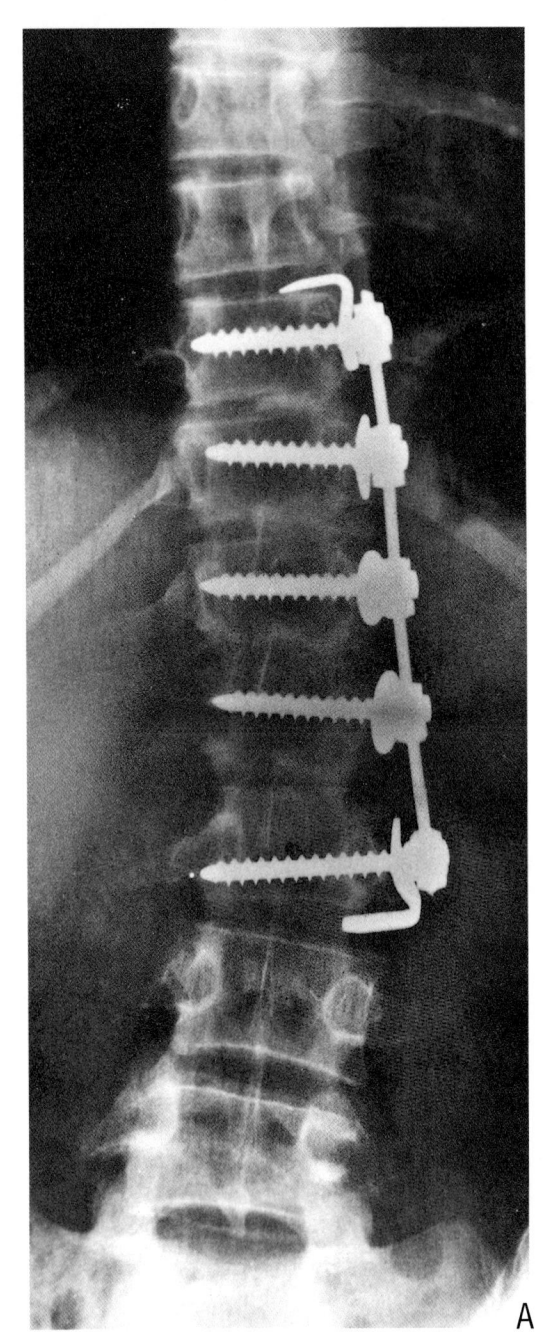

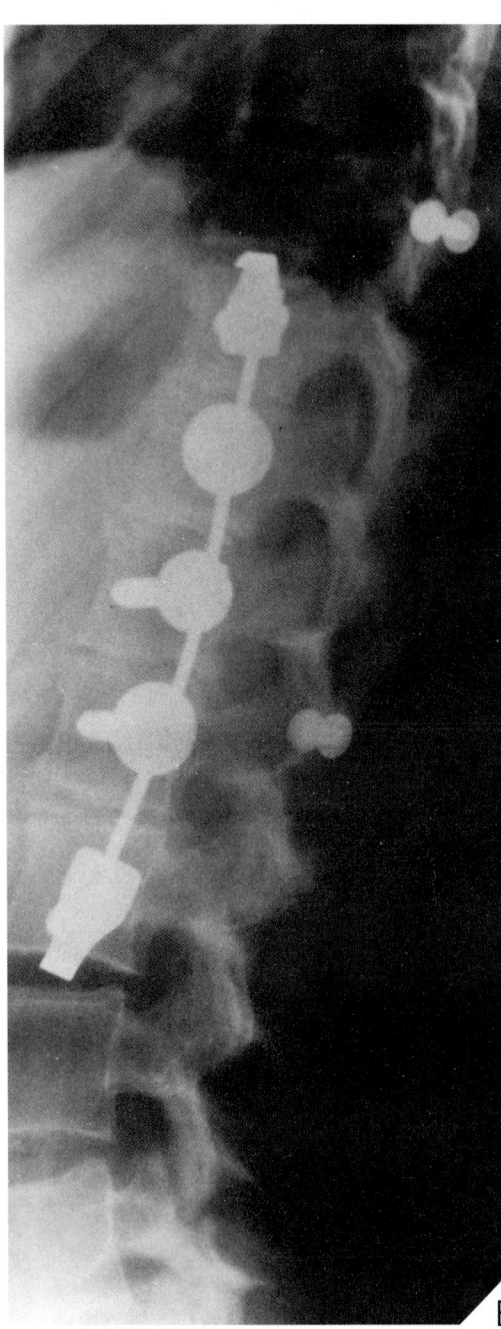

FIGURE 19.22 (A,B) A 14-year-old girl with a progressive idiopathic lumbar scoliosis that measured 46° has been treated with Zilke instrumentation. The treatment resulted in correction of the curve to 15°.

The postoperative radiographic evaluation of internal fixation should focus on: (1) whether the hooks of the rods are properly anchored, with their brackets on the laminae of the superior and inferior vertebrae of the fused segment; (2) whether a hook has separated or been displaced (Fig. 19.23); and (3) whether the rods and wires are intact. Moreover, evidence of pseudoarthrosis of the fused vertebrae should be sought when the postoperative loss of correction exceeds 10°; a range of 6° to 10° loss of correction is ordinarily seen. The evaluation of pseudoarthrosis may require conventional tomography in addition to the standard projections. Tomography may also be needed within 6 to 9 months after surgery to demonstrate suspected nonunion of the bone engrafted on the concave side of the curve. Union of the graft with the spinal segment should appear solid; tomography may demonstrate radiolucent defects suggesting nonunion. Other complications involving the instrumentation may occur, such as fracture of a distraction rod, a wire cable, or a screw, or excessive bending of the rods. Usually these are easily demonstrated on standard radiograms (Fig. 19.24).

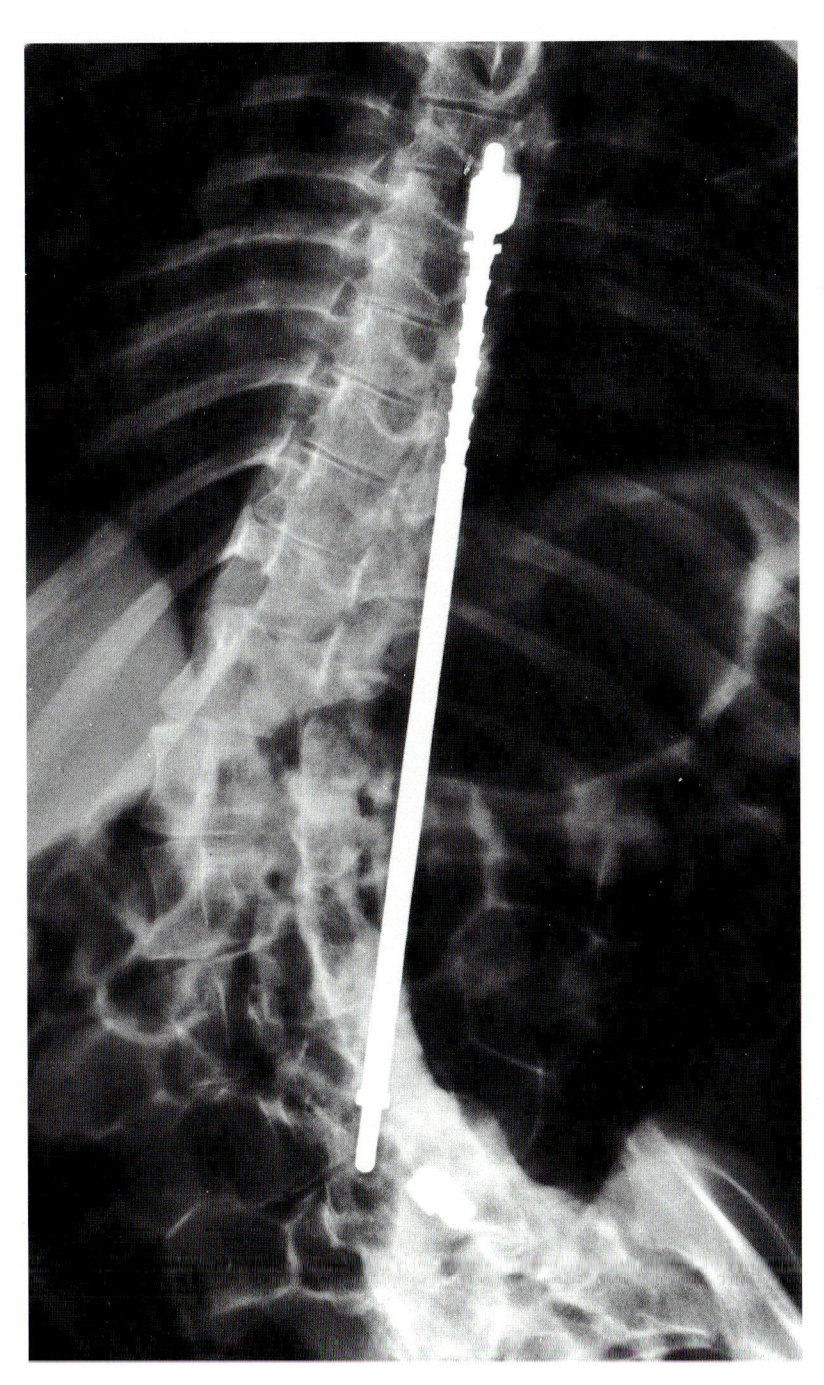

FIGURE 19.23 Anteroposterior view of the spine following vertebral fusion and internal fixation using Harrington instrumentation shows separation of the lower hook from the rod. A defect in the graft material on the concave side of the curve is also evident.

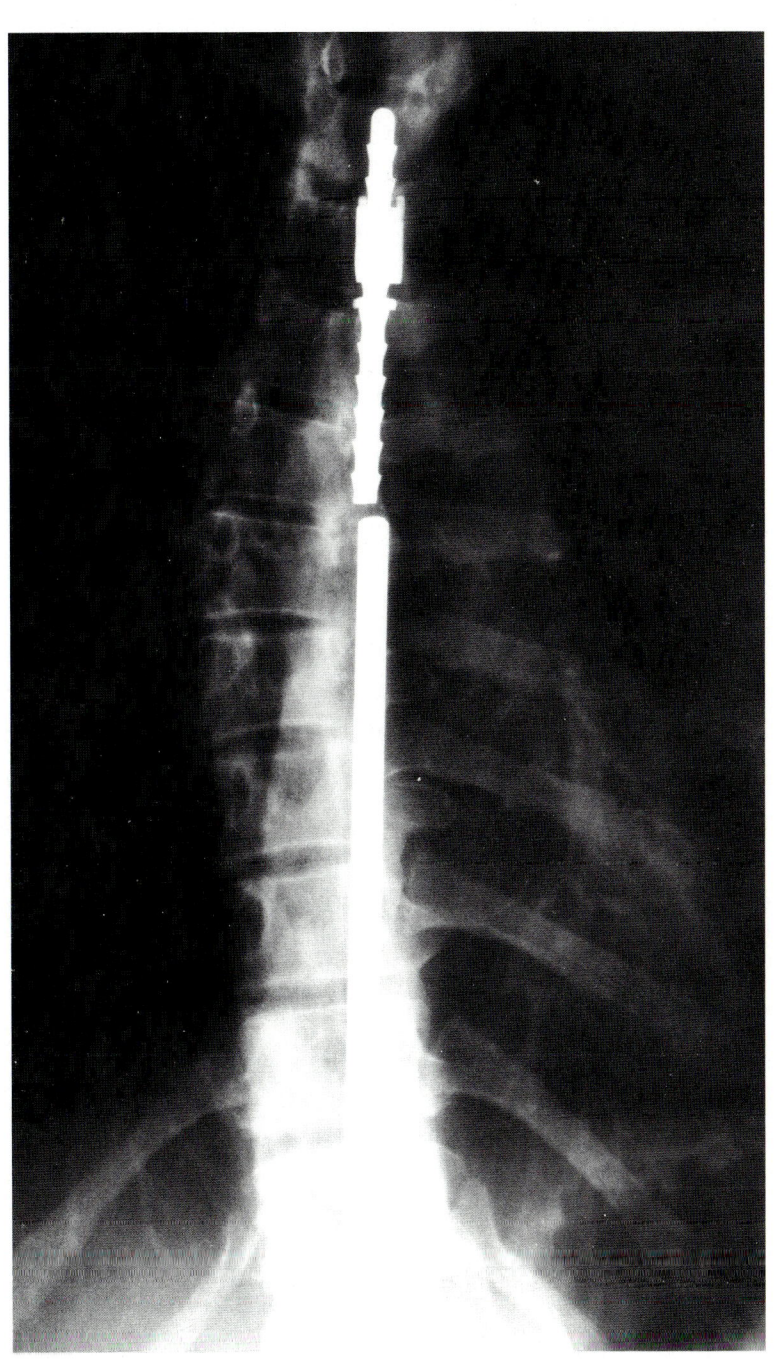

FIGURE 19.24 Anteroposterior view of the thoracic spine demonstrates a fracture of the Harrington rod. The break occurred at the junction of the solid and notched segments, the usual site of this complication.

Anomalies with General Effects on the Skeleton

Neurofibromatosis

Originally considered a disorder of neurogenic tissue (nerve trunk tumors), neurofibromatosis (also called *von Recklinghausen disease*) is now believed to be a hereditary dysplasia that may involve almost every organ system of the body. It is transmitted as an autosomal-dominant trait with variable penetrance and expression; more than 50% of patients report a family history of neurofibromatosis. Sessile or pedunculated skin lesions (mollusca fibrosa) are a consistent finding in symptomatic patients and café-au-lait spots are present in more than 90%. The latter lesions have a smooth border that has been likened to the coast of California; this distinguishes them from the café-au-lait spots seen in fibrous dysplasia, which have rugged "coast of Maine" borders. Plexiform neurofibromatosis is a diffuse involvement of the nerves, associated with elephantoid masses of soft tissue (elephantiasis neuromatosa) and localized or generalized enlargement of a part or all of a limb. Patients with these manifestations are particularly prone to develop malignant tumors.

Skeletal abnormalities are often encountered in neurofibromatosis; at least 50% of patients demonstrate some bone changes, most commonly extrinsic, pit-like cortical erosions resulting from direct pressure by adjacent neurofibromas; these erosions are common in long bones and ribs. The long bones often exhibit bowing deformities, and pseudoarthroses, observed in about 10% of cases, usually occurring in the lower tibia and fibula.

The spine is the second most frequent site of skeletal abnormalities in neurofibromatosis. Scoliosis or kyphoscoliosis, which characteristically involves a short segment of the vertebral column with acute angulation, commonly occur in the lower cervical or upper thoracic spine (Fig. 19.25A,B). Widening of the intervertebral foramina in the cervical segment may also occur, caused by dumbbell-shaped neurofibromas arising in spinal nerve roots (Figs. 19.25C, 19.26). In the thoracic and lumbar segments, scalloping of the posterior border of vertebral bodies is another characteristic feature (Fig. 19.27; see also Fig. 17.3). Although most of

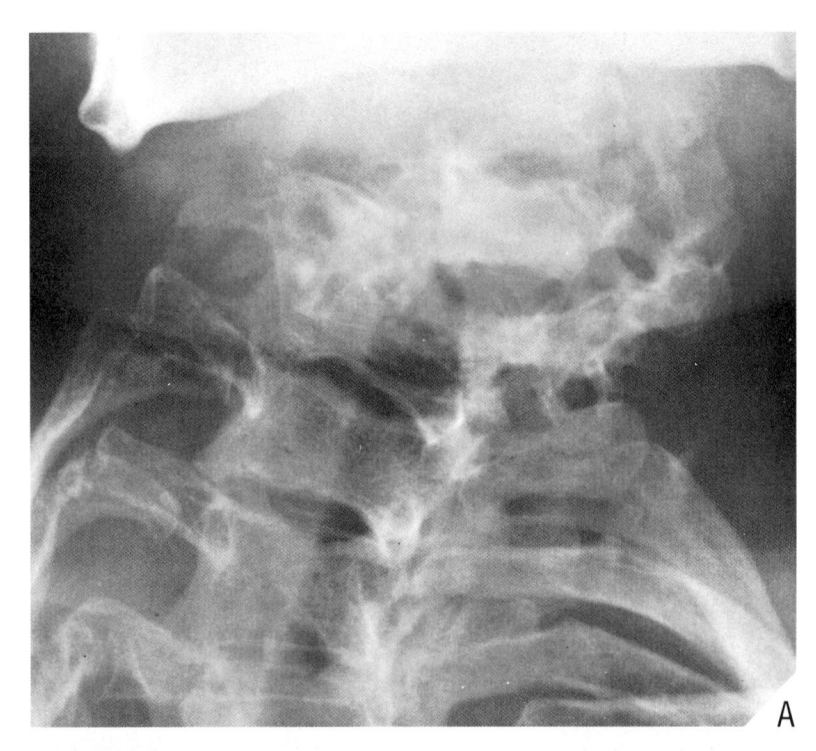

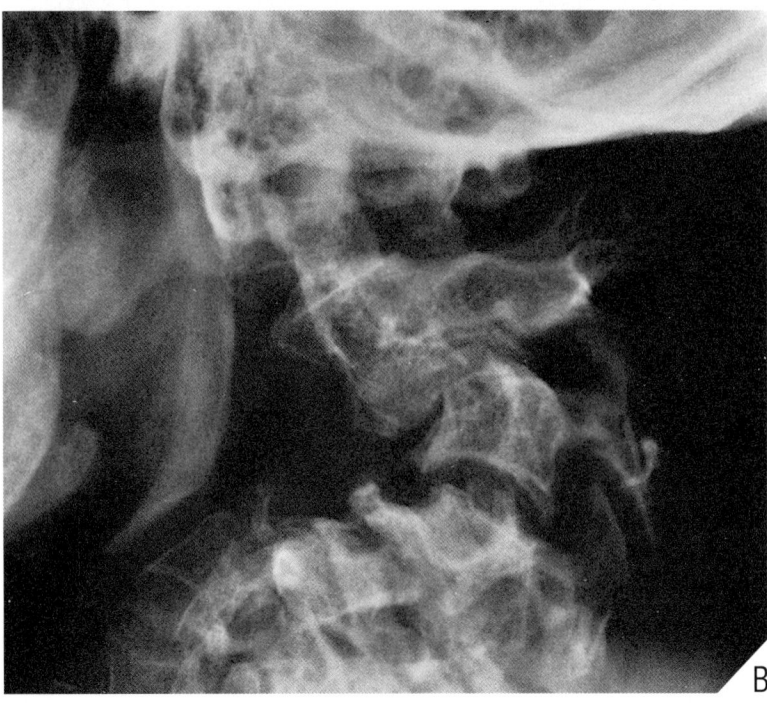

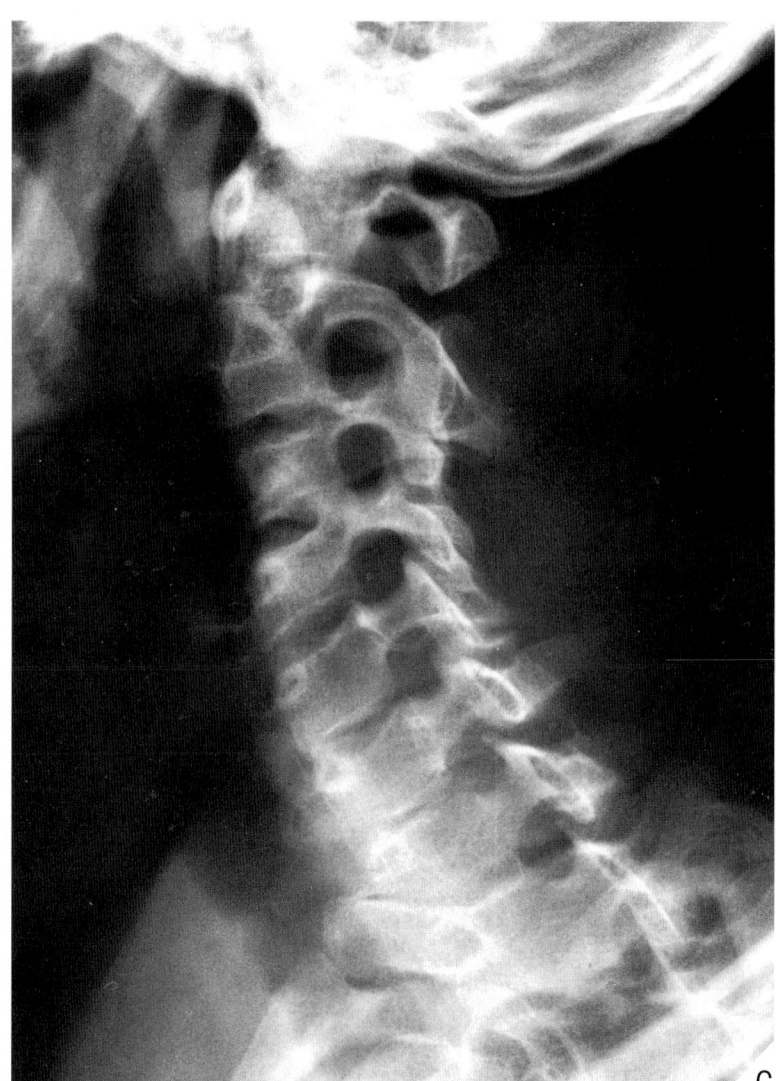

FIGURE 19.25 Anteroposterior **(A)** and lateral **(B)** radiographs of the cervical spine of a 39-year-old woman with neurofibromatosis demonstrate severe degree of kyphoscoliosis. Note the acute angle of the cervical curve typical for this abnormality. **(C)** Oblique view of the cervical spine in a 26-year-old man with congenital neurofibromatosis demonstrates widening of the neural foramina secondary to "dumbbell" neurofibromas arising in the spinal nerve roots.

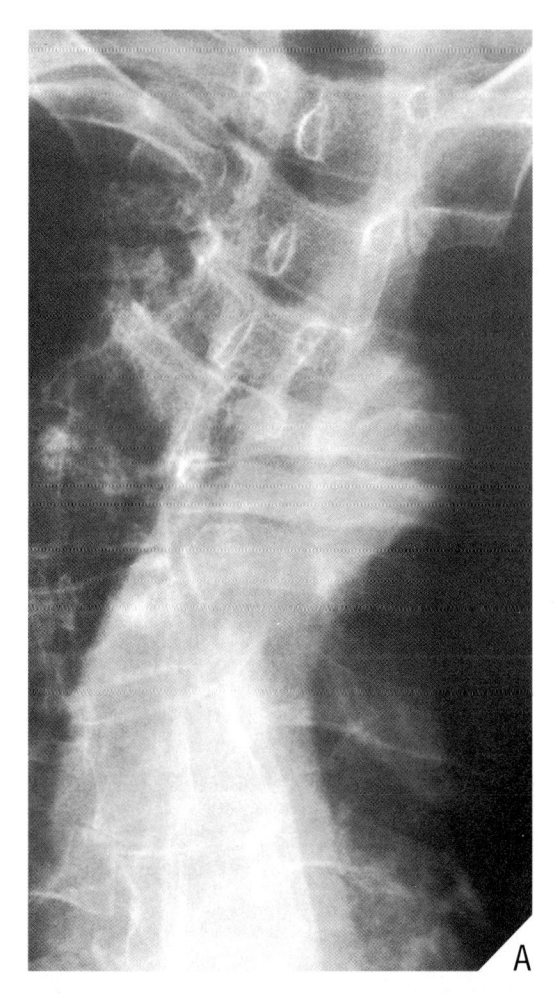

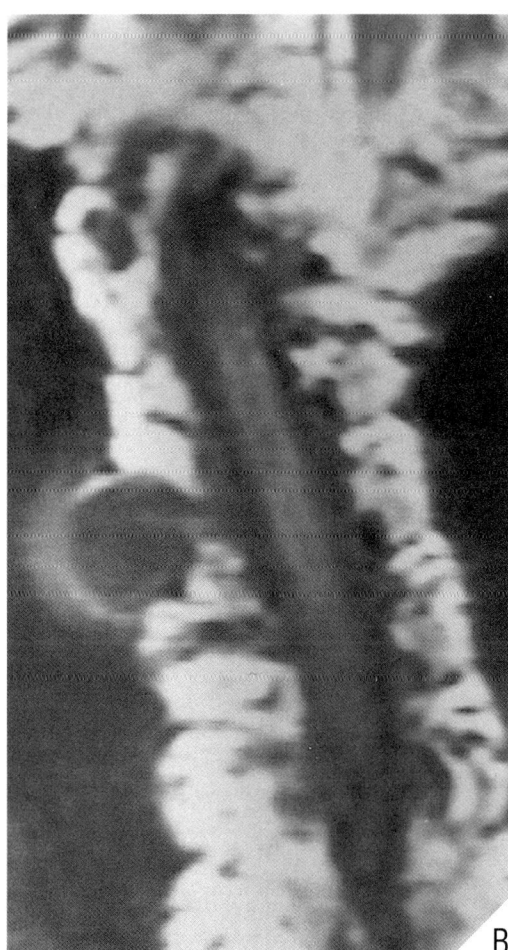

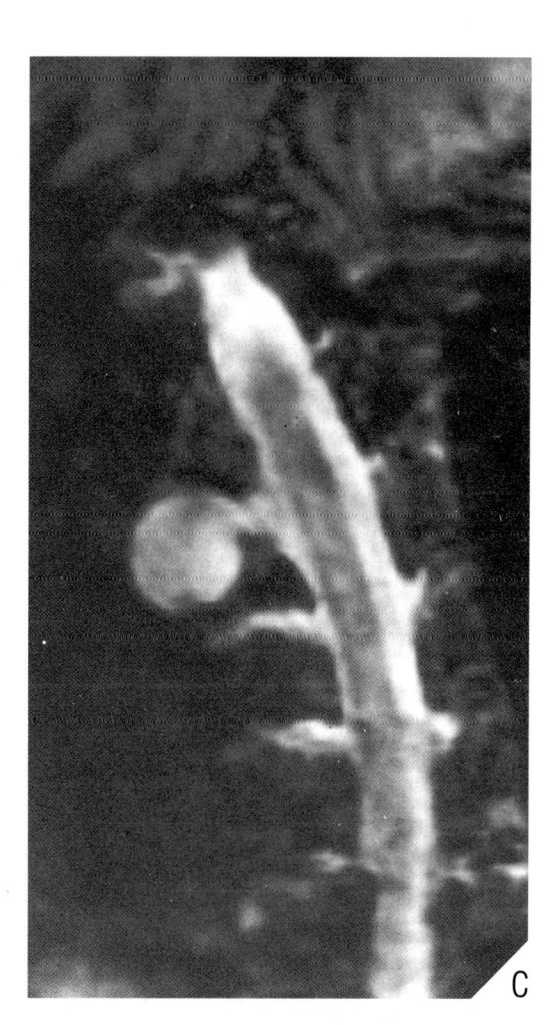

FIGURE 19.26 (A) Anteroposterior radiograph of the thoracic spine shows scoliosis in the middle segment convexity to the right in this 53-year-old woman with neurofibromatosis. T1-weighted spin-echo **(B)** and T2*-weighted gradient-echo (MPGR) **(C)** coronal MRI demonstrate dumbbell-shaped neurofibroma arising in spinal nerve root.

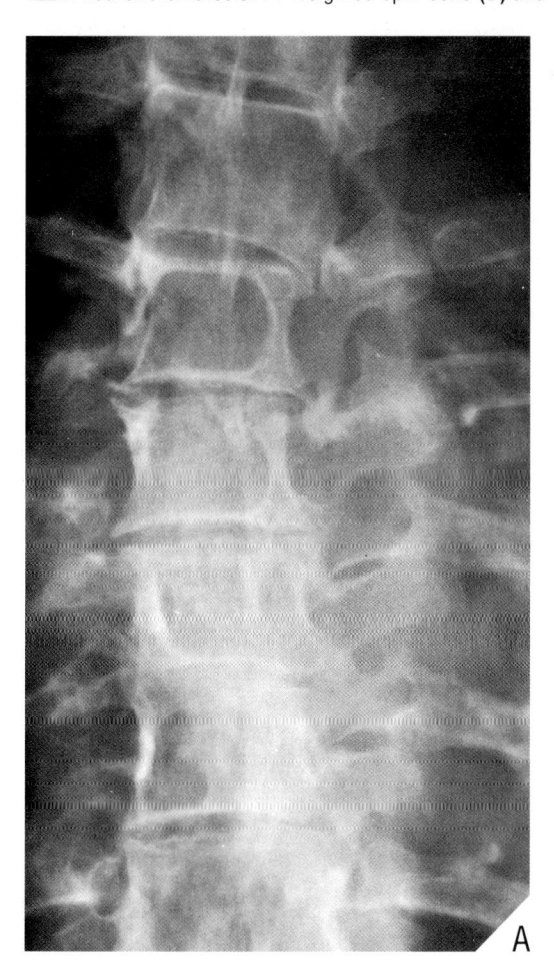

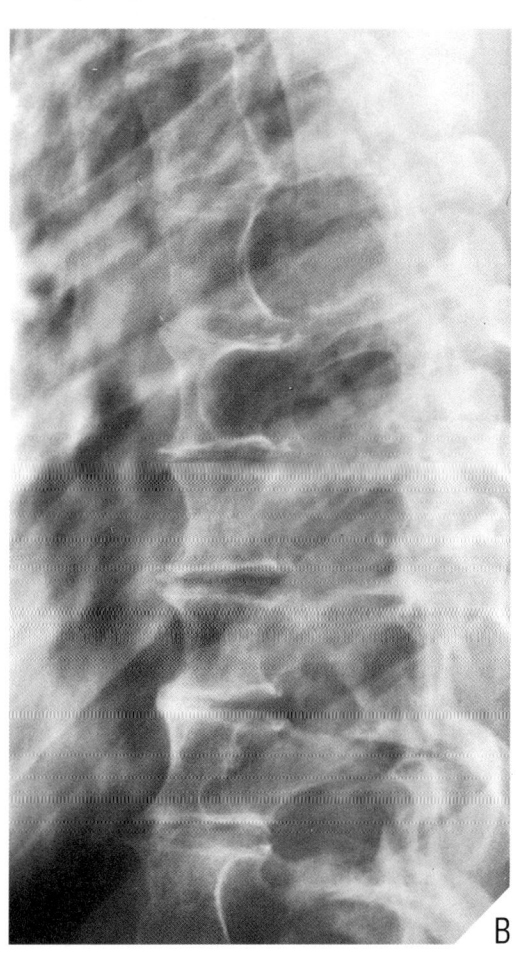

FIGURE 19.27 Anteroposterior **(A)** and lateral **(B)** radiography of the thoracic spine in a 26-year-old woman with neurofibromatosis show scalloping of the posterior vertebral borders, a common manifestation of this condition.

Scoliosis and Anomalies with General Effects on the Skeleton

these abnormalities can easily be diagnosed with conventional radiography, some ancillary techniques may be useful. Myelography is particularly valuable for demonstrating the cord compression associated with kyphoscoliosis, demonstrating increased volume of the enlarged subarachnoid space, and to localize dural ectasia extending into the scalloped defects in the vertebral bodies. With introduction of MRI, this modality has become more prevalent in investigation of the above-mentioned abnormalities (Fig. 19.28).

Osteogenesis Imperfecta

Osteogenesis imperfecta, also known as *fragilitas ossium,* is a congenital, hereditary disorder that manifests in the skeleton as a primary defect in the bone matrix. It is characterized by bone fragility resulting from abnormal quality and/or quantity of type I collagen. Depending on the type of osteogenesis imperfecta, the inheritance of the disorder can be autosomal dominant, autosomal dominant with new mutation, or autosomal recessive. Looser, in 1906, divided this condition into two forms, "congenita" and "tarda," and suggested that they are expressions of the same disease. Osteogenesis imperfecta congenita (Vrolik disease) has been classified as the more severe form, which is evident at birth and is marked by bowing of the upper and lower extremities in an infant who is either stillborn or does not survive the neonatal period. The more benign osteogenesis imperfecta tarda (Ekman–Lobstein disease), in which there is a normal life expectancy, may exhibit fractures at birth, but more often, fractures appear later in infancy. This condition is also associated with other manifestations, such as deformities of the extremities, blue sclerae, laxity of ligaments, and dental abnormalities.

CLASSIFICATION

In general, four major clinical features characterize osteogenesis imperfecta: osteoporosis with abnormal bone fragility; blue sclerae; defective dentition (dentinogenesis imperfecta); and presenile onset of hearing impairment. Other clinical features also may be seen, including ligamentous laxity and hypermobility of joints, short stature, easy bruising, hyperplastic scars, and abnormal temperature regulation. The earlier classification of osteogenesis imperfecta into two types, congenita and tarda, failed to reflect the complexity and heterogenous nature of this disorder. The new classification, proposed by Sillence and colleagues in 1979 and later revised, is based on phenotypic features and the mode of inheritance. At present, four major types of osteogenesis imperfecta and their subtypes are recognized.

Type I This most common type of the disorder is a relatively mild form, with autosomal-dominant inheritance. Bone fragility is mild to moderate and osteoporosis is invariably present. Sclerae are distinctly blue. Hearing loss or impairment is a common feature. Stature is normal or near normal. Wormian bones are present. The two subtypes are distinguished by the presence of normal teeth (subtype IA) or dentinogenesis imperfecta (subtype IB).

Type II This is the fetal or perinatal lethal form of the disorder which demonstrates an autosomal dominant inheritance with new mutation. The very severe nature of generalized osteoporosis, bone fragility, and severe intrauterine growth retardation results in death during the fetal or early perinatal period. Of those infants who survive, 80% to 90% die by 4 weeks of age. All of these patients have radiologic features typical of

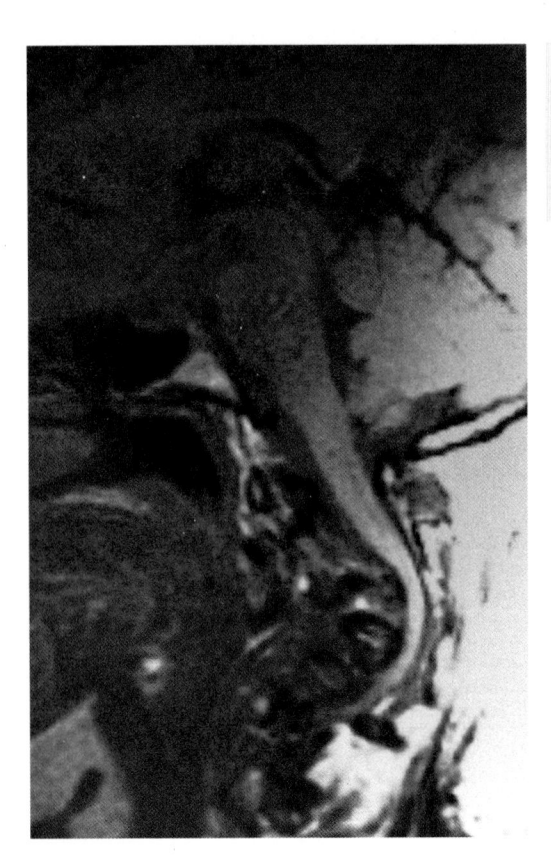

FIGURE 19.28 Sagittal MRI of the cervical spine of the patient shown in Figure 19.25 exhibits compression of the spinal cord by posteriorly displaced vertebrae.

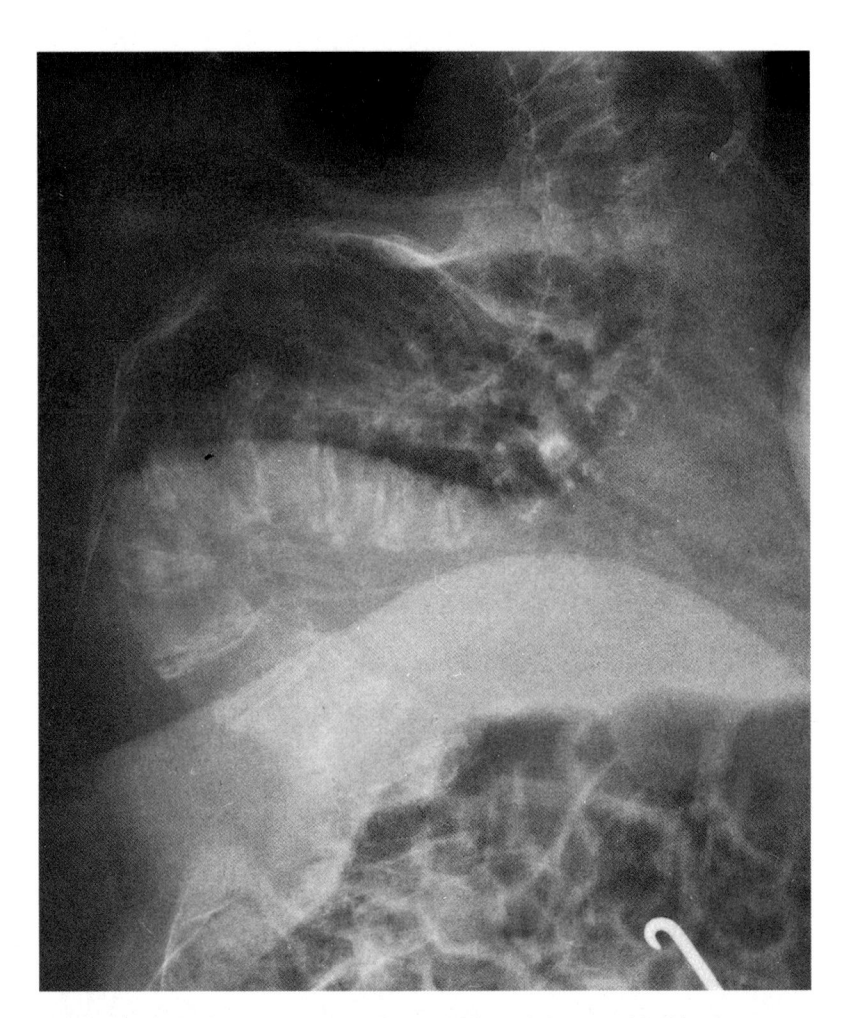

FIGURE 19.29 Anteroposterior radiograph of an adolescent girl with osteogenesis imperfecta shows severe spinal deformity and marked osteoporosis. (Reproduced with permission from Bullough PG, Boachie-Adjei O: *Atlas of Spinal Diseases.* New York, Gower, 1988)

osteogenesis imperfecta. In addition, the sclerae are blue and the face has a triangle shape caused by soft craniofacial bones and a beaked nose. The calvaria is large relative to the face, and the skull shows a marked lack of mineralization as well as the presence of wormian bones. Limbs are short, broad, and angulated. The three subtypes—A, B, C—are marked by differences in the appearance of the ribs and the long bones. In subtype A the long bones are broad and crumpled and the ribs are broad, with continuous beading. In subtype B the long bones also are broad and crumpled, but ribs show either discontinuous beading or no beading. Subtype C is characterized by thin, fractured long bones and ribs that are thin and beaded.

Type III This is a severe, progressive form and represents a rare autosomal-dominant inheritance with new mutations. Bone fragility and osteopenia are considerable, leading with age to multiple fractures and severe progressive deformity of the long bones and spine. Bone abnormalities are generally less severe than in Type II and more severe than in Types I or IV. Sclerae are normal, although pale blue or gray at birth, but the color changes through infancy and early childhood until it is normal by adolescence or adulthood. The calvaria is large, thin, and poorly ossified; wormian bones are also present.

Type IV This is also a rare type of osteogenesis imperfecta and is inherited as an autosomal-dominant trait. Characteristically, osteoporosis, bone fragility, and deformity are present, but they are very mild. Sclerae are usually normal. The incidence of hearing impairment is low, and is even lower than in Type I.

Radiologic Evaluation

The radiographic features of osteogenesis imperfecta are easily identified on standard radiographs. Severe osteoporosis, deformities of the bones, and thinning of the cortices are consistently observed. The bones are also attenuated and gracile, with a trumpet-shaped appearance to the metaphysis. Other typical skeletal abnormalities are seen in the skull, where wormian bones are a recognizable feature, and in the spine, where severe scoliosis or kyphoscoliosis may develop from a combination of osteoporosis, ligamentous laxity, and post-traumatic deformities (Figs. 19.29, 19.30). The pelvis is invariably deformed, and acetabular protrusion is a frequent finding.

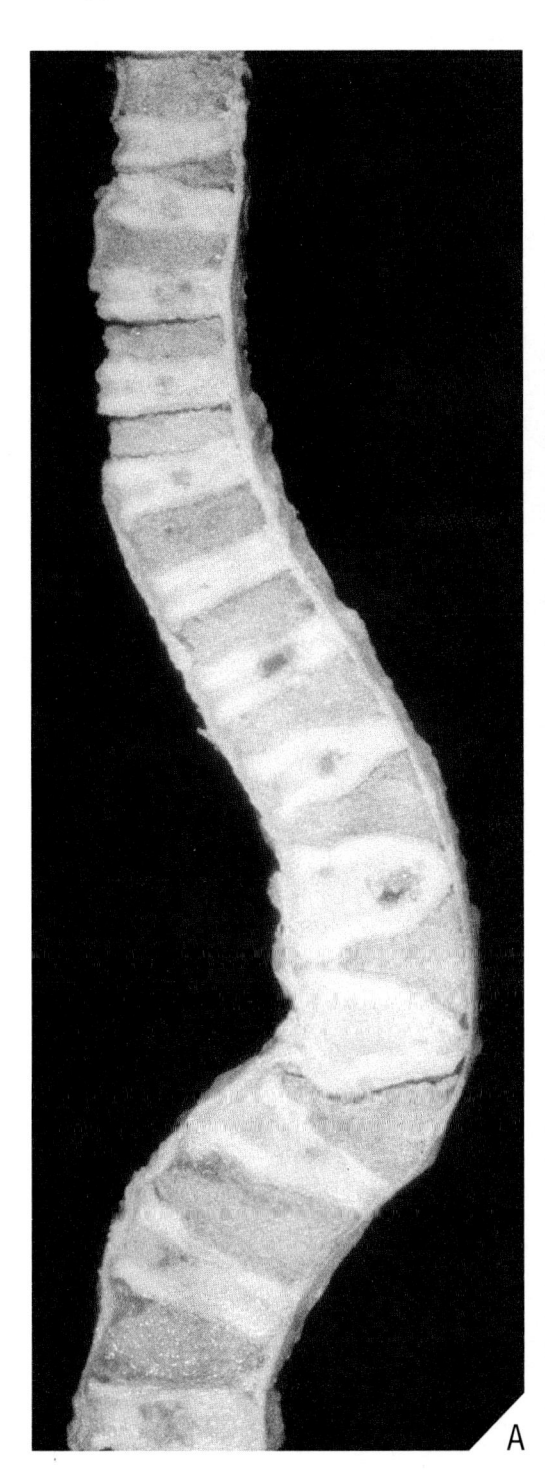

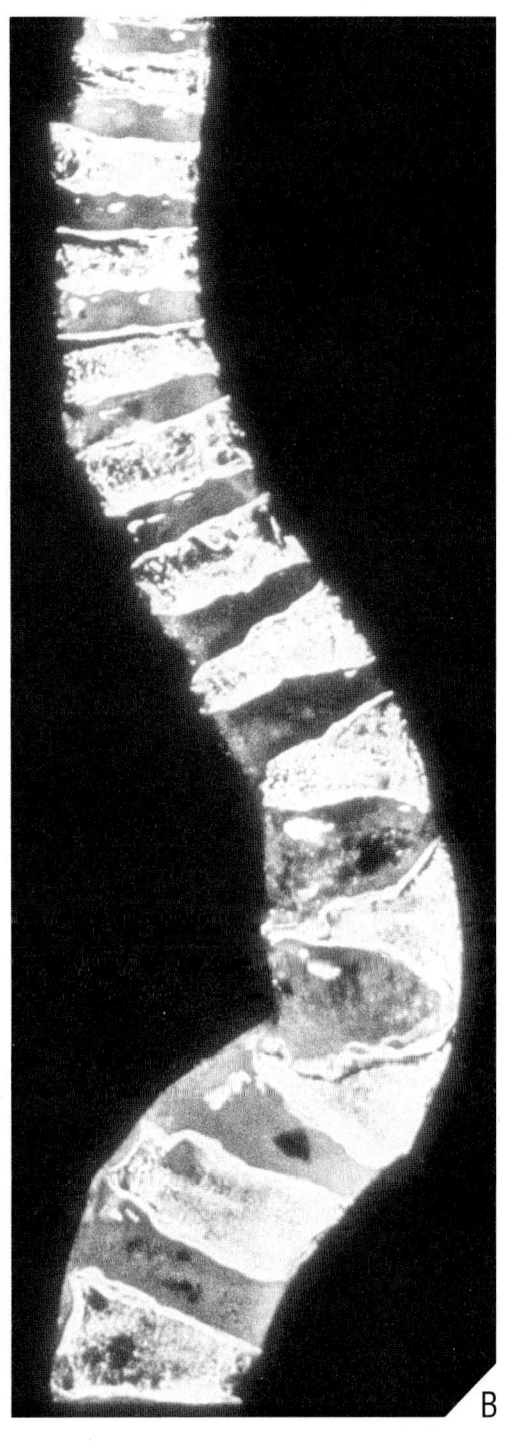

FIGURE 19.30 (A) A photograph of a coronal section through the spine of a patient with osteogenesis imperfecta, and **(B)** a specimen radiograph of the same spine shows scoliotic deformity secondary to multiple compression fractures. Note also severe vertebral osteoporosis. (Reproduced with permission from Bullough PG, Boachie-Adjei O: *Atlas of Spinal Diseases*. New York, Gower, 1988)

DIFFERENTIAL DIAGNOSIS

Occasionally, osteogenesis imperfecta may be misdiagnosed as child abuse, and vice versa. Patient and family histories, physical examination, diagnostic imaging, and the clinical course of the abnormalities all contribute to the distinction of this condition from child abuse. The keys to distinguishing osteogenesis imperfecta from child abuse are as follows: the presence of blue sclerae or abnormal teeth in osteogenesis imperfecta (OI); investigation of clinical and family history (invariably positive in OI); physical examination; and radiologic examination for detection of wormian bones and osteoporosis in OI, and metaphyseal corner fractures and "bucket handle" fractures, which are highly specific and virtually pathognomonic features of child abuse. Several other features are also specific for child abuse, including: multiple rib fractures, especially posterior rib fractures near or at the costovertebral junction; multiple fractures and/or multiple fractures showing different stages of healing; and sternal or scapular fractures, especially of the acromion. Transverse, oblique, or spiral fracture of a long bone with normal mineralization in the absence of any prior history, especially in a nonambulatory infant, are also highly suggestive of child abuse. The key to diagnosis of either condition is the correlation of clinical history, physical examination, family history, and radiologic findings.

TREATMENT

There is no specific treatment for osteogenesis imperfecta other than correction of the deformities it produces and the prevention of fractures. However, the condition tends to improve spontaneously at puberty, with cessation or a decrease in the number of fractures.

Achondroplasia

Achondroplasia is a hereditary autosomal-dominant anomaly. It begins in utero due to a failure in endochondral bone formation that affects the growth and development of cartilage. Its most prominent effect is short-limbed, rhizomelic (disproportional) dwarfism. The hands and feet are short and stubby. The trunk is relatively long, with the chest flattened in the anteroposterior dimension. The lower limbs are often bowed, producing a characteristic waddling gait. The head is large, with prominent frontal bossing, a depressed nasal bridge, and a "scooped-out" facial appearance.

Radiographically, achondroplasia has distinct features. As with rhizomelic dwarfism, the tubular bones of the limbs are shortened, with the proximal segments (humeri and femora) more severely affected than the distal portions of the extremities (radius, ulna, tibia, and fibula); the growth plates are V-shaped. The fingers are short and stubby, with the middle one separated from the others, giving the hand a "trident" appearance. Identifying features of this disorder may also be seen in the spine and pelvis. The spine shows a characteristic narrowing of the interpedicular distance and short pedicles, often resulting in spinal stenosis; scalloping of the posterior vertebral aspect is also a common finding (Fig. 19.31).

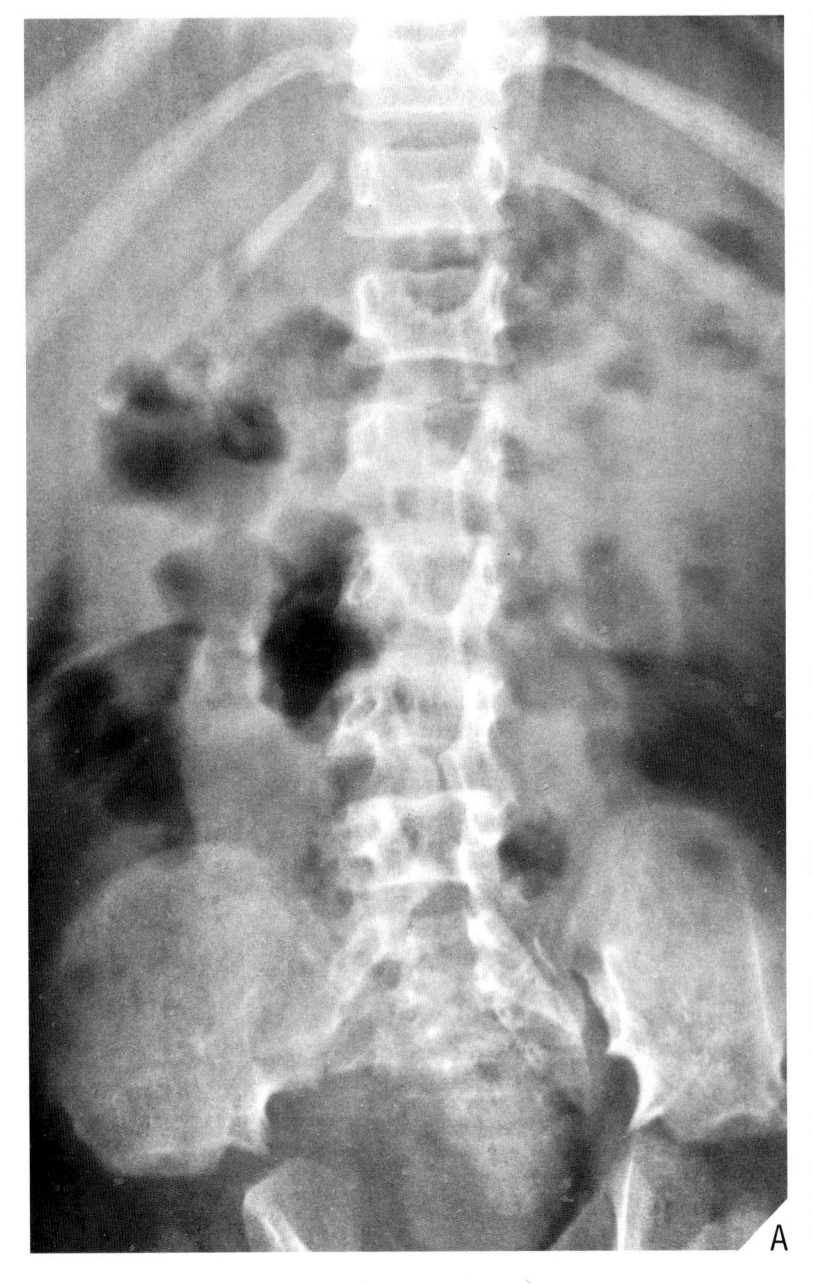

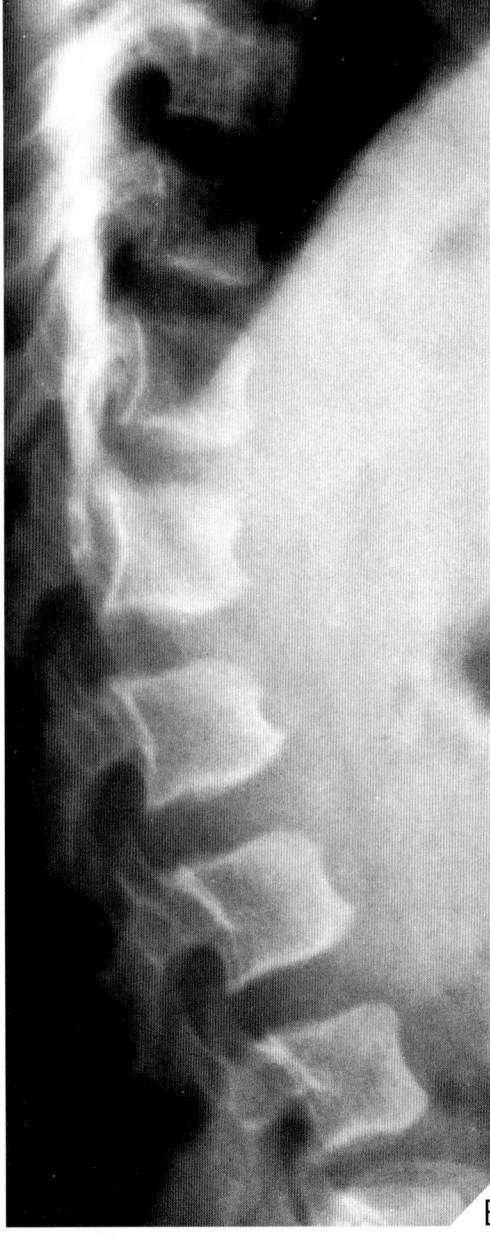

FIGURE 19.31
(A) Anteroposterior view of the thoracolumbar spine in a 2-year-old boy with achondroplasia shows progressive narrowing of the interpedicular distance of the lumbar vertebrae in a caudal direction. **(B)** Lateral view reveals the short pedicles and posterior vertebral scalloping.

In the pelvis, which is short and broad, the iliac bones are rounded, lacking the normal flaring; the acetabular roofs are horizontally oriented, and the sciatic notches are small. These features, taken together, give the hemi-pelvis the appearance of a table tennis paddle. The shape of the inner contour of the pelvis has also been likened to a champagne glass (Fig. 19.32).

The most serious complication of achondroplasia is related to the spinal stenosis secondary to the typically short pedicles and congenitally small foramen magnum. CT and MRI are procedures of choice for confirming this complication (Fig. 19.33). Patients with the disease also occasionally develop herniation of the nucleus pulposus.

It is important to note that two other conditions resemble achondroplasia but can be distinguished by the severity of their symptoms and by their radiographic presentation. *Hypochondroplasia* is a mild form of chondrodystrophy, in which the skeletal abnormalities are less severe than in achondroplasia. The skull is unaffected. *Thanatophoric dwarfism*,

FIGURE 19.32 Anteroposterior radiograph of the pelvis of the 13-year-old boy with achondroplasia shows the classic manifestations of this condition. The iliac bones are rounded, lacking their normal flaring, and the acetabular roofs are horizontal—features rendering the appearance of a table tennis paddle. Note also the "champagne glass" inner contour of the pelvic cavity and decrease in the interpedicular distances in the lower lumbar vertebrae.

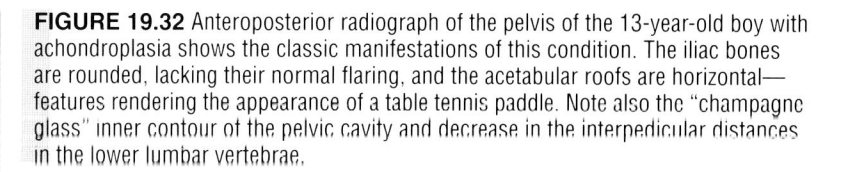

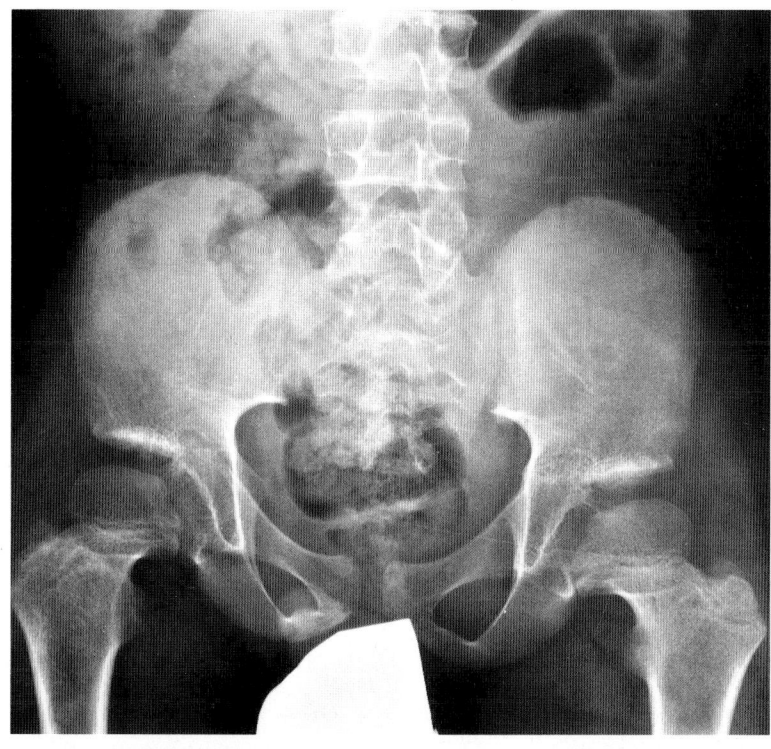

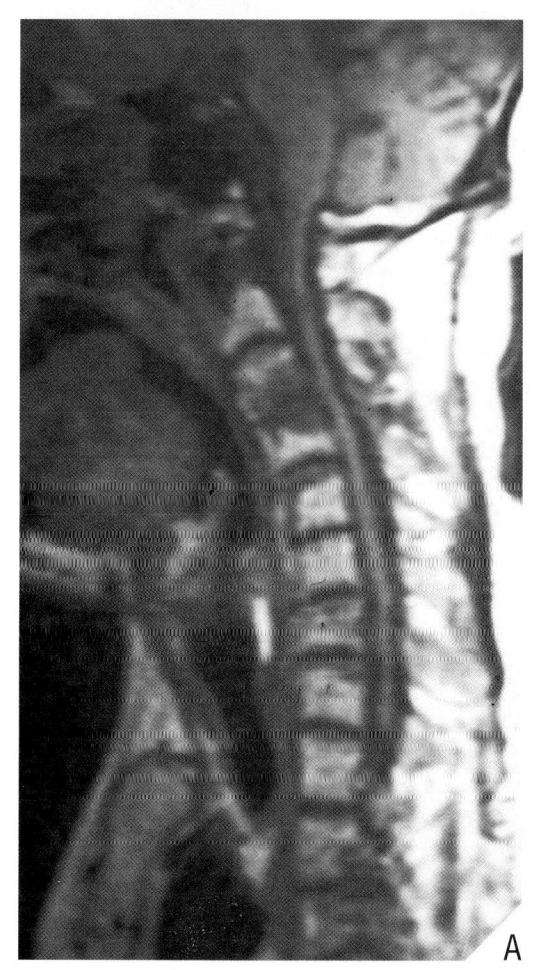

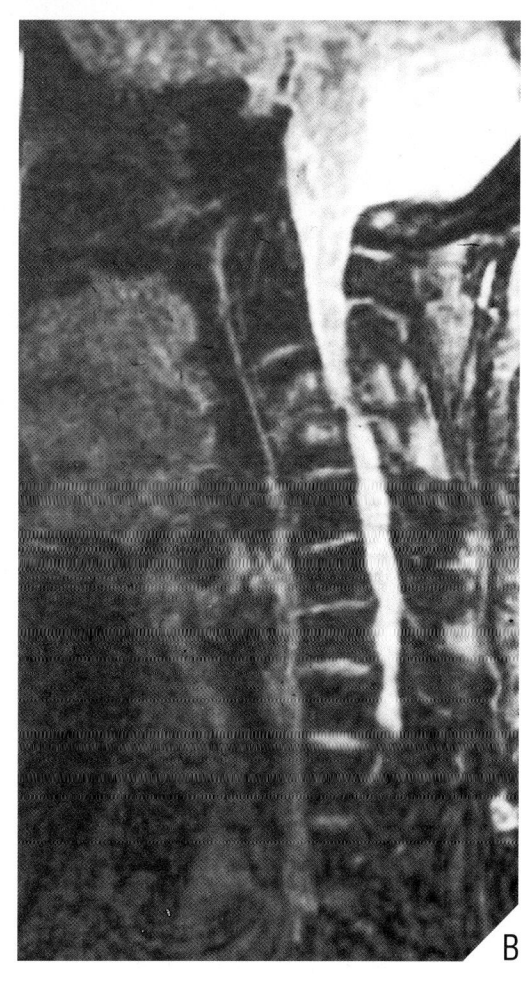

FIGURE 19.33 T1-weighted spin-echo **(A)** and T2*-weighted gradient-echo **(B)** sagittal MR images of the cervical spine in a patient with achondroplasia demonstrate crowding of the craniocervical junction by a congenitally small foramen magnum. The thecal sac is narrowed, particularly at the C3–C4 level. There is a reversal of the normal lordotic curve. (Reproduced with permission from Beltran J: *MRI: Musculoskeletal System*. New York, Gower, 1990).

on the other hand, is believed to represent a severe form of achondroplasia. It is lethal either in utero or within hours to days after birth.

Mucopolysaccharidoses

The mucopolysaccharidoses constitute a group of hereditary disorders having in common an excessive accumulation of mucopolysaccharides secondary to deficiencies in specific enzymes. Although several distinctive types of mucopolysaccharidosis have been delineated (Fig. 19.34), each with distinctive clinical and radiologic features, a specific diagnosis of any of these conditions is made on the basis of the patient's age at onset, the level of neurologic stunting, the degree of corneal clouding, and other clinical features. With the exception of Morquio–Brailsford disease, all of the mucopolysaccharidoses are marked by excessive urinary excretion of dermatan and heparan sulfate.

The mucopolysaccharidoses exhibit common radiographic findings. These include osteoporosis, oval or hook-shaped vertebral bodies, and an abnormal configuration of the pelvis, with overconstruction of the iliac bodies and wide flaring of the iliac wings (Fig. 19.35). The tubular bones are shortened, and dysplastic changes are evident in the proximal femoral epiphyses. The mucopolysaccharidoses, however, do exhibit variations in these radiographic abnormalities; Hurler syndrome, for example, shows a

FIGURE 19.34 CLASSIFICATION OF THE MUCOPOLYSACCHARIDOSES (MPS)

DESIGNATED NUMBER	EPONYM	GENETIC AND CLINICAL CHARACTERISTICS
MPS I-H	Hurler syndrome (gargoylism)	Autosomal-recessive Corneal clouding, mental retardation, hepatosplenomegaly, cardiomegaly Urinary excretion of dermatan and heparan sulfates Deficiency of α-L-iduronidase enzyme
MPS I-S	Scheie syndrome	Autosomal-recessive Corneal clouding, normal mental development, near-normal skeleton, aortic valve disease
MPS I-H/S	Hurler–Scheie compound	Urinary excretion of same product as in MPS I-H, and same enzyme deficiency
MPS II	Hunter syndrome (mild and severe variants)	Sex-chromosome-linked recessive disorder (males only) Mild mental retardation, absence of corneal clouding Urinary excretion of same product as in MPS I-H Deficiency of iduronate sulfatase
MPS III	Sanfilippo syndrome (A, B, and C variants)	Autosomal-recessive Progressive mental retardation, motor overactivity, coarse facial features Urinary excretion of heparan sulfate Deficiency of heparan-N-sulfatase
MPS IV	Morquio–Brailsford disease (type A, classic; type B, milder abnormalities)	Autosomal-recessive Short-trunk dwarfism; characteristic posture with knock knees, lumbar lordosis, and severe pectus carinatum; corneal opacities; impaired hearing, hepatosplenomegaly Urinary excretion of keratan sulfate Deficiency of galactosamine-6-sulfate sulfatase
MPS V	Redesignated MPS I-S	
MPS VI	Maroteaux–Lamy syndrome	Autosomal-recessive Normal intelligence, short stature, lumbar kyphosis, hepatosplenomegaly, joint contractures Urinary excretion of dermatan sulfate Deficiency of arylsulfatase B
MPS VII	Sly syndrome	Autosomal-recessive Growth and mental retardation; hepatosplenomegaly, pulmonary infections Urinary excretion of heparan and dermatan sulfates Deficiency of β-glucuronidase
MPS VIII	DiFerrante syndrome	Probably genetic trait Short stature Urinary excretion of keratan and heparan sulfates Deficiency of glucosamine-6-sulfate sulfatase

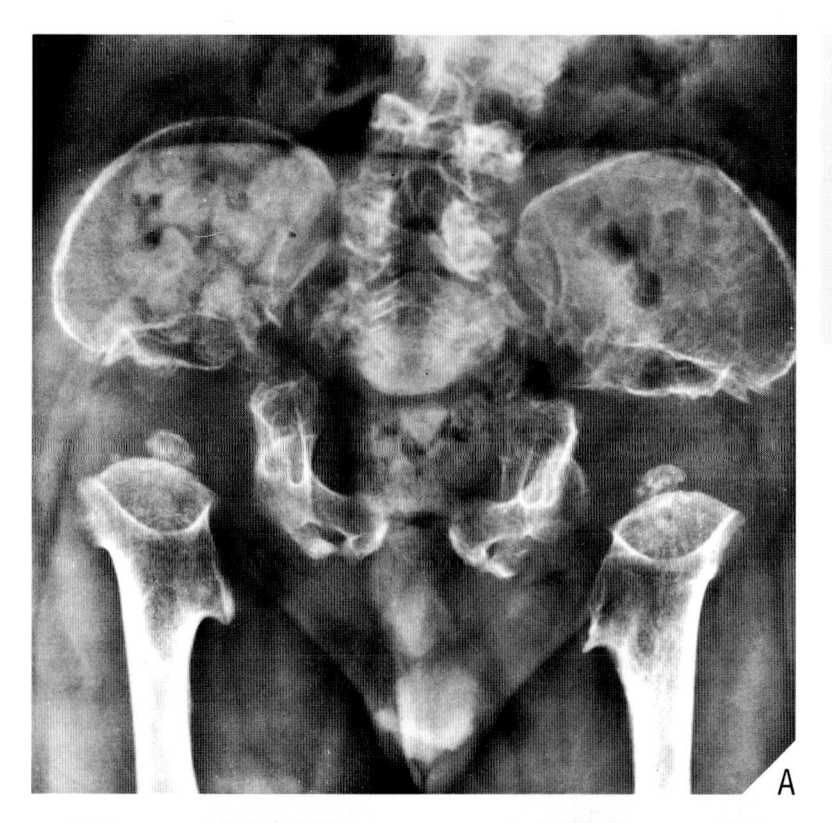

FIGURE 19.35 The classic features of Morquio–Brailsford disease are exhibited in these radiographic studies of a 3-year-old boy. **(A)** Anteroposterior view of the pelvis and hips shows flaring of the iliac wings and constriction of the iliac bodies. The narrowing of the pelvis at the level of the acetabulae, which are distorted, produces a characteristic "wine-glass" appearance. **(B)** Anteroposterior view of the spine shows marked kyphoscoliosis. The vertebrae are grossly deformed and flat (platyspondyly), and the ribs are wide but with narrow vertebral ends, giving them a characteristic "canoe-paddle" appearance. Note the pronounced osteoporosis. **(C)** Lateral radiograph of the spine shows hyperlordosis in the lumbar segment and kyphosis at the thoracolumbar junction. Note the shape of the vertebral bodies, with the characteristic irregular outline of the endplates and central, tongue-like or beak-like projections in the lumbar vertebral bodies.

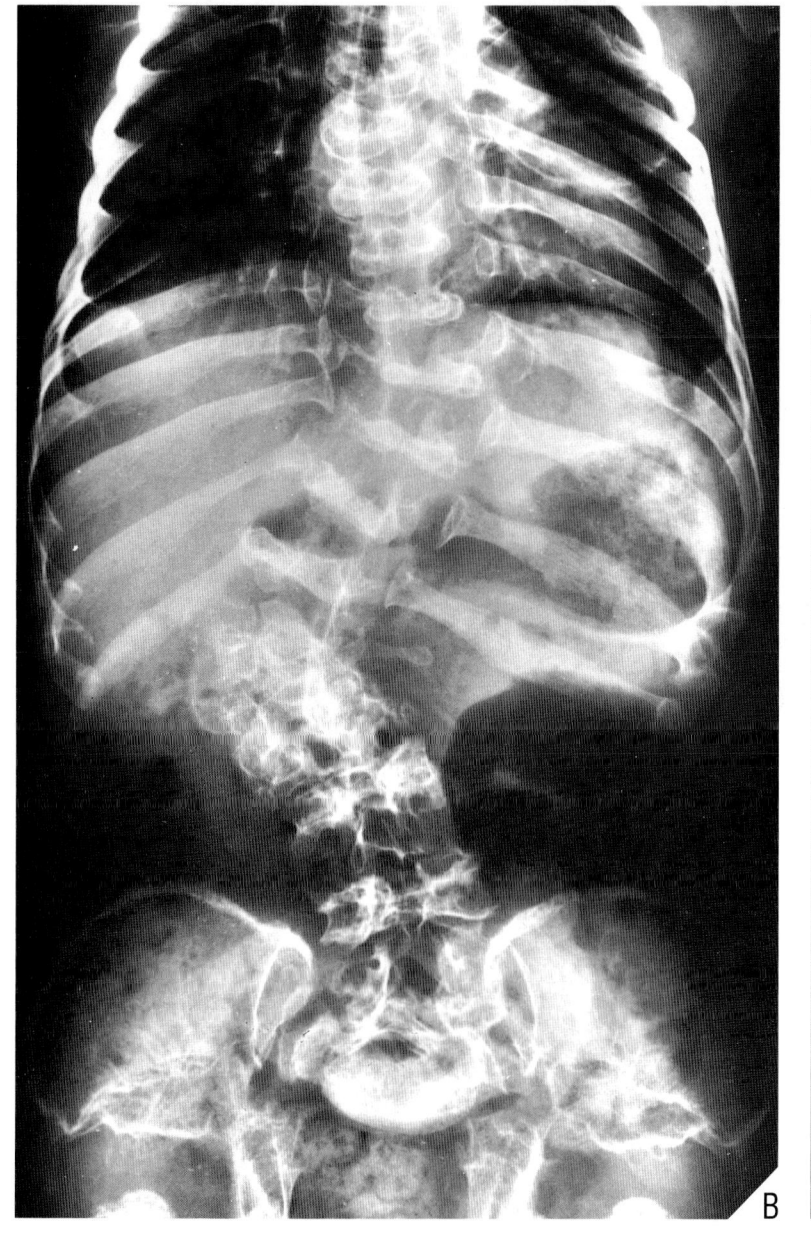

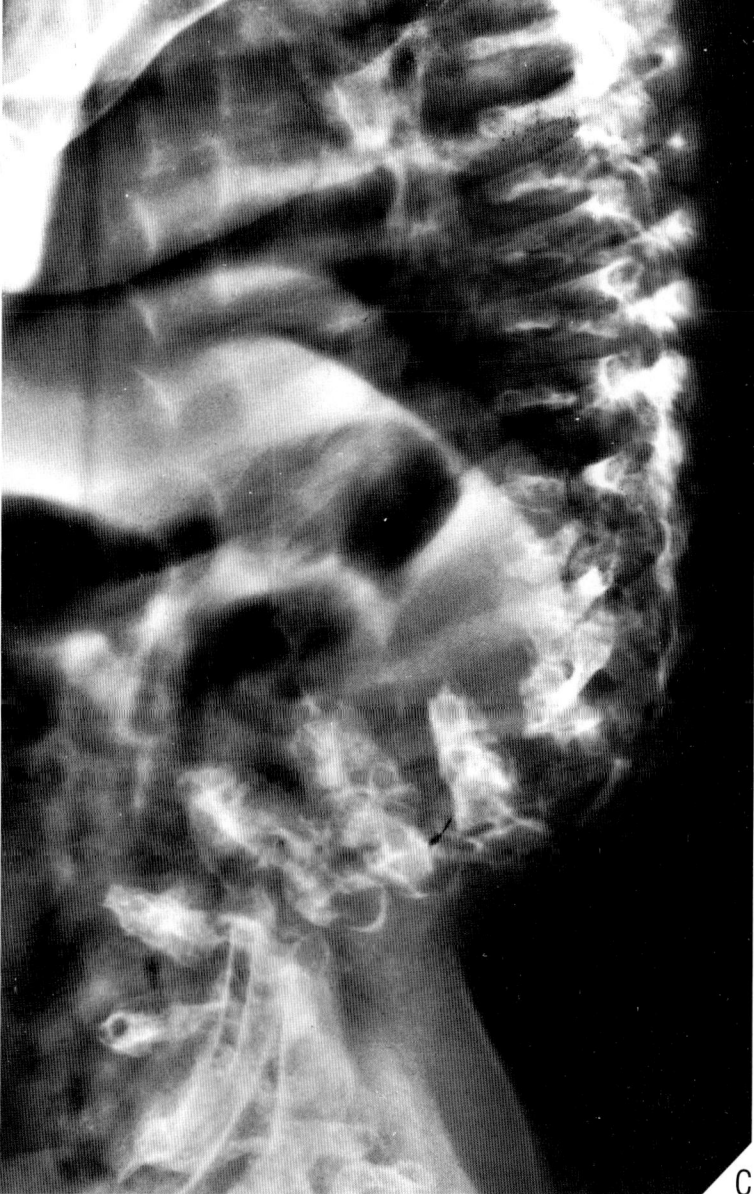

characteristic rounding of the vertebral endplates on the lateral projection; the vertebral bodies appear oval, but often there is a dorsolumbar gibbous with a hypoplastic hook-shaped, recessed vertebral body.

Fibrodysplasia Ossificans Progressiva (Myositis Ossificans Progressiva)

Fibrodysplasia ossificans progressiva is a rare, systemic autosomal-dominant disorder with a primary histopathologic abnormality of the connective tissues. Most patients are affected early in life (from birth to 5 years), and there is no sex predominance. The earliest clinical symptom is the appearance of painful nodules and masses in the subcutaneous tissue, particularly around the head and neck, with associated stiffness and limitation of movement. Subsequently, excessive ossification of muscles, ligaments, and fascia occurs, with the predominant sites of involvement being the head and neck, the dorsal paraspinal muscles, the shoulder girdles, and the hips (Fig. 19.36). Involvement of intercostal musculature interferes with respiration.

Clinically, the condition progresses from the shoulder girdle to the upper arms, spine, and pelvis. The natural history is one of remissions and exacerbations, with an almost inevitable outcome of death secondary to respiratory failure caused by constriction of the chest wall. No effective treatment is known to date.

RADIOGRAPHIC EVALUATION

Abnormalities of the thumb and great toe are present at birth and precede the soft tissue ossification. The characteristic radiologic findings include agenesis, microdactyly (Fig. 19.37), or congenital hallux valgus, occasionally with fusion at the metacarpophalangeal or metatarsophalangeal joints. Short great toes and short thumbs may be associated with clinodactyly of the fifth finger and with brachydactyly. In the soft tissues,

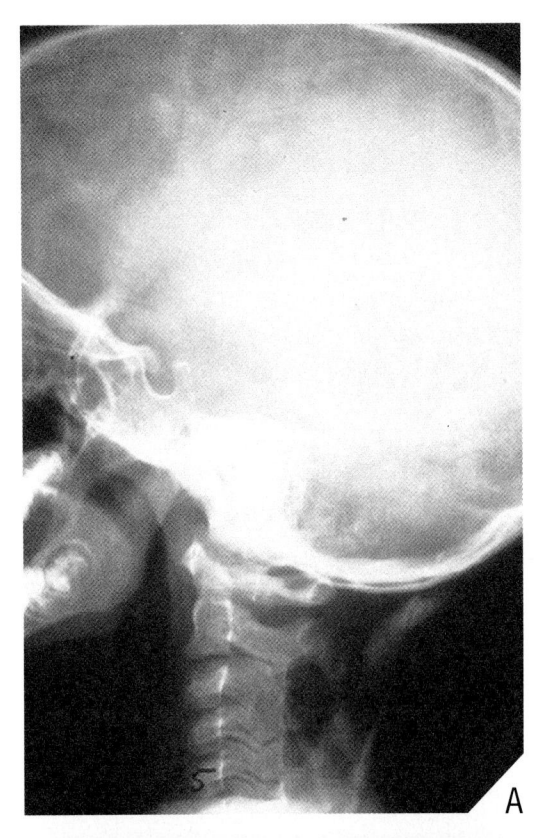

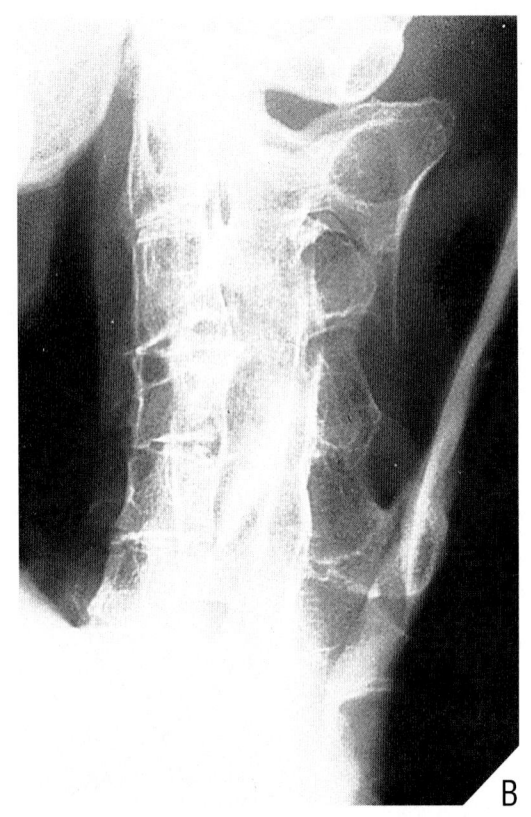

FIGURE 19.36 A 6-year-old girl presented with typical clinical and radiographic findings of fibrodysplasia ossificans progressiva. **(A)** A lateral radiograph of the skull and upper cervical spine shows mature ossifications extending caudally from the occiput along the spine. **(B)** A lateral film of the cervical spine demonstrates the ossifications in the posterior soft tissues of the neck and fusion of the lower vertebrae.

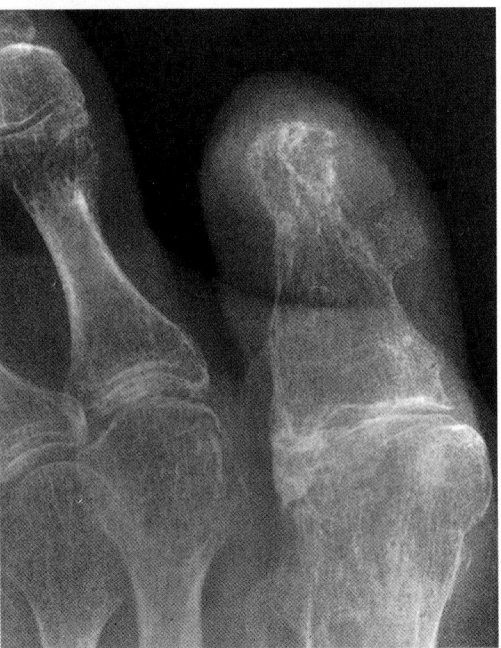

FIGURE 19.37 Microdactyly of the great toe is present in this 28-year-old man with fibrodysplasia ossificans progressiva, diagnosed at age three.

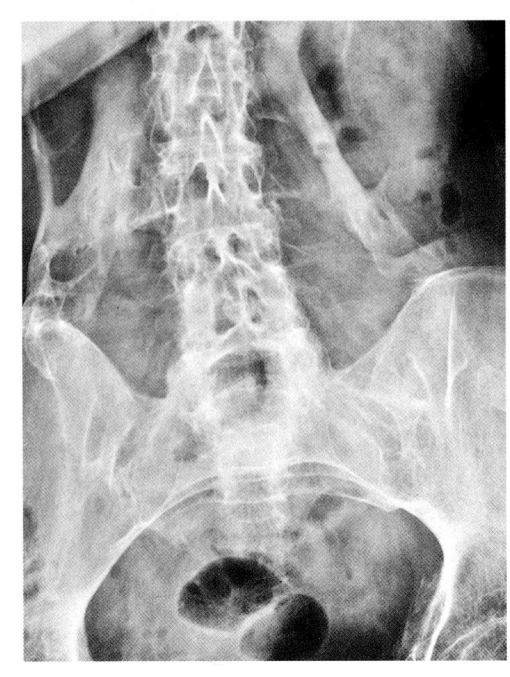

FIGURE 19.38 A 19-year-old woman with classic changes of fibrodysplasia ossificans progressiva. Note paraspinal ossifications, scoliosis, and fusion of sacroiliac joints.

extensive ossifications are seen, along with bridging bone masses in the cervical and thoracic spine, the thorax, and the extremities (Fig. 19.38). Involvement of the insertions of ligaments and tendons occasionally produces bony excrescences mimicking exostoses. Joint ankylosis most often results from ossification of the surrounding soft tissue, but a true intra-articular fusion may occur.

HISTOPATHOLOGY

The pathologic abnormalities are similar to those of myositis ossificans circumscripta, but the zoning phenomenon of centripetal ossification is absent. The earliest histologic changes are edema and inflammatory exudate, followed by mesenchymal proliferation and formation of a large mass of collagen. This collagen is capable of accepting the deposition of calcium salts. Eventually, the lesion is transformed into irregular masses of lamellar and woven bone.

Sclerosing Dysplasias of Bone

The sclerosing bone dysplasias are a group of developmental anomalies that reflect disturbances in the formation and modeling of bone, usually as a result of inborn errors in metabolism. A common defect in many of these disorders is characterized by the failure of cartilage and/or bone to resorb during the process of skeletal maturation and remodeling. One defect, in many cases, involves the resorption capabilities of osteoclasts in the presence of normal osteoblastic activity. In other instances the defect lies in excessive bone formation by osteoblasts, which may occur in the presence of normal or diminished osteoclastic activity. These basic errors in metabolism most commonly arise during the processes of endochondral and intramembranous ossification. All sclerosing dysplasias share the common feature of excessive bone accumulation, leading to the radiographic appearance of increased bone density. Norman and Greenspan have developed a classification of these disorders based on the site of failure, whether endochondral or intramembranous, in skeletal development and maturation. Recently, Greenspan (1991) expanded and modified this classification (Fig. 19.39). The approach reflected in this classification is focused on target sites of involvement and on the pathologic mechanisms of these dysplasias.

OSTEOPETROSIS

An inherited disorder, osteopetrosis (also called *Albers–Schönberg disease* or *marble-bone disease*) involves a failure in resorption and remodeling of bone formed by endochondral ossification. The result is an excessive accumulation of primary spongiosa (calcified cartilage matrix) in the medullary portion of flat bones and in long and short tubular bones, as well as in the vertebrae. Until recently, two variants have been described. The infantile "malignant" autosomal recessive form is recognized at birth or in early childhood, and if not treated by bone marrow transplantation is frequently fatal as the result of severe anemia secondary to overgrowth of the marrow cavity by substantial quantities of cartilage and immature bone. The "benign" autosomal-dominant adult form, which is marked by sclerosis of the skeleton, is compatible with a long lifespan. More recent reports describe what appear to be additional variants of this developmental anomaly, which illustrate the heterogeneity of inheritance of osteopetrosis: intermediate recessive type and autosomal recessive type with renal tubular acidosis. The radiographic hallmark of this disorder, as of all sclerosing bone dysplasias, is increased bone density. The radiographic examination also reveals a lack of differentiation between the cortex and the medullary cavity and, occasionally, a bone-in-bone appearance (Fig. 19.40). The long and short tubular bones exhibit a club-like deformity and splaying of their ends secondary to a failure in remodeling. The same failure in the spine results in a characteristic sandwich-like appearance of the vertebral bodies (Fig. 19.41). Osteopetrosis may occur in a cyclic pattern, with intervals of normal growth. This produces alternating bands of normal and abnormal bone in a ring-like pattern, which is particularly well demonstrated in the metaphyses of long bones and in flat bones, such as the pelvis and scapula.

Fractures are a frequent complication of osteopetrosis owing to the brittleness of the bones.

FIGURE 19.39 CLASSIFICATION OF SCLEROSING DYSPLASIAS OF BONE

I. DYSPLASIAS OF ENDOCHONDRAL BONE FORMATION
- Affecting primary spongiosa (immature bone)
  - Osteopetrosis (Albers–Schönberg disease)
    - Autosomal-recessive type (lethal)
    - Autosomal-dominant type
    - Intermediate-recessive type
    - Autosomal-recessive type with tubular acidosis (Sly disease)
  - Pycnodysostosis (Maroteaux–Lamy disease)
- Affecting secondary spongiosa (mature bone)
  - Enostosis (bone island)
  - Osteopoikilosis (spotted bone disease)
  - Osteopathia striata (Voorhoeve disease)

II. DYSPLASIAS OF INTRAMEMBRANOUS BONE FORMATION
- Progressive diaphyseal dysplasia (Camurati–Engelmann disease)
- Hereditary multiple diaphyseal sclerosis (Ribbing disease)
- Endosteal hyperostosis (hyperostosis corticalis generalisata)
  - Autosomal-recessive form
    - van Buchem disease
    - Sclerosteosis (Truswell–Hansen disease)
  - Autosomal-dominant form
    - Worth disease
    - Nakamura disease

III. MIXED SCLEROSING DYSPLASIAS (AFFECTING BOTH ENDOCHONDRAL AND INTRAMEMBRANOUS OSSIFICATION)
- Affecting predominantly endochondral ossification
  - Dysosteosclerosis
  - Metaphyseal dysplasia (Pyle disease)
  - Craniometaphyseal dysplasia
- Affecting predominantly intramembranous ossification
  - Melorheostosis
  - Progressive diaphyseal dysplasia with skull base involvement (Neuhauser variant)
  - Craniodiaphyseal dysplasia
- Coexistence of two or more sclerosing bone dysplasias (overlap syndrome)
  - Melorheostosis with osteopoikilosis and osteopathia striata
  - Osteopathia striata with cranial sclerosis (Horan–Beighton syndrome)
  - Osteopathia striata with osteopoikilosis and cranial sclerosis
  - Osteopathia striata with generalized cortical hyperostosis
  - Osteopathia striata with osteopetrosis
  - Osteopoikilosis with progressive diaphyseal dysplasia

PYCNODYSOSTOSIS

Pycnodysostosis (Maroteaux–Lamy disease) is an inherited autosomal recessive disorder whose skeletal manifestations are caused by a failure of resorption of primary spongiosa. Patients with this disease, such as the French artist Toulouse–Lautrec, have a disproportionately short stature, which becomes evident in early childhood. Unlike patients with osteopetrosis, however, those with pycnodysostosis are usually asymptomatic; often the condition is discovered incidentally to a pathologic fracture.

Radiographically, pycnodysostosis presents with the increased bone density common to all sclerosing bone dysplasias. Moreover, in the skull there is persistence of the anterior and posterior fontanels, wormian bones, and an obtuse angle to the ramus of the mandible. The features that distinguish this disease from osteopetrosis are hypoplasia of the distal phalanges of the fingers and toes and resorption of the terminal tufts of the distal phalanges. However, the latter feature, known as *acroosteolysis*, may also be seen in a variety of other conditions.

ENOSTOSIS, OSTEOPOIKILOSIS, AND OSTEOPATHIA STRIATA

When endochondral ossification proceeds normally but mature bone trabeculae coalesce and fail to resorb and remodel, the resulting developmental anomalies are referred to as *enostosis* (bone island), *osteopoikilosis*, or *osteopathia striata*. The exact mode of inheritance of each is not known, but the latter two are probably transmitted as autosomal-dominant traits. The most common and mildest of the three is enostosis (Fig. 19.42), which is asymptomatic; it is important, however, to differentiate this condition from an osteoid osteoma (see Chapter 9) or from osteoblastic bone metastasis (see Chapter 10). Osteopoikilosis (osteopathia condensans disseminata, or "spotted-bone" disease) is also an asymptomatic disorder, is

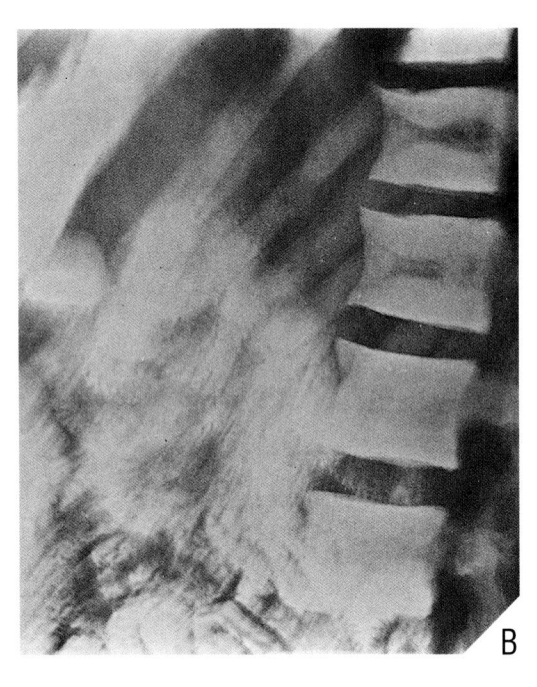

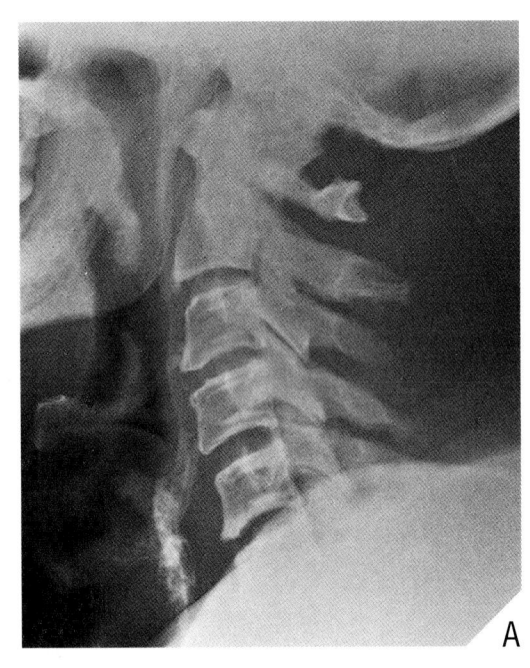

FIGURE 19.40 (A) "Bone-in-bone" appearance in osteopetrotic cervical spine. (Courtesy of Harold G. Jacobson, M.D., Bronx, NY). **(B)** In another patient, a different type of "bone-in-bone" appearance is seen in the thoracic vertebrae.

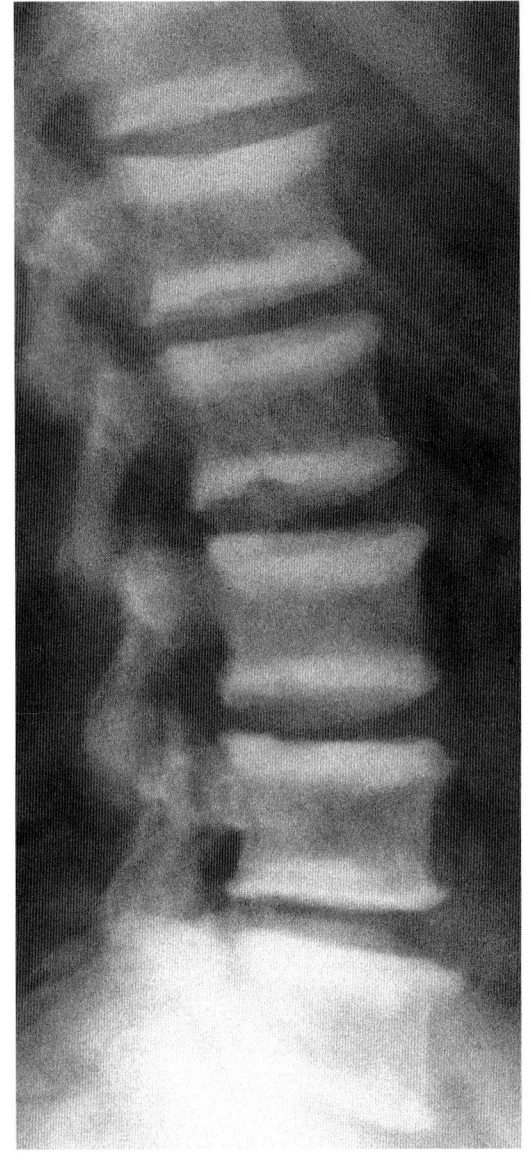

FIGURE 19.41 Lateral radiograph of the thoracolumbar spine in a 14-year-old boy with osteopetrosis demonstrates the characteristic "rugger-jersey" appearance seen in this disorder. Note the overall increase in bone density.

Imaging of the Spine in Clinical Practice

characterized by multiple bone islands symmetrically distributed and clustered near the articular ends of a bone. Although plain film radiography is usually sufficient to make a diagnosis, questionable cases may require radionuclide imaging, which is diagnostic. In osteopoikilosis, the bone scan is relatively normal, unlike the case with metastatic disease in which the bone scan invariably exhibits increased uptake of the radiopharmaceutical agent.

Histologically, both enostoses and the lesions of osteopoikilosis are characterized by foci of compact bone scattered in the spongiosa, with prominent cement lines and occasionally a Haversian system. Clinically, osteopoikilosis must be distinguished from more severe disorders such as mastocytosis and tuberous sclerosis, as well as from osteoblastic metastatic lesions.

Osteopathia striata, the least common disorder in this group, is an asymptomatic lesion marked by fine or coarse linear striations, chiefly in the long bones and at sites of rapid growth such as the knee and shoulder. Several authors postulate a relationship between this disorder and osteopoikilosis, some suggesting that it actually represents a variant of osteopoikilosis. Although bone island can occasionally be seen in the vertebral body, changes of osteopoikilosis and osteopathia striata have not been reported in the spine.

Progressive Diaphyseal Dysplasia

Failure of bone resorption and remodeling at the sites of intramembranous ossification (eg, as the cortex of tubular bones, the vault of the skull, the mandible, the midsegment of the clavicle) is the abnormality typically noted in progressive diaphyseal dysplasia, also called Camurati–Engelmann disease. Like osteopoikilosis and osteopathia striata, this is an autosomal dominant disorder with considerable variability of expression. Clinically, it is characterized by growth retardation, muscle wasting, pain and weakness in the extremities, and a waddling gait.

Because of its striking tendency towards symmetric involvement of the extremities, with characteristic sparing of the epiphysis and metaphysis (the sites of endochondral ossification), progressive diaphyseal dysplasia is recognized radiographically by symmetric fusiform thickening of the cortices of the long bone shafts, particularly in the lower extremities. Involvement of the spine has not been reported.

Melorheostosis

A rare condition of unknown etiology, melorheostosis (Leri disease) shows no evidence of hereditary features. It belongs to a group of bone disorders called the *mixed sclerosing dysplasias,* which combine characteristics of both endochondral and intramembranous failure of ossification. The presenting symptom is pain intensified by activity. Limitation of joint motion and stiffness are common, and are caused by contractures, soft tissue fibrosis, and periarticular bone formation in the soft tissues. The condition can be monostotic *forme fruste* or polyostotic, affecting an entire limb.

Standard radiography is sufficient to make a diagnosis. The lesion is characterized by a wavy hyperostosis that resembles melted wax dripping down the side of a candle, the feature from which the disease derives its name (Greek *melos* = member, *rhein* = flow); moreover, only one side of the bone is usually involved. Associated joint abnormalities are also well delineated on standard radiographs. Radionuclide bone scan can determine other sites of skeletal involvement by demonstrating abnormal uptake of radiopharmaceutical.

Other Mixed Sclerosing Dysplasias

The most common of the other mixed sclerosing dysplasias is the coexistence of melorheostosis, osteopathia striata, and osteopoikilosis. The radiographic features of this "overlap syndrome" are a combination of each of these three dysplasias, a phenomenon suggesting a common pathogenetic mechanism.

The discussion of other sclerosing dysplasias is beyond the scope of this text.

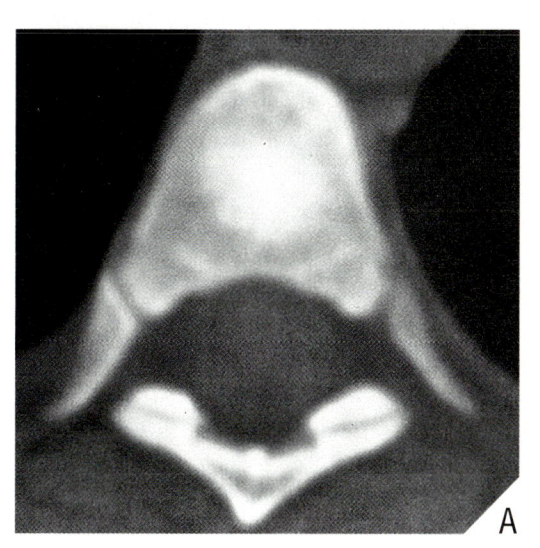

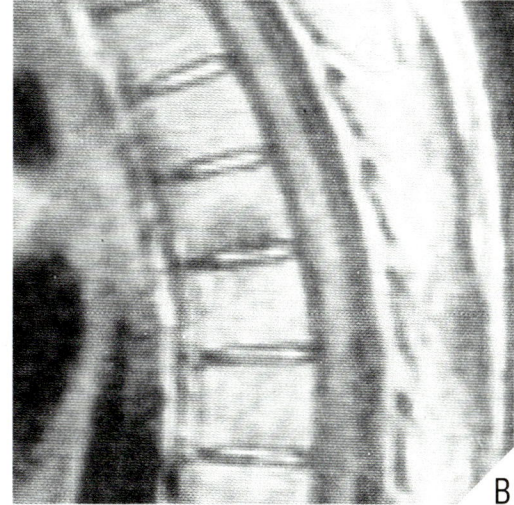

FIGURE 19.42 (A) Axial CT section of the thoracic vertebra shows a giant bone island located in the cancellous portion of the vertebral body. **(B)** Sagittal T1-weighted MRI demonstrates the bone island to display a low signal intensity. Note ragged borders of the lesion, typical of enostosis. (Courtesy of L.L. Seeger, M.D., and J. Eckardt, M.D., Los Angeles, CA)

Suggested Reading

Ablin DS, Greenspan A, Reinhart M, et al: Differentiation of child abuse from osteogenesis imperfecta. *AJR* 154:1035, 1990.

Abrahamson MN: Disseminated asymptomatic osteosclerosis with features resembling melorheostosis, osteopoikilosis and osteopathia striata. *J Bone Joint Surg* 50A:991, 1968.

Andersen PE Jr, Bollerslev J: Heterogeneity of autosomal dominant osteopetrosis. *Radiology* 164:223, 1987.

Bailey JA II: Orthopedic aspects of achondroplasia. *J Bone Joint Surg* 52A:1285, 1970.

Bauze RJ, Smith R, Francis JO: A new look at osteogenesis imperfecta. *J Bone Joint Surg* 57B:2, 1975.

Beighton P: *Inherited Disorders of the Skeleton*. Edinburgh, Churchill-Livingstone, 1978.

Beighton P, Cremin BJ: *Sclerosing Bone Dysplasias*. New York, Springer-Verlag, 1984.

Beighton P, Cremin BJ, Hamersma H: The radiology of sclerosteosis. *Br J Radiol* 49:934, 1976.

Bradford DS, Lonstein JE, Moe JH, et al: *Moe's Textbook of Scoliosis and Other Spinal Deformities*, 2nd ed. Philadelphia, W B Saunders, 1987.

Cobb JR: Outline for the study of scoliosis. Instructional Course Lectures. *Am Acad Orthop Surg* 5:261, 1948.

Connor J, Evans DA: Genetic aspects of fibrodysplasia ossificans progressiva. *J Med Genet* 19:35, 1982.

Connor J, Evans DA: Fibrodysplasia ossificans progressiva. *J Bone Joint Surg* 64B:76, 1982.

Cremin B, Connor J, Beighton P: The radiological spectrum of fibrodysplasia ossificans progressiva. *Clin Radiol* 33:499, 1982.

D'Agostino A, Soule E, Miller R: Sarcomas of the peripheral nerves and somatic tissue associated with multiple neurofibromatosis (von Recklinghausen's disease). *Cancer* 16:1015, 1963.

Eggli KD: The mucopolysaccharidoses. In Taveras JM, Ferrucci JT (eds): *Radiology—Diagnosis, Imaging, Intervention*. Philadelphia, J B Lippincott, 1986.

Elmore SM: Pycnodysostosis. A review. *J Bone Joint Surg* 49A:153, 1967.

Fairbank HAT: *An Atlas of General Affections of the Skeleton*. Edinburgh, Livingstone, 1951.

Falvo KA, Root L, Bullough PG: Osteogenesis imperfecta: Clinical evaluation and management. *J Bone Joint Surg* 56A:783, 1974.

Felson B: Dwarfs and other little people. *Semin Roentgenol* 8:133, 1973.

Gehweiler JA, Bland WR, Carden TS Jr, et al: Osteopathia striata—Voorhoeve's disease: Review of the roentgen manifestations. *Am J Roentgenol* 118:450, 1973.

George K, Rippstein JA: A comparative study of the two popular methods of measuring scoliotic deformity of the spine. *J Bone Joint Surg* 43A:809, 1961.

Gertner JM, Root L: Osteogenesis imperfecta. *Orthop Clin North Am* 21:151, 1990.

Goldstein LA, Waugh TR: Classification and terminology of scoliosis. *Clin Orthop* 93:10, 1973.

Greenspan A: Sclerosing bone dysplasias—A target sites approach. *Skel Radiol* 20:561, 1991.

Greenspan A, Pugh JW, Norman A, et al: Scoliotic index: A comparative evaluation of methods for the measurement of scoliosis. *Bull Hosp Joint Dis Orthop Inst* 39:117, 1978.

Greenspan A, Steiner G, Knutzon R: Bone island (enostosis): Clinical significance and radiologic and pathologic correlations. *Skel Radiol* 20:85, 1990.

Harrington PR, Dickson JM: An eleven-year clinical investigation of Harrington instrumentation: A preliminary report on 578 cases. *Clin Orthop* 93:113, 1973.

Hoppenfeld S: *Scoliosis: A Manual of Concept and Treatment*. Philadelphia, J B Lippincott, 1967.

Hundley JD, Wilson FC: Progressive diaphyseal dysplasia. Review of the literature and report of seven cases in one family. *J Bone Joint Surg* 55A:462, 1973.

Jacobson HG: Dense bone—too much bone: Radiological considerations and differential diagnosis. Part I. *Skel Radiol* 13:1, 1985.

Kaftori JI, Kleinhaus U, Naveh Y: Progressive diaphyseal dysplasia (Camurati–Engelmann): Radiographic follow-up and CT findings. *Radiology* 164:777, 1987.

Klatte EC, Franken EA, Smith JA: The radiographic spectrum in neurofibromatosis. *Semin Roentgenol* 11:17, 1976.

Kleinman PK: Differentiation of child abuse and osteogenesis imperfecta: Medical and legal implications. *Am J Roentgenol* 154:1047, 1990.

Lagier R, Mbakop A, Bigler A: Osteopoikilosis: A radiological and pathological study. *Skel Radiol* 11:161, 1984.

Langer LO Jr, Baumann PA, Gorlin RJ: Achondroplasia. *AJR* 100:12, 1967.

Lonstein JE: Patient evaluation. In Bradford DS, Lonstein JE, Moe JH, et al: *Moe's Textbook of Scoliosis and Other Spinal Deformities*, 2nd ed. Philadelphia, W B Saunders, 1987.

MacEwen GD, Conway JJ, Miller WT: Congenital scoliosis with a unilateral bar. *Radiology* 90:711, 1968.

McKusick V: *Hereditary Disorders of Connective Tissue*, 4th ed. St. Louis, C V Mosby, 1972.

Nash C, Moe J: A study of vertebral rotation. *J Bone Joint Surg* 51A:223, 1969.

Norman A: Myositis ossificans and fibrodysplasia ossificans progressiva. In Taveras JM, Ferrucci JT (eds): *Radiology—Diagnosis, Imaging, Intervention*, vol. 5. Philadelphia, J B Lippincott, 1986.

Norman A, Greenspan A: Bone dysplasias. In Jahss MH (ed): *Disorders of the Foot*, vol. 1. Philadelphia, W B Saunders, 1982.

Norman A, Greenspan A: Sclerosing dysplasias of bone: In Taveras JM, Ferrucci JT (eds): *Radiology—Diagnosis, Imaging, Intervention*, vol 5. Philadelphia, J B Lippincott, 1986.

Norman A, Greenspan A: Bone dysplasias. In Jahss MH (ed): *Disorders of the Foot and Ankle. Medical and Surgical Management*, vol I. Philadelphia, W B Saunders, 1991.

Ozonoff M: *Pediatric Orthopaedic Radiology*. Philadelphia, W B Saunders, 1979.

Paul LW: Hereditary, multiple, diaphyseal sclerosis (Ribbing). *Radiology* 60:412, 1953.

Resnick D, Nemcek AA Jr, Haghighi P: Spinal enostoses (bone islands). *Radiology* 147:373, 1983.

Ribbing S: Hereditary, multiple, diaphyseal sclerosis. *Acta Radiol* 31:522, 1949.

Riccardi VM: von Recklinghausen's neurofibromatosis. *N Engl J Med* 305:1617, 1981.

Risser JC: The iliac apophysis: An invaluable sign in the management of scoliosis. *Clin Orthop* 11:111, 1958.

Rubin P: *Dynamic Classification of Bone Dysplasias*. Chicago, Year Book Medical Publishers, 1964.

Schwartz A, Ramos R: Neurofibromatosis and multiple nonossifying fibromas. *AJR* 135:617, 1980.

Sillence DO: Osteogenesis imperfecta: An expanding panorama of variants. *Clin Orthop* 159:11, 1981.

Sillence DO, Senn A, Danks DM: Genetic heterogeneity in osteogenesis imperfecta. *J Med Genet* 16:101, 1979.

Silverman BJ, Greenbarg PE: Internal fixation of the spine for idiopathic scoliosis using square-ended distraction rods and lamina wiring (Harrington–Luque technique). *Bull Hosp Joint Dis Orthop Inst* 44:41, 1984.

Spranger JW, Langer LO Jr, Wiederman HR: *Bone Dysplasias. An Atlas of Constitutional Disorders of Skeletal Development*. Philadelphia, W B Saunders, 1974.

Stevenson R, Howell R, McKusick V, et al: The iduronidase deficient mucopolysaccharidoses: Clinical and roentgenographic features. *Pediatrics* 57:111, 1976.

Taitz LS: Child abuse and osteogenesis imperfecta. *Br Med J* 295:1082, 1987.

Walker GF: Mixed sclerosing bone dystrophies. *J Bone Joint Surg* 46B:546, 1964.

Whyte MP, Murphy WA, Fallon MD, et al: Mixed-sclerosing-bone-dystrophy: Report of a case and review of the literature. *Skel Radiol* 6:95, 1978.

Whyte MP, Murphy WA, Siegel BA: ^{99m}Tc-pyrophosphate bone imaging in osteopoikilosis, osteopathic striata and melorheostosis. *Radiology* 127:439, 1978.

Winter RB, Moe JH, Eilers VE: Congenital scoliosis. A study of 234 patients treated and untreated. *J Bone Joint Surg* 50A:1, 1968.

Wynne-Davies R, Fairbank TJ: *Fairbank's Atlas of General Affections of the Skeleton*, 2nd ed. New York, Churchill-Livingstone, 1976.

Yaghmai I: Spine changes in neurofibromatosis. *Radiology* 6:261, 1986.

INDEX (NUMBERS IN BOLD TYPE INDICATE FIGURES.)

Achondroplasia, 19.22–19.24
    pelvic contour in, 19.23, **19.32**
    scalloping of vertebrae in, 19.22, **19.31**
    spinal stenosis in, 19.23, **19.33**
Acromegaly, 17.2–17.4
    arthritis in, **4.1**, 4.2
    scalloping of vertebrae in, 17.3, **17.3**
Age
    skeletal, determination of, 19.8, 19.10, 19.11, **19.15–19.17**
    and tumor incidence, 8.8, **8.9**
AIDS, arthritis in, 7.5
Albers–Schönberg disease. *See* Osteopetrosis
Alkaptonuria, **7.1**, 7.2
Anatomy
    of cervical spine, **2.1–2.2**, 2.2–2.3
        ligaments in, 2.17, **2.21**
    of thoracolumbar spine, 3.2–3.10
Aneurysmal bone cyst, 9.8–9.9
    myelography in, 8.5, **8.6**, 9.8, **9.12**
    plain films of, 8.11, **8.15**, 9.8, **9.10–9.11**
    thecal sac compression in, 8.5, **8.6**, 9.8, **9.12**
    treatment of, 9.9
Angiography, 1.3–1.4, 8.4, **8.5**
    radionuclide, 1.7–1.8
    in tumors, 8.2, 8.4, **8.5**
Ankylosing spondylitis, **4.1**, 4.2, 6.3–6.8
Arthritides and arthropathies, 4.2–4.11
    classification of, **4.1**, 4.2
    clinical findings in, 4.3
    computed tomography in, **4.2–4.4**, 4.3–4.4
    distribution of lesions in, 4.10–4.11, **4.14**
    magnetic resonance imaging in, 4.4–4.5, **4.5–4.6**
    morphology of lesions in, 4.6–4.9, **4.7–4.13**
    plain films in, 4.3
    scintigraphy in, 4.4
Arthritis
    in AIDS, 7.5
    enteropathic, **4.1**, 4.2, 6.10, **6.14**
    gouty. *See* Gout
    infectious, **4.1**, 4.2, 7.5, 12.2
    inflammatory, **4.1**, 4.2, 6.2–6.11
    in metabolic and endocrine disorders, **4.1**, 4.2
    mutilans, 6.9
    psoriatic, **4.1**, 4.2. *See also* Psoriatic arthritis
    rheumatoid, **4.1**, 4.2. *See also* Rheumatoid arthritis
Arthropathy, connective tissue, **4.1**, 4.2
Articular pillars, 2.2
Atlantal-dens interval, 2.2
Atlas, 2.2
Axis, 2.2

Back pain, differential diagnosis of, 11.2
Bamboo spine, in ankylosing spondylitis, 4.6, **4.7**, 4.8, 4.9, **4.12**, 6.4, 6.5, **6.5**
Bekhterev disease. *See* Spondylitis, ankylosing
Biopsy, aspiration
    CT-guided, 1.3, 1.4, **1.5**
    in infections, 12.6
    in metastatic lesions, 10.13, **10.17**
Block vertebrae, scoliosis in, 19.5, **19.6**
Blood pool scans, 1.8
Bone
    composition and production of, **14.1**, 14.2
    cortical thickness measurements, 14.2, 14.3, **14.3–14.4**
    cyst of, aneurysmal. *See* Aneurysmal bone cyst
    density abnormalities in metabolic and endocrine disorders, **14.2**, 14.3

destruction in tumors, 8.11, 8.12, **8.15–8.17**
sclerosing dysplasias of, 19.27–19.29, **19.39–19.42**
tumor bone appearance, 8.10, 8.11, **8.13**
Bridging of vertebrae, in Reiter syndrome, 6.9, **6.12**
Brown tumor of hyperparathyroidism, 9.12–9.13
Burst fracture
    cervical, 2.29, **2.36**
        treatment of, 2.29
    thoracolumbar, 3.13–3.16, **3.17–3.19**
        treatment of, 3.13–3.19, **3.19–3.23**

Calcifying enchondroma, 9.6
Calcium metabolism, 15.5
Calcium pyrophosphate dihydrate crystals, 4.3, 7.4
Cartilage in tumors, 8.11, **8.14**
    in osteochondroma, 9.5
Cellulitis, 12.2
Cervical spine, 2.2–2.37
    anatomy of, **2.1–2.2**, 2.2–2.3
    anteroposterior view of, 2.6–2.8, **2.8**, 2.16, **2.18**
    burst fracture, 2.29, **2.36**
        treatment of, 2.29
    clay-shoveler's fracture, 2.33, **2.43**
    computed tomography of, 2.12, 2.13, **2.14**, 2.16, **2.19**
    diskography of, 2.16, **2.19**
    dislocation of C1-C2, 2.22, **2.26**
    Fuchs view of, 2.7, 2.9, **2.10**, 2.16, **2.18**
    hangman's fracture, 2.26–2.29, **2.33–2.35**
        treatment of, 2.26, 2.29
    injuries of
        in C1 and C2 vertebrae, 2.20–2.29, **2.24–2.35**
        classification of, 2.15–2.17, **2.20**
        in mid and lower region, 2.29–2.36, **2.36–2.48**
    Jefferson fracture, 2.20–2.22, **2.24–2.25**
    lateral view of, **2.2–2.3**, 2.3–2.6, 2.16, **2.18**
    ligaments of, 2.17, **2.21**
    locked facets
        bilateral, 2.34, 2.35–2.36, **2.45–2.48**
        unilateral, 2.36
    magnetic resonance imaging of, 2.13, 2.15, **2.15**, 2.16, **2.17**, **2.19**
    measurement of odontoid process migration, **2.4–2.7**, 2.6–2.7
        Chamberlain's line in, **2.4**, 2.6
        McGregor's line in, **2.6**, 2.7
        McRae's line in, **2.5**, 2.6
        Ranawat's method in, 2.7, **2.7**
    myelography of, 2.14, 2.15, **2.16**, 2.16, **2.19**
    oblique view of, 2.7, 2.10–2.11, **2.11**, 2.16, **2.18**
    occipital condyle fractures, 2.17–2.19, **2.22**
    occipito-cervical dislocations, 2.19–2.20, **2.23**
    odontoid process fractures, 2.22–2.25, **2.27–2.29**
        treatment of, 2.25–2.26, 2.27, **2.30–2.32**
    open-mouth view of, 2.7, 2.9, **2.9**, 2.16, **2.18**
    osteoarthritis, 3.3–3.4, **5.3–5.4**
    perched facets, bilateral, 2.36
    pillar view of, 2.11, **2.12**, 2.16, **2.18**
    plain films of, 2.6–2.12, **2.8–2.13**, 2.16, **2.18**
    rudimentary odontoid process, 18.3, **18.4**
    scintigraphy of, 2.16, **2.19**
    swimmer's view of, 2.11, 2.12, **2.13**, 2.16, **2.18**
    teardrop fracture, 2.29–2.32, **2.37–2.39**
        treatment of, 2.30–2.32, **2.40–2.42**
    tomography of, 2.16, **2.19**
    wedge fracture, 2.33–2.35, **2.44**
Chamberlain's line for measurement of odontoid process migration, **2.4**, 2.6, 6.3

Chance fractures, lumbar, 3.19–3.21, **3.24–3.26**
    treatment of, 3.21–3.23, **3.27–3.28**
Chondroblastoma, 9.7
Chondrocalcinosis, 4.3, 7.4
Chondroma, 9.6
Chondromyxoid fibroma, 9.7
Chondrosarcoma, 8.11, **8.14**
    dedifferentiated, 10.6
    development from osteochondroma, 9.5, 10.4, **10.5**
    differential diagnosis and treatment of, 10.6
    periosteal, 10.5, **10.6**
Chordoma
    complications and treatment of, 10.11
    physaliphorous cells in, 10.11
    radiographic appearance of, 8.12, **8.17**, 10.11, 10.12, **10.14–10.15**
Clay-shoveler's fracture, 2.33, **2.43**
Clivus-odontoid line, **2.3**, 2.5, 2.20
Cobb spinous-process method for rotation determination, 19.8, 19.9, **19.13**
Coccidioidomycosis, 13.7–13.8, **13.13**
Codman tumor, 9.7
Colitis, ulcerative, arthropathy in, 6.10, **6.14**
Compression fractures
    cervical, 2.33–2.35, **2.44**
    in Gaucher's disease, 17.4, **17.5**
    in osteoporosis, 15.3, 15.4, **15.4**
    in Paget disease, 16.3, **16.3**
    thoracolumbar, 3.10, 3.13, **3.16**
        treatment of, 3.13
Computed tomography, 1.2–1.3, **1.3**, 19.6, **19.7**
    in arthritides, **4.2–4.4**, 4.3–4.4
    aspiration biopsy with, 1.3, **1.5**
    in bone mineral analysis, 14.4–14.5, **14.6**
    of cervical spine, 2.12, 2.13, **2.14**, 2.16, **2.19**
    in giant-cell tumor, 9.9, **9.13**
    in hemangioma, 9.11, 9.12, **9.16–9.17**
    in infections of spine, 12.3, **12.3**
    of lumbar spine, myelography with, 3.7, 3.9, **3.11**
    in metastatic lesions, 10.14, **10.18**
    in osteoblastoma, 9.3, **9.5**
    in osteosarcoma, 10.4, **10.4**
    in plasmacytoma, 10.9, **10.12**
    single photon emission, 1.8
    in tuberculosis of spine, 13.8, **13.12**
    in tumors, 8.2, 8.4, **8.4**, 8.9
Congenital and developmental anomalies
    absence of bone in, **18.1**, 18.2
    achondroplasia, 19.22–19.24, **19.31–19.33**
    fibrodysplasia ossificans progressiva, 19.26–19.27, **19.36–19.38**
    imaging modalities in, 18.2–18.3
    mucopolysaccharidoses, 19.24–19.26, **19.34–19.35**
    myelography in, 18.2, 18.2–18.3
    neurofibromatosis, 19.18–19.20, **19.25–19.28**
    osteogenesis imperfecta, 19.20–19.22, **19.29–19.30**
    sclerosing dysplasias of bone, 19.27–19.29, **19.39–19.42**
    scoliosis in, 19.2–19.17
Connective tissue arthropathy, **4.1**, 4.2
Corduroy pattern in hemangiomas, 8.3, **8.3**, 8.4, **8.5**, 9.11, 9.12, **9.15**
Cotrel–Dubousset technique in scoliosis, 19.13, 19.14–19.15, **19.20–19.21**
CPPD crystal deposition disease, 4.3, 7.4
Crankshaft phenomenon in scoliosis, 19.10
Crohn disease, arthropathy in, 6.10, **6.14**

Index i.1

Crystal-induced arthritis, **4.1**, 4.2, 7.4
Cyst of bone, aneurysmal. *See* Aneurysmal bone cyst

Degenerative diseases, 5.2–5.12
    diffuse idiopathic skeletal hyperostosis, 5.6, 5.7, **5.10**
    disk disease, 5.3, 5.6, **5.8**
    morphology of, 4.6, **4.7**, 4.8, **4.11**
    osteoarthritis, **5.2**, 5.3, 5.4–5.5, **5.3–5.7**
    spinal stenosis in, 4.4, **4.4**, 5.9, 5.10–5.11, **5.14–5.16**
    spondylolisthesis in, 5.6–5.10, **5.11–5.14**
    spondylosis deformans, 5.6, **5.9**
    treatment of, 5.11–5.12
Dens, 2.2
Denis classification of burst fractures, 3.17
Diaphyseal dysplasia, progressive, 19.29
Diastematomyelia, myelography in, 18.2, **18.2**
DiFerrante syndrome, 19.24, **19.34**
Differential diagnosis of back pain, 11.2
Diphosphonates in scintigraphy, 1.7–1.8
Disk conditions
    anatomy, 3.43
    degenerative disease, 5.3, 5.6, **5.8**
    herniations, 3.31, 3.35–3.36, **3.43–3.44**
        anterior, 3.31, 3.37, **3.45**
        intravertebral, 3.31, 3.37–3.39, **3.46–3.50**
        posterior and posterolateral, 3.39–3.45, **3.51–3.57**
    staging of disk abnormalities, 3.41, **3.51**
Diskography, 1.4–1.6, **1.8**
    cervical, 2.16, **2.19**
    in infections of spine, 12.4, 12.5, **12.6**
    lumbar, 3.7, 3.9, **3.10**
Duchenne muscular dystrophy, scoliosis in, 19.11
Dwarfism, thanatophoric, 19.23–19.24
Dysplasia of bone
    fibrodysplasia ossificans progressiva, 19.26–19.27, **19.36–19.38**
    progressive diaphyseal, 19.29
    sclerosing, 19.27–19.29, **19.39–19.42**
        classification of, 19.27, **19.39**
        mixed, 19.29, **19.42**

Ekman–Lobstein disease, 19.20
Enchondroma, 9.6
    calcifying, 9.6
    complications of, 9.6
    treatment of, 9.6
Enchondromatosis, 9.6–9.7, **9.9**
    complications of, 9.7
Endocrine disorders. *See* Metabolic and endocrine disorders
Enostosis, 19.28, 19.29, **19.42**
Enteropathic arthropathies, **4.1**, 4.2, 6.10, **6.14**
Eosinophilic granuloma, 9.12, 9.13, **9.18–9.19**
    pathologic fractures in, 8.12, 8.13, **8.20**
Erlenmeyer flask deformity
    in Gaucher disease, 17.4
Ewing sarcoma, 10.6, 10.7, **10.7**
    differential diagnosis and treatment of, 10.7
Exostoses, osteocartilaginous, 9.4
    multiple, 9.6

Fibrodysplasia ossificans progressiva, 19.26–19.27, **19.36–19.38**
Fibroma, chondromyxoid, 9.7
Fibrosarcoma, 10.10–10.11
    treatment of, 10.11
Forestier disease, 5.6, 5.7, **5.10**
Fractures
    compression. *See* Compression fractures
    pathologic, in eosinophilic granuloma, 8.12, 8.13, **8.20**
    in hemangioma, 9.12

    in Paget disease, 16.3, **16.3**
    traumatic
        cervical. *See* Cervical spine
        thoracolumbar. *See* Thoracolumbar spine
Fracture dislocations, 3.24–3.29
Fungal infections, 13.7–13.8, **13.13**

Gargoylism, 19.24, **19.34**
Gaucher cells, 17.4
Gaucher disease, 17.4–17.5
    compression fractures in, 17.4, **17.5**
Giant-cell tumor, 9.9–9.11
    complications and treatment of, 9.10–9.11
    computed tomography of, 9.9, **9.13**
    differential diagnosis of, 9.10
    in Paget disease, 9.10, **9.14**
    plain films of, 9.9, **9.13**
Gout, **4.1**, 4.2, 7.3–7.4
    clinical features of, 4.3
    hyperuricemia in, 7.3–7.4
    radiographic features of, 7.4
    tophi in, 7.4
Granuloma, eosinophilic, 9.12, 9.13, **9.18–9.19**
    pathologic fractures in, 8.12, 8.13, **8.20**

Hangman's fracture, 2.26–2.29, **2.33–2.35**
    treatment of, 2.26, 2.29
Harrington–Luque technique in scoliosis, 19.12–19.13, **19.18–19.19**
Hemangioma, 9.11–9.12
    computed tomography in, 9.11, 9.12, **9.16–9.17**
    corduroy pattern in, 8.3, **8.3**, 8.4, **8.5**, 9.11, 9.12, **9.15**
    differential diagnosis of, 9.12
    plain films in, 9.11, **9.15–9.16**
    treatment of, 9.12
Hemochromatosis, 7.4–7.5
    arthritis in, **4.1**, 4.2
Histiocytic lymphoma. *See* Lymphoma of bone
HIV infection, arthritis in, 7.5
HLA antigens
    in ankylosing spondylitis, 6.4
    in arthritic disorders, 4.3
    in hemochromatosis, 7.4
    in psoriatic arthritis, 7.5
    in Reiter syndrome, 6.8, 7.5
Hunter syndrome, 19.24, **19.34**
Hurler–Scheie compound, 19.24, **19.34**
Hurler syndrome, 19.24, **19.34**
Hyperostosis, diffuse idiopathic skeletal, 5.6, 5.7, **5.10**
Hyperparathyroidism, 15.5–15.6, **15.7–15.8**
    arthritis in, **4.1**, 4.2, **7.2**, 7.2–7.3
    brown tumor of, 9.12–9.13
    calcium metabolism in, 15.5
    complications of, 15.6
    osteopenia in, 14.4, **14.5**, 15.6, **15.7**
    pathophysiology of, 15.5
    rugger-jersey spine in, 15.6, **15.8**
Hyperphosphatasia, familial idiopathic
    differential diagnosis of, 16.3
    picture-frame appearance in, **17.1**, 17.2
    platyspondylisis in, 17.2, **17.2**, 17.3
Hypochondroplasia, 19.23

Iliac apophysis ossification, and skeletal maturity, 19.10, 19.11, **19.16–19.17**
Infections, 12.2–12.7, **12.2–12.8**
    arthritis in, **4.1**, 4.2, 7.5, 12.2
    cellulitis in, 12.2
    computed tomography in, 12.3, **12.3**
    diskography in, 12.4, 12.5, **12.6**
    fungal, 13.7–13.8, **13.13**
    magnetic resonance imaging in, 12.4, 12.6, **12.7**
    myelography in, 12.4, **12.5**

    osteomyelitis in, 12.2
    plain film radiography in, 12.2–12.3, **12.2–12.3**, 13.2, **13.2**
    pyogenic, 13.2–13.4
    routes of, **12.1**, 12.2, **13.1**, 13.2
    scintigraphy in, 12.3–12.4, **12.4**, 13.2, 13.3, **13.3**
    treatment of, 12.6–12.7, **12.8–12.9**
    tuberculous, 13.5–13.7, 13.8, **13.6–13.12**
Inflammatory arthritides, **4.1**, 4.2, 6.2–6.11
    ankylosing spondylitis, 6.3–6.8
    enteropathic arthropathies, 6.10, **6.14**
    morphology and distribution of lesions in, **6.1**, 6.2
    psoriatic arthritis, 6.9, **6.13**
    Reiter syndrome, 6.8–6.9, **6.11–6.12**
    rheumatoid arthritis, 6.2–6.3
Injuries of spine. *See* Trauma
Isotope bone scanning, three-phase, 1.7–1.8

Jefferson fracture, 2.20–2.22, **2.24–2.25**

Kidney disease
    in congenital scoliosis, 19.4, 19.5, **19.6**
    osteodystrophy in, 15.5, 15.6, **15.6**
    osteomalacia in, 15.4
Kyphoscoliosis, 19.2
    in neurofibromatosis, 19.18, **19.25**
Kyphosis, 19.2, **19.2**, 19.3
    juvenile thoracic, 3.39, **3.50**

Leri disease, 19.29
Limbus vertebra, 3.47
    differential diagnosis of, 3.38, **3.48**
Lipoma, 9.12
Lippman–Cobb measurements of scoliotic curves, 19.7, 19.8, **19.9**, 19.11
Lordosis, 19.2, **19.2**, 19.3
Lumbar spine
    ancillary imaging techniques, 2.16, **2.19**
    anteroposterior view of, 3.2, **3.3–3.4**, 3.4–3.5, 3.12, **3.13**
    computed tomography of, 3.7, **3.8**
        myelography with, 3.7, 3.9, **3.11**
    diskography of, 3.7, 3.9, **3.10**
    fractures. *See* Thoracolumbar spine
    lateral view of, 3.2, 3.5, **3.5**, 3.12, **3.13**
    magnetic resonance imaging of, 3.7, 3.10, 3.11, **3.12**
    myelography of, 3.7, 3.8, **3.9**
        computed tomography with, 3.7, 3.9, **3.11**
    oblique view of, 3.2, 3.6, **3.6–3.7**, 3.12, **3.13**
    osteoarthritis of, **5.2**, 5.3
    plain films of, 3.2–3.6, **3.3–3.7**, 3.12, **3.13**
    "Scotty dog," 3.2, 3.7
Lupus erythematosus, arthropathy in, **4.1**, 4.2, 4.3
Luque rods in scoliosis, 19.12–19.13, **19.18–19.19**
Lymphangioma, 9.12
Lymphoma of bone, 10.6, 10.7–10.8
    differential diagnosis of, 10.8
    ivory-like vertebra in, 10.7, **10.10**
    moth-eaten bone pattern in, 8.11, **8.16**
    osteolytic lesion in, 10.6, 10.7, **10.8–10.9**
    treatment of, 10.8

Maffucci syndrome, 9.7
Magnetic resonance imaging, 1.8–1.11, **1.10–1.11**
    in arthritides, 4.4–4.5, **4.5–4.6**
    of cervical spine, 2.13, 2.15, **2.15**, 2.16, **2.17**, **2.19**
    in infections of spine, 12.4, 12.6, **12.7**, 13.2, 13.4, **13.4–13.5**
    of lumbar spine, 3.7, 3.10, 3.11, **3.12**
    in meningomyelocele, 18.3, **18.3**
    in osteoblastoma, 9.3, **9.5**
    in rudimentary odontoid process, 18.3, **18.4**

Imaging of the Spine in Clinical Practice

in scoliosis, 19.6, **19.7**
in tumors, 8.2, 8.5–8.7, **8.7**, 8.9
Marie–Strümpell disease. *See* Spondylitis, ankylosing
Maroteaux–Lamy syndrome, 19.24, 19.28, **19.34**
Maturity, skeletal, determination of, 19.8, 19.10, 19.11, **19.15–19.17**
McGregor's line for measurement of odontoid process migration, **2.6**, 2.7, 6.3
McRae's line for measurement of odontoid process migration, **2.5**, 2.6, 6.3
Melorheostosis, 19.29
Meningomyelocele, magnetic resonance imaging in, 18.3, **18.3**
Metabolic and endocrine disorders
 acromegaly, 17.2–17.4, **17.3–17.4**
 arthritis in, **4.1**, 4.2
 bone density abnormalities in, **14.2**, 14.3
 cortical thickness measurements in, 14.2, 14.3, **14.3–14.4**
 Gaucher disease, 17.4–17.5, **17.5**
 hyperparathyroidism, 15.5–15.6, **15.7–15.8**
 hyperphosphatasia, familial idiopathic, **17.1–17.2**, 17.2, 17.3
 mineral content of bones in, 14.4–14.5, **14.6**
 osteoporosis, **15.1–15.5**, 15.2–15.3, 15.4
 Paget disease, 16.2–16.5
 renal osteodystrophy, 15.5, 15.6, **15.6**
 rickets and osteomalacia, 15.4–15.5
 scintigraphy in, 14.5–14.6, **14.7**
Metastases to spine, 8.5, 8.6, **8.7–8.8**, 10.12, 10.13–10.14, **10.16–10.17**
 complications of, 10.14, **10.18**
 incidence of, **11.1**, 11.2
 treatment of, **11.2–11.4**, 11.3–11.5
Morquio–Brailsford disease, 19.24, 19.25, **19.34–19.35**
Mucopolysaccharidoses, 19.24–19.26
 classification of, 19.24, **19.34**
Muscular atrophy, spinal, scoliosis in, 19.11
Muscular dystrophy, Duchenne, 19.11
Myelodysplasia, treatment of scoliosis in, 19.11
Myelography, 1.4, **1.6–1.7**
 in aneurysmal bone cyst, 8.5, **8.6**, 9.8, **9.12**
 of cervical spine, 2.14, 2.15, 2.16, **2.16**, **2.19**
 in diastematomyelia, 18.2, **18.2**
 in infections of spine, 12.4, **12.5**
 of lumbar spine, 3.7, 3.8, **3.9**
  computed tomography with, 3.7, 3.9, **3.11**
 in metastatic lesions, 10.14, **10.18**
 in scoliosis, 19.6, **19.7**
 in tuberculosis of spine, 13.8, **13.12**
 in tumors, 8.2, 8.5, **8.6**
Myeloma, 10.8–10.9
 complications and treatment of, 10.9
 differential diagnosis of, 10.9
 radiographic appearance of, 10.8, 10.10, **10.11**, **10.13**
 solitary, 10.8, 10.9, **10.13**
Myositis ossificans progressiva, 19.26–19.27, **19.36–19.38**

Napoleon's (inverted) hat sign, 3.40
Nash–Moe pedicle method for rotation determination, 19.8, 19.9, **19.14**
Neurofibromatosis, 19.18–19.20
 kyphoscoliosis in, 19.18, **19.25**
 scalloping of vertebrae in, 19.19, **19.27**
 scoliosis in, 19.19, **19.26**
 spinal cord compression in, 19.20, **19.28**

Occipital condyle fractures, 2.17–2.19, **2.22**
Occipito-cervical dislocations, 2.19–2.20, **2.23**
Ochronosis, **7.1**, 7.2
Odontoid process, 2.2
 in clivus-odontoid line, **2.3**, 2.5, 2.20
 fractures of, 2.22–2.25, **2.27–2.29**
  treatment of, 2.25–2.26, 2.27, **2.30–2.32**
 migration measurements, **2.4–2.7**, 2.6–2.7
 rudimentary, 18.3, **18.4**
Ollier disease, 9.6–9.7, **9.9**
 complications of, 9.7
Osteitis deformans. *See* Paget disease
Osteoarthritis, **4.1**, 4.2, 5.3
 apophyseal, 5.3, 5.5, **5.5**
 cervical, 5.3–5.4, **5.3–5.4**
 clinical features of, 4.3
 distribution of lesions in, 4.10–4.11, **4.14**, **5.1**, 5.2
 lumbar, **5.2**, 5.3
 morphology of, **5.1**, 5.2
 sacroiliac, 5.3, 5.5, **5.6–5.7**
Osteoblastoma, 8.10, **8.12**, 9.3–9.4
 computed tomography in, 9.3, **9.5**
 differential diagnosis of, 9.4
 magnetic resonance imaging of, 9.3, **9.5**
 tomography in, 9.3, **9.4**
 treatment of, 9.4
Osteochondroma, 9.4–9.6
 complications of, 9.5–9.6
 malignant transformation of, 9.5, **9.8**, 10.4, **10.5**
 multiple, 9.6
 plain films of, 9.5, **9.7**
 treatment of, 9.6
Osteoclastoma, 9.9. *See also* Giant-cell tumor
Osteodystrophy, renal, 15.5, 15.6, **15.6**
Osteogenesis imperfecta, 19.20–19.22
 classification of, 19.20–19.21
 congenita, 19.20
 differential diagnosis of, 19.22
 radiologic evaluation of, 19.20, 19.21, **19.29–19.30**
 tarda, 19.20
 treatment of, 19.22
 types I–IV, 19.20–19.21
Osteoma, osteoid
 complications of, **9.1**, 9.2
 computed tomography in, 9.2, **9.3**
 differential diagnosis of, 9.3
 periosteal reaction in, 8.12, **8.18**
 plain films in, **9.1**, 9.2
 tomography in, 9.2, **9.2**
 treatment of, 9.3
Osteomalacia, 14.4, **14.5**, 15.4–15.5
Osteomyelitis, 12.2
 aseptic, 17.4
Osteopathia striata, 19.29
Osteopenia, 14.4, **14.5**
Osteopetrosis, 19.27, 19.28, **19.40–19.41**
Osteopoikilosis, 19.28–19.29
Osteoporosis, 14.4, **14.5**, 15.2–15.3
 causes of, **15.1**, 15.2
 circumscripta, 16.3
 codfish vertebrae in, 15.3, **15.3**
 empty box appearance of, 15.2, **15.2**
 iatrogenic, 15.3, 15.4, **15.4–15.5**
 involutional, 15.2
 in osteogenesis imperfecta, 19.20, 19.21, **19.29–19.30**
 pathologic fractures in, 15.3, 15.4, **15.4**
 Schmorl's nodes in, 3.38, **3.49**
Osteosarcoma, 8.10, **8.13**, 10.2–10.5
 classification of, **10.1**, 10.2
 complications and treatment of, 10.5
 computed tomography in, 10.4, **10.4**
 multicentric, 10.5
 periosteal reaction in, **10.2–10.3**, 10.3
 plain films in, **10.2–10.3**, 10.3
 primary, 10.3–10.5
 secondary, 10.5
 tumor bone formation in, **10.2–10.3**, 10.3

Paget disease, 16.2–16.5
 complications of, 16.3–16.5
 cool phase in, 16.3
 differential diagnosis of, 16.3
 giant-cell tumors in, 9.10, **9.14**
 intermediate or mixed phase in, 16.3
 juvenile, 16.3
 management of, 16.5
 osteolytic or hot phase in, 16.2–16.3
 pathologic fractures in, 16.3, **16.3**
 picture-frame appearance of, **16.1**, 16.2, 16.3
 radiographic appearance of, **16.1–16.2**, 16.2–16.3
 scintigraphy in, 14.6, **14.7**
 spinal stenosis in, 16.4, **16.4**, 16.5, **16.5**
Periosteal response in tumors, 8.10, 8.11–8.12, **8.13**, **8.18**
 in osteosarcoma, **10.2–10.3**, 10.3
Photodensitometry, 14.4
Physaliphorous cells in chordomas, 10.11
Picture-frame appearance
 in familial idiopathic hyperphosphatasia, **17.1**, 17.2
 in Paget disease, **16.1**, 16.2, 16.3
Pillars, articular, 2.2
Plain film radiography, **1.1**, 1.2
 in arthritides, 4.3
 of cervical spine, 2.6–2.12, **2.8–2.13**, 2.16, **2.18**
 in giant-cell tumor, 9.9, **9.13**
 in hemangioma, 9.11, **9.15–9.16**
 in infections of spine, 12.2–12.3, **12.2–12.3**, 13.2, **13.2**
 of lumbar spine, 3.2–3.6, **3.3–3.7**, 3.12, **3.13**
 in metastatic lesions, 10.12–10.14, **10.16–10.18**
 in myeloma, 10.8, **10.11**
 in osteoid osteoma, **9.1**, 9.2
 in osteosarcoma, **10.2–10.3**, 10.3
 in scoliosis, 19.6, **19.7**
 of thoracic spine, **3.1–3.2**, 3.2–3.3, 3.12, **3.13**
 in tumors, 8.2, 8.3, **8.3**, 8.7
Plasmacytoma, 10.8, 10.9, **10.12**
Platyspondylisis in familial idiopathic hyperphosphatasia, 17.2, **17.2**, 17.3
Podagra, 7.3
Pseudogout, 7.4
 clinical features of, 4.3
Pseudospondylolisthesis, 3.27, 3.30–3.31, 3.32, **3.37–3.39**
Psoriatic arthritis, **4.1**, 4.2, 6.9, **6.13**
 in AIDS, 7.5
 clinical features of, 4.3
 distribution of lesions in, 4.10–4.11, **4.14**
 morphology of, 4.6, **4.7**, 4.8, 4.9, **4.13**
Pycnodysostosis, 19.28
Pyelography, intravenous, in scoliosis, 19.5, **19.6**, 19.7
Pyogenic infections, 13.2–13.4

Radiation-induced sarcoma, 10.11
Radiographic plain films. *See* Plain film radiography
Radionuclide bone scans. *See* Scintigraphy
Ranawat method for measurement of odontoid process migration, 2.7, **2.7**, 6.3
Reiter syndrome, **4.1**, 4.2, 6.8–6.9, **6.11–6.12**
 in AIDS, 7.5
 bridging of vertebrae in, 6.9, **6.12**
 clinical features of, 4.3
 distribution of lesions in, 4.10–4.11, **4.14**
 epidemic, 6.8
 morphology of, 4.6, **4.7**
 sporadic, 6.8
Rheumatoid arthritis, **4.1**, 4.2, 6.2–6.3
 cervical, 4.5, **4.5**, **6.2**, 6.3
  treatment of instability in, 6.3
 clinical features of, 4.3

distribution of lesions in, 4.10–4.11, **4.14**
  juvenile, 4.8, **4.10**
    distribution of lesions in, 4.10–4.11, **4.14**
  morphology of, 4.6, 4.7–4.8, **4.7–4.9**
  seronegative, 6.2
Rheumatoid factors, 4.3, 6.2
Rickets, 15.4
Risser–Ferguson measurements of scoliotic curves, 19.7, **19.10**
Rotation determinations, 19.8, 19.9, **19.13–19.14**
Rugger-jersey spine
  in hyperparathyroidism, **7.2**, 7.3, 15.6, **15.8**
  in renal osteodystrophy, 15.6, **15.6**

Sacroiliac joints
  osteoarthritis of, 5.3, 5.5, **5.6–5.7**
  in Reiter syndrome, 6.9, **6.11**
Sanfilippo syndrome, 19.24, **19.34**
Sarcoma
  chondrosarcoma, 10.5–10.6, **10.5–10.6**
  Ewing, 10.6, 10.7, **10.7**
  fibrosarcoma, 10.10–10.11
  osteogenic. See Osteosarcoma
  in Paget disease, 16.4–16.5
  radiation-induced, 10.13
  reticulum cell. See Lymphoma of bone
Scalloping of vertebrae
  in achondroplasia, 19.22, **19.31**
  in acromegaly, 17.3, **17.3**
  causes of, 17.4, **17.4**
  in neurofibromatosis, 19.19, **19.27**
Scheie syndrome, 19.24, **19.34**
Scheuermann disease, 3.38–3.39, **3.50**
Schmorl's nodes, 3.38–3.39, 3.44, **3.49–3.50**
Scintigraphy, 1.6–1.8, **1.9**
  in arthritides, 4.4
  of cervical spine, 2.16, **2.19**
  diphosphonate, 1.7–1.8
  gallium-67, 1.8
  indium, 1.8
  in infections of spine, 12.3–12.4, **12.4**, 13.2, 13.3, **13.3**
  in metabolic disorders, 14.5–14.6, **14.7**
  nanocolloid, 1.8
  in tumors, 8.6, 8.7, **8.8**
Scleroderma, connective tissue arthropathy in, **4.1**, 4.2
Sclerosing dysplasias of bone, 19.27–19.29, **19.39–19.42**
  classification of, 19.27, **19.39**
  mixed, 19.29
Scoliosis, **19.2**, 19.2–19.17
  classification of, **19.1**, 19.2
  clinical features of, 19.7
  congenital, 19.4–19.6
    block vertebrae in, 19.4, 19.5, **19.6**
    classification of, 19.4, **19.4**
    in failure of vertebral formation, 19.4, 19.5, **19.5**
    renal disorders in, 19.4, 19.5, **19.6**
    treatment of, 19.10
  crankshaft phenomenon in, 19.10
  idiopathic, 19.3, **19.3**, 19.4
  imaging modalities in, 19.6, 19.7, **19.7**
  measurements of curvature in, 19.7–19.10
    Lippman–Cobb method, 19.7, 19.8, **19.9, 19.11**
    Risser-Ferguson method, 19.7, **19.10**
    scoliotic index in, 19.8, **19.12**
  in neurofibromatosis, 19.19, **19.26**
  postoperative findings in, 19.17, **19.23**
  radiographic appearance of, **19.3**, 19.4, 19.7
  rotation determinations in, 19.8, 19.9
    Cobb spinous-process method, 19.8, 19.9, **19.13**
    Nash–Moe pedicle method, 19.8, 19.9, **19.14**
  skeletal maturity determinations in, 19.8, 19.10, 19.11, **19.15–19.17**
    iliac apophysis ossification in, 19.10, 19.11, **19.16–19.17**
    vertebral ring apophysis ossification in, 19.10, **19.15**
  terminology describing curves in, 19.6, **19.8**
  treatment of, 19.10–19.17, **19.18–19.23**
    complications of, 19.17, **19.24**
    Cotrel–Dubousset technique, 19.13, 19.14–19.15, **19.20–19.21**
    Harrington–Luque technique, 19.12–19.13, **19.18–19.19**
    Zielke technique, 19.13, 19.16, **19.22**
Single photon emission computed tomography, 1.8
Sly syndrome, 19.24, **19.34**
Soft tissue extension of tumors, 8.12–8.13, **8.19**
Spinous process sign, in spondylolisthesis, 3.27, 3.30, **3.38**, 5.6
Spondylitis, ankylosing, **4.1**, 4.2, **6.3–6.4**, 6.3–6.8
  bamboo spine in, 4.6, **4.7**, 4.8, 4.9, **4.12**, 6.4, 6.5, **6.5**
  clinical features of, 4.3
  morphology of, 4.6, **4.7**
  treatment of, 6.4, 6.6–6.8, **6.6–6.10**
    cervical osteotomy in, 6.4, 6.6
    in lumbar kyphosis, 6.6–6.7, **6.7–6.8**
    in lumbar lordosis, 6.7, 6.8, **6.9–6.10**
Spondylolisthesis, 3.27, 3.30–3.32, 3.32–3.35, **3.37–3.42**
  degenerative, 3.27, 3.30–3.31, 3.32, **3.37–3.39**, 5.6–5.10, **5.11–5.14**
  in Paget disease, 16.4, **16.4**
  treatment of, 5.12
  grading (Meyerding), 3.41
  pars interarticularis defect in, 3.31, 3.32–3.35, **3.39–3.42**
  spinous process sign in, 3.27, 3.30, **3.38**, 5.6
  slip angle, 3.42
  treatment of, 3.31
Spondylolysis, 3.27
  treatment of, 3.31
Spondylosis deformans, 5.6, **5.9**
Stenosis, spinal, 4.4, **4.4**, 5.9, 5.10–5.11, **5.14–5.16**
  in achondroplasia, 19.23, **19.33**
  in Paget disease, 16.4, **16.4**, 16.5, **16.5**
  treatment of, 5.12
Synovial fluid in arthritic disorders, 4.3

Teardrop fracture, cervical, 2.29–2.32, **2.37–2.39**
  treatment of, 2.30–2.32, **2.40–2.42**
Thanatophoric dwarfism, 19.23–19.24
Thecal sac compression
  in achondroplasia, 19.23, **19.33**
  in aneurysmal bone cyst, 8.5, **8.6**, 9.8, **9.12**
  in metastatic lesions, 10.14, **10.18**
Thoracic spine
  ancillary imaging techniques, 2.16, **2.19**
  anteroposterior view of, **3.1**, 3.2–3.3, 3.12, **3.13**
  lateral view of, 3.2, **3.2**, 3.3, 3.12, **3.13**
  plain films of, **3.1–3.2**, 3.2–3.3, 3.12, **3.13**
Thoracolumbar spine, 3.2–3.46
  anterior column of, 3.10, 3.12, **3.14**
  burst fracture, 3.13–3.19, **3.17–3.19**
    treatment of, 3.14–3.19, **3.19–3.23**
  Chance fractures, 3.19–3.21, **3.24–3.26**
    treatment of, 3.21–3.23, **3.27–3.28**
  compression fracture, 3.10, 3.13, **3.16**
    treatment of, 3.13
  disk herniations, 3.31, 3.35–3.36, **3.43–3.44**
    anterior, 3.31, 3.37, **3.45**
    intravertebral, 3.31, 3.37–3.39, **3.46–3.50**
    posterior and posterolateral, 3.39–3.45, **3.51–3.57**
  vacuum phenomenon, 3.31, 3.37, **3.46**
  fracture dislocations, 3.24–3.27, **3.29–3.33**
    treatment of, 3.27–3.29, **3.34–3.36**
  injuries of, 3.10–3.27, 3.28–3.29, **3.14–3.36**
    classification of, 3.10, 3.12, **3.15**
  ligaments of, 3.10
  middle column of, 3.10, 3.12, **3.14**
  posterior column of, 3.10, 3.12, **3.14**
  radiographic projections for, **3.1–3.7**, 3.2–3.6, 3.12, **3.13**
  spondylolisthesis, 3.27, 3.30–3.31, 3.32–3.35, **3.37–3.42**
  spondylolysis, 3.27
  three-column concept in classification of injuries, 3.12
Tomography
  of cervical spine, 2.16, **2.19**
  computed. See Computed tomography
  in hemangioma, 9.11, **9.16**
  in osteoblastoma, 9.3, **9.4**
  in osteoid osteoma, 9.2, **9.2**
  trispiral, 1.2, **1.2**
Tophi in gout, 7.4
Trauma
  cervical, 2.2–2.37. See also Cervical spine
  thoracolumbar, 3.10–3.29. See also Thoracolumbar spine
Trispiral tomography, 1.2, **1.2**
Tuberculosis
  arthritis in, **4.1**, 4.2
  of spine, 13.5–13.7, 13.8, **13.6–13.12**
    cold abscess in, 13.5, 13.6, 13.7, **13.10–13.11**
    complications of, 13.5–13.7, 13.8, **13.9–13.12**
    computed tomography in, 13.7, **13.11**
    gibbous formation in, 13.5, 13.6, **13.9**
    myelography in, 13.8, **13.12**
    radiographic appearance of, 13.5, 13.6, **13.6–13.8**
Tumor bone formation, 8.10, 8.11, **8.13**
  in osteosarcoma, **10.2–10.3**, 10.3
Tumors and tumor-like lesions, 8.2–8.13
  age incidence of, 8.8, **8.9**
  algorithm for evaluation of, 8.9, **8.10**
  aneurysmal bone cyst, 8.5, 8.6, 8.11, **8.15**, 9.8–9.9, **9.10–9.12**
  angiography of, 8.2, 8.4, **8.5**
  bone destruction in, 8.11, 8.12, **8.15–8.17**
  borders of, 8.10–8.11, 8.12, **8.12, 8.17**
  cartilage in, 8.11, **8.14**
  chondroblastoma, 9.7
  chondroma, 9.6
  chondromyxoid fibroma, 9.7
  chondrosarcoma, 10.5–10.6, **10.5–10.6**
  chordoma, 8.12, **8.17**, 10.11–10.12, **10.14–10.15**
  classification of, **8.1–8.2**, 8.2, 8.3
  complications of, 8.13
  computed tomography of, 8.2, 8.4, **8.4**, 8.9
  diagnostic approach in, 8.7–8.13, 11.2
  differential diagnosis of, 11.2
  distribution of, 8.10, **8.11**
  enchondroma, 9.6
  enchondromatosis, 9.6–9.7, **9.9**
  Ewing sarcoma, 10.6, 10.7, **10.7**
  fibrosarcoma, 10.10–10.11
  giant-cell tumor, 9.9–9.11
  hemangioma, 9.11–9.12
  imaging modalities in, 8.2–8.7, **8.3–8.8**
    choice of, 8.7–8.10
  lipoma, 9.12
  lymphangioma, 9.12
  lymphoma of bone, 8.11, **8.16**, 10.6, 10.7–10.8, **10.8–10.10**
  magnetic resonance imaging of, 8.2, 8.5–8.7, **8.7**, 8.9

management of, 8.13
metastasis to spine, 8.5, 8.6, **8.7–8.8**, 10.12, 10.13–10.14, **10.16–10.18**
myelography of, 8.2, 8.5, **8.6**
myeloma, 10.8–10.10, **10.11–10.13**
osteoblastoma, 9.3–9.4, **9.4–9.6**
osteochondroma, 9.4–9.6, **9.7–9.8**
osteoid osteoma, 8.12, **8.18**, **9.1–9.3**, 9.2–9.3
osteosarcoma, 10.2–10.5
in Paget disease, 16.4–16.5
pathologic fractures in, 8.12, 8.13, **8.20**
periosteal response in, 8.10, 8.11–8.12, **8.13, 8.18**
plain film radiography of, 8.2, 8.3–8.4, **8.3–8.4**
radiation-induced sarcoma, 10.13
scintigraphy of, 8.6, 8.7, **8.8**
simulations of, 9.12–9.13
soft tissue extension of, 8.12–8.13, **8.19**
treatment of, 11.2–11.5
tumor bone in, 8.10, 8.11, **8.13, 10.2–10.3**, 10.3

Ulcerative colitis, arthropathy in, 6.10, **6.14**
Ultrasonography, 1.6
Urate crystals in gout, 4.3
Uremic osteopathy, 15.5
Uric acid levels in gout, 7.3–7.4

Vacuum phenomenon
　in degenerative spondylolisthesis, 5.6, **5.8**
　in disk herniations, 3.31, 3.37, **3.46**
　in osteoarthritis of lumbar apophyseal joints, 5.3, 5.5, **5.5**
Vertebral ring apophysis ossification, and skeletal maturity, 19.10, **19.15**
Von Recklinghausen's disease, 19.18–19.20, **19.25–19.28**
Vrolik disease, 19.20

Wedge fracture, cervical, 2.33–2.35, **2.44**

Yaws, arthritis in, **4.1**, 4.2

Zielke technique in scoliosis, 19.13, 19.16, **19.22**